A HISTORY OF DENTISTRY IN THE US ARMY TO WORLD WAR II

by
JOHN M. HYSON, JR, DDS
JOSEPH W.A. WHITEHORNE, PhD
JOHN T. GREENWOOD, PhD

Office of The Surgeon General
United States Army
Falls Church, Virginia

Borden Institute
Wallter Reed Army Medical Center
Washington, DC

2008

Borden Institute
Martha K. Lenhart, MD, PhD, FAAOS
Colonel, MC, US Army
Director and Editor in Chief

Editorial Staff: Joan Redding
Senior Production Manager

Ronda Lindsay
Editor, Photo Researcher

Douglas Wise
Layout Editor

The opinions or assertions contained herein are the personal views of the authors and are not to be construed as doctrine of the Department of the Army or the Department of Defense.

Published by the Office of The Surgeon General at TMM Publications
Borden Institute
Walter Reed Army Medical Center
Washington, DC 20307-5001

Library of Congress Cataloging-in-Publication Data

For sale by the Superintendent of Documents, U.S. Government Printing Office
Internet: bookstore.gpo.gov   Phone: toll free (866) 512-1800;   DC area (202) 512-1800
Fax: (202) 512-2104 Mail: Stop IDCC, Washington, DC 20402-0001

ISBN 978-0-16082159-2

Contents

Foreword

We have special reason for congratulation also in the fact that the Congress of these United States was the first legislative body in the world to formally recognize the value and need of the beneficent services of our specialty as a department of military medical practice, and that we have been given an opportunity to prove the wisdom of its action to our country and the world.

- John Sayre Marshall, 1901

The words of civilian contract dental surgeon John Sayre Marshall in 1901 were a celebration of one victory in a long struggle by the civilian dental profession to gain recognition for dentistry as a unique area of medicine, not just in the Army but in the world. Dr Marshall's challenge was that we, the dentists who were granted the privilege of military service, must prove our value. I am honored to claim Captain Marshall as my professional forefather. I also celebrate the accomplishments of our Corps in the past and challenge the Army Dental Corps and the dental services of all US forces and all nations to serve military personnel in the same selfless spirit that our forefathers have. We have made progress. When Marshall made this 1901 statement in a message to the profession, the debate was whether there was any value in military dental surgeons having rank. I believe that in the subsequent 105 years, we have put that debate to rest.

With the exception of *A History of the United States Army Dental Service in World War II* by George F Jeffcott, there has been a void in the written history of US Army dentistry from its beginnings until today. Printing and distributing this volume admirably fills a significant part of that void and I am extremely privileged to be associated with this project. This detailed and scholarly history brings into focus many issues of current interest to the Army Dental Corps by clarifying the origins of the policies and practices of military dentistry. It brings to light the selfless dedication with which civilian dentists and organized dentistry supported the military when there was no official program for oral health. It took decades of persistent political effort to establish official dental service for soldiers, sailors, marines, and airmen, and that hard work is chronicled in detail in these pages.

Beginning before the birth of the Republic, this book explores the requirements for dental service the wars of the 19th century and first half of the 20th century, through the role of the dentist in the nascent Army Air Corps, and up to the advent of the Second World War. The need for military dental care was first recognized, interestingly enough, in the 18th century, when it was critical for the European and American musketeer to possess strong front teeth to pull the cap off wooden gunpowder tubes before bringing the charge to the musket's muzzle. Arms manuals of the day show that little had changed 250 years later as America became caught up in civil war. At that time, infantrymen needed enough strong teeth to tear open the paper cartridge that contained musket ball and powder. We see also that it was an able-bodied sailor who could hold tools or rope in his teeth when climbing to set or adjust sails, and dental requirements were reflected in the recruitment standards of the time. As weaponry progressed, the US military recognized that more destructive power could tear apart faces and jaws, making the unique skills of the dental profession essential in the preservation of life and restoration of deforming wounds. As the general health and nutrition of the soldier gained importance of the years, the US military also began to focus its attention on oral health and its influence on fitness to fight.

This book is an extremely valuable medium through which our traditions and heritage can be shared and preserved. For those interested in developing leadership and management of dental personnel, this history also will serve as a textbook. For policy makers, I expect it will be a reference book to analyze and compare our past experience with today's issues. I challenge dental officers, especially dental commanders, to use this book to illustrate the value of documenting the events and issues of today through records, anecdotes, and written analysis of current operations, so that historians of the future will have an accurate picture of what happened and why. I encourage you to read of our achievements and progress—we have great reason for our pride. However, do not overlook the stories and records that demonstrate our challenges and sometimes failure. There are ample anecdotes, both inspiring and discouraging, to keep the military dental community on its game.

Although I have the privilege of launching this publication, it should be recognized that it was the vision and support of MG Thomas R Tempel, MG John J Cuddy, and MG Patrick D Sculley that contributed the resources and encouraged the interest needed for such a monumental task. On behalf of the Dental Corps, I especially extend thanks to the authors, Doctors Hyson and Whitehorne, for their meticulously researched account. No thread was overlooked in their very successful quest to weave a definitive history. Certainly we should acknowledge the untiring efforts of Dr John Greenwood at the Center for Military Medical History of the Office of the Surgeon General and COL Martha Lenhart at the Borden Institute. I offer my heartfelt congratulations for their efforts in concluding this masterful work. And finally, I would like to thank my friend, COL John King, who, for the past twenty-five years, has been the unofficial "Dental Corps Historian" and driving force behind capturing and publishing our history.

Major General Joseph Webb
Deputy Surgeon General
US Army

Washington, DC
September, 2006

Preface

As the 25th Chief of the US Army Dental Corps, it is my distinct honor and tremendous privilege to join Major General Joseph G Webb, Jr, in introducing this comprehensive, descriptive look at the fascinating evolution of the art and science of dentistry, titled *A History of Dentistry in the US Army to World War II*. The publication of this book is an obvious labor of love that comes after many years of hard work and effort on the part of many, but especially the authors, John Hyson, Jr, DDS; Joseph Whitehorne, PhD; and John Greenwood, PhD.

This publication pays tribute to those who laid the foundation on which the dental profession is built. It documents the origins of dentistry in the Army and depicts the close relationship between organized dentistry and the founding of the US Army Dental Corps. It fills a void in the literature concerning the importance of establishing, sustaining, and continually transforming the dental profession in our military. It was only through close cooperation and mutual support between civilian dental organizations and the US Army Dental Corps that the dental profession was able to mature and flourish over time. We owe a great debt of gratitude to those involved in civilian dentistry for their many inventions and innovations, from the use of anesthesia for surgical procedures to the ability to use teeth for postmortem identification.

Oral health plays an integral part in the overall general health of individuals, and the dental profession is an integral part of the overall healthcare profession. Current research on how oral health–or, more importantly, poor oral health–can negatively affect the overall well being of an individual only strengthens the importance of the dental profession. The extreme value of good oral health is documented in this publication, from early critical soldier skills of opening wooden gunpowder tubes and grenade fuses, to ripping paper cartridge pouches with opposing teeth in order to load gunpowder into the muzzle of a musket. Also noted is the importance of having a healthy maxillofacial substructure for proper protective mask fit, as well as the potential it provides for a better postsurgical outcome for reconstruction of facial injuries from war wounds.

Knowledge of history provides us a means to better understand the challenges of the present, and to set the best conditions for the future. I challenge all dental providers, military and civilian, to read, enjoy, and learn from this publication. It is important to recognize that what transpires within the healthcare of the military during a given period is representative of the overall state of healthcare systems of the nation during that time. Such a relationship is a valuable tool in understanding the evolution of national healthcare. This perspective of history will be of interest to everyone.

As Major General Webb, Jr, points out, many of my predecessors were influential in initiating and sustaining the effort to bring this publication to fruition. My sincere gratitude goes to them, the authors, and to all others who contributed to this publication. I especially want to thank those who had a part in our history: our former Corps Chiefs, general officers, officers, noncommissioned officers, enlisted soldiers, and civilians who are the inspiration for this book. Special thanks to the Center for Military Medical History of the Office of The Surgeon General and Colonel Martha Lenhart at the Borden Institute for assuring this work is published, and to Colonel (RET) John King who served as the unofficial Dental Corps historian throughout much of his career.

Major General Russell J. Czerw
Chief, Dental Corps
US Army

Fort Sam Houston, Texas
October 2008

Introduction

This is an account of the many American dentists both in and out of uniform who believed fervently that their profession could contribute significantly to the health and readiness of the American soldier. After the years of struggle that are well documented in this book, initial success was achieved on February 2, 1901, when Congress authorized the employment of 30 contract dental surgeons for the US Army. During this long struggle, the American dental profession, its journals, and its most influential professional associations (the National Dental Association and its successor, the American Dental Association), were ever present in the halls of Congress, the War Department, and the Office of The Surgeon General promoting the cause and the benefits of modern dentistry for soldiers of the US Army. The years between 1901 and 1911 were marked by the constant efforts of those both inside and outside the Army to create a Dental Corps of commissioned officers. Despite repeated setbacks, John Sayre Marshall, the senior supervising and examining contract dental surgeon during these years, never waned in his efforts to secure a commissioned dental service.

While John Marshall most definitely earned his title as the father of the US Army Dental Corps, Robert T Oliver, another of the original three supervising and examining contract dental surgeons, led the Dental Corps through some of its most demanding times on the battlefields of France while serving as the chief dental surgeon for the American Expeditionary Forces during World War I. It was in the trenches of the Western Front that the officers and enlisted technicians of the Dental Corps won the respect and admiration of their medical department colleagues, the commanders they served, and the soldiers they cared for. As chief of the Dental Division in the surgeon general's office, Oliver oversaw some very significant developments for the Dental Corps during the most difficult years of postwar retrenchment and reductions, late 1919 to mid-1924. While trying years in many respects, the 1920s and 1930s were also years of significant professional growth and maturity. For the first time in peace, Dental Corps officers were fully integrated into medical department field training at the new Medical Field Service School at Carlisle Barracks, Pennsylvania. In addition, the opening of the Army Dental School in Washington, DC, in 1922 allowed the Dental Corps to create its own professional education and development program that greatly enhanced the technical and clinical skills of the Army's dentists and the quality of their service. The hard years of the Depression steeled the dental officers and enlisted dental technicians for the enormous challenges that another world war would bring.

The origins of this volume can be traced to October 1998 when I joined the Office of The Surgeon General, US Army/Headquarters, US Army Medical Command, as the chief of its new Office of Medical History. During my initial meeting with Major General John J Cuddy, then the deputy surgeon general and Dental Corps chief, he expressed his desire to someday see published a comprehensive history of the US Army Dental Corps. With his support and that of his successor in both positions, Major General Patrick D Sculley, my office was able to contract with John M Hyson, Jr, DDS, and Joseph WA Whitehorne, PhD, to research and write a history of dentistry in the US Army from its origins to the beginning of

World War II. John Hyson and Joe Whitehorne had worked on previous projects together, and both of them had proven records as authors.

The manuscript that John and Joe produced was based on extensive original research that John had undertaken during the 1980s and 1990s in the records of the US Army and the Office of the Surgeon General, US Army, in the main building of the National Archives and Records Administration in Washington, DC, and those then located at the Washington National Record Center at Suitland, Maryland (subsequently moved to Archives II at College Park, Maryland). After review by personnel at the US Army Dental Command at Fort Sam Houston, Texas, the now retired Major General Pat Sculley reviewed the entire manuscript and met with John to provide additional comments and recommendations. Based on these comments, John and Joe revised the manuscript and submitted it to my office in October 2005.

Early in 2006, I began my review of the manuscript and realized that additional textual material was needed to fill gaps in the narrative and make the final volume more pertinent to the current members of the Dental Corps, historians, and the general public. In this process, I have relied heavily upon the generous support of Colonel John King, US Army Dental Corps, retired, himself a historian of the Dental Corps in the Vietnam era. He has provided candid and expert advice and professional perspectives that have allowed me to enhance this volume. Using the copious documentation that John and Joe provided from their work and additional research, I have added to their text and produced a more comprehensive coverage of the events and personalities that have shaped the history of dentistry in the US Army and the Dental Corps after its establishment on March 3, 1911.

Without the exceptional work of John Hyson and Joe Whitehorne, this volume would not have been possible. In addition, I wish to thank Ms Emily Court, Ms Yvetta White, and Mr Patrick Walz of the Armed Forces Medical Library for their unstinting and always smiling support in handling my numerous interlibrary loans requests for obscure dental publications. Ms Lisa Wagner and Mr William Edmondson, the Office of Medical History's archivists, did exceptional work in tracking down even more documents for me in the National Archives and Records Administration II at College Park, Maryland, that have added substantial and important details to the this story.

To Colonel Martha Lenhart, MC, director of the Borden Institute, and Colonel Dave E Lounsbury, MC, her predecessor, go my appreciation for their patience and support during the seemingly endless revision and writing process. Equally, Ms Joan Redding and the editorial staff at the Borden Institute deserve much credit for the creation of another exceptional volume.

Finally, my appreciation gratitude must be extended to Major General Joseph G Webb, Jr, the recently retired deputy surgeon general and chief, Dental Corps, who continued, in the tradition of his predecessors, to support and encourage the completion and publication of this volume.

John T Greenwood, PhD
Chief, Office of Medical History 1998–2007
Headquarters, US Army Medical Command

Annandale, Virginia
September 2008

x

Chapter I

The Beginnings of Military Dentistry, 1617–1860

Introduction

After European armies adopted firearms, soldiers used their teeth to bite open gunpowder tubes and later paper cartridges, making dental health essential to performing infantry duties until after the American Civil War. Despite this requirement for healthy teeth, dentistry was a neglected aspect of military medicine. Armies expected medical surgeons to provide needed dental care until February 1901, when Congress authorized the US Army's Medical Department to hire 30 contract dental surgeons.[1]

The earliest recorded acknowledgement of the dental needs of British soldiers occurred in 1617, when John Woodall, the surgeon general of the East India Company, listed the contents of the typical company surgeon's medical chest in his *Surgion's* [*sic*] *Mate*. This chest was the first military dental supply issued in any army, and it soon became the standard for the British. In 1626 King Charles I authorized it as a "free issue" to surgeons who joined his expeditionary forces against France. Included in the chest were the following eight dental instruments for the scaling and extraction of teeth: paces (crown forceps), pullicans (dislocating forceps), forcers (elevators), punches (chisels), crowes bills (root forceps), flegmes (periosteal elevators), gravers (scalers), and small files. The instruments were described and illustrated in Woodall's *Viaticum, Being the Pathway to the Surgeon's Chest* (1617), in which he states:

> All these recited instruments, and each of them, are needfull in the surgeons chest, and cannot bee well forborne for the drawing of teeth, forasmuch as the cleansing of the teeth and gums, and the letting of the gums' bloud are often no small things for keeping men in health, and sometimes doe save the lives of men both at sea and land. For we see that from an Apostume begun under a rotten or hollow tooth, for want of drawing of the same, sometimes proceedeth great swellings in the face, or in the Amygdals and throat, and the party is suffocated and dieth.[2(p149)]

In this early army, the surgeon and his mate were completely responsible for the soldiers' dental care, including both preventive and surgical procedures.

The Soldiers' Teeth: Biting the Cartridge

Before the formation of a standing British army in 1660, soldiers and their accompanying medical staff were "raised under a system of contract for the duration" of the campaign, meaning that soldiers were selected for the various arms of the period according to their physiques. Each infantry company was allowed a surgeon and his apprentice mate. The surgeon received an additional 2 pence a month pay per patient for furnishing his own instrument chest.[2]

The standard infantry unit in the early 17th century British army was the company, which consisted of 100 to 300 men. One-third of these soldiers were pikemen, who each carried an 18-foot, metal-tipped pike, and the rest were musketeers. The musketeers carried bandoliers, which were suspended from a shoulder strap and contained gunpowder charges in 4-inch wooden tubes. To load the gunpowder into the musket barrel, it was necessary to remove the tube cap; the easiest way to do this was to use the front teeth to pull it off, making the incisors and canines essential. On the command, "open them with your teeth," the musketeer brought the charge to his mouth and pulled off the cap with his teeth and thumb. At "charge with powder," he brought the charge to the musket's muzzle, turned it up, and poured the powder down the barrel.[2]

Grenadiers, introduced in 1678, were required to have sufficient incisor and canine teeth to bite open the fuse of a grenade. At the command "open your fuse," the grenadier brought the grenade to his mouth, counted to two, and opened the fuse with his teeth.[2]

Pikemen largely disappeared from the military by the end of the 17th century because of the introduction of the bayonet. The paper cartridge, which combined the bullet and powder, replaced the bandoleer tubes. Now the infantryman simply bit the cartridge. At the command "handle cartridge," the soldier drew the cartridge from his box, brought it to his mouth, and bit off the top.[2,3]

At this time, dental standards began appearing in European armies. Although intentionally removing the front teeth of a man of military age, rendering him unfit for military service, was a punishable offense, for some the prospect of war was worth the risk. French conscripts frequently resorted to self-mutilation by filing off their incisors below the gum, destroying them with acid, or extracting them. Other drafted soldiers tried to destroy their teeth with caustics and simulate "sponginess of the gums"—a symptom of scurvy. As a result, medical examiners had to "pass the finger along the jaw" prior to granting an exemption from service because of tooth loss.[4]

In the Continental Army of the Revolutionary War (1775–1783), Baron Friedrich von Steuben's 1778 drill manual described the technique of loading the flintlock musket in one motion under the title "Handle Cartridge":

> Bring your right hand short round to your pouch, flapping it hard, seize the cartridge, and bring it with a quick motion to your mouth, bite the top off down to the powder, covering it instantly with your thumb, and bring the hand as low as the chin, with the elbow down.[5(p18)]

Soldiers needed to possess teeth capable of performing such techniques until the mid 19th century in Europe and after the Civil War in America, when the pinfiring mechanism and the metallic cartridge were introduced in infantry firearms. This advancement in firearms technology ended the need for soldiers to use their teeth to load weapons.[3,6]

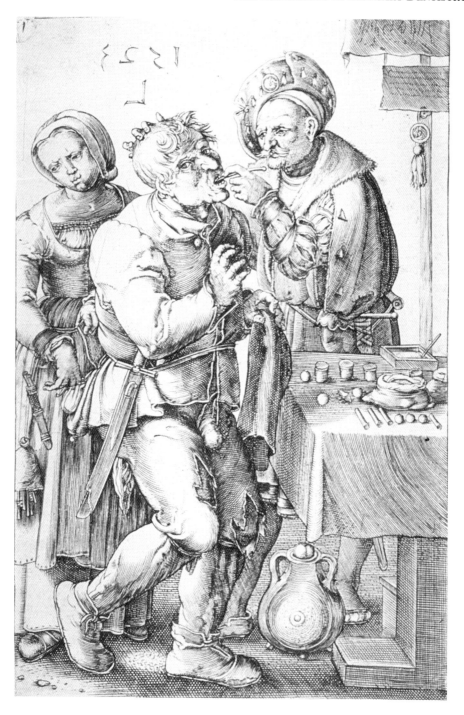

Public Toothdrawer.
Reproduced from: http://wwwihm.nlm.nih.gov/ihm/images/A/21/200.jpg.
Courtesy of the National Library of Medicine.

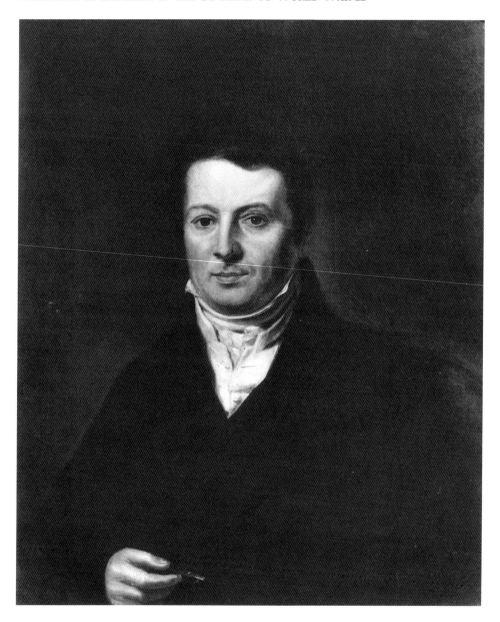

*James (Jacques) Gardette, a French naval surgeon who was
the first dentist to treat military personnel on a regular basis.
Courtesy of Baltimore College of Dental Surgery.*

In October 1777 Gardette, an enthusiastic supporter of the American Revolution, sailed with a group of volunteers bound for Boston aboard the French brig-of-war, *La Barquaize de St Jean de Luz*. During the voyage, Gardette's ship was involved in a conflict with two British warships, and the 21-year-old naval surgeon helped treat the casualties. After the ship arrived in Plymouth, Massachusetts, in January 1778, Gardette promptly resigned from the French navy and adopted America as his home.[9]

In 1780 when Newport, Rhode Island, became the headquarters of the Comte de Rochambeau's newly arrived 6,000-man French army, Gardette rejoined his countrymen as a civilian dentist. Rochambeau's command contributed substantially to the American victory at Yorktown, but it is not known whether Gardette was present at the battle. However, he was reported to have been with the command during their 1781–1782 winter encampment in Providence, Rhode Island. During that time, he became acquainted with a young American soldier, Josiah Flagg (1763–1816), whom he is thought to have instructed in the art of French dentistry. Flagg became the patriarch of an illustrious line of American dentists.[9,10]

Gardette remained in America after the war, establishing a practice first in New York City and then in Philadelphia in 1784. In late 1795 or early 1796, he made a set of ivory (hippopotamus) dentures for George Washington just before the famous Gilbert Stuart portrait sittings, which took place that spring. When asked about the teeth, Gardette claimed it was "impossible to distinguish them from the natural ones," and that a person could "take them out and fix them again themselves with the greatest ease." However, others disagreed, describing them as "too large and clumsy." In 1859 Rembrandt Peale (1778–1860) stated that Gardette's dentures caused Washington's "mouth to be changed." Stuart said that when he painted Washington, "he had just had a set of false teeth inserted, which accounts for the constrained expression so noticeable about the mouth and lower part of the face." Regardless of the success of Washington's dentures, Gardette can be given credit for introducing the advanced techniques of Fauchard into American dentistry.[11-14] In 1829, at age 73, Gardette returned to France, where he later died from gout.[9]

Another French dentist, Jean Pierre Le Mayeur, also provided dental service in Revolutionary America. Le Mayeur was a London surgeon before he came to America in 1781, and in 1782 he was living in British-occupied New York, where he was well known for his ability to transplant teeth. Le Mayeur became one of the many dentists consulted by George Washington, who held him in high regard and recommended him to the Marquis de Lafayette. Le Mayeur treated Washington at the Army headquarters in New Windsor, New York. Over the next 5 years, Le Mayeur was a frequent visitor to Mount Vernon on both social and professional calls. After settling in Mount Pleasant, Virginia, he became an American citizen in 1789, and died in May 1806.[11,15]

In addition to Gardette and Le Mayeur, other foreign-born dentists arrived in the new nation and established themselves in major American cities. Mostly French or English, these immigrants advertised such services as cleaning, extraction, and replacement. Their advertisements often included thanks to long-term patients, indicating the growing use and acceptance of dentistry by the end of the century. At the same time, the increasing professionalism of dentistry was reflected in the growing amount of literature on dental topics. The English immigrant dentist Richard Cortland Skinner published *A Treatise on the Human Teeth* in 1801—the first American book on a dental topic. A year later, BT Longbotham, who advocated filling root canals to save teeth, published *Treatise of Dentistry Explaining the Diseases of the Teeth and Gums with the Most Effectual Means of Prevention and Remedy.* Other practitioners of the time patented improved dental instruments and prosthetic devices.[7,16,17]

American Practitioners in the Revolutionary Period

At least one American contributed to the history of military dentistry during the Revolutionary War era. While Paul Revere (1735–1818), the Revolutionary patriot, is not often thought of as a dentist, he did practice dentistry in Boston for about 6 years. He apparently studied the craft under John Baker (1732–1796), a dentist who

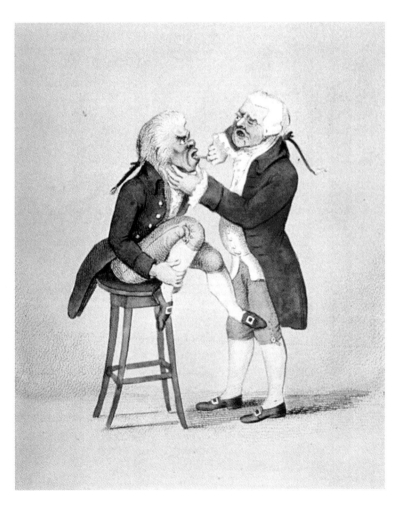

"Easing the Tooth-Ach." 1796.
Reproduced from: http://wwwihm.nlm.nih.gov/ihm/images/A/21/943.jpg.
Courtesy of the National Library of Medicine.

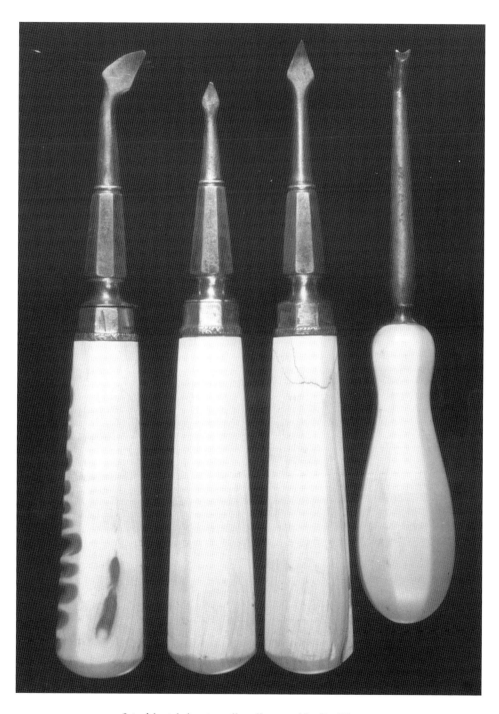

Set of dental elevators allegedly owned by Paul Revere.
Photograph: Courtesy of the National Museum of Health and Medicine,
Armed Forces Institute of Pathology. NCP 1331.

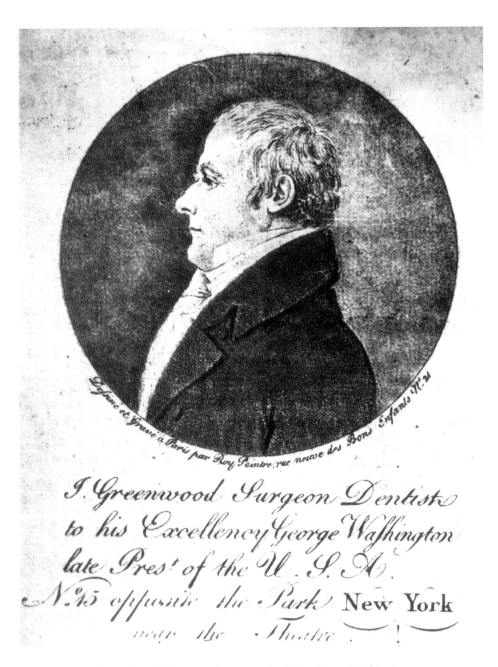

Engraving of J Greenwood, surgeon dentist to George Washington.
Courtesy of the National Museum of Health and Medicine,
Armed Forces Institute of Pathology. NCP 3282.

worked in Boston before 1766 and later provided services to George Washington while working in Williamsburg, Virginia, from 1771 to 1773.[11,18]

Revere, an expert goldsmith, silversmith, and engraver, concerned himself mainly with prosthetics, but after 1774 he lost interest in making artificial teeth. However, in 1776, he played a large part in one of the earliest cases of forensic dentistry on record. At the battle of Bunker Hill the year before, Dr Joseph Warren (1741–1775), a physician and major general in the Massachusetts militia, was the first American general officer to be killed in action. His body was buried in a mass grave. A year later, Massachusetts wanted to honor Warren and planned to exhume his body for reburial in a private plot, but his body could not be immediately identified. Finally, after recognizing a prosthetic dental appliance (bicuspid tooth) he had made for Warren, Revere was able to identify him.[11,19]

Revere was one of an estimated 79 professional dentists who were practicing at some level in the years before the Revolution. Newspaper advertisements of the period reveal that John Baker of Boston, Revere's mentor, and Robert Wooffendale (1742–1828) of Philadelphia were offering their services as early as 1767. Both were trained in Britain and offered extraction and cleaning; Baker also sold a simple dentifrice.[20,21] Between 1768 and 1773, numerous advertisements appeared for Michael Poree, a "surgeon dentist" practicing in New York, Boston, and Philadelphia. Moving among the cities because of the limited volume of business, Poree claimed to be able to treat "various complaints incidental to the teeth and gums: as well as to provide prosthetic devices." Poree was the first dentist in America to publish a lay article on dentistry, which appeared in the *New York Gazette* and the *Weekly Mercury* in December 1769.[17,22]

A number of veterans of the Revolutionary War went on to careers in dentistry, many rising to social and professional prominence. One of these, John Greenwood (1760–1819), established himself in New York City in 1786 after working briefly in the South.[13] Greenwood made and maintained several sets of dentures for George Washington between 1789 and 1798, carving them out of hippopotamus ivory and setting them using beeswax molds. He employed spiral springs—invented by the Frenchman Nicholas Dubois de Chemant—to keep the upper and lower plates in place and functioning.[14,23,24]

The War of 1812

Relatively little is known about dental care or the prevalence of oral disease among American soldiers during the War of 1812. Available information is derived from incomplete administrative and hospital records, medical reports, and archeological discoveries and analysis. These sources show that, despite the increasing acceptance and modest growth of the dental profession, little thought was given to soldiers' oral health when the United States entered its second war with Great Britain. In fact, the country was vastly unprepared for war overall. During the first year, one surgeon and two surgeon's mates were authorized for each regiment, with a few others allowed for hospitals. Given little authority or respect, these men were forced to work mostly on their own, and good medical care was hard to come by. In March 1813 Congress approved the positions of surgeon general and apothecary general, which brought order and accountability to military medicine.[25]

Fortunately for the dental surgeons, the newly appointed apothecary general, Francis Le Baron, provided medical supplies surprisingly efficiently. However, poorly trained physicians often overused some of the medications, resulting in serious injury to some patients. The most damaging example of this was the overly generous use of calomel (mercurous chloride), a popular treatment of the day used to remedy intestinal afflictions and repel insects. Calomel caused caries of the jaw, tooth loss, and even death in at least three cases at the Army hospital in Lewiston, New York, on the Niagara frontier.[26,27]

One case of calomel poisoning involves 17-year-old Private Thomas Broughton, 6th Regiment, US Infantry. In 1813 Broughton was being treated for dysentery with large doses of calomel when his physician, Dr Joshua B Whitridge, reported that he had developed mercurial poisoning:

> Mortification had taken place in the buccinator muscle of his right cheek, and under his jaw, and had been progressing several days. The hole in his cheek, occasioned by the sloughing, (when I first saw him,) was about three quarters of an inch in diameter, perfectly round, and had the appearance of being cut out with a knife, or some sharp instrument.[28(p82),29]

The surgeon ordered that the wound be kept clean by using a syringe to inject it with warm water and diluted brandy. Fowler's solution (potassium arsenite) was also used to irrigate the wound five or six times a day, and Broughton steadily recovered.[28]

Archeological investigations have provided more detailed information on the oral health of American soldiers. In 1987 construction at Fort Erie, Ontario, uncovered the remains of 28 US enlisted soldiers killed during the operations there from August to October 1814. These soldiers came from regular and militia units with origins in rural areas of Massachusetts, Vermont, eastern and central New York, and southwest Pennsylvania. In studying the remains, "dentitions from 25 mandibles and 24 maxillae were analyzed, totaling nearly 600 teeth." The remains showed traits such as Carabelli's cusp, which is evidence of European origins, and of early dietary deficiencies revealed in hypoplastic enamel losses. Further analysis showed a strikingly low rate of dental caries when compared to other 19th century military groups. The soldiers' diet was low in cariogenic items and included large amounts of salted meats, which may account for their dental health. Although many of the corpses did show evidence of antemortem tooth loss, there had been little abscessing. The dental condition of this small group suggests that the modest physical requirements for recruits, coupled with a soldiers' diet, made for relatively good dental health, aided only occasionally by extraction.[30]

Josiah Flagg was one of the few dentists recorded as having served in any capacity during the War of 1812. He had received his early training from James (Jacques) Gardette during the Revolutionary War and later, at the age of 49, enlisted in the Navy. After brief service, he was captured by the British and sent to England as a prisoner of war. He was later paroled and allowed to practice dentistry in London from 1813 to 1815. On September 14, 1815, after the conclusion of the war, Flagg was granted a passport to return home. Unfortunately, a few hours before docking, he was shipwrecked in New York Harbor. After suffering from exposure, he finally reached Boston. He decided to seek a warmer climate for his health and went to Charleston, South Carolina, where he contracted yellow fever and died on September 30, 1816.[11,31,32]

Despite the obvious need for better medical organization, Congress was, overall, slow to react once the War of 1812 was over. At first, the surgeon general's position was eliminated in the initial flurry of force reductions in 1815. However, it was reestablished in April 1818, and in 1821 Army Regulations finally listed sets of "Teeth Instruments" among the Medical Department's supply tables.[33]

Horace Hayden: The First Dental College

Dentist Horace Hayden (1769–1844) served in the War of 1812 as a soldier and assistant surgeon. Hayden was born on October 13, 1769, in Windsor, Connecticut, into a military family. One of his ancestors, William Hayden, had saved his captain's life in the Pequot War of 1637. Horace's grandfather, Daniel Hayden, was a lieutenant in the French and Indian War, and his father, Thomas Hayden, served as a sergeant and then first lieutenant in the Revolutionary War. Hayden began a career in architecture, his father's trade, but a professional visit to Dr John Greenwood in New York influenced him to change his vocation. In 1800 he moved to Baltimore, established a dental office, and began to study medicine, especially anatomy, making a solid reputation for himself. On August 16, 1813, after the first British threat to Baltimore, he enlisted as a private in Captain Christian Andreon's infantry company, in the 39th Regiment (Fowler's) of the Maryland militia. He served for only 8 days (for which he was paid $2.06) before Major General Samuel Smith, aware of Hayden's medical skills, ordered him to serve as an assistant surgeon at the hospital.[34,35]

In 1819 Hayden delivered a course of lectures on dental surgery to the medical students at the University of Maryland. This was the first time a dentist lectured in a medical school in the United States. Together with Chapin A Harris (1806–1860), Hayden founded the Baltimore College of Dental Surgery in March 1840, the world's first institution dedicated to dental education (today known as the Baltimore College of Dental Surgery, Dental School, University of Maryland, Baltimore). Before that time, apprentice dentists were trained by preceptors—experienced dentists who took young students into their offices for anywhere from 3 months to 5 years and taught them the rudimentary facts of dentistry. But because the majority of the early 19th century dentists were itinerant practitioners, moving from town to town in search of profit, standards were difficult to maintain. Progressive dentists such as Hayden and Harris realized that a formal education, either by itself or in conjunction with a medical education, would give dentistry professional credibility. In 1839 Hayden organized the first dental journal ever published, the *American Journal of Dental Science,* which Harris edited until his death in September 1860.[36] Hayden was also instrumental in founding the first national dental society in America, the American Society of Dental Surgeons, in 1840. (In addition to his work in dentistry, Hayden wrote the first general work on geology published in the United States, *Geological*

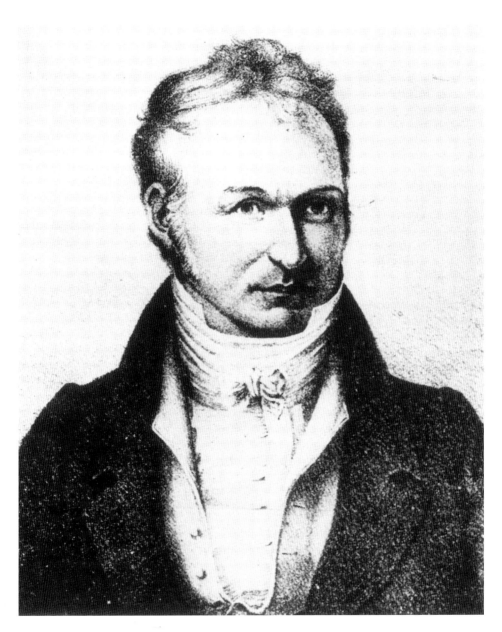

Engraving of Horace Hayden, MD, DDS (1769–1844).
Courtesy of the National Museum of Health and Medicine,
Armed Forces Institute of Pathology. NCP 3300.

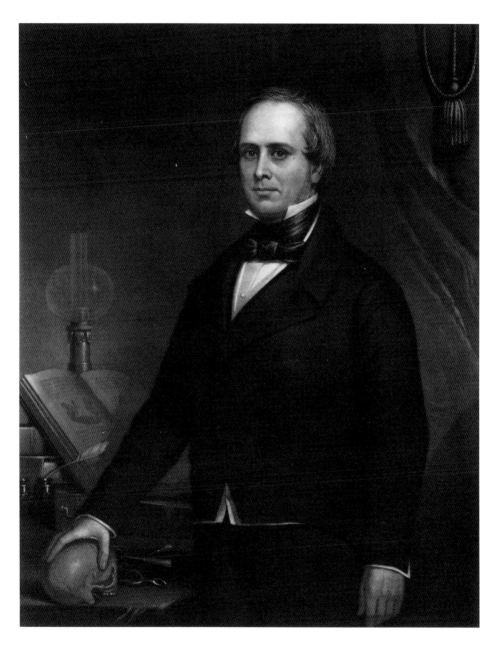

Chapin Harris, AM, MD.
Reproduced from: http://wwwihm.nlm.nih.gov/ihm/images/B/13/841.jpg.
Courtesy of the National Library of Medicine.

Essays or, An Inquiry into some of the Geological Phenomena to be Found in Various Parts of America, and Elsewhere, in 1820). Hayden died on January 26, 1844, in Baltimore.[34,36]

From the War of 1812 to the War with Mexico (1846–1848)

The establishment of a formal training institute was only one of several advances in dentistry in the decades after the War of 1812. Professional societies, such as Hayden's American Society of Dental Surgeons, proliferated at the state level by the mid 1840s. The first state dental society, the Virginia Society of Surgeon Dentists, was organized in 1842 in Richmond.[37] By the end of the decade, several of the societies had formed regional associations to assure better professional standards and to exchange information. The Mississippi Valley Association of Dental Surgeons, which was organized in Cincinnati in 1844, established its own influential dental periodical in 1847, *Dental Register of the West* (later *Dental Register*). This publication was produced until 1923, well after the association itself had disappeared. According to Milton Asbell, author of *Dentistry, a Historical Perspective* (1988), increased activity in dental literature inspired the publication of "about 60 books and pamphlets" during this time, which covered topics as diverse as tooth preservation, anatomy, and tips for parents.[7(p124),38]

Clinical improvements also advanced after the war. For example, dentists began urging the correction of dental bite problems (malocclusion) in young people before they became critical—the first hint of simple orthodontia. Perhaps the most significant discovery was Horace Wells's use of nitrous oxide as an anesthetic in 1844. During an operation at Massachusetts General Hospital in 1846, another dentist, William TG Morton (1819–1868), built on Wells's discovery and demonstrated the successful use of sulphuric ether as a general anesthetic.[7,39] In a letter to Morton that same year, Oliver Wendell Holmes (1809–1894), a professor of anatomy at Harvard Medical School, poet, writer, and father of Supreme Court Justice Oliver Wendell Holmes, Jr, defined the term "anesthesia" as the absence of all sensibility.[40] Inhalation anesthesia has since been called dentistry's greatest gift to humankind.

In 1844 Samuel Stockton White (1822–1879) established a dental supply house in Philadelphia called Jones, White & Company (later SS White Dental Manufacturing Company). White carved his own metal tooth molds and ground the porcelain materials in a hard mortar. He was a master mold maker, so his porcelain teeth looked real and dentists were quick to recognize the quality. In October 1847 he began publishing *Dental News Letter*, which became another leading publication in the field. In August 1859 it became *Dental Cosmos*, which eventually merged with the *Journal of the American Dental Association*.[36,41] In 1849 Chapin Harris first described a crude "pivot crown" (an artificial tooth designed to be applied to the root of a natural tooth by means of what is usually termed a pivot, but more properly a dowel or tenon) in *A Dictionary of Dental Science, Biography, Bibliography, and Medical Terminology*.[42]

Despite the emerging professionalism of American dentistry, a growing body of specialized knowledge, and skilled dental practitioners, the Army surgeon general remained confident that his surgeons could deal with the dental requirements of the soldiers in the ranks. The 1841 Army Regulations continued to carry "teeth-extracting" instrument sets in the Medical Department supply table for the doctors' use, but no further accommodation was considered necessary. In fact, at the time of the Mexican-American War (1846–1848), many of the surgeons discounted the use of ether as unnecessary and potentially harmful to blood flow.[43,44]

Many dentists volunteered their service at the outbreak of the war, and some probably provided their comrades-in-arms with dental care unofficially. Among the first to volunteer was Joseph Hassell (1828–1901) of Lexington, Missouri, who had just completed his dental apprenticeship with Dr Clark of Saint Louis. On May 18, 1846, he enlisted to serve 6 months as a private in Company G, 1st Regiment,

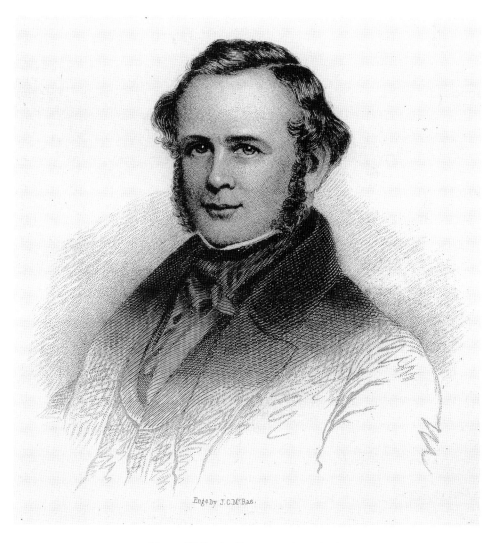

Horace Wells, the discoverer of anesthesia.
Courtesy of the National Museum of Health and Medicine,
Armed Forces Institute of Pathology. NCP 1327.

17

Saint Louis Legion, Missouri Infantry. (Captain Henry JB McKellops [1823–1901], a prominent dentist in Saint Louis and later a leader in the fight for Army dentists, organized and commanded this infantry company, called the Morgan Riflemen, during the war.)[31,45] Hassell was discharged on September 2, 1846, at Jefferson Barracks, Missouri. He then returned to Lexington, established a dental practice, and later received his dental degree from the Missouri Dental College in Saint Louis. During the Civil War, he served in the Confederate army. After that, he resumed his practice in Lexington until his death at age 73. He was one of the earliest dentists to practice west of the Mississippi River.[46-48]

The Amalgam War

In 1805 WH Pepys of London first introduced a fusible metal filling material to seal decaying teeth, but melting the metal required an impractical amount of heat. In 1818 Regnart, a French chemist, overcame this problem by adding mercury to the mix, inventing amalgam (an alloy of mercury combined with another metal).[39,49,50] But in the 1840s and 1850s, the "Amalgam War" divided the dental profession into two distinct groups: the dentists who endorsed amalgam as an alternative restorative material to gold (which was then the accepted standard) and those who did not. This divisive issue fractured the nascent American Society of Dental Surgeons and led to the establishment of both the American Dental Convention and the American Dental Association in 1859 (these two groups became the principal advocates of dentistry in the Army). The issue also spurred the development of new dental amalgams, techniques, and denture technology that influenced the future of American dentistry.

The amalgam conflict began in 1833, when the Crawcour brothers came to New York from Europe with a coin-silver amalgam they called "royal mineral succedaneum." Their dental business boomed, and practitioners who used gold and tin lost patients. The Crawcour brothers' amalgam was a soft, plastic mix of impure material, which they thumbed into cavities without removing the decay. This technique was painless, but the fillings fell out and, because of the amalgam's expansion, caused tooth fractures. As the public became aware of the amalgam's failure, the Crawcours retreated to Europe, leaving amalgam with a bad reputation despite the fact that, if used properly, it was an excellent filling material.[50]

In 1841 the American Society of Dental Surgeons (then the only national dental organization) appointed a committee to study the amalgam problem. Although they had not tested amalgam, the committee reported 2 years later that "the use of amalgam constituted malpractice."[50(p66)] In 1844 the society required its members to sign a pledge never to use amalgam or risk expulsion. In response, many members resigned and, by 1847, only five of New York's 200 dentists remained in the society. The society eventually rescinded the pledge, but the organization folded in 1856.[50,51]

In 1855 Dr J Foster Flagg (1828–1903), professor of dental pathology and therapeutics at the Philadelphia College of Dental Surgery, began testing different amalgam formulas for bicuspid and molar fillings. Flagg modified the then–popular formula of 60% tin to 40% silver, reversing it to 60% silver and 40% tin, and added combinations of other metals, such as copper, zinc, antimony, gold, platinum, and cadmium. In 1881 he published a book on amalgams called *Plastic and Plastic Fillings* (amalgam fillings were popularly referred to as "plastic fillings" at the time).[50] His cavity preparation and instrumentation techniques were meticulous, and Flagg was convinced he could "save teeth with amalgam which I could not save with gold." In 1861 he presented his findings to the Pennsylvania Association of Dental Surgeons, who decided that silver amalgam was "an excellent filling material," and expanded dentistry's "ability to save teeth."[50]

A major breakthrough in denture construction technology also took place in 1855 with the introduction of vulcanite (named after the Roman god of fire and metal working). Vulcanite was a hard, rubber denture base material, patented by Nelson Goodyear in 1851. His brother, Charles Goodyear, had secured a patent in 1844 for his discovery of the "vulcanization" process, in which a rubber-sulphur mixture was heated into a hard, ebony-like compound. Vulcanite was inexpensive, relatively easy to make, and accurately fit a patient's jaw, bringing an end to the practices of carving ivory or pounding out (swaging) gold or silver denture bases. Other porcelain, cheoplastic metal, celluloid, and aluminum bases were tried during this period, but none could compete against vulcanite, which remained dentists' denture material of choice until the advent of the acrylic resins in the late 1940s.[39]

The Presidents' Dentist: Edward Maynard

The first dentist to make an effort to convince the US War Department that the Army needed dental surgeons was Dr Edward Maynard (1813–1891) of Washington, DC. A former West Point cadet, Maynard was internationally renowned for his dental proficiency and his ordnance inventions, which included a new priming system to replace the percussion cap, a breech-loading rifle, and a metallic center-fire cartridge. These and his many other inventions revolutionized firearms technology prior to the Civil War. Maynard's dental office, located near the White House, catered primarily to a wealthy clientele, including several presidents, cabinet officers, congressmen, Army and Navy officers, and foreign diplomats.[31]

A July 1859 editorial (presumably by Chapin Harris) in the *American Journal of Dental Science* noted that Maynard had personally brought the matter of the need for Army dental surgeons to the attention of President Millard Fillmore during Fillmore's 1850–1853 tenure. The president then "brought it before the cabinet in council," but the secretaries of war and the Navy failed to accomplish any dental legislation.[52]

Later, during the Franklin Pierce administration (1853–1857), Secretary of War Jefferson Davis "received the proposition [for Army dentists] as one of great value." Maynard was well known to Davis because in 1853 the War Department had purchased the right to use his "improved system of firing" for 100,000 firearms. Maynard had also discussed the matter with the surgeon general of the Army, Colonel Thomas Lawson, who "was willing to advocate the establishment of a corps of army dental surgeons of six to begin with, to be entirely distinct from the corps of surgeons in their duties, examinations, promotions and rank." However, no official action was taken. Because a bill affecting the "corps of surgeons of the army" had been pending before Congress for quite some time, many thought it

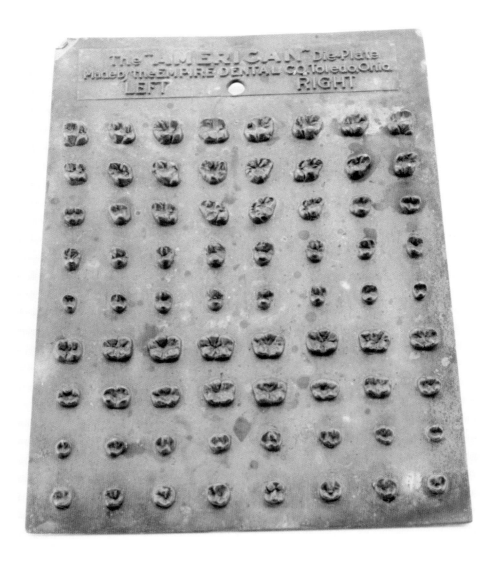

Die plate, circa 1875. This die plate was used to swage (pound into shape)
the occlusal surface of a shell crown made of 22K plate gold.
By 1955 this technique was superseded by cast gold crowns.
Photograph: Courtesy of the National Museum of Health and Medicine, Armed Forces Institute of
Pathology. NCP 3278.

best "not to propose anything that might defeat that bill."[52,53]

At President Pierce's direction, Secretary of the Navy John P Kennedy became involved in the matter. On February 16, 1853, Kennedy addressed the chief of the Naval Bureau of Medicine and Surgery, Dr Thomas Harris, to report on the "propriety of enlarging the requisitions upon Candidates for admission into the Medi-

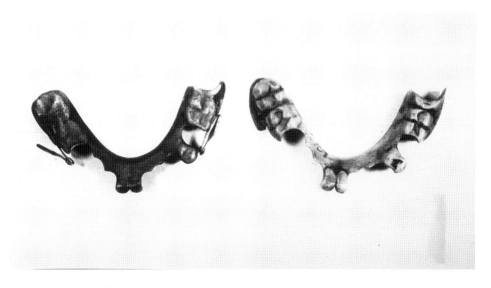

Teeth carved in Paris from hippopotamus tusk before 1854.
Worn by a French naval [undetermined] officer.
Reproduced from: http://wwwihm.nlm.nih.gov/ihm/images/A/23/308.jpg.
Courtesy of the National Library of Medicine.

cal Corps, so far as to demand from them a more full knowledge of the science and practice of Dentistry in preparing them for the duties of the Naval service."[54] Upon hearing this report, Maynard wrote Kennedy's successor, James Dobbin, on April 13, 1853, to ask for a copy. Dobbin replied that he "heartily approved the proposition [dental surgeons for the Navy]," and thanked Maynard "for bringing to his notice a project which his own sufferings from his teeth and benefit from their proper surgical treatment, convinced him was a most humane suggestion." However, once again, no official action was taken. Maynard died on May 4, 1891, at age 78, 10 years before his efforts were finally realized.[31]

Antebellum Legislative Efforts: The McKellops Resolution, 1858–1859

Despite a lengthy and distinguished civilian career, as well as military service in the Saint Louis Legion and Missouri National Guard during the 1840s and 1850s, Henry JB McKellops is best known for his efforts to lobby Congress for Army dental surgeons. A prominent dentist in the Mexican-American War, McKellops undoubtedly witnessed the dental sufferings of his fellow volunteer soldiers, who rarely had the opportunity to see a qualified dentist. Many soldiers went to Mexico "with sound and beautiful teeth, and returned within a year or two with them almost destroyed, and in some cases entirely so, and almost all much diseased."[31,56] On July 21, 1858, at a meeting of the Western Dental Society in Quincy, Illinois, McKellops offered the following preamble and resolution:

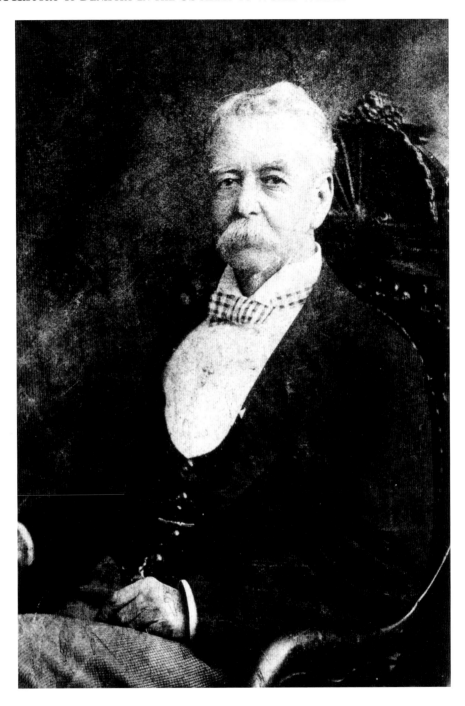

*Henry JB McKellops, a distinguished civilian dentist who also served in the
Saint Louis Legion and Missouri National Guard during the 1840s and 1850s.
McKellops is best known for his efforts to lobby Congress for Army dental surgeons.
Photograph: Courtesy of the American Dental Association.*

Whereas, Owing to the great inconvenience of the officers and soldiers in procuring competent dentists, when necessarily required, and knowing the difficulty in which they are placed, being stationed at distant posts, where it is absolutely impracticable for a regular practitioner of dentistry to visit them; therefore,

Resolved, That this Society appoint a committee of five, for the purpose of memorializing Congress on the necessity of appointing dentists to be attached to the regular army, and that we recommend the same to the consideration of the American Dental Convention [which replaced the nearly defunct American Society of Dental Surgeons as the national dental association in 1855], and ask their co-operation with us.[38,55]

The society adopted his resolution and formed a committee consisting of Drs McKellops, Christopher W Spalding, Isaiah Forbes, IB Branch, Lewis, and WW Allport.[31,56]

At the American Dental Convention meeting in August, another committee was formed after McKellops repeated the proposal.[57] Apparently the committees met with little success, for no congressional action was taken. In April 1859 Dr John R McCurdy, the coeditor of *Dental News Letter*, commented on the subject:

The soldier has as much need for a dentist as for a surgeon, and that in the aggregate, he suffers as much or more from diseases of the teeth as from any cause incident to his profession. He certainly has as much use for his teeth as for his limbs, and we are quite sure he does more eating than fighting, and should, therefore, be as well furnished with the needful appliances for the effective performance of the former, as he is for the latter, and as his occupation is a hard one at best, he is deserving and entitled to as many comforts and as much exemption from annoyance and suffering as it is possible to afford him.[58(p206)]

When the American Dental Convention met the next year, McKellop's proposed committee admitted that their report was not ready, and they were directed to continue their efforts.[59]

Foreign Influences

In its efforts to secure dentistry for the US military forces during the 1850s, the American dental profession did not let the health and sanitary problems of the recent Crimean War (1854–1856) go unnoticed. The war, which involved Imperial Russia, Turkey, Great Britain, France, and several other European countries, had drawn attention to the "sad misfortunes" endured by the British army because of poor sanitary conditions. British soldiers' and sailors' teeth were known to be in "deplorable condition," but all attempts to provide dental surgeons for them failed. French soldiers were at least supplied with toothbrushes and obliged to clean their teeth.[60]

The dental requirements for recruits were similar for all armies of the time. In the French army, the manual for the recruiting service, the *Aide Memoire*, listed the following dental causes for rejection of an applicant: "Loss of the whole or part of either jaw-bone; Deformities of either jaw bone, interfering with mastication, speech, or the tearing of the cartridge; Anchylosis of the jaws; Loss of the incisor and canine teeth of both jaws." The British army regulations mention the "loss of many teeth, or teeth generally unsound," and "extensive deficiency, particularly of the front teeth." In 1859 Sir Charles Trevelyan, then governor of Madras, India, recommended that European medical officers should be "instructed in dental surgery, that the teeth of all soldiers . . . be examined, and operative assistance rendered to such as require it." Commenting on this recommendation, the *British Journal of Dental Science* suggested "a dentist should be appointed to every division of the [British] army." Although gunshot wounds of the face and jaws would come under a dentist's care, "diseases of the teeth and necessary artificial work would be his special province."[61]

US Army Dental Care Before the Civil War

In his 1856 medical manual, *Hints on the Medical Examination of Recruits for the Army*, Dr Thomas Henderson writes, "extensive loss of teeth, particularly the incisors (front teeth), is good cause for refusing a certificate. The teeth should be amply sufficient for healthy mastication, and for distinct enunciation. The front cutting teeth are especially necessary to tear the cartridge." The US Army Medical Department's official 1857 supply table included one instrument set, "teeth extracting (key and 3 claws, gum lancet, straight and curved forceps)," in its list for each military post.[62–64]

Unfortunately, the growing support for military dental service in the late 1850s meant little to the soldier in the field. Sergeant Percival Lowe of the US Dragoons recalled that, "in my whole five years of service [1849–1854] while on the plains, every summer on a long campaign and always expecting it, we never had a doctor." According to Lowe, only one fellow soldier, who had joined the unit with his dental instruments in hand, performed dental work on the soldiers. Unfortunately, this man later deserted. The advent of the Civil War in 1861 raised hopes among dentists that the crisis would bring formal recognition of the need for dental care in the military.[65]

References

1. *Congressional Record, 56th Cong, 2nd Sess*. Act of Feb 2, 1901. Sec 18, 31 Stat 752. Vol 34. Washington, DC: Government Printing Office.

2. Woods SH. An outline of dentistry in the British army, 1626-1938. *Proc R Soc Med*. Cited in: *Br Dent J*. 1939;66:147–152.

3. Allen WGB. *Pistols, Rifles and Machine Guns*. 2nd ed. London, UK: English Universities Press Ltd; 1961: 12–13.

4. Gavin H. Dental information for drafted men. *On Feigned Diseases*. Cited in: *NY Dent J*. 1863;6:187–188.

5. Von Steuben FWA. *Regulations for the Order and Discipline of the Troops of the United States*. Philadelphia, Pa: Styner and Cist; 1779. Reprint. Philadelphia, Pa: Ray Riling Arms Book Co; 1966.

6. Godden LJ, ed. *History of the Royal Army Dental Corps*. Aldershot, UK: Royal Army Dental Corps; 1971.

7. Asbell MB. *Dentistry: A Historical Perspective*. Bryn Mawr, Pa: Dorrance and Co; 1988.

8. Weinberger BW. Dentistry in America up to the middle of the nineteenth century, I. *Dent Items Interest*. 1943;65:681.

9. Gardette EB. Biographical notice of the late James Gardette, surgeon dentist, of Philadelphia. *Am J Dent Sci*. 1850:375–376.

10. Viau G. French dentistry in the United States: James Gardette, 1756–1831. *Dental Cosmos*. 1925;67:389–390.

11. Weinberger BW. *An Introduction to the History of Dentistry in America*. Vol 2. St Louis, Mo: CV Mosby Co; 1948: 137–150.

12. Greenwood IJ. Remarks on the portraiture of Washington. *Magazine Am Hist*. 1878;2:37–38.

13. Manchester HH. Post-Revolutionary dental announcements. *Dent Dig*. 1925;31:764.

14. Brown L. The antiquities of dental prosthesis, part III, section II, eighteenth century. *Dental Cosmos*. 1934;76:1156–1160.

15. Weinberger BW. Jean Pierre Le Mayeur in America: no longer the man of mystery. *Dental Cosmos*. 1934;76:573–574.

16. Asbell MB. First article on dentistry published in America. *Outlook Bull South Dent Soc N J*. 1964;33:49–52.

17. Robinson B. *The Foundations of Professional Dentistry*. Baltimore, Md: Waverly Press Inc; 1940: 27–34.

18. FitzPatrick, JC, ed. *The Diaries of George Washington 1748-1799*. Vol 2. Boston, Mass: Houghton Mifflin Co; 1925.

19. Brown, RK. *Fallen in Battle: American General Officer Combat Fatalities*. New York, NY: Greenwood Press; 1988.

20. Manchester, HH. The first dentists in America. *Dent Dig*. 1925;31:162–63.

21. Historical review of the progress of dental surgery in the United States, with reflections upon the causes that have accelerated it, and the means necessary for its further advancement. *Am J Dent Sci*. 1851;2:97.

22. Manchester HH. Dentists notices of the Revolutionary period. *Dent Dig*. 1925;31:687–689.

23. DeLessert CG. The origins of spiral springs. *Br J Dent Sci*. 1870;13:550.

24. Hayden HH. An opening address. *Am J Libr Dent Sci*. 1841;2:23–24.

25. Duncan LC. The medical service in the War of 1812, II. *Milit Surg*. 1932;71:542.

26. Duncan LC. Sketches of the medical service in the War of 1812. *Milit Surg*. 1932;71:439.

27. Anderson FJ. Medical practices in Detroit during the War of 1812. *Bull Hist Med*. 1944;16:267.

28. Mann J. *Medical Sketches of the Campaigns of 1812, 13, 14*. Dedham, Mass: H Mann & Co; 1816: 82.

29. Edgar J. The Army Medical Department in the War of 1812. *Milit Surg*. 1927;60:307.

30. Pfeiffer S, Williamson RF. *Snake IIill, an Investigation of a Military Cemetery from the War of 1812*. Toronto, Ontario, Canada: Dundurn Press; 1991: 226-234.

31. Thorpe BL. Biographies of pioneer American dentists and their successors. In: Koch C. *History of Dental Surgery*. Vol 3. Ft Wayne, Ind: National Art Publishing Co; 1910: 223.

32. Lockley F. Impressions and observations of the Journal Man. *The Oregon Journal*. 1936 (March).

33. US War Department. *General Regulations for the Army: or, Military Institutes*. Philadelphia, Pa: M Cary and Sons; 1821: 293–294.

34. Thorpe BL. A biographical review of the careers of Hayden and Harris. In: *Transactions of the Fourth International Dental Congress* [1904]. Vol 3. Philadelphia, Pa: The SS White Dental Mfg Co; 1905: 413-416.

35. National Archives and Records Administration. Compiled Military Service Record. Record Group 94. 39th Regiment (Fowler's) Maryland Militia (War of 1812).

36. Lufkin AW. *A History of Dentistry*. Philadelphia, Pa: Lea & Febiger; 1948: 198–203 .

37. Powell H, ed. *100 Years of Dentistry in Virginia*. Richmond, Va: Virginia State Dental Association; 1969: 10–11.

38. McCluggage RW. *A History of the American Dental Association: A Century of Health Service*. Chicago, Ill: American Dental Association; 1959.

39. Taylor JA. *History of Dentistry*. Philadelphia, Pa: Lea & Febiger; 1922.

40. Tilton EM. *Amiable Autocrat. A Biography of Dr. Oliver Wendell Holmes*. New York, NY: Henry Schuman; 1947: 187.

41. SS White Dental Mfg Co. *A Century of Service to Dentistry*. Philadelphia, Pa: The SS White Dental Mfg Co; 1944: 3–4.

42. Harris CA. *A Dictionary of Dental Science, Biography, Bibliography, and Medical Terminology*. Philadelphia, Pa: Lindsay and Blakiston; 1849: 595.

43. US War Department. *General Regulations for the Army of the United States, 1841*. Washington, DC: J and GS Gideon, Printers; 1841: 313.

44. Duncan LC. Medical history of General Scott's campaign to the city of Mexico in 1847. *Milit Surg.* 1920.

45. Obituary, Dr. Henry J.B. McKellops. *Dental Cosmos.* 1901;43:704.

46. Obituary, Dr. Joseph F. Hassell. *Dental Cosmos.* 1901;43:963.

47. National Archives and Records Administration. Compiled Military Service Record. Record Group 94. JF Hassell. First Regiment, St Louis Legion, Missouri Infantry.

48. National Archives and Records Administration. Compiled Military Service Record. Record Group 15. JF Hassell. Pension file. First Missouri Volunteers. Certificate no. 19521.

49. Prinz H. *Dental Chronology: A Record of the More Important Historic Events in the Evolution of Dentistry*. Philadelphia, Pa: Lea & Febiger; 1945: 87.

50. Sweet PA. Amalgam and the "New Departure." *Dent Radiogr Photogr.* 1959;32:66–69.

51. Allen C. A society of dental surgeons in New York. *NY Dent Rec.* 1847;2:2.

52. [Harris CA]. Importance of Army and Navy dentists. *Am J Dent Sci.* 1859;9:444.

53. Dunbar R, ed. *Jefferson Davis Constitutionalist: His Letters, Papers and Speeches*. Vol 2. Jackson, Miss: Mississippi Department of Archives and History; 1923: 281.

54. Hodgkin WN. Edward Maynard, a progenitor of the United States Army and Navy Dental Corps. *J Am Dent Assoc.* 1941;28:1970.

55. Meeting of the western dental society. *Quincy Whig and Republican.* Cited in: *Dental News Letter.* 1858;12:37–38.

56. Taft J. The influence of camp life upon the teeth. *Dental Register of the West.* 1861.

57. American Dental Convention, fourth annual session [proceedings]. *Dental News Letter.* 1858;12:6.

58. McCurdy JR. The employment of dentists in the Army. *Dental News Letter.* 1859;12:206.

59. Barker G. American Dental Convention [proceedings]. *Dental Cosmos.* 1859;1:81.

60. Roberts W. Remarks on dentistry in the Army. *American Medical Times.* Cited in: *Dental Cosmos.* 1861;3:51–52.

61. Dental reform in the Indian army. *Friend of India.* Cited in: *Br J Dent Sci.* 1859;3:45–46.

62. Taft J. The teeth of Army recruits. *Dental Register of the West.* 1861;15:435.

63. Henderson T. *Hints on the Medical Examination of Recruits for the Army; and on the Discharge of 60 Soldiers from the Service on Surgeon's Certificate.* New rev ed. Philadelphia, Pa: JB Lippincott & Co; 1856: 99.

64. US War Department. *Regulations for the Army of the United States, 1857.* New York, NY: Harper & Brothers; 1857: 250.

65. Lowe PG. *Five Years A Dragoon ('49–'54) and Other Adventures on the Great Plains.* Norman, Okla: University of Oklahoma Press; 1965: 34,100–101

Chapter II

THE CIVIL WAR:
DENTAL CARE IN THE UNION ARMY,
1861–1865

Introduction

Many American dentists in the Union states believed the Civil War provided the opportunity for the military to finally admit its need to care for soldiers' dental health. Not only did the US Army enter the war without dental surgeons, but the federal government did not supply toothbrushes for its troops. Dentists hoped the new call to arms would make the military aware of its dental shortcomings.

The Soldiers' Dental Requirements

Many potential enlistees were rejected during the war because of dental deficiencies. As part of the physical examination given to drafted men or their substitutes (the 1863 conscription act allowed a drafted man to hire someone else to perform his military service), the surgeon was to determine "whether he has a sufficient number of teeth in good condition to masticate his food properly, and to tear his cartridge quickly and with ease." Revised regulations were even more specific, stating that "total loss of all the front teeth, the eye-teeth, and first molars, even if only of one jaw" was cause for rejection.[1(p429)]

By the middle of the 19th century many more Americans appeared to be experiencing serious dental problems. This was attributed at least in part to the increased use of refined sugar in foods and a greater consumption of fresh, rather than salted, meats. Recent archaeological studies show evidence of increased antemortem tooth losses and abscesses, which may also be an indicator of unskilled dental intervention.[2] For example, 5% of the remains of 30 Confederate soldiers buried in Glorietta, New Mexico, had sustained tooth loss through alveolar abscessing, and 30% had abscessed teeth at their time of death. Only 4 of the 30 had no carious teeth, and 3 of the 30 had gold fillings. A study of a small sample of the skulls of Virginia soldiers held at the Armed Forces Institute of Pathology showed similar care, with fillings made of tinfoil, amalgam, or thorium.[3,4]

Just as in early European armies, some drafted Americans had their teeth extracted to be exempted from service. Dr David Noble of Ohio reported "one man exhibited twelve sound teeth that had been recently extracted, thus settling the question that a man may stand the steel, but fear the powder and lead." Some Army surgeons said that they "refused to exempt any whose alveolar processes were not absorbed, or whose gums indicated that the teeth had been recently extracted."[1(p429)]

The conscription records of 1863–1864 show that a large number of recruits were rejected because they failed to meet the dental requirements. In the draft of 1863 nearly one fifteenth of all physical exemptions were from "loss of teeth." In 1864 nearly one tenth of the total exemptions were dental.[5(p240)]

Dr Roberts Bartholow's *Manual of Instructions for Enlisting and Discharging Soldiers* (1863) called for rejection of recruits for "loss of a sufficient number of teeth to prevent proper mastication of food and tearing the cartridge," and "incurable deformities or loss of part of either jaw, hindering biting the cartridge, or proper mastication, or greatly injuring speech; anchylosis of lower jaw." It also cited "a carious condition of the teeth, and loss of the incisors and canines" as causes for rejection.[6]

In his *Manual of Instructions for Military Surgeons on the Examination of Recruits and Discharge of Soldiers* (1863), Dr John Ordronaux listed the following causes for rejection:

> shrinking of the gums, giving rise to loosening of the teeth; loss or decay of the four incisors of the same jaw; loss or decay of the two lateral incisors or cuspids of each jaw; loss or caries of several incisors or cuspids in either jaw (five at least); and, where the other teeth are not in a state of soundness.[7]

He also advised the surgeon to look for loss of teeth "concealed by the introduction of artificial ones." Other conditions such as temporomandibular articulation, anchylosis, harelip, stomatitis, "gangrene" of the mouth, facial paralysis, gingivitis, congenitally missing teeth, dental anomalies, supernumerary teeth, and diastemas were also mentioned. However, some recruits slipped through without meeting the requirements. Dr Daniel Holt, an assistant surgeon with the 121st New York Volunteer Regiment from August 1862 to October 1864, mentions seeing "grandfathers without teeth" serving in the line.[7,8]

In July 1861 Dr Jonathan Taft (1820–1903), the coeditor of *Dental Register of the West*, had already commented extensively on the subject of a soldier's dental requirements:

> The soldier requires a sufficient number of teeth in good condition, to enable him to masticate his food properly. Hard bread, tough beef, and salt pork, require good molars for this purpose. The incisor and canine teeth are not adapted to this end, *i.e.*, without the aid of some of the molars. . . . The soldier must again have teeth of some description, strong enough to tear his cartridge. This is usually done with the incisor and canine teeth. But if the bicuspid and two of the molars in both jaws upon the right side remain and are sound, we think this may be done as conveniently as with the incisor and canine. The instructions for tearing the cartridge in the infantry tactics, merely prescribe that it is to be put between the teeth, without specifying the particular teeth by which it is to be torn.

> If, then, the front teeth have been lost by accident, as sometimes happens, we should not reject the man on that account, provided the double teeth, or a sufficient number of them, remain sound in both jaws, and upon the right side. But if the front teeth have been lost from caries, and the double teeth are unsound to any extent, the man should be rejected. If the front teeth remain and the molars are gone, we think rejection is again demanded, because the man is evidently incapable of properly masticating the food he must subsist upon in the field.

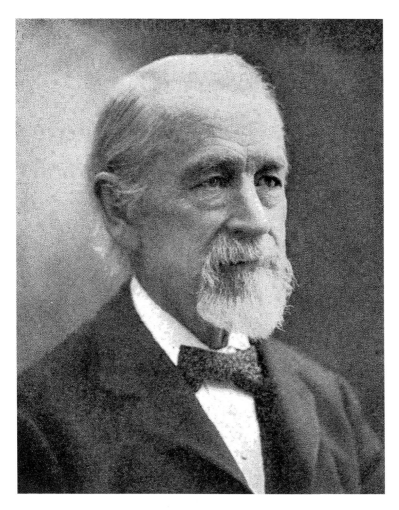

Jonathan Taft (1820–1903), coeditor of Dental Register of the West.
Photograph: Courtesy of the American Dental Association.

31

"Fetid breath" is sometimes a reason for rejection. If merely a sign of temporary de-
rangement of the digestive organs or the like, it is of no consequence. But if it depend
upon extensive caries of the teeth, chronic ozoena, scorbutic, syphilitic, scrofulous, or
mercurial cachexia, it demands rejection as well from its own offensiveness as from its
being one of the indications of grave disqualifying disease.[9(pp435–436)]

Taft then concluded that "if good teeth are so important for the soldier, would
it not be well to adopt some means by which they can receive the attention necessary for their preservation?" Commenting on the government's apparent disinterest in providing dental care for the thousands of volunteers pouring into
Army camps, he noted that not even "tooth-brushes, dentifrices, tooth-picks,
etc.," were supplied by the civilian provisioners (sutlers) in the large encampments. In the US Army of the day, as in those of the rest of the world, however,
advice such as Taft's was ignored, and still nothing was done to maintain the
soldiers' dental health.[10]

Army Surgeons and Hospital Stewards: A Muscular Right Arm

Any dental care the soldier received once in the Army was either paid for by
the individual or received from an Army surgeon, hospital steward, or a trained
dentist serving in another capacity in the same unit. Dental care from the surgeon
or steward was usually less than satisfactory. Dr John Sayre Marshall (1846–1922),
a veteran of the 2nd New York Volunteer (Harris) Cavalry and often referred to as
the "founding father of the Dental Corps" later said:

In the Union armies the only dental service rendered was that of lancing a "gum boil"
and the extraction of teeth. The latter service was usually performed by a hospital
steward, whose only qualification for this service was generally the fact that he possessed a muscular right arm. The victims, God rest their souls, after one experience
with the hospital steward were not usually willing to submit to such treatment a
second time.[11(p138)]

Brigadier General William Hammond, the Army surgeon general from April
1862 to August 1864, began reforming the Army Medical Department during the
first year of his tenure. He acknowledged the value of good oral health in his *Treatise on Hygiene* (1863), in which he stressed the need for healthy gums and strong,
caries-free teeth. "The importance of these points is, we think, liable to be overlooked. No one can be healthy whose teeth are deficient or in bad condition; and
soldiers, of all other classes of men, require that these organs should be sound."
When an American Dental Convention committee conferred with Surgeon General Hammond sometime after his appointment in April 1862, it was reported that
"the matter [commissioning dentists for the Army] was very favorably received by
him." However, Hammond believed that unhealthy gums were often indicators of
other medical problems, and insisted that Army surgeons already in service could
meet any required dental minimums.[12(p59)] He never took action to add dental surgeons to the Medical Department.[13]

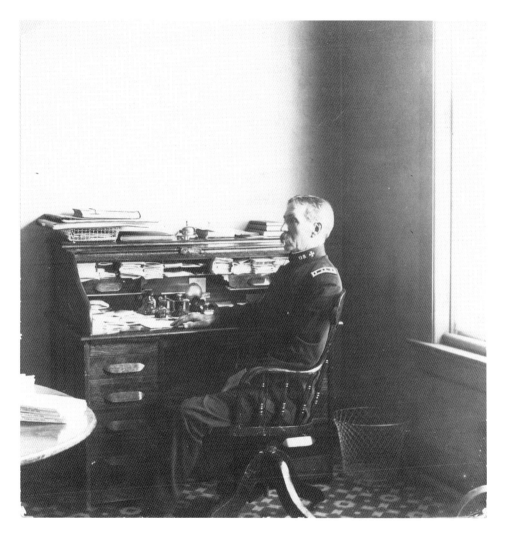

John Sayre Marshall.
Photograph: Courtesy of US Army Medical Department Museum. DCC01 Marshall-02.

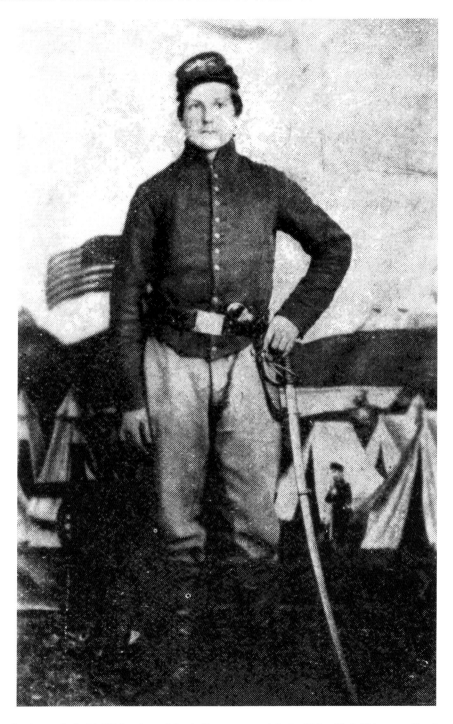

John S Marshall, Civil War photo. Marshall, a veteran of the 2nd New York Volunteer Cavalry, is often called the founding father of the Army Dental Corps.
Photograph: Courtesy of: the American Dental Association

For dental operations, the government provided the Army surgeons with the following set of instruments: "one turn-key, two pairs of straight forceps, one pair of lower molar forceps [beaks half an inch wide], one gum lancet, one stump screw [occasionally]." This limited instrumentation, coupled with a lack of training and experience, made an extraction by an Army surgeon quite an adventure for the patient. Writing in the March 1862 issue of the *New York Dental Journal*, its editor, Dr William Roberts, noted that "the army surgeon is generally not only utterly incompetent to the proper care of the teeth, but he is also entirely averse to it, and when forced to its consideration, hastens his disagreeable task as much as possible." Roberts thought that dentists attached to the Army, carrying along their own sets of instruments, would solve the problem and save the government "a useless and illy-regulated expense."[14]

William Roberts's 1861 Concept for a Dental Department of the US Army

In July 1861 Roberts proposed a thoughtful solution to the dental situation already confronting Union soldiers. In his *New York Dental Journal*, he argued that "a corps of dentists, or dental staff, should be attached to the United States Army, similarly organized with the surgical department, who would act in connection with and as an efficient aid to that department, besides performing their own duties in a proper manner." He further proposed that the newly formed US Sanitary Commission, organized in June 1861 to provide civilian assistance to Union army casualties and their dependents, direct its efforts to lobby Congress on this "humane" and "economical" measure at the next congressional session.[15,16]

Roberts also presented a plan in which he recommended that the secretary of war form a "Dental Department of the United States Army." This group would be headed by a "Dental Surgeon-General," appointed by the secretary, who in turn would appoint qualified dental surgeons to be "Dental Inspectors." The inspectors were to be assigned to posts of two to four regiments, and their duties would include quarterly oral health inspections and statistical reporting. His plan also implied that the inspectors would supervise dental personnel working at the regimental level.[15] A "Board of Dental Surgeons," also appointed by the secretary, would examine and approve the qualifications of candidates for appointment to the dental department and would examine those eligible for promotion. Those selected would be ranked as either "Dental Surgeons" or "Assistant Dental Surgeons." A dental surgeon would be assigned to each regiment and would be responsible for the dental care of all of its members, as well as for the maintenance of individual dental records to be shown to the inspectors. An assistant dental surgeon would be appointed to each regiment to assist the dental surgeon as directed. Roberts suggested that applicants to this latter position be between 21 and 28 years old and become eligible for promotion after 5 years service and examination by the dental board.[15]

Furthermore, he recommended that dental supplies be issued the same way they were in the Medical Department, with dental inspectors drawing all medicines and materials and distributing them to the dental surgeons at each post. Pay and fiscal matters would also conform to the scales and practices of the Medical Department.

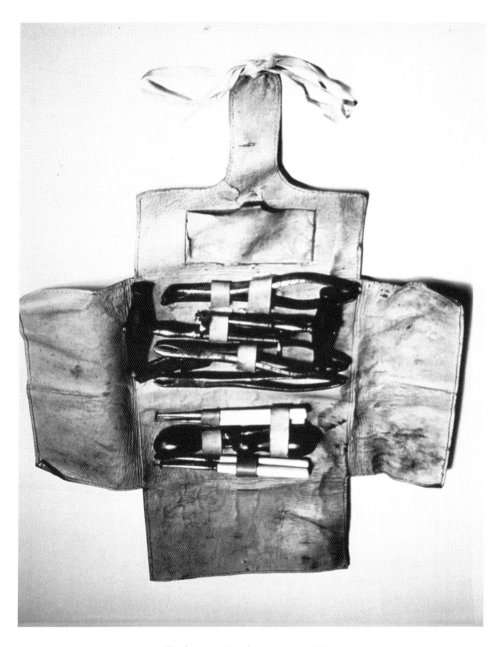

Tooth extracting forceps, circa 1850.
Reproduced from: http://wwwihm.nlm.nih.gov/ihm/images/A/23/323.jpg.
Courtesy of the National Library of Medicine.

Roberts concluded with a strong recommendation:

> Thus, by some such system as the above attached to the United States Army, every recruit would be inspected by the Dental Surgeon on entering the army, and his mouth put into a healthy and proper condition, in which condition it would be kept during his time of service; a judicious series of regulations would compel every soldier to keep his teeth carefully brushed and cleansed, and this of itself would greatly lessen the chances of disease.[15(p186)]

In 1863 Roberts revised his dental plan to reflect the changing situation. He proposed that the War Department authorize qualified dentists to practice among the troops in the field at their own expense, receiving compensation through reasonable fees. If that was not acceptable, he urged that one dentist and one assistant be appointed to each brigade with the equivalent rank and pay of their medical counterparts. If the government was unwilling to assume that expense, Roberts suggested that the Sanitary Commission appoint qualified dentists who would practice among the forces for fees first approved by the commission. He believed that "plenty of excellent dentists" would respond to the call, and that the "comfort and well being" of the soldier would be greatly improved if this plan was adopted.[14,21]

Remarkably, Roberts's plans came very close to the system adopted by the Army when contract dental surgeons were finally authorized in February 1901. In 1861 and 1863, however, his ideas were not viewed favorably.

John Hugh McQuillen: Army Surgeons are not Dentists

In December 1861 Dr John Hugh McQuillen (1826–1879), coeditor of *Dental Cosmos*, commented on some of the problems inherent in establishing a dental service for the Army. He noted that with the federal government already spending approximately $1.5 million daily on the war, it was unlikely that the secretaries of the Army and Navy would "recommend to Congress the propriety of establishing an entirely new department, which will be attended by a very large additional outlay per annum."[17]

McQuillen also foresaw insurmountable problems with "furnishing the materials, gold-foil, plate, teeth, etc., demanded in the performance of dental operations." He did not think the government, with all its other obligations, would provide such items, but neither could dentists on their small salary. This meant that the cost of treatment would pass to the soldiers, whose low pay and other obligations made that expense nearly impossible to manage. McQuillen anticipated further problems with poor working conditions and unit deployments, which would prevent any conscientious follow-up. These roadblocks would "reduce the operations of the dentist simply to the treatment of exposed nerve pulps, alveolar abscesses, and the extraction of teeth—operations which the *thoroughly* educated surgeon should be prepared to meet."[17]

McQuillen went on to observe that:

The education of the surgeon, however, in this direction, it must be admitted, has not heretofore been sufficiently attended to, and it is extremely doubtful whether one out of ten can diagnose between an aching and sound tooth, an exposed pulp and acute periostitis, the course of treatment demanded in each case, or, when extraction is demanded, perform that operation as it should be done. Indeed, it is difficult to conceive how it could be otherwise in the latter operation, as the surgeon is only provided, by a regulation of the service, with two pair of forceps, one straight and one curved. With these he is expected to meet every emergency that may arise.[17]

McQuillen insisted that his remarks were not meant to demean the Army surgeons, but merely to emphasize the fact that physicians were not educated in the dental sciences. He recommended that the medical bureaus of the services take steps to correct this deficiency in surgeons' education. He also observed that some medically trained dentists had given up their dental practices and been accepted by the Army as surgeons or assistant surgeons. Among this group were Dr John McGrath of Philadelphia, Dr William M Wright of Pittsburgh, and Dr Joseph Richardson of Cincinnati.[25]

As the war progressed, McQuillen and *Dental Cosmos* continued to track developments in the Union army and to editorialize on the most pressing dental issues. In October 1862 the coeditor of *Dental Cosmos* noted that:

It is a constant source of complaint on the part of many army and navy surgeons, both in the regular and volunteer service, that the instruments supplied by the medical bureaus for the extraction of teeth are inadequate to meet the most ordinary contingencies of practice. The justice of this complaint must be apparent when it is known that only two pair of forceps, one straight and one curved, are all that the departments furnish. It is not surprising, therefore, that aching teeth, which could be readily removed with properly-constructed forceps, are frequently allowed to remain after several abortive attempts have been made to extract them. Under such circumstances, the poor soldier or sailor is, of course, compelled to submit to that "Hell o' pains, the toothache," with no prospect of relief, from the surgeon at least. Notwithstanding these facts, and the great improvements that have been made during the past twenty-five years in extracting instruments, some of the older surgeons, wedded, of course, to bygone days, regard the instruments furnished as all-sufficient.[2]

Regarding forceps, McQuillen thought that "while six pair, perhaps, would answer ordinary contingencies, *at least twelve pair* were demanded to meet every contingency that might arise." He recommended that Army and Navy surgeons be supplied with the proper instruments and textbooks to meet every emergency.[17,18]

In the fall of 1862 some Army surgeons complained about the "small cap" worn by the troops. They thought that it provided little protection from the weather elements as winter approached, and that it was partially responsible for so many soldiers suffering from "neuralgia in the head." In December 1862 McQuillen and the editors of *Dental Cosmos* suggested that these "neuralgic affections" could often be traced to dental diseases and were curable with proper dental treatment. It was possible that a dentist could cure in minutes what might cause the "poor fellows" to suffer for several weeks.[19]

The Legislative Efforts of the American Dental Convention's Military Committee in 1861–1862

When Taft, editor of *Dental Register of the West*, had noted the government's disinterest in the soldiers' dental care in July 1861, he also pointed out that the American Dental Convention committee made "little or no effort" to secure the appointment of dentists in the Regular Army. While he surmised that perhaps the committee found the "difficulties to be so great, as to render any effort in that direction impracticable," he believed that the "welfare of the soldiers" dictated that increased efforts continue toward that goal.[20]

On August 9, 1861, at the American Dental Convention meeting in New Haven, Connecticut, the Committee on Appointing Dentists in the Army and Navy reported that more time was needed to consider this important matter than the present session would allow. A five-person committee was appointed to address the government about admitting dental surgeons to the Army and Navy.[21,22] The committee consisted of Dr WH Atkinson, Dr George H Perine, and Dr BW Franklin, all of New York City; Dr JD White of Philadelphia; and Dr IJ Wetherbee of Boston.[3] In January 1862 the committee urged members of the dental and medical professions to submit any recommendations or suggestions on how this could be accomplished "for the benefit of our volunteers."[23(p312)]

In the April 1862 issue of *Dental Cosmos*, John McQuillen noted that early in the year, the War Department established new military hospitals in New York, Philadelphia, Saint Louis, Cincinnati, and other northern cities to prepare for upcoming offensive operations. These hospitals were placed under the charge of "visiting" and assistant surgeons selected from among the local practitioners of each city. While nothing was "left undone to contribute to the comfort and welfare of the patients, on the part of the medical officers," visiting dental surgeons were not appointed, nor was provision made for dental care for those patients suffering "from a deranged condition of the teeth."[24]

On August 5, 1862, a letter from Surgeon General Hammond to Dr JD White of Philadelphia was read at the American Dental Convention meeting in Trenton Falls, New York. Dated July 28, it addressed the addition of dentists to the Army Medical Department:

> Nothing would give me greater satisfaction than to have a corps of accomplished dentists added to the medical department of the army. I shall recommend it in my report to Congress. Nothing can be done, however, but by law, and I would suggest to you the propriety of agitating the subject through the public prints.[25]

In the discussion that followed, Dr William Dwinelle of New York City said that Hammond had personally expressed to him his "sympathy with and appreciation of the movement." Other dentists urged the committee to "increased action" and more individual effort in conjunction with exerting the committee's "influence." Jonathan Taft of Cincinnati argued that if dentists were given the opportunity to exhibit their value to the Army, the need for a dental department would soon be recognized; in this manner, both the Army and the dental profession would benefit—the latter by the "advancement and elevation of the profession." He also claimed that he had received a request from a "military division" for the "permanent services of a dentist." After Dr Burras of Buffalo, New York, joined the committee, the members voted to continue it for another year.[25,26]

The American Dental Association and Continuing Efforts to Secure Dentists in the Union Army

On July 28, 1863, at the Philadelphia meeting of the American Dental Association, McQuillen, coeditor of *Dental Cosmos* and a frequent commentator on the lack of dentists in the Union army, proposed the following resolution:

> That a committee of five be appointed by this Association to confer with Surgeon-General Hammond relative to the appointment of dentists to the military hospitals of the United States, and also to secure, if possible, prompt and successful action on the part of Congress, by having petitions prepared, signed, and sent to that body from all parts of the country in favor of the measure.[27]

After some discussion, the resolution was adopted and a committee appointed, consisting of McQuillen, Taft, and Drs CW Spalding, CP Fitch, and HN Wadsworth. Again, another resolution for Army dental surgeons was on the table, but apparently little was accomplished after that.[27]

A year later, on July 26, 1864, at the American Dental Association's meeting in Niagara Falls, New York, McQuillen, the chairman of the committee lobbying to appoint dentists to military hospitals, reported that he had written to Surgeon General Hammond, who was in the midst of an ugly court-martial, but did not receive a reply. He also contacted the acting surgeon general, Colonel Joseph Barnes, and received an "unfavorable response." He urged members to engage in a "more vigorous" effort because of the "importance of the subject."[28]

As the discussion continued, Dr Samuel White of the SS White Dental Manufacturing Company in Philadelphia said that he had spoken to President Abraham Lincoln personally and asked his advice on the "direction" that efforts would have to take to secure a dental service for the soldiers. The president suggested that White talk to Secretary of War Edmund Stanton. However, when White called at the War Department, the secretary was absent. Instead, he, too, spoke to Barnes, who said that he was fully aware of the situation and had already concluded that nothing could be done while the armies were engaged in battle. If the war lasted until winter and the armies went into winter quarters, Barnes said, perhaps something could be worked out. He added that the Medical Department could issue the necessary regulations without congressional action. The only thing White actually accomplished was to get his company an order for a supply of dental forceps for use by the Army surgeons.[28,29]

Following some spirited discussion, McQuillen reminded the meeting members that the subject was the introduction of dental surgeons into the "military hospitals" and not into the Army, as it would seem from the trend of the speakers' comments. The committee then discussed congressional action, the problem of fees or salaries for Army dental surgeons, seeking gubernatorial or Medical Department approval for visiting Army camps, independent action by individuals, establishment of a "dental bureau," enlisting Army support and influence, and the humane nature involved in dental work with the soldiers. Eventually McQuillen's report was approved, the committee was voted to be continued, and the meeting was adjourned. [29]

The Wartime Service of Dentists

While their colleagues unsuccessfully lobbied the Medical Department and Congress, many dentists served in the Union army and contributed to the war effort in a variety of ways, despite the government's reluctance to give them military status within their profession. In fact, any dental service these soldiers performed was strictly unofficial, and the activities of some dentists contributed to a misconception, perpetrated in earlier literature, that there were dentists appointed by the federal government serving the various Army units. Actually, none were officially designated until 1872, well after the Civil War, when Dr William Saunders, a US Army hospital steward, was named the official dentist for the cadets at the US Military Academy at West Point, New York. A few dentists were appointed unofficially by the commanders of state volunteer regiments to serve their respective units, but this practice must have been rare because only occasional references to such appointments were made in the dental literature of the time.[30]

Despite the national government's refusal to recognize the need for dental care for its soldiers, many dentists made substantial contributions in the course of the war. Some dentists carried their dental instruments as part of their field kits, doing what they could for their fellow soldiers as time permitted. For example, Dr Charles Koch (1844–1916) of Chicago, Illinois, served as an enlisted soldier and officer from August 1862 until March 1866, and commanded the 49th Regiment (US Colored Troops), held staff positions, and was a provost marshal in Mississippi. While serving as an infantry officer during the Civil War, he carried "a small satchel, in which he kept dental instruments and medicines to relieve the tortures of the mouth" for the duration of his service.[31]

During the Civil War, some dentists enlisted as privates in the various state volunteer regiments, some received commissions as line officers in these same regiments, and some became hospital stewards to take advantage of their medical training. Others who had medical degrees (it was quite common at that time for a physician to practice dentistry) received appointments as surgeons or assistant surgeons in volunteer regiments or the Regular Army. Dr Royal Varney joined the Army as assistant surgeon in the 31st Ohio Volunteer Infantry, but his dental skills were never used; instead, his duties required him to staff a dressing station for the walking wounded, mostly wrapping bandages.[32]

Some civilian dentists voluntarily offered their professional services to the various training camps and on the battlefield. Dr William Morton, who had successfully demonstrated the use of sulphuric ether as a general anesthetic during surgery in 1846, volunteered his services to administer ether in the Wilderness Campaign of 1864. News that May led him to volunteer, first in Fredericksburg, then around Spotsylvania, roving informally among field hospitals and delivering anesthesia. When the Army continued southward, Morton remained in Freder-

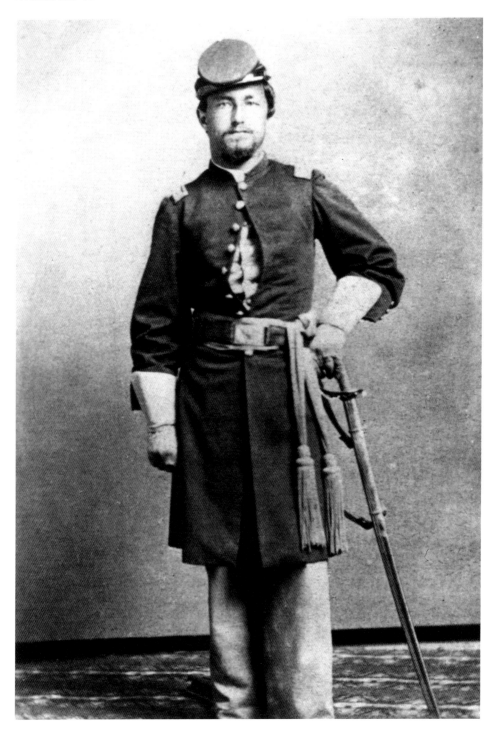

Charles RE Koch, Civil War, 72nd Illinois Infantry, 58th US Colored Troops.
Photograph: Courtesy of Illinois State Historical Library, Springfield.

icksburg and assisted in the evacuation of patients to the Washington area before returning to private practice.[33] Morton died in poverty in 1868.[34]

Dr George Watt (1820–1893), coeditor of *Dental Register of the West*, was an 1848 graduate of the Medical College of Ohio at Cincinnati and an 1854 graduate of the Ohio College of Dental Surgery. On May 9, 1864, he joined the service as a major and surgeon of the 154th Regiment of Ohio Infantry (National Guard) for 100 days at Camp Dennison, Ohio. He was subsequently stationed with his regiment at New Creek (now Keyser), West Virginia, an area noted for its guerrilla activities. In August 1864 Jonathan Taft, his coeditor of the *Dental Register*, quoted a letter from Watt:

> He reports that his health has very much improved. Has not had sick headache (with which he was very much afflicted before) since he has been in the service; has "consolidated from 211 lbs. to 180! laying off his pomposity." Says he has been shot at several times but not hit.[35–38]

Watt was discharged from the service on September 1, 1864, as a result of a spinal injury that caused locomotor ataxia, and he resumed his dental practice in Xenia, Ohio, where he lived until his death.[35–38]

Another dentist serving as a surgeon was Clark Smith (1832–1899), of Washington County, New York, who was a practicing dentist with a medical degree (MD). On July 29, 1862, he signed a contract as an assistant surgeon for the US Army and was issued a medical field case, medical pocket case, and one "teeth extracting" set from the medical purveyor's office in New York. Smith was assigned as the assistant surgeon to the 169th New York Volunteers.[39]

One physician-dentist, John Randolph Lewis (1834–1900), became the colonel of his regiment, the 5th Vermont Infantry. Lewis had received his DDS in 1858 from the Pennsylvania College of Dental Surgery, and later his MD from the University of Vermont.[40] On May 2, 1861, Lewis was called up as a private in Company H, 1st Vermont Infantry, where he served for 3 months. He saw action at Big Bethel, Virginia, in June 1861, and was mustered out with his regiment on August 15. He was then commissioned a captain in Company I, 5th Vermont Infantry, on September 12. Rapid promotions followed. He was promoted to major over five senior captains (at their request) on July 16, 1862. Lewis was promoted to lieutenant colonel on October 6, 1862, and to colonel on June 5, 1864.[40–42]

Lewis saw action in all the battles in which his regiment participated except Mine Run and Antietam until May 1864. On June 30, 1862, he was wounded in the right leg by a shell fragment at White Oak Swamp, Virginia. While commanding his regiment at the "dreary wasteland fringing the south bank of the Rapidan River" during the Wilderness Campaign, he was wounded early in the first day's fighting; his left arm was "shattered by a musket ball, which entered just below the shoulder.[43] That evening the arm was amputated at the shoulder (exsection of the humerus) at the division field hospital. The next day Lewis was taken to Fredericksburg by field ambulance, a journey that took 3 days. Lewis convalesced in Buffalo, New York, under his wife's care, and was honorably discharged from active duty on September 11, 1864. The next day, he was appointed a colonel in the 1st Regiment, Veteran Reserve Corps.[41,44,45]

Subsequently Lewis served on the Veteran Reserve Corps' Examining Board in Washington, DC; guarded Confederate prisoners at Elmira, New York; served as the inspector general on the staff of Brigadier General Clinton Fiske at Nashville; and was a member of the Bureau of Refugees, Freedmen and Abandoned Lands for the state of Tennessee. Lewis was mustered out on March 31, 1867, at Macon, Georgia. The same year, he accepted an appointment as a major in the 44th Infantry Regiment, US Army, at the personal request of General Ulysses S Grant. Grant was aware that Lewis's amputation kept him from "taking up his profession, that of a Dentist." Service on the staff of Colonel Caleb C Sibley in Georgia, as inspector general, and on the Freedmen Bureau followed. Finally on April 28, 1870, Lewis was retired with the rank of colonel, under section 22 of the Act of July 28, 1866, after almost 9 years of active duty. [42,46,47]

On June 6, 1863, Dr John Patten (1826–?), a former captain in the 50th New York Engineers who had resigned his commission because of ill health the previous July, wrote to Brigadier General Henry Benham, the commander of the Engineer Brigade, Army of the Potomac. He asked for permission to "follow the Brigade" at his own risk and expense in order to provide dental care to its members. [47,48] The request was endorsed by Lieutenant Colonel William Pettes, the commanding officer of the 50th New York Engineers, with the recommendation that Patten's "professional services would be of much service" to the regiment. Benham agreed to Patten's request subject to the approval of the provost marshal general. Also on June 6, Brigadier General Marsena Patrick, the provost marshal general of the Army of the Potomac, authorized Patten's presence until further orders. [48] At the very least, this was a tacit admission of the need for professional dental care for soldiers.

Consequences of Serving without Dental Service

In March 1863, 2 years after the war began, William Roberts, the coeditor of the *New York Dental Journal* who had proposed the "Dental Department" for the Army, offered this comment on the soldiers' continuing dental plight:

> If the soldier could only take reasonable care of his teeth himself, he would get on much better, but a tooth-brush is an article not in the regulations and sutlers don't supply them. If they did, it would be at a cost far beyond the soldier's purse and inclination. People can stand paying high prices for luxuries, but not for necessities; they would sooner go without. But if there were a dentist in the brigade, with good tooth-brushes, at the usual prices, every *decent* soldier would have one and use it, and there would be one great gain over the enemy.
>
> Next, supposing the soldier's teeth decay, which they are almost sure to; he cannot ask for a furlough, to go home and get his teeth filled; and, probably, if he got a furlough, would readily find some other way to spend it. There is no dentist in the army, so all the tooth has to do is to rot away at its earliest convenience, when the soldier goes to the surgeon, and the surgeon draws the tooth as expeditiously and as painfully as he knows how. [13(p145)]

After the 2 days of fighting at Little Round Top at Gettysburg, First Lieutenant Ziba Graham of the 16th Regiment, Michigan Volunteer Infantry, described his dental visit to the regimental surgeon on Friday, July 3, 1863, in his diary:

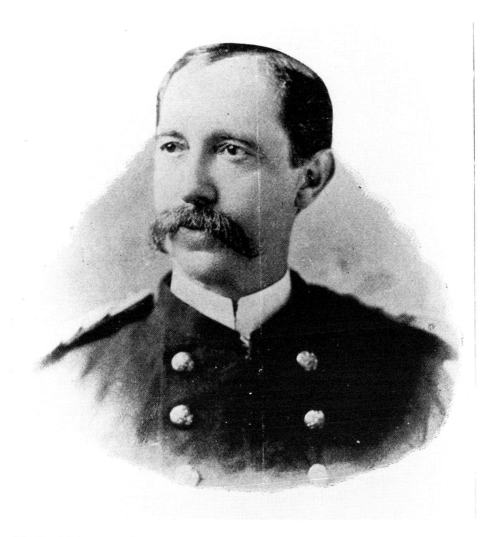

John Randolph Lewis, a dentist and physician, saw action during the Civil War and was wounded during the Wilderness Campaign. Later, Lewis accepted an appointment as a major in the 44th Infantry Regiment, US Army, at the personal request of General Ulysses S Grant. Photograph: Courtesy of Massachusetts Commandery, Military Order of the Loyal Legion, and US Army Military History Institute.

All being quiet in our front I received permission to go back to the hospital to get an ugly tooth extracted that had kept me dancing all the night before. Our surgeon, Doctor [Robert] Everett, who had been hard at work all night at the amputation table, made but short work and little ado about one tooth. He laid me on the ground, straddled me, and with a formidable pair of nippers pulled and yanked me around until either the tooth had to come out, or my head off. I was glad when the head conquered. I then made up my mind never to go to a surgeon for a tooth-pulling matinee the day after a fight.[49(p12)]

Regardless of one's rank, dental problems drew little sympathy from the medical establishment. Twice in 1863 Brigadier General Albion Howe, commanding the 2nd Division, VI Corps, required a surgeon's certificate stating he was unfit for duty because of "several defective teeth" before he could go on leave and get treatment at his own expense.[50] Soldiers experiencing trauma to the face and jaw were also in for a hard time. Sergeant Asa Smith of the 16th Massachusetts Volunteer Infantry sustained a severe jaw wound at Glendale in 1862 and was considered walking wounded. The first surgeon he encountered declared his wound fatal and refused to treat him. Finally, after 2 days, one of his regimental officers, himself wounded, persuaded a doctor at one of the medical collecting points to operate on Smith. Two men held him while the physician removed 18 pieces of bone without anesthesia, then sewed up the wound, leaving part of it open to drain. Smith was still considered walking wounded and fended for himself for 2 more days before another sympathetic doctor cleaned his wound and bandaged it to keep the flies off. A few days later he was evacuated by boat to a hospital at the Naval Academy. He received a medical discharge in July 1862 and made his own way home, where he eventually recovered.[51]

The nature of the war and types of ordnance used meant that many soldiers sustained injuries to the jaw similar to Sergeant Smith's. Final federal statistics reported in the US Army Medical Department's 6-volume *Medical and Surgical History of the War of the Rebellion* showed that 4,502 soldiers sustained gunshot fracture wounds to the face, of which 3,700 patients were known to have recovered, 404 died, and 398 outcomes were undetermined. Thus, only 9.8% died (primarily due to secondary hemorrhage) in the course of treatment, thanks in part to the voluntary efforts of civilian dentists contributing their expertise.[52,53]

Ironically, when Dr James Garretson (1828–1895), considered to be the "father" of oral surgery, volunteered his services for the Union cause, the surgeon general's office rejected him. On July 29, 1862, Dr Hayes Agnew of Philadelphia had recommended to the surgeon general that Garretson be appointed "visiting physician" to the military hospital at the corner of 16th and Filbert Streets in Philadelphia.[54] On August 12, 1862, Garretson himself applied to Surgeon General Hammond to be appointed as the surgeon-in-charge of the contemplated military hospital at Red Bank, New Jersey. On August 14 the surgeon general's office replied, "your request cannot be granted, as the Red Bank hospital is to be placed in charge of an Ass[istant] Surgeon of the regular service." Thus, the Army Medical Department failed to utilize Garretson's unique talents in plastic and oral surgery. Later, Garretson was the first surgeon to successfully use Dr WGA Bonwill's dental engine, an early foot-powered drill, in surgical operations, and his textbook, *A Treatise on*

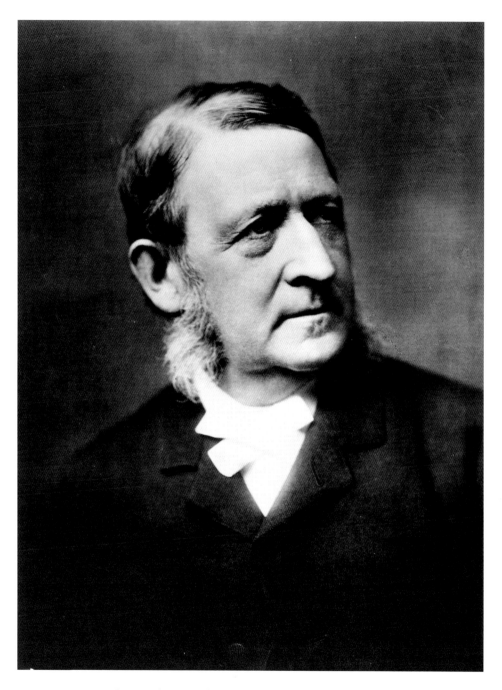

James E Garretson (1825–1895), plastic and oral surgeon.
Photograph: Courtesy of the American Dental Association.

the Diseases and Surgery of the Mouth, Jaws and Associated Parts (1869), went through six editions as *A System of Oral Surgery* (1873–1895). In 1872 the Medical Department finally adopted the book in the supply table as the official standard reference for its surgeons.[55–57]

In the "Dental Gossip" section of the January 1864 edition of the *Dental Times*, the following item appeared on the need for Army dental surgeons:

> I have been told by a military officer that dentists are greatly needed in the army. That he had repeated occasions to give men furloughs to go to Washington to have teeth filled and otherwise treated; for very many in our army are sufficiently intelligent to know that troublesome or decayed teeth may be saved, and are therefore unwilling to have them sacrificed by extraction, which is all the army surgeon can do; therefore, the want of an intelligent dentist is apparent, who, I have no question, could make it mutually advantageous, (as he would charge for his operations,) by remaining with the army, which, no doubt, he would be permitted to do on making proper representations to those in immediate authority. I trust this hint may be acted upon, to the advantage of both soldier and dentist. Such a procedure would furnish an unanswerable argument in favor of what the profession has been long contending for, Governmental employment of dentists in the army.[58(p126)]

Such arguments did not prevail, although many officers of the line recognized the need for good dental health. For example, a participant in the Vicksburg campaign of Ulysses S Grant noted the general's priorities in *Dental Cosmos* in October 1864:

> In starting on the movement the General disencumbered himself of everything, setting an example to his officers and men. He took neither a horse nor a servant, overcoat nor blanket, nor tent nor camp-chest, nor even a clean shirt. *His only baggage consisted of a tooth-brush.* He always showed his teeth to the Rebels. *He shared all the hardships of the private soldier, sleeping in the front and open air, and eating hard tack and salt pork* [emphasis in original].[59(p176)]

In April 1870 Dr Findley Y Clark (1829-1903), a local dentist who would play a leading role in the postwar push for military dentists, commented on the wretched dental condition of General William T Sherman's troops as they marched into Savannah in December 1864:

> When the steamer "Water Witch" was captured, and the prisoners brought to Savannah, we learned there was a Dentist among the number; and that he had quite a supply of material. From this we were led to believe that the Government recognized our profession, and that Dentists were appointed in the army and navy. Shortly after, however, when General Sherman and his hundred thousand men entered Savannah, we were by practical demonstration better informed. From daylight until dark our dental offices were besieged. The cry was, relief from present suffering, "Do something for my teeth that will keep them from aching." We remember one fellow coming to us a few days after having one or two nerves destroyed in his teeth, who wished, as he said, "to buy a good smart quantity of that white, creamy stuff," for, said he, "when the boys get on the march, and have the tooth-ache, I can get their last dollar with it."[60]

Some Small Steps, No Giant Leaps

The continuing pressure and concerted lobbying from American dental groups during the Civil War produced only small gains in the struggle to establish dental care in the Army. Many soldiers and officers understood the need from personal experience, but little real change took place in the status of military dentistry. The war ended in April 1865 with dentists just where they were 4 years earlier—the Army had no trained dentists officially serving the troops. In the Union army, the surgeon general was seriously impeded by the presence of an established bureaucracy, including his own physicians, who were jealous of its prerogatives and quick to defend its interests. As a result, scant formal change occurred.

However, the knowledge and expertise of dentists was repeatedly validated by the benefits of dental hygiene, as well as in the treatment of maxillofacial wounds and injuries. The dentists' specialized mechanical and metallurgical knowledge made them even more desirable assets in both the North and South. The wartime generation, with its many Union and Confederate veterans, could speak with greater authority and practical wisdom when the drive for military dentists was renewed. By the end of the war, the defeated Confederate forces had adopted a significantly different approach to dental care for its soldiers, which provided an important counterpoint to the bleak Union experience.

References

1. Bumgardner E. Disqualification for military service in the Civil War on account of loss of teeth. *Dental Cosmos*. 1894;36:429.

2. Sledzik PS, Moore-Jansen PH. Dental diseases in nineteenth century military skeletal samples. Cited in: *Advances in Dental Anthropology*. Kelley MA, Larsen CS, eds. New York, NY: Wiley-Liss; 1991: 218,223.

3. Owsley DW. *Bioarchaeology on a Battlefield: the Abortive Confederate Campaign in New Mexico*. Located at: Museum of New Mexico, Office of Archaeological Studies, Santa Fe; 1994: 25.

4. Glenner RA, Willey P, Seldzik PS, Junger E. Dental fillings in Civil War skulls: what do they tell us? *J Am Dent Assoc*. 1996;127:1676.

5. Lewis JR. Exemptions from military service on account of loss of teeth. *Dental Cosmos*. 1865;7:240.

6. Bartholow R. *Manual of Instructions for Enlisting and Discharging Soldiers: with Special Reference to the Medical Examination of Recruits, and the Detection of Disqualifying and Feigned Diseases*. Philadelphia, Pa: JB Lippincott & Co; 1863: 54–55.

7. Ordronaux J. *Manual of Instructions for Military Surgeons, on the Examination of Recruits and Discharge of Soldiers*. New York, NY: D Van Nostrand & Co; 1863.

8. Greiner JM, Coryell JL, Smither JR, eds. *A Surgeon's Civil War: the Letters and Diary of Daniel M. Holt, M.D.* Kent, Ohio: Kent State University Press; 1994: 24.

9. Taft [J]. The teeth of Army recruits. *Dental Register of the West*. 1861;15:435–36.

10. Taft [J]. The influence of camp life upon the teeth. *Dental Register of the West*. 1861;15:432,436.

11. CRE Koch, ed. *History of Dental Surgery*. Vol 1. Fort Wayne, Ind: National Art Publishing Co; 1910: 138.

12. Hammond WA. *Treatise on Hygiene with Special Reference to the Military Service*. Philadelphia, Pa: JB Lippincott & Co; 1863: 59.

13. Perine GH. The necessity of dental appointments in the Army and Navy. *DentalCosmos*. 1880;22:467.

14. [Roberts WB]. Twenty-five days in the Sanitary Commission. *NY Dent J*. 1863;6:145–47.

15. [Roberts WB]. Dentistry in the Army. *NY Dent J*. 1861;4:184.

16. Faust PL, ed. *Historical Times Illustrated Encyclopedia of the Civil War*. New York, NY: Harper & Row; 1986: 656.

17. McQ[uillen] [JH]. Dentists in the Army and Navy of the United States. *Dental Cosmos.* 1861;3:268–269.

18. McQ[uillen] [JH]. Instruments furnished for the extraction of teeth to Army and Navy surgeons. *Dental Cosmos.* 1862;4:148–151.

19. Neuralgia in the Army. *Dental Cosmos.* 1862;4:262.

20. T[aft] [J]. Dentists in the Army. *Dental Register of the West.* 1861;15:430.

21. Barker GT, comp. American Dental Convention [proceedings]. *Dental Cosmos.* 1861;3:85.

22. Notice [American Dental Convention Committee]. *Dental Cosmos.* 1862;3:312.

23. The American Dental Convention to be held at Trenton Falls, N.Y. *Dental Cosmos.* 1862;3:312.

24. McQ[uillen] [JH]. Dentists in military hospitals. *Dental Cosmos.* 1862;3:498–99.

25. Ellis GW, comp. Proceedings of the American Dental Convention. *Dental Cosmos.* 1862;4:79–80.

26. Enthusiastic war meeting. *Utica Herald.* Quoted in: *Dental Cosmos.* 1862;4:100.

27. Ellis GW, comp. Proceedings of the American Dental Association. *Dental Cosmos.* 1863;5:76,91.

28. Ellis GW, comp. American Dental Association [proceedings]. *Dental Cosmos.* 1864;6:65,69,70–72.

29. Dentists in the Army and Navy. *Dental Headlight.* 1890;11:206.

30. Marshall JS. Fracture and diastasis of the superior maxillae and upper bones of the face . . . *Dental Cosmos.* 1891;33:180.

31. Cigrand BJ. Abraham Lincoln and dentists. *Am Dent J.* 1913;10:344.

32. Callahan K. A backward glance at Civil War surgery. *Bull Cleve Dent Soc.* 1966;22:15.

33. Morton WTG. The first use of ether as an anesthetic, at the battle of the wilderness in the Civil War. *J Am Med Assoc.* 1904;42:1068–1073.

34. Kelly HA, Burrage WL. *American Medical Biographies.* Baltimore, Md: Norman Remington Co; 1920.

35. Teacher, editor, pioneer dental chemist [George Watt, MD, DDS]. *Dent Radiogr Photogr.* 1965.

36. T[aft] [J]. Gone to the war. *Dental Register of the West*. 1864;18:285.

37. T[aft] [J]. Personal [letter from Dr Watt]. *Dental Register of the West*. 1864;18:380.

38. National Archives and Record Administration. Compiled Military Service Record. Record Group 94. G Watt, 154th Ohio Infantry (National Guard).

39. National Archives and Record Administration. Record Group 94. C Smith, medical officer's file. Box 532. Entry 561.

40. TGL. Colonel John R Lewis. *Dental Cosmos*. 1864;6:124–125.

41. National Archives and Record Administration. Compiled Military Service Record. Record Group 94. JR Lewis, 1st, 5th Vermont Infantry.

42. Vermont Adjutant & Inspector General's Office. *Revised Roster of Vermont Volunteers and Lists of Vermonters Who Served in the Army and Navy of the United States During the War of the Rebellion, 1861-66*. Montpelier, Vt: Watchman Publishing Co; 1892: 751.

43. Steere E. *The Wilderness Campaign*. Mechanicsburg, Pa: Stackpole Books; 1960: 1.

44. National Archives and Record Administration. Record Group 94. Report, Board of Examination for Officers, appointment, commission and personal branch, January 30, 1867. No. 2423: 1881. Box 722. Entry 297.

45. Benedict GG. *Vermont in the Civil War: a History of the Part Taken by the Vermont Soldiers and Sailors in the War for the Union, 1861-5*. Vol 1. Burlington, Vt: The Free Press Association; 1886: 196.

46. National Archives and Record Administration. Record Group 15. Pension record, JR Lewis. Certificate no. 509425.

47. National Archives and Record Administration. Compiled Military Service Record. Record Group 94. JER Patten, 50 NY Engineers.

48. John ER Patten to BG Benham, June 6, 1863. Personal collection of John M Hyson, Jr.

49. Graham ZB. *On to Gettysburg: Ten Days from my Diary of 1863*. Detroit, Mich: Winn & Hammond; 1893: 12.

50. National Archives and Records Administration. Albion P Howe Papers, May 15, December 31, 1863.

51. Catton B, ed. Asa Smith leaves the war. *Am Herit*. 1971;22(no. 2):55,59,104–105.

52. Woodward JJ. *Medical and Surgical History of the War of the Rebellion, III*. Vol 2. Washington, DC: Government Printing Office; 1879: 688.

53. Marshall JS. Fracture and diastasis of the superior maxillae and upper bones of the face, treated by the aid of the interdental splint and cranial support; with three cases in illustration. *Dental Cosmos*. 1891;33:180.

54. National Archives and Record Administration. Record Group 94. D Hayes Agnew to Surgeon General Hammond, July 20, 1862. Letter. Box 211. Entry 561.

55. National Archives and Record Administration. Record Group 112. Letter Book No. 32, July 25, 1862 to Sept 30, 1862, surgeon general's office. Charles H Alden, assistant surgeon to Garretson, August 14, 1862, 243. Letter. Entry 2.

56. National Archives and Record Administration. Record Group 112. Letter Book No. 50, Dec 16, 1871 to Dec 31, 1872, surgeon general's office. JS Billings, assistant surgeon, to Garretson, December 4, 1872, 582–583. Letter. Entry 2.

57. Obituary, Dr. James E. Garretson. *Dental Cosmos*. 1895;37:977–979.

58. Dentists in the Army. *Dental Times*. 1864;1:126.

59. Lieutenant-General U.S. Grant. *Dental Cosmos*. 1864;6:176.

60. Clark FY. The employment of dentists in the Army and Navy. Cited in: *Transactions of the Southern Dental Association*. Cincinnati, Ohio: Wrightson & Co, Printers; 1870: 71.

Chapter III

Dentistry in the Confederacy: 1861–1865

Introduction

Military dentistry seemed to be more appreciated in the Confederate army than in its Union counterpart. Records show that as early as May 13, 1861, the Confederate army commissioned Dr JB Deadman as a post dentist. Perhaps this was because Confederate President Jefferson Davis, in favor of dental surgeons for the US Army when he was the secretary of war (1853–1857), was sympathetic to the dental cause.[1–3] More importantly though, the challenges of fighting against the heavily populated and industrialized Union forced the Confederacy to adopt unique approaches to organizing its army and conducting a war. One of these innovations was the introduction of dentists and dental care in military hospitals, which resulted in the conservation of much-needed personnel and the swift return of soldiers with dental problems to their units. Although dentistry in the Confederacy suffered severely from a shortage of trained dentists and a lack of supplies, the military medical leadership displayed a consistent willingness to employ dentists in new and creative ways.

Early Confederate Support for Dentistry

An example of early Confederate interest in military dentistry can be seen in the 1861 *Regulations for the Medical Department of the CS Army*, which required that the standard medical supply table for both field service and hospitals include teeth extracting sets. The regulations allowed one set for commands of 100 to 500 soldiers and two sets for commands of a thousand. For field service, the regulations called for a single set per unit.[4,5] However, few surgeons were familiar with the instruments or their use. In 1863 Lieutenant George J Huntley wrote home about an extraction he experienced: "It took seven pulls to fetch it [his tooth] and I was pretty certain my head would come with it." The operation, which was done in the open, did not attract additional customers.[6(p102)]

In 1861 Southern civilian dental offices were also busy taking care of the army's dental needs; when they were able, soldiers often visited dentists in the towns near their encampments. For example, in July 1861, just before the opening of the First Battle of Bull Run (Manassas), Sergeant Samuel Buck of Company H, 13th Virginia Infantry, asked Colonel Ambrose Powell (AP) Hill for permission to go to Winchester "to have a tooth filled" by a civilian dentist. Hill replied: "No, Sergeant, wait until tomorrow. You may have it filled with lead before night."[7(p22)]

Problems of Secession

Approximately one fifth of the country's 5,000 dentists (1860 estimate) were in the South, but they were almost entirely dependent on the North for their contacts with organized dentistry, supplies, and professional development. The war isolated them from both materiel resources and professional interchange. One contemporary source estimated that by 1864, there were only 250 to 300 dentists in the entire Confederacy.[8,9] Virginia, for example, had only 40.[1]

Dr Findley Clark compared the dental resources between the two adversaries:

> At the North almost every State had its society. The American Association and American Convention were in full operation; besides three or four Dental colleges, and as many Dental journals. . . .

> With us in the South it was very different. We had no dental society or journal, and owing to the irregularity of the mails, and stringency of conscription, we could not act collectively but had to do what we could individually. As the war went on, and the call for men was renewed and the conscription increased to fifty, we were thinned to almost a corporal's guard. Many towns, of several thousand inhabitants, had no Dentist.[10]

Actually, the South did have one dental society, the Georgia State Dental Society, founded in 1859 with 11 members. Although the Virginia Society of Surgeon Dentists was the first state dental society organized in the United States in 1842, it had held its last meeting in 1846.[8,11]

Furthermore, the Confederacy lacked a fully accredited and functioning dental school of its own. The later shortage of Southern dentists can be attributed directly to the war, which curtailed the steady stream of dental graduates from the Baltimore College of Dental Surgery and the Pennsylvania College of Dental Surgery in Philadelphia. The Baltimore College of Dental Surgery was the primary source of prewar dental degrees for Southern students (49% of its students were from the South). A total of 59 students, 24 graduates and 35 future graduates, served in the Confederate forces with distinction.[8,12,13]

The only dental school in the Confederate States, the New Orleans Dental College, was chartered in March 1861, but students did not start classes until that November. However, the war disrupted its curriculum, and the first graduates (four regular and five honorary) did not receive their diplomas until after the war, in 1868. Consequently, the school was not a factor in Southern dental education nor a source of dentists during the war.[14,15]

The South's Only Dental Journal: The Southern Dental Examiner

The first issue of the only dental journal in the South, the *Southern Dental Examiner*, appeared in May 1860 with a message that the dentists of the South needed "a medium" through which they could "express and interchange their views to their mutual benefit." The firm of Brown and Hape of 30 Whitehall Street, Atlanta, Georgia, coincidentally the South's only dental supply house, published the periodical. Dr JPH Brown, one of the firm's proprietors, served as head editor, while

Dr George S Fouke of Westminster, Maryland, was the corresponding editor.[16,17]

The war had a dramatic effect on this sole source of dental journalism. Most of the other professional journals in the South had already suspended publication by July 1861, when the *Southern Dental Examiner* informed its readers that it would publish only every other month.[18] By January 1862 the journal experienced difficulties in obtaining "suitable paper" for its press, and publication was delayed.[19] The March issue turned out to be the journal's last. The following editorial appeared in that issue and made an appeal for dentists to be included in the Confederate military:

> We think it strange that no effort has, to our knowledge, been made to add to the efficiency of the Medical and Surgical Staffs of the army, by the appointment of dentists competent to treat and relieve the sufferings of hundreds of poor soldiers afflicted with neuralgia, fistulous discharges about the jaws, periodontitis, etc. Such cases instead of being treated for weeks and months by physicians and surgeons, without affording the slightest relief to the patients, would at once be referred to the dentist for advice and assistance. In England the staffs of some of the hospitals have included, for nearly a century, dentists in addition to the physicians and surgeons.
>
> Physicians as a general thing do not make the teeth and their relation to the body a matter of sufficient study and importance, hence it can not be expected that they should be very successful in treating the diseases of the dental organs and their appendages.
>
> We have thrown out the above views suggestively, trusting they may meet a favorable response, and if such a movement should be deemed practicable, that it may be the means of extending the sphere of usefulness of the dental profession.[20(p127)]

The South's Only Dental Supply House: Brown and Hape in Atlanta

In 1860 Brown and Samuel Hape of Hapeville, Georgia, foreseeing a protracted war and subsequent shortage of dental materials, founded the South's only dental supply company. In October 1860 Brown and Hape informed their customers that they had received an assortment of teeth and dental instruments as well as materials from the North, "all of which we offer at New York and Philadelphia prices."[21,22(p95)]

Because of the uncertainty of the Southern currency, the company advised its customers of a new payment policy in January 1861:

> Owing to the great political excitement in our country, nearly all paper money, except Georgia, is taken at a discount in Atlanta. Therefore, dentists, when ordering goods, should remit in Georgia funds, or in gold or silver.
>
> The profits upon gold foil being so very small, we cannot stand to be shaved upon uncurrent money; hence we are compelled to sell it "gold for gold," or its equivalent in bankable funds.
>
> For the same reason we are obliged to decline sending goods with bill to be *collected on delivery* by Express, unless persons will agree to pay in funds which are *par here*.[23(p152)]

In addition to the currency problem, Brown and Hape also faced the problem of obtaining dental supplies for its customers because of the Union blockade. Surgical instruments and medicines had been declared contraband by the US government, and running the blockade was a dangerous and uncertain business. Consequently, a shortage of dental supplies developed early in the war. The manufacture of gold foil, porcelain teeth, and other necessary supplies was soon affected by the scarcity of materials. Brown resorted to melting down scraps of platinum (essential to the manufacture of porcelain teeth) to get the metal he needed. For this process, he invented a special oxyhydrogen blowpipe. Needing feldspar, he prospected with "pick and shovel" and located excellent sources in Madison County, Georgia, and in Greenville, South Carolina, near the Saluda River. He carved tooth molds by hand and cast them out of gun metal. Brown also chemically refined gold foil in his own laboratory.[21,24]

In July the company assured its customers that it was still in business by announcing in the *Southern Dental Examiner*:

> Although we are represented in the army, we have not suspended, nor have we any intention of doing so, but shall continue to supply the profession with gold foil, teeth and materials just as low as they can be sold.[18(p52)]

In November 1861 Brown and Hape used the *Southern Dental Examiner* once again to notify their customers of revised fees for dental materials, especially gold:

> We are continually receiving letters from every portion of the Confederacy, asking: "How are you off for material? Do you sell Gold Foil, Teeth, etc., at the old rates?" To all we will say, that we have a large stock of material, and that we sell teeth, and nearly every other article, at the old rates. On some things we have been compelled to make a small advance. Gold Foil we sell at the old rate, when paid in gold, but when paid in paper we have been forced, from the advance of gold, and the increased price of all articles used in its manufacture, to add 5 per cent to the old price of $28 per oz. We are the pioneers in the Confederacy in the manufacture of Foil, and are determined to increase and extend our manufactory just as soon as the times will admit.[25(p85)]

Problems of Dental Care for the Confederate Soldier

Dental care was extremely expensive for Confederate soldiers, who were usually in the field, far from home, and earned only about $18 a month. After the war Dr Watkins Leigh Burton (1830–1892), a dentist in Richmond, Virginia, wrote of the problem:

> During the progress of the late unhappy war, it soon became apparent that the soldiers of the Confederate armies stood sadly in need of the services of dentists. Most of them being from extreme sections of the country, without means, being cut off from all communications with their homes, and their pay being totally inadequate to meet the most ordinary and pressing wants, it was out of the question for them to attempt to pay for dental operations. Particularly when it is remembered the price of one gold filling in the depreciated currency of the Confederacy, was more than six months pay of a private! The price demanded for gold foil in 1864 and the beginning of 1865 was sixty-four dollars per oz. in gold coin. This

amount in confederate money would be, three thousand eight hundred and forty dollars, for the prevailing price of gold was sixty for one. Having to pay so enormously for materials—the value being enhanced from the fact of their having to run the blockade—the charges of dentists were proportionally high. The charge for a gold filling was $120.00, for extracting a tooth $20.00, and for an upper set of teeth on gold or vulcanite base, from $1800.00 to $4000.00. Let it not be understood that high prices were confined to dentistry alone. It was no uncommon thing to pay $1800.00 for a coat, $300.00 for shoes, $1000.00 for cavalry boots, and from $300.00 to $500.00 for an ordinary felt hat.[26]

Dental treatment was a luxury far beyond the financial means of the average Confederate soldier. Dr LD Carpenter, an Atlanta dentist who had been in practice since 1858, said that in the month of April 1865, he did "one million dollars' worth of work in Confederate money value." Dr WH Morgan of Tennessee commented on one of the consequences of this unfortunate situation, saying that "a large amount of suffering was occasioned by a low class of men following the army and pretending to practice Dentistry," and he mentioned "One case . . . of a man preparing his cement, by the wholesale quantity, in a tin cup, enough to last all day, and filling the teeth of the soldiers indiscriminately with the same."[26–28]

In addition, the majority of Confederate troops had been serving for years without a dental examination. Their poor oral hygiene, lack of toothbrushes, and the "miserable and scanty" food that made up their field rations all contributed to the "wretched condition" of their teeth. On August 27, 1862, when the Confederate troops captured the railroad yard at Manassas Junction, Virginia, an observer noted that among the items the hungry soldiers stuffed in their haversacks and pockets were "ground coffee, tooth-brushes, condensed milk…." In Stonewall Jackson's infantry, the "tooth-brush was a button-hole ornament." One Confederate's 1864 prescription for a toothache was: "1 Grain of Arsenic, 1 Grain of Morphine, Kresote [creosote] enough to make a paste of it, then put a piece the size of a pin's head in the cavity & confine it there with a little wax or cotton."[26,29,30]

On July 16, 1863, 30 of the officers and medical staff of the Army of Northern Virginia encamped near Martinsburg addressed a petition to Confederate Secretary of War James Seddon. They argued that the "health comfort" of the soldiers would be greatly improved by "the services of a good Practical Dental Surgeon." Furthermore, they recommended that Dr Robert E Grant be selected and allowed to "practice his profession" in the army.[31,32] A former captain in the 37th Virginia Infantry, Grant had attended the Baltimore College of Dental Surgery but had not received a degree. Seddon approved the request on August 3.[32,33]

The high fees during the war also affected civilian dentistry. All dental home care products, such as toothbrushes, dentifrices, and toothpicks, were scarce and expensive. Mary Boykin Chesnut of Mulberry Plantation near Camden, South Carolina, mentioned in her diary that a toothbrush cost $10 and a visit to the dentist for a "look" at teeth "the whitest and most regular" cost $350 in Confederate money. Old toothbrushes were rethreaded with hog bristles from slaughtered animals, while twigs became popular tools for cleaning teeth. Homemade toothpicks were carved from bone or wood, and ground charcoal was often used as a dentifrice.[34,35]

Conscription of Dentists: Dentists as "Special Practitioners"

To alleviate the chronic personnel shortages in the army, the Confederate congress passed the first universal conscription law for men in American history on April 16, 1862. The law applied to all men in the Confederacy between the ages of 18 and 35 and called them up for 3 years of service, but it also included a number of exemption categories. Physicians and hospital personnel were specifically exempt to assure the continued healthcare of the civilian population. In September 1862 the act was extended to include men to the age of 45, and a final conscription act in February 1864 broadened the call to all men from 17 to 50. In an effort to alleviate the costs of dental care for enlisted soldiers, dentists were included in the conscription laws.[26]

Under the conscription law, physicians who had practiced at least 7 years were exempt from service, and some dentists tried to argue that the exemption should apply to them as well, claiming that they were practicing a medical specialty. One such dentist (referred to as "Mr. Benton, the dentist" by John Beauchamp Jones, a Baltimore native who served as a clerk under five Confederate secretaries of war) attempted to avoid conscription. Benton's attorney, George W Randolph, was the former Confederate secretary of war (1862) who had originally convinced President Jefferson Davis to sign the 3-year conscription bill. In 1863 Randolph defended Benton's exemption under the medical clause. However, Benton was eventually drafted and served as a hospital steward.[36–38]

Finally, to clarify this contentious issue, on December 29, 1863, a petition signed by 13 Virginia dentists, including Burton of Richmond, was presented to the Confederate congress. It recommended that dental surgeons who had practiced at least 10 years be exempt from military service. The petitioners argued that dentistry was a medical specialty outside the training of general medical practitioners, and that knowledge of dental and oral problems required years of training and experience. Therefore, there were few men who possessed the necessary specialized skills throughout the South, and not including them under the physicians' draft exemption would cause considerable hardship to the general population.[39,40]

The group included a testimonial with the petition that was endorsed by 35 prominent Confederate army surgeons, including Dr William A Carrington, the medical director of the Confederate hospitals in Virginia, and several civilian physicians. It argued that the "professional services" of dental surgeons were "essential and necessary to the health, comfort and well being of every community," and, therefore, they should be "exempted from military service." Confederate army Surgeon General Samuel Preston Moore (1813–1889) and Surgeon James Harrison, the chief of the Confederate navy's Office of Medicine and Surgery, approved the petition. However, the War Department ultimately overruled all arguments for exemptions for dentists and ordered conscription to continue.[26,40]

Unsatisfied with the decision, Dr John Hunter (1826–1902) of Salem, North Carolina, an 1856 graduate of the Pennsylvania College of Dental Surgery, decided to carry the matter to the Supreme Court of North Carolina. Hunter had been advised by a friend, Dr Benjamin Arrington (1827–1907), a prominent Raleigh dentist, to refuse conscription. Arrington wrote the brief, which claimed that dentistry was "an exact specialty of medicine," and loaned Hunter the money (nearly $100) to carry the case to the higher court. The judge, Chief Justice Richard Pearson, ruled in favor of Hunter's exemption, saying "I am satisfied not only that regular, educated dentists are physicians, but that the human family are much indebted to them." This was "the first decision of the kind ever rendered in the United States giving to dentistry the legitimate right to professional distinction." After the verdict, the Confederate congress changed the wording in the draft exemption clause to "the term physicians *not to include* dentists." The Hunter decision finally settled the matter.[26,41–43]

Once the wording in the clause was changed, Moore immediately made provision to assign the newly conscripted dentists to hospital duty. Because neither the Confederacy nor the Union ever established a commissioned corps of dental officers during the war, drafted dentists on both sides of the line continued to serve in military hospitals as stewards throughout the conflict.[26]

The Perils of Conscription: the Case of Dr Watkins Leigh Burton

The most descriptive accounts of the Confederate dental service were provided by Dr Watkins Leigh Burton, whose experience illustrated the problems of dentists trying to establish their status under the conscription law. Burton was born on February 5, 1830, in Chelsea, near Richmond. He attended the Hanover Academy and worked as a clerk until becoming interested in dentistry. He began an apprenticeship with Dr John Wayt in Richmond, and at age 22 he enlisted in Company F, 21st Regiment, Virginia Infantry, which served at Harpers Ferry during John Brown's raid.[44]

On April 30, 1861, the governor of Virginia recommended Burton for appointment as a captain and assistant quartermaster in the Virginia militia, which was stationed at Fredericksburg. On March 13, 1862, Burton applied for a similar position in the provisional army of the Confederate States, but never received the appointment.[45,46] However, Burton was inducted into the Confederate army on June 28, 1863, under the provisions of the draft. A week later, his attorneys began legal proceedings for his exemption. A writ of habeas corpus granted him temporary release from the army, and he returned to his dental practice to await a higher ruling on the case, which was delayed, apparently to await the decision on the Hunter case pending in North Carolina. Meanwhile, Burton's status came to the attention of the Confederate adjutant and inspector general's office. On February 12, 1864, the office wrote the Bureau of Conscription, saying Burton had a very weak claim for exemption and should be drafted immediately; additionally, it did not feel that dentists were included under the medical clauses of the conscription law.[44] A few days later, Surgeon General Moore intervened on Burton's behalf. On February 15, he wrote Major TG Peyton, who was in charge of conscription at Camp Lee in Richmond, and asked him to defer drafting Burton until the secretary of war decided on his application for special duty.[44]

The same day, Surgeon General Moore also wrote General Samuel Cooper, the adjutant and inspector general, requesting that Burton be appointed a hospital steward and assigned to the surgeon general's office:

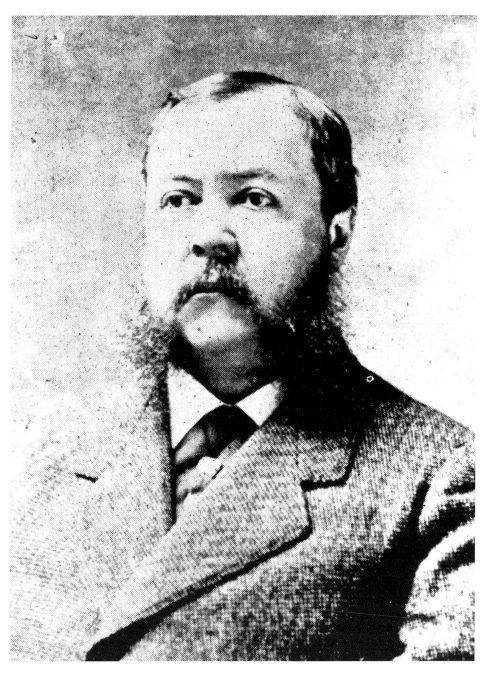

Watkins Leigh Burton, a dentist appointed a hospital steward by the Confederacy.
Reproduced from: Annals of Dentistry. 1946;5-6:55.

The Surgeons in charge of hospitals in this City state that patients frequently require the aid of a Dentist and it is thought that the services of Dr. Burton can be made very useful in the performance of such Dental operations as the soldiers may require.

Surgeons in the field have also made statements on this subject to the effect that Officers and Soldiers in the Army of Northern Virginia are frequently granted leaves of absence for the purpose of having Dental Operations performed; the assignment to duty in this City of a Dentist would render a protracted absence from their commands unnecessary.

The large size of Dr. Burton (his weight being upwards of 240 lbs) incapacitates him for the duties of a soldier and it is thought the interests of the Service will be promoted by his appointment to this duty.[44(p57)]

On February 17, 1864, the same day that the Confederate congress ruled that dentists were eligible for conscription, Burton was appointed a hospital steward and ordered to report to the surgeon general for duty. However, the Bureau of Conscription was still unsatisfied; Colonel JW Preston wanted Burton's status better defined. On February 21 he complained to the War Department that Burton seemed to be conducting his personal business as usual from his home and doing little military work.[44,47]

In order to clarify the situation, on February 25 Moore informed Dr Carrington, the Richmond medical director, that Burton was to be assigned as follows:

Dr. W. Leigh Burton, Dentist, has been appointed Hospital Steward, and will be stationed in Richmond. Information will be given to the Surgeons in charge of hospitals to have their patients who require dental operations to be collected on certain days in the week at some convenient place in each hospital, and Dr. Burton to be notified so that he can visit the hospital at the specified time, and perform the necessary operations.

To save time and to permit Dr. B[urton] to carry his instruments, an ambulance should be furnished him.[44,48]

Burton's status underwent several administrative alterations over the next few weeks; however, he continued to function in some official capacity as a military dentist. On June 13, 1864, he was assigned by the Bureau of Conscription to "perform Dental operations" at hospitals in Richmond.[48] The same day, Moore repeated his advice to Carrington about Burton's administrative requirements.[44,49–51] The next day, Carrington told the Richmond hospital chiefs:

You are directed to have the patients in the hospital under your charge who require dental operations collected on one day in each week & to some convenient place & to notify Dr. Burton corner 8th & Franklin St[reet]s so that he can attend at the time specified & perform the necessary operations.[52]

Burton performed these duties until the end of the war.[44] Finally, systematic dental care was established in the Confederacy's largest medical complex in Richmond and soon spread to all of its general hospitals.

Dental Surgeons and Hospital Duty, 1863–1865

Even before the conscription laws were clarified, the Confederates were pulling soldier-dentists from their units and contracting civilian dentists to serve the military. For example on March 20, 1863, Carrington told James McCaw (1823–1906), the medical officer in charge of Chimborazo Hospital in Richmond:

> You are resp[ect]f[ully] requested to state (after consultation with your Division Surgeons) your opinion as to the advisability of a Surgeon Dentist making visits to your Hosp[ita]l at stated times say 2 or 3 weekly for such simple operations on the teeth (principally extraction) as may be required. The services of a Dentist very skillful in extraction can be procured on contract.[53]

McCaw replied, "I have always required [dental] surgeon to extract teeth." Two days later, on March 22, Carrington asked the Confederate medical purveyor whether or not Chimborazo Hospital could be supplied with the necessary dental forceps. The medical purveyor replied that although there was a supply of dental instruments within the Confederate lines, there were none available at his depot. However, he hoped that McCaw would receive the forceps within a week.[53]

The first conscripted hospital dentist was assigned to duty in March 1864. Dentists were given the rank of hospital steward because Surgeon General Moore could find "no authority of law" to appoint them to a higher grade. They received the pay equivalent for their grade, plus "extra duty pay" amounting to about $10 a day. (For example, a typical month could look like this: extra duty pay at $4 per diem for 30 days, $120; commutation for room, $40; company pay, $18; monthly rations at $125; clothing, two suits worth $15 per month, $15; monthly total: $318.)[26,40,54]

Dental patients admitted to the military hospitals were divided into three categories: the front line emergency cases, the convalescents, and the sick. The soldiers from the front received priority treatment so that they could return to their units. They were sent to the hospital for a particular dental operation and discharged as soon as possible. Burton made these comments on the problem of dental malingerers:

> If it was argued by some officers that men from the front made the requirement of dental operations a pretext for absence from their commands, in order to have a day's relaxation in the city, they generally paid for it by the loss of one or more teeth. And even if they relished the operation, there was but little opportunity afforded them for any other enjoyment. After being discharged from the hospital they were conveyed, under guard, to the "Soldier's Home," where they remained until the "Provost Guard" escorted them to their commands. These measures appear harsh, and while no doubt they were very necessary in some cases, many men were deterred from having the benefit of dental operations rather than submit to them.[24(p445),55]

Officers and enlisted soldiers not registered as patients in the hospitals were not entitled to dental treatment unless they had a special order signed by the medical director of their departments, which was rarely granted except in emergency cases.[24]

Dentists were not allowed to "mess or lodge" at the hospitals. The uniform of the hospital steward was similar to that worn by an orderly or first sergeant in the Confederate army, except that the chevrons on the coat sleeves and the stripe down the trousers were black, the color indicating the medical department. The cap emblem was a gold "MS" embraced in two olive branches.[40,56]

The surgeons in charge were usually cooperative and accommodating to the needs of an assigned dentist. Dental materials and appliances were paid for from hospital funds.[57] Burton described a typical hospital dental operating room:

> A room with a good light, cold and warm water, soap and towels, and a servant or soldier, were invariably provided. The making of the operating chair was entrusted to the hospital carpenter, and generally constructed by a [c]rude design drawn in pencil. A tin basin placed upon a bench or stool answered for a spittoon. In cold weather a good fire was kept constantly burning in the room—that is to say, when the hospital was supplied with wood.[24(p444)]

However, army dentists were provided with a special privilege: ambulance transportation to their respective hospitals, which caused some jealousy among their medical colleagues. Without this assistance, many dentists would have had to walk several miles to hospitals located outside the city, carrying their heavy instrument cases and dental materials. Some of the assistant medical surgeons, having to walk to their posts, made complaints to the medical department to have the service discontinued. Burton recalls the following incident:

> In a case of the writer's, the ambulance having failed to call for him at the usual hour, and being compelled to walk to the hospital, he was of course behind time. This apparent dereliction of duty was reported promptly to the surgeon in charge, and eventually went the rounds of all official papers until it became at last so filled with endorsations that it was positively frightful to behold. The point made against the offender was, that as many of the surgeons were in the daily habit of *walking* to the hospital, the non-arrival of the ambulance could not be received as an excuse for not being in place at the proper time.[24(445-446)]

Despite the physicians' complaints, the dental ambulance service continued up to the "last days of the Confederacy." Dentists may not have had the rank, but they did get to ride to work.[24(p446)]

The following orders from Medical Director Carrington to the senior surgeon of the Lynchburg hospitals, dated September 6, 1864, detail the duties of Dr Steward Bidgood and are an example of the typical itinerary of a hospital steward-dentist:

> In accordance with the enclosed order Hosp[ital] Steward Bidgood, will be re- quired to visit in rotation, and at stated times, the Hospitals at Lynchburg, Va. and perform such operations on the teeth and mouth as are found necessary. Suit- able place should be provided for him and all facilities required furnished. I have furnished him with amalgam and some files and he has his own instruments. If he requires them or any such articles they should be procured on requisition or if not so much procurable purchased with the Hosp[ital] Funds of some of the Hos- pitals. It will be inconvenient for him to quarter or mess at any of the Hospitals and consequently should commute his quarters, rations & fuel. I have applied for extra pay for the dentists reporting to me and will inform you of the result of my

application. In addition to plugging cleaning and extracting teeth, the Dentists have been serviceable in adjusting fractures of the jaw and in operating on the mouth and fauces.[40,58]

Other dentists were assigned to a single hospital. For example, on November 3, 1864, Carrington advised Surgeon Davis of the Harrisonburg General Hospital that "Private J.W. Harris is detailed for duty at Gen[eral] Hosp[ita]l Harrisonburg, Va. and assigned to duty as Dentist to that Hosp[ita]l."[40]

Some dentists were even assigned to hospitals near their homes and commuted, like Dr William Thackston (1820–1899) of Farmville, Virginia, an 1842 graduate of the Baltimore College of Dental Surgery. On April 20, 1864, Thackston enlisted as a private in Company D, 3rd Regiment (Booker's Regiment), Virginia Reserves. On March 3, 1865, he was assigned by Carrington as the "Dentist" to the general hospital at Farmville with the following remark:

> Detailed from the Reserves as Dentist at Hosp[i]t[a]l Farmville. Will be allowed to reside at his residence near Burkeville, Va. and visit the Hosp[ita]l once weekly or as often as necessary.[40,59,60]

This arrangement solved the problem of providing quarters for the dentist, saving the government money.

Finally, after a trial period of several months, on November 4, 1864, Carrington issued the following directive (Army Medical Department Circular 15):

> I. As far as practicable in future, the operations of dentistry required in General Hospitals in Virginia, will be performed by officers, soldiers or conscripts assigned to those duties, who are dentists by profession.

> II. Examinations will be made, at such times as may be fixed by the surgeon in charge, of each officer and soldier admitted into hospitals, and the necessary operation performed with the concurrence of the attending Medical officer.

> III. Dentists are expected to be provided with their own instruments, but the necessary materials and files will be purchased with the hospital funds, and requisition made for other instruments thought necessary.

> IV. Dentists will have the rank, pay and perquisites which their position in the army entitles them, and in addition, such extra duty pay for extraordinary skill and industry, as the Surgeon General will allow, in accordance with general order, No. 66, A & IG [Adjutant and Inspector General], office, current series.

> V. Monthly reports of Dental operations and accompanying registers in accordance with forms furnished, will be forwarded through the Surgeon in charge and through this office, to the Surgeon General by the 5th of the month succeeding.[26(pp183–185)]

Once this program was underway, the dental surgeons were kept busy with the backlog of restorations (fillings), extractions, dental prophylaxis (cleanings), and maxillofacial fractures and wounds. According to Burton, amalgam was the most popular filling material at the time because it was inexpensive and simple to use. A typical day's work for a hospital dentist consisted of "from twenty to thirty fillings, the preparation of the cavities included, the extraction of fifteen or twenty teeth, and the removal of the tartar *ad libitum*!"[26(pp184–185)]

Dentists also practiced some endodontic (root canal) treatment, saving many teeth that would otherwise have been extracted. Most commonly, these problems were treated with a paste containing arsenic, morphine sulphate, and creosote. While prosthetic work (dentures) was not allowed, dowel crowns (pivot teeth) were permissible.[26]

In addition to the orders in Circular 15, hospitals kept monthly records that showed each date, patient's name, rank, regiment, company, and operation performed. Consolidated monthly returns listed the number of patients operated on and the number of extractions; fillings, prophylaxis, fractures, and miscellaneous operations; and the total number of operations. These reports were forwarded through the hospital's medical director to the surgeon general's office by the fifth of each month.[24,26]

Toward the end of the war, almost all of the larger Confederate hospitals had a dental surgeon assigned to the staff, and the results of the dental hospital practice were so productive that support for regiment-level dentists grew. Findley Clark quotes one supportive source as follows:

> Our own experience with soldiers, in and around Richmond during the last year, in connection with the statements of some of the most intelligent physicians and officers in the service, fully convinces us that out of every one hundred men sent to the hospital, or those on the sick list—exclusive of those wounded in battle—five, at least can be traced directly, or indirectly, to some derangement of the teeth; that might have been remedied in a few minutes, or hours. Thus we have of one hundred thousand men *five thousand* unnecessarily off duty. Now, this five thousand in every hundred thousand, might be returned to active duty, or prevented from leaving it, by the appointment of a few Dentists, say one to every army division.[10(p73),54]

Dr Samuel Stout, the medical director of the general hospitals of the Confederate army and Department of Tennessee, explained his use of dentists and their future in the Confederate service in the September 1899 issue of *The Texas Medical Journal*:

> In my administration as hospital director, I early directed the purchase of dental materials and instruments with the hospital funds, to be used by dentists detailed for that service in the hospital under the supervision of the surgeons. After, on several occasions, pressing the subject upon the attention of the Surgeon General, he issued a circular authorizing the employment of dentists of qualifications approved and vouched for by the medical directors, with the rank and pay of hospital stewards. . . . Thus you will see that I am the first army medical officer in high authority, who ever recognized the importance of the services of dental surgeons, and the first to use them in army practice. Had the Confederacy survived the conflict of arms with the U.S. government, I doubt not the regulations of its army and navy would have contained provisions for the utilization of the services of dentists, in both field and hospital service and aboard war vessels.[57(pp133-134)]

Stout's idea of adding uniformed dentists to the army in the field died with the Confederacy in April 1865. Had the war continued another year, it is likely that "provision would have been made for the recognition by law of the office of Dentist in the Confederate service."[10,54]

Dentists in the Line

While the majority of Confederate dentists served in the medical departments of hospitals, many others joined front line units as ordinary soldiers because there was no dental service in the field. As in the Union army, some of the graduate dentists serving in the line did whatever dental work they could for their fellow soldiers. Those who had completed their dental training undoubtedly cared for their comrades; others, some of whom had their dental apprenticeships interrupted by the war, did not begin their formal dental education until after the conflict.

One such soldier-dentist was Dr Theodore Francis Chupein (1830–1901), a Charleston, South Carolina, dentist who began his dental apprenticeship at 17 and opened his own practice in 1852. He served in the Confederate army as a sergeant in the (South Carolina) Washington Artillery for the duration of the war, but still managed to practice dentistry. When General Shanks Evans heard of Chupein's dental training, he sent him to Charleston to pick up his case of dental instruments and assigned him to perform dentistry on the soldiers during a lull in the fighting. Because Chupein could not replace his instruments, he was forced to repair them and improvise new ones at the camp forge. Chupein did much to relieve suffering and prevent tooth loss until the soldiers could get back to their own dentists. He stressed oral hygiene to the point that the men of his company began carrying their toothbrushes in the button holes of their uniforms, a practice that spread throughout the army.[61,62]

Another Confederate soldier, Dr William Hoffman (1836–1916), an 1861 graduate of the Baltimore College of Dental Surgery, served as a sergeant in Company M, 16th Regiment, North Carolina Infantry. Hoffman carried a kit of dental instruments with him throughout the war and created his own dental chair by driving a sharpened, forked stick into the ground to serve as a headrest and placing a cracker box or a log against the stick for a chair. Hoffman was captured on April 6, 1865, at Harper's Farm, Virginia, and taken to the prisoner-of-war camp at Point Lookout, Maryland. He continued to practice dentistry there on his fellow prisoners until he was released on June 3.[42,63–65]

Fracture Wounds of the Jaw: Dr James Baxter Bean

Because much of the fighting in the Civil War was done from behind earthen field fortifications ("breastworks") in which the head was the most frequently exposed part of the body, many soldiers sustained jaw fractures. Surviving Confederate records show that hospitals in the South treated at least 3,312 gunshot fractures of the bones of the face, 1,604 of which were of the lower jaw. All but 340 patients were reported to have survived.[66]

In 1864 the most common treatment for a fractured jaw was reduction and fixation by means of a gutta-percha splint. For example, James Hutchinson, Company

C, 53rd Georgia Regiment, 2nd Division, had incurred a fracture of the left maxilla, involving the first and second premolar teeth. At Jackson Hospital in Richmond, Burton wrote:

> After forcing the fracture into its proper position, gutta percha—having been soft-ened in warm water—was pressed on the teeth included in the fractured portion and extended to the firm teeth, the lower jaw closed and the teeth embedded in the lower portion. It was then carefully removed, placed in cold water to harden and readjusted afterwards. This accomplished all that could be desired. The fracture was held perfectly firm, the material afforded a pleasant rest to the jaw, and left an open-ing through which food might be received, and at the same time, it was not affected by the secretions of the mouth, or by discharges from the wound.[26(pp185–186)]

In more complicated fracture cases that involved displacement and fragmen-tation, an "outer splint" of gutta-percha, which conformed to the "shape of the jaw," was applied in addition to the interdental splint and held in place by a head bandage.[26(p186)] Some surgeons also used splints made of pasteboard and softened with vinegar and water.[26,67]

The best-known Confederate dentist was Dr James Baxter Bean (1834–1870). Born in Tennessee on July 19, 1834, Bean was an 1860 graduate of the Baltimore College of Dental Surgery and had practiced medicine in Micanopy, Florida, be-fore receiving his dental degree. In September 1861, Bean published the first part of his article "Plaster and Its Manipulations" in the *Southern Dental Examiner*. In part three (January 1862), he described his technique of making a pair of calipers to measure the vertical dimension (space between the jaws), and his design for a simple, inexpensive articulator. [68–71]

In May 1862 Bean moved to Atlanta, where he first worked at the dental sup-ply firm of Brown and Hape. The following year he developed an interdental splint made of vulcanized India-rubber (vulcanite), which he used successfully in treating jaw fracture wounds.[21,68]

During the winter of 1863, Samuel Stout was requested to administer anes-thesia (chloroform) to a Confederate commissary officer's wife who was having several teeth extracted by Bean at his dental office on Marietta Street. Of his first meeting with Bean, Stout wrote:

> Dr. B[ean], then a stranger, excited my admiration by the dexterity and skill with which he extracted the lady's teeth, upon which I sincerely complimented him. This drew us into a protracted conversation in regard to Dentistry and Surgery in general. Dr. B[ean] tendered his services at least one day in every week to perform operations upon the teeth of soldiers in hospitals in Atlanta, which I gladly accepted, as I found him high-ly intelligent and benevolently disposed. I directed the Post Surgeon, Dr. J.P. Logan, now Professor of Theory and Practice in Washington University, Baltimore, to inform the surgeons in charge of hospitals in the city of the tender made by Dr. B[ean]. Soon Dr. B[ean]'s visits to the hospital suggested to Dr. W[illis] F[urman] Westmoreland, now Prof[essor] of Surgery in the Atlanta Medical College, then Surgeon in charge of the Medical College Hospital, that Dr. B[ean]'s skill in Mechanical Dentistry might be made use of in the treatment of gun shot fracture of the inferior maxilla. The result of the suggestions of Dr. W[estmoreland] and the ingenuity of Dr. B[ean] was the pro-duction of a splint, which might be said to have been a perfect success.[54,57]

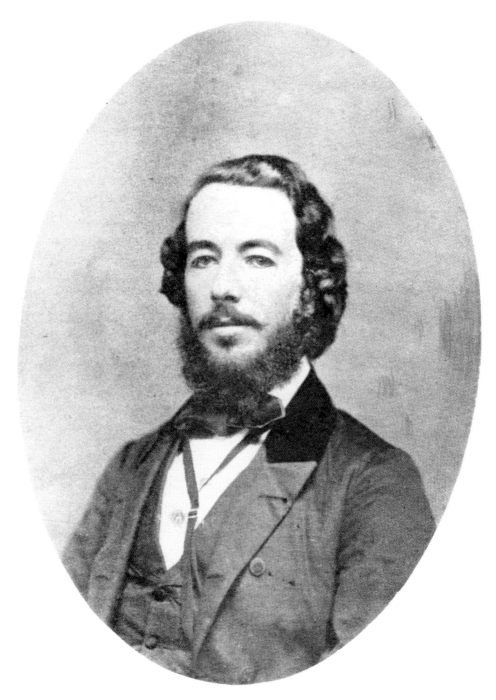

*James Baxter Bean, a Confederate dentist who developed
an effective interdental splint made of vulcanite.
Courtesy of the National Library of Medicine.*

In his capacity as medical director, Stout had already shown strong support for dental care. He made it a practice to assign all soldiers with dental training to dental duties long before doing so was required. His hospital directors determined the men's qualifications and, if satisfactory, appointed them to the rank and pay of hospital stewards. Stout used part of his hospital funds to buy dental materials and instruments and continually pressed for formal recognition of dental needs.[57]

In June 1864 Dr Edward Covey, a medical inspector for Surgeon General Moore and a former US Army assistant surgeon (served 1856–1861), while on a tour of inspection of the Department of Tennessee, observed Bean's work in Atlanta. Covey and Stout were so impressed with Bean's method of treating jaw fractures that a special ward devoted to the task was established in the medical college hospital in Atlanta, and all cases in the area were to be sent there for treatment by Bean. Results in the ward were so good that during the evacuation of Atlanta in the summer of 1864, the patients in the ward were transferred to the Blind Asylum Hospital in Macon, Georgia, so that Bean could continue treating them. Over 40 cases were treated successfully in a 6-month period. These two hospitals were probably the first medical facilities in history to have special wards devoted exclusively to the treatment of maxillofacial war injuries.[40,54,72]

Covey offered the following description of Bean's technique:

> The instrument consists of an interdental splint . . . made of vulcanized india-rubber, having on both horizontal surfaces cup-shaped depressions, sufficiently deep to embrace the crowns of the teeth. In the adjustment of the instrument, the teeth are placed in their corresponding indentations in the splint, and kept in position, by the mental compress and occipito-frontal bandage, to be described. This compress and bandage have advantages over all others I have seen used.[72(p83)]

One of Bean's patients was Major General James Patton Anderson of the Army of Tennessee, who was wounded on August 31, 1864, in the battle at Jonesboro, Georgia. Anderson sustained a compound fracture of the mandible when he was hit by a minié ball and was left unable to speak. After consulting with several surgeons, Bean decided to leave the wound alone for several days to allow the swelling to subside. Within 3 days it had gone down enough to allow Anderson to take liquid nourishment, and Bean began to take wax impressions and measurements necessary to make the splint. Three days later Bean inserted the interdental splint, forcing it into place, then carefully syringed the wound to remove more fragments and debris. Within days it was evident the operation had been a success. The swelling was gone, the jaw and teeth were properly aligned, and Anderson was comfortable enough to be released from the hospital on September 28. A follow-up visit on November 1 indicated full healing and only the need for some artificial teeth to replace those shattered by the bullet.[72,73] Covey said that Anderson's fracture had "united with such little deformity, and with such perfect antagonism of his teeth, that the closest inspection does not detect that his inferior maxilla had ever been broken."[72(p91)]

Another (future) Confederate general who sustained a jaw wound was Colonel John Brown Gordon. During the battle of Antietam (Sharpsburg), Maryland, on September 17, 1862, he was hit in the face by a minié ball, which "passed through his left cheek" and exited through his jaw, resulting in his fifth wound of the day. After being hit, Gordon fell forward into his cap, unconscious, and would have drowned in his own blood, except that a hole had been shot through the hat earlier in the battle. After being removed from the battlefield by litter, he was taken to a barn and treated by a surgeon. Attended to by his wife, Gordon recovered, and on November 1, 1862, was promoted to brigadier general. It is likely that his fracture was reduced and treated by means of an interdental splint, probably gutta-percha.[74]

Meanwhile, reports of Bean's successful treatments were sent to Moore, who ordered Bean to Richmond to show his splint to the Confederate army medical board. At a meeting of the board, held in Burton's dental office, Bean presented his drawings and models and explained his splint. The board members argued that "the principles of it were not entirely new," but unanimously recommended its adoption for general use. Army dentists were to be "instructed in its construction," and a ward set up at the Robertson Hospital, at the corner of Third and Main Streets, Richmond, for the "exclusive treatment" of jaw injuries.[26,75]

Apparently, some maxillofacial patients were also sent to Receiving and Wayside Hospital, on the corner of Franklin and 19th Streets in Richmond, which treated transient "sick and wounded soldiers, on furlough or honorably discharged from the service." Carrington ordered surgeons in charge at all Richmond and Petersburg hospitals to send the cases "for treatment of fractures of the maxillary bones" to a ward in this hospital, where at least one dentist was assigned. Listed on a roster report for the month ending February 15, 1865, there appears the following: "W.S. Wilkinson, Hospital Steward, date of commission November 4, 1862. On duty as dentist."[40,75]

Moore officially confirmed Bean's duties on February 6, 1865, in Circular 24, which he issued to the medical directors of the various Richmond hospitals. The directors were ordered to set up well-lit wards within their hospital systems to which all jaw injury patients would be transferred. The use of Bean's apparatus would be supervised by the assigned hospital dentist. Once the ward was established, Bean would visit it to train personnel on the preparation and use of his splint, and patients could not be furloughed until treatment was complete.[76] The surgeon general, recognizing Bean's value, ordered him to be ready to go to any hospital requiring his expertise.[77] Two days later, Carrington told Moore that Receiving and Wayside Hospital had been set up to receive jaw injury patients from all Richmond and Petersburg hospitals. He asked that Bean be sent to train the "resident dentist" and surgeons.[78] That day, Carrington also notified the surgeons in charge of the Richmond and Petersburg hospitals to begin to transfer patients to the special facility and invited all medical officers to "call and examine the cases under treatment."[79]

Following the war, Bean returned to Baltimore and established a highly lucrative civilian practice. He published several articles, but none on his interdental vulcanite splint. Dr Thomas Brian Gunning (1813–1899) of New York, Bean's Union counterpart, claimed to be the inventor of the interdental splint. Gunning had mended fractured jaws since 1840 and had successfully treated Secretary of State William H Seward (1801–1872) for a broken jaw with an interdental splint in 1865. It seems likely that both men developed the splint almost simultaneously, but be-

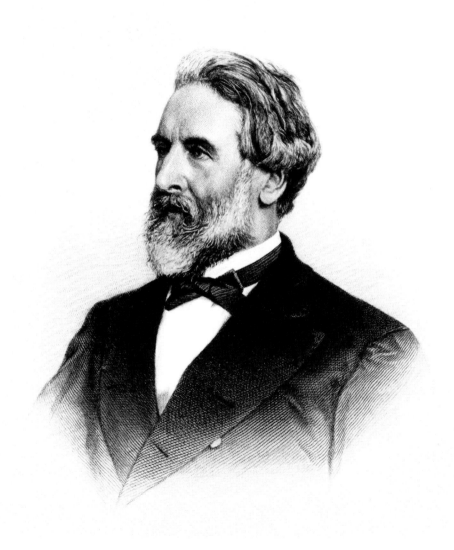

*Dr Thomas Brian Gunning, a Union dentist who
developed an interdental splint during the Civil War.
Courtesy of Department of Special Collections,
the Joseph Regenstein Library, University of Chicago.*

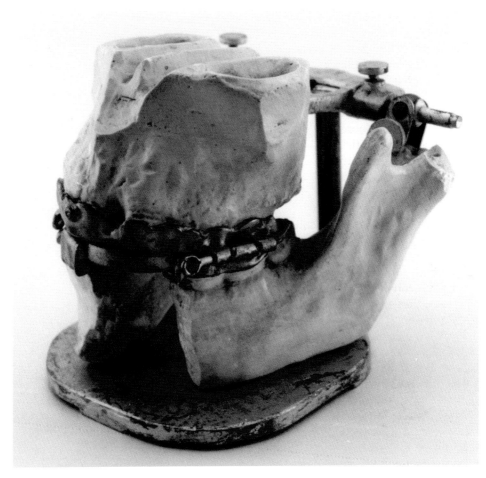

Gunning Mandible Splint, circa 1918. This splint was created to treat a jaw fracture that healed in the wrong position. The mandible was cut and fixed to the maxilla with the splint and gap in the jaw was filled with a bone graft. The horizontal pin, which may be removed quickly by the patient in case of nausea, locks the jaws together. The metal is an alloy of 80 parts silver and 20 parts copper (Maxillor) developed by the French Army Dental Corps.
Photograph: Courtesy of the National Museum of Health and Medicine, Armed Forces Institute of Pathology. NCP 3272.

cause of the war, neither was aware of the other's work. While Bean never published a single article on his splint, Gunning published a series of articles describing his invention in the *American Journal of Dental Science* in 1868. However, Bean's accomplishments are well documented in the Confederate military records.[80]

Bean also developed a method of casting aluminum denture bases, invented an apparatus for the manufacture and administration of nitrous oxide gas, and was one of the founders of the Maryland State Dental Society in 1866, serving as its president in 1868. He died in September 1870, the victim of an avalanche while climbing Mont Blanc in Switzerland. Dr Bean is regarded as one of the pioneer dental surgeons in treating wartime maxillofacial wounds. As late as 1900, the *Chicago Times-Herald* credited Bean's interdental splint as "the means of saving scores of Southern wounded from disfigurement, if not death, from gunshot wounds in the jaw."[68,81,82]

Through his support of Bean's work as well as military dentistry, in general, Surgeon General Moore was the first American official to incorporate the emerging profession of dentistry into military medicine. Some observers, such as Burton, were so impressed with Moore's official recognition of the role of dentistry that they concluded that dentists owed more to Moore "than to any man of modern times." Moore and others, such as Samuel Stout, reflected a willingness to change, innovate, and improve the health care of the soldiers, a spirit that was sadly lacking in the Union army and its medical department.[38]

A Clear Need for Military Dental Support

By the end of the Civil War the need for military dental support was obvious to the soldiers who had fought on both sides of the front lines. Perhaps because the Confederacy was, in essence, creating new institutions, it was more willing to acknowledge a need for improvements. The 1863 conscription call-up left civilians lacking dental care, making people more aware of the service they had begun to take for granted. Assigning dentists to military hospitals was so beneficial to soldiers, ultimately reducing their time away from their duties, that the need for dentists appeared fully justified. After the Civil War the formation of the Southern Dental Association was a direct by-product of the first-hand experience dentists had gained during the conflict. Findley Clark was the first person in the postwar era to urge the creation of a permanent military dental corps; however, it would take another generation of effort before his vision could be realized.[8,10]

References

1. [Harris CA]. Importance of Army and Navy Dentists. *Am J Dent Sci*. 1859;9:444.

2. Freeman DS. *A Calendar of Confederate Papers with a Bibliography of Some Confederate Publications*. 1908. Reprint. New York, NY: Kraus Reprint Co; 1969: 288.

3. National Archives and Records Administration. War Department Collection of Confederate Records, 1850-1852. Record Group 109. Printed regulations for the medical department of the CS Army. Microfilm Publication M 253, roll 120.

4. National Archives and Records Administration. Collected Record Books of Various Executive, Legislative, and Judicial Offices, 1860–1865. Record Group 109. Vol 582. Chapter 6. Medical department medical purveyor's office. Entry 3.

5. *Regulations for the Medical Department of the Confederate States Army*. Richmond, Va: Ritchie & Dunnavant; 1861.

6. Taylor MW, ed. *The Cry is War, War, War: the Civil War Correspondence of Lts. Burwell Thomas Cotton and George Job Huntley, 34th Regiment North Carolina Troops*. Dayton, Ohio: Morningside House, Inc.; 1994: 102.

7. Buck SD. *With the Old Confeds: Actual Experiences of a Captain in the Line*. 1925. Reprint. Gaithersburg, Md: Butternut Press; 1983: 22.

8. Schwartz LL. War problems of dentistry: the South in the Civil War. *J Am Dent Assoc*. 1945;32:37–42.

9. National Archives and Records Administration. Record Group 109. Dr W Leigh Burton to Porter Miles. January 5, 1864. Letter. Microfilm Publication M 331, roll 42.

10. Clark FY. The employment of dentists in the Army and Navy. Cited in: *Transactions of the Southern Dental Association*. Cincinnati, Ohio: Wrightson & Co, Printers; 1870: 72–73, 151–152.

11. Koch CRE, ed. *History of Dental Surgery*. Vol 2. Fort Wayne, Ind: National Art Publishing Co; 1910.

12. Foley GPH, comp. Compilation of Civil War veterans who attended the Baltimore College of Dental Surgery. 1992. Located at: National Museum of Dentistry Archives, University of Maryland, Baltimore, Md.

13. Callcott GH. *A History of the University of Maryland*. Baltimore, Md: Maryland Historical Society; 1966.

14. American Academy of Dental Science. *History of Dental and Oral Science in America*. Philadelphia, Pa: Samuel S White; 1876.

15. New Orleans Dental College. *Dental Cosmos*. 1861;2:558.

16. [Brown JPH]. Objects and aims. *Southern Dental Examiner*. 1860;1:1.

17. Obituary, Dr. George S. Fouke. *Dental Cosmos*. 1896;38:446.

18. [Brown JPH], Hape [S]. A word with our subscribers. *Southern Dental Examiner*. 1861;2:52.

19. [Brown JPH]. To our readers. *Southern Dental Examiner*. 1862;2:107.

20. [Brown JPH]. Dental surgery in the army. *Southern Dental Examiner*. 1862;2:127.

21. Georgia Dental Association. *History of Dentistry in Georgia*. Macon, Ga: Southern Press, Inc.; 1962.

22. Brown [JPH], Hape [S]. Business notice. *Southern Dental Examiner*. 1860;1:95.

23. Brown [JPH], Hape [S]. Business notice. *Southern Dental Examiner*. 1861;1:152.

24. Burton WL. Dental notes on the late Civil War. *Am J Dent Sci*. 1868;3:441,443–446.

25. Brown JPH, Hape S. Our policy. *Southern Dental Examiner*. 1861;2:85.

26. Burton WL. Dental surgery as applied in the armies of the late confederate states. *Am J Dent Sci*. 1867;3:181–188.

27. National Dental Association, Southern Branch [proceedings]. *Dental Cosmos*. 1911;53:1052.

28. Minutes [second annual meeting]. Cited in: *Transactions of the Southern Dental Association*. Cincinnati, Ohio: Wrightson & Co; 1870: 10.

29. Henderson GFR. *Stonewall Jackson and the American Civil War*. New York, NY: Longmans, Green & Co; 1936: 169.

30. Hotchkiss J. *Make Me a Map of the Valley: the Civil War Journal of Stonewall Jackson's Topographer*. Dallas, Tex: Southern Methodist University Press; 1973: xxviii, 271.

31. National Archives and Records Administration. Record Group 109. Petition, officers of Army of Northern Virginia to Seddon, July 16, 1863. Microfilm Publication M 437. No. G-319.

32. Stout WC. *The First Hundred Years: a History of Dentistry in Texas*. Dallas, Tex: Egan; 1969: 288.

33. National Archives and Records Administration. Compiled Military Service Record. Record Group 109. RE Grant. Company H, 37th Virginia Infantry. Microfilm Publication M 324, roll 834.

34. Massey ME. *Ersatz in the Confederacy: Shortages and Substitutes on the Southern Homefront.* Columbia, SC: University of South Carolina Press; 1952.

35. Chesnut MB. *A Diary from Dixie.* Boston, Mass: Houghton Mifflin Co; 1949.

36. Jones JB. *A Rebel War Clerk's Diary.* Baton Rouge, La: Louisiana State University Press; 1993: 354.

37. Faust PL, ed. *Historical Times Illustrated Encyclopedia of the Civil War.* New York, NY: Harper and Row, Publishers; 1986: 613–614.

38. Cunningham HH. *Doctors in Gray. The Confederate Medical Service.* Baton Rouge, La: Louisiana State University Press; 1958: 243–246.

39. National Archives and Records Administration. Printed Records Relating to Confederate Congress. Record Group 109. Petition of dental surgeons of ten years' practice, for exemption from military service, December 29, 1863.

40. Hodgkin WN. Dentistry in the Confederacy. *J Am Dent Assoc.* 1955;50:648–654.

41. Obituary, Dr. J.W. Hunter. *Dental Cosmos.* 1903;45:70.

42. Fleming JM. *The History of the North Carolina Dental Society: with Biographies of its Founders.* Raleigh, NC: North Carolina Dental Society; 1939.

43. Walker JM. An interesting Supreme Court decision. *Dental Brief.* 1899;4:573.

44. Schwartz LL. American dentists: Watkins Leigh Burton (1830–1892). *Ann Dent.* 1946–1947;5–6:54–59.

45. US War Department. *The War of the Rebellion: A Compilation of the Official Records of the Union and Confederate Armies, II.* Vol 51. Washington, DC: Government Printing Office; 1897: 54–55.

46. National Archives and Records Administration. Record Group 109. WL Burton to Secretary of War John P Benjamin, March 13, 1862. Letter. Microfilm Publication M 331, roll 42.

47. [Confederate States of America, War Department]. *Special Orders of the Adjutant and Inspector General's Office, Confederate States, 1864.* No 40; par 26: 93, 95. No 100; par 22, 29: 266, 268.

48. National Archives and Records Administration. Record Group 109. Surgeon General Moore to Surgeon Carrington. February 25, 1864. Letter. Microfilm Publication M 331, roll 42.

49. National Archives and Records Administration. Record Group 109. Pay voucher, WL Burton. May 5, 1864. Microfilm Publication M 331, roll 42.

50. National Archives and Records Administration. Record Group 109. Surgeon General Moore to Surgeon Carrington. June 13, 1864. Letter. Microfilm Publication M 331, roll 42.

51. National Archives and Records Administration. Collected Record Books of Various Executive, Legislative, and Judicial Offices, 1860–1865. Record Group 109. Vol 364. Letter. Carrington to various hospital directors. June 14, 1864. Entry 3.

52. National Archives and Records Administration. Collected Record Books of Various Executive, Legislative, and Judicial Offices, 1860–1865. Record Group 109. Vol 364. Letters sent and received, medical director's office, Richmond, Va, 1864–1865. Carrington to various hospital directors. June 14, 1864. Letter. Entry 3.

53. National Archives and Records Administration. Collected Record Books of Various Executive, Legislative, and Judicial Offices, 1860–1865. Record Group 109. Vol 708. Carrington to McCaw. March 20, 1863. Letter. No 73 3.

54. Stout SH. Correspondence [WH Morgan]. *Dent Reg.* 1869;23:162–164.

55. Macaulay JG. Dentistry in the Confederate Armies. *SC Dent J.* 1950;8:13.

56. Thomson H. *Prisons and Hospitals.* Vol 7. In: Miller F, ed. *The Photographic History of the Civil War.* New York, NY: The Review of Reviews Co; 1912: 350.

57. Stout SH. Dental surgeons in the armies and navies. *Tex Med J.* 1899;15:132–134.

58. National Archives and Records Administration. Collected Record Books of Various Executive, Legislative, and Judicial Offices, 1860–1865. Record Group 109. Vol 364. Carrington to the senior surgeon, Lynchburg hospitals. September 6, 1864. Entry 3.

59. National Archives and Records Administration. Record Group 109. WWH Thackston, Company D, 3rd Virginia Reserves. Microfilm Publication M 324, roll 400.

60. 'He lent charm and dignity to his calling,' (William WH Thackston, MD, DDS). *Dent Radiogr Photogr.* 1953;26(no. 1):ii.

61. Obituary, Dr. Theodore Francis Chupein. *Dental Cosmos.* 1901;43:563.

62. Macaulay NW. *History of the South Carolina Dental Association: Centennial Edition 1869–1969.* Columbia, SC: the South Carolina Dental Association; 1969: 14.

63. Foley GPH, ed. *Proceedings of the 125th anniversary celebration of the Baltimore College of Dental Surgery, March 4, 5 and 6, 1965, Baltimore, Maryland.* Baltimore, Md: Alumni Association & Faculty of the Baltimore College of Dental Surgery, Dental School, University of Maryland; 1966: 177.

64. Baltimore College of Dental Surgery. *79th Annual Catalogue of the Baltimore College of Dental Surgery, Baltimore, Maryland, 1918–1919.* Baltimore, Md; 1918: 19.

65. National Archives and Records Administration. Record Group 109. WH Hoffman, Company M, 16th North Carolina Infantry. Microfilm Publication M 270, roll 244.

66. Jones LL. Dentistry under the stars and bars. [DDS thesis]. Baltimore College of Dental Surgery, Dental School, University of Maryland; 1960: 10.

67. Bolton J. A simple interdental splint. *Richmond Med J.* 1866;1:318–319.

68. Obituary, James Baxter Bean, D.D.S., M.D. *Am J Dent Sci.* 1870;4:287–288.

69. Bean JB. Plaster and its manipulations. *Southern Dental Examiner*. 1861;2:53–57.

70. Bean JB. Plaster and its manipulations. *Southern Dental Examiner*. 1861;2:69–76.

71. Bean JB. Plaster and its manipulations. *Southern Dental Examiner*. 1862;2: 91–92, 93–95.

72. Covey EN. The interdental splint. *Richmond Med J.* 1866;1:81,83,88–91.

73. Warner EJ. *Generals in Gray: Lives of the Confederate Commanders*. Baton Rouge, La: Louisiana State University Press; 1959: 7, 111.

74. Eckert RL. *John Brown Gordon: Soldier, Southerner, American*. Baton Rouge, La: Louisiana State University Press; 1989.

75. Blanton WB. *Medicine in Virginia in the Nineteenth Century*. Richmond, Va: Garrett & Massie, Inc.; 1933.

76. National Archives and Records Administration. Collected Record Books of Various Executive, Legislative, and Judicial Offices, 1860-65. Record Group 109. Vol 741. Letters, orders, and circulars sent, surgeon general's office, Richmond, Virginia, June 1864–April 1865, II. No. 502, 508. Entry 3.

77. National Archives and Records Administration. Collected Record Books of Various Executive, Legislative, and Judicial Offices, 1860–1865. Record Group 109. Vol 741. Chap 6. Medical Department. Letters, orders, and circulars sent, surgeon general's office, Richmond, Virginia, June 1864–April 1865, II. Surgeon General Moore to Bean, February 18, 1865. Letter no. 508. Entry 3.

78. National Archives and Records Administration. Collected Record Books of Various Executive, Legislative, and Judicial Offices, 1860–1865. Record Group 109. Vol 364. Carrington to Surgeon General Moore, February 20, 1865. Letter. Entry 3.

79. National Archives and Records Administration. Collected Record Books of Various Executive, Legislative, and Judicial Offices, 1860–1865. Record Group 109. Vol 364. Carrington to surgeon-in-charge, Richmond hospitals, and to Dr Smith, Petersburg, February 20, 1865. Entry 3.

80. Gunning TB. Treatment of fracture of the lower jaw by interdental splints, I. *Am J Dent Sci.* 1868;2:53–65.

81. Gunning TB. Treatment of fracture of the lower jaw by interdental splints, II. *Am J Dent Sci.* 1868;2:106–120.

82. Gunning TB. Treatment of fracture of the lower jaw by interdental splints, III. *Am J Dent Sci.* 1868;2:214–220.

83. Hyson JM Jr, Foley GPH. Thomas Brian Gunning and his splint for jaw fractures. *MSDA J.* 1997;40:35–38.

84. Schwartz LL. The development of the treatment of jaw fractures. *J Oral Surg.* 1944;2:193–220.

85. Pioneer military dentist [James Baxter Bean, MD, DDS]. *Dent Radiogr Photogr.* 1957;30:20.

86. Dental surgeons in the Army. *Chicago Times-Herald.* Cited in: *Dental Brief.* 1900;5:280.

Chapter IV

THE QUEST FOR DENTISTS IN THE US ARMY, 1865–1898: "THE LAW MAKES NO PROVISION FOR THE EMPLOYMENT OF DENTISTS"

Introduction

From the end of the Civil War through the turn of the century, American dentists never ceased their efforts to win recognition of soldiers' dental needs. Whether decorated veterans or ordinary civilian dentists who wanted the best for the troops, practitioners were frustrated by the opposition of the Army surgeon general and the Medical Department. Their petitions, letters, and inquiries to the Army surgeon general concerning dental hygiene, the lack of professional dentists in the service, the possibility of commissioning or employment, and other issues pertaining to dentistry received responses such as "the law makes no provision for the employment of dentists."[1,2] That answer only further fueled their efforts to bring the benefits of modern dentistry to the American soldier.

Continuing Efforts for Dental Legislation

In 1868, 3 years after the end of the Civil War, Senator Hannibal Hamlin of Maine drafted a bill authorizing the appointment of dentists in the Army and Navy.[3,4] The bill was passed to the committee on military and naval affairs, where it subsequently died, likely because of the presumed financial requirement. On December 29, 1869, Findley Clark, undeterred by the indifference of the legislators, proposed a resolution at the annual meeting of the Georgia State Dental Society in Savannah, ordering "that this society instruct their delegates to the American and Southern Dental Association to request said Association to appoint Dentists in the army and navy of the United States." After some debate, it passed.[5]

At the second annual meeting of the Southern Dental Association in New Orleans, on April 13, 1870, Clark read a paper titled, "The Employment of Dentists in the Army and Navy," that began with his resolution. Clark made it clear that his experience with Sherman's troops in Savannah in December 1864 had prompted his strong support for military dentistry:

> The innumerable quantity of broken teeth and fractured jaws, produced by bungling instruments and unfamiliar hands, along with stories of rheumatic and neuralgic suffering, caused by exposed pulps and diseased teeth, which we were obliged to listen to during the sojourn of the army in Savannah, were disheartening; and we determined then, should an opportunity ever occur, to contribute our mite [sic] towards a remedy.[5(pp71–72)]

Clark strongly advocated that dentists be appointed to the military, stating:

> No military school; no army post, or station; no naval ship, or foreign port where ships are stationed, should be without a dentist. Our sailors and soldiers are no more able to pay for dental operations than they are for medical attention; therefore, if we value their services, we should, as a humane and enlightened nation, value their lives. . . . But it is no easy matter to convince the appointing power. No doubt, could we make them look on the broken teeth and fractured jaws, and force them to listen to the stories of suffering, above mentioned; and better still, experience a little of the pain, there alluded to, away from the means of relief, it would not be long before this vacuum in our army and navy would be filled. But as we can not do this we must do what is next best, we must keep telling them until they do believe us.[1,6]

The majority concurred with Clark's viewpoint, and the association passed a resolution declaring dentists essential to the military. The resolution also established a committee to work with the American Dental Association (ADA) and other state associations to bring the subject to the notice of their congressmen. Clark, along with SJ Cobb of Tennessee, was appointed to represent the Southern Dental Association.[6] While little immediate action came from Clark's speech and resolution, it set the tone American dentists would take for the remainder of the century.

Army Dentistry in the 1870s

Following the Civil War, the Army continued to expect its surgeons to perform all dental duties in addition to their medical and surgical functions. In April 1871 the Army was supplying post surgeons in the West with a "teeth extracting case" issued by the SS White Company of Philadelphia. On November 14, 1871, the surgeon general's office notified Dr James Garretson of Philadelphia that it wanted to add his book, *A System of Oral Surgery*, to the supply table when the second edition came out, if funds were available. In February 1872 the Army Medical Department ordered 150 copies of Garretson's book and issued it to the same posts that had been supplied with the extracting instruments, which were considered post property and were not to be taken when an individual was transferred.[7–10] Apparently, the surgeons were expected to read the book and, using the tools, apply its principles. On December 4, 1872, the department ordered 50 more copies through the chief medical purveyor in New York. In January 1881 the surgeon general's office ordered 25 copies of Dr JW White's book, *The Teeth: Natural and Artificial*, also for the surgeons to use as reference.[10]

During these years, many dentists continued to serve in a variety of military positions in the Regular Army and the militia or National Guard, but not as dentists. For example, Dr Charles Parmele Graham (1839–1904) of Middletown, Connecticut, who began his dental apprenticeship in the office of Dr Luther Parmele in 1858, enlisted in the 2nd Regiment, Connecticut National Guard, on December 8, 1871. He was commissioned a lieutenant within 9 months. In 1885 he was promoted to brigadier general and served until March 1890. When Governor O Vincent Coffin assumed office in 1895, Graham was appointed his adjutant general.[11]

Another dentist, Dr N Malon Beckwith (1845?–1894) of New York City, served in Company B, 7th Regiment, New York National Guard, for 17 years, while Dr John Meyer (18??–1918) of New York City enlisted in the 9th Regiment, New York National Guard, in 1871 and served until 1884 as an orderly sergeant. Dr Wilbur Litch (1840–1912) of Philadelphia, who received his DDS in 1861 from the Pennsylvania College of Dental Surgery and his MD in 1865 from Jefferson Medical College, served several years in the US Army Medical Department. His last assignment was as post surgeon at Fort Yuma, California, after which he resumed his civilian dental practice in Philadelphia, was editor of *Dental Brief*, and frequently commentated on Army dentistry issues.[12–14]

Dentistry in the Frontier Army

Colonel George Adair, who served in the Army Medical Department from 1874 to 1909, told of his experiences practicing dentistry in the isolated, Indian-fighting garrisons on the Western frontier. Recalling his early days as an assistant surgeon in the Department of Texas in the 1870s, he wrote:

> In an humble way, I raised the status of dentistry in the army. I had extracted a few teeth in civil practice before entry into the service; but was by no means an expert. At the time, by general custom, the Hospital Stewards extracted the teeth. Observing their operations, I felt convinced that the ancient barbers did better work. An inward reaction prevented me from assigning to a steward, work that I could do better myself. It was not conscience. To see a steward shutting his eyes when he pulled, and listen for the expected crunch or snap of a crushed or broken molar—to use expressive modern speech—got on my nerves. Did I not sacrifice many teeth that might have been preserved for several years of usefulness by filling? Yes. Dentists were scarce on the frontier. An annual visit by a traveling dentist was all that could be expected, and that was uncertain. The dentist was always welcome and an office provided for him at the hospital. A busy week in the garrison showed that I had left some business for him. Upon the whole, I believe that I did more good than harm with my inexpert dentistry. . . .[15(pp108–109)]

The frontier soldier's lack of access to dental care guaranteed extended dental problems and discomfort. Examination of the remains of soldiers killed at the 1876 Battle of Little Big Horn indicated a wide spectrum of dental problems, largely because of poor hygiene. Almost all the remains showed heavy tobacco use, substantial antemortem tooth loss, carious lesions, and alveolar resorption.[16]

The Townsend Bill of 1872

In 1872 a group of academic and private dentists submitted a petition to the 42nd Congress, urging the appointment of dental surgeons at the two service academies. These surgeons would meet a long-standing need and encourage substantial health and morale gains among the cadets and midshipmen. Having dentists on staff would assure expert treatment, save duty time currently lost at private dentist visits, and reduce the incidence of deferred treatment. A number of prominent civilian dentists put their names to the petition, including professors Williard

Parker, James Wood, John Metcaff, William Van Buren, Frank Hamilton, Fordyce Barker, and Alexander Mott, and doctors John Peters, George Peters, Charles Mc-Millian, Edward Bradley, and Leroy Milton Yale.[4]

As a direct result of this petition, on April 1, 1872, Congressman Dwight Townsend of New York introduced a bill (HR 2140) that created professorships of dental surgery at the US Military Academy in West Point and the US Naval Academy in Annapolis. The bill was read twice and referred to the House Committee on Military Affairs.[17]

On April 19, after studying the proposed bill, Secretary of War William Belknap asked Colonel Thomas Ruger, West Point's superintendent, about the need for a dental surgeon and why dental duties could not be performed by the medical officer on the post. On April 23 Ruger replied:

> There is no necessity therefor [*sic*], as the Academy is now provided with a thoroughly competent Dentist [William Saunders], who is a Hospital Steward on Special service for the purpose. A moderate charge is allowed for service for Cadets, which when approved by the Superintendent of the Academy is entered against their accounts with the Treasurer and paid as are other charges. The present arrangement gives entire satisfaction.[18,19]

Ruger also argued that the cadets should pay their share of the cost of their dentistry, and when and if the "present arrangement" had to be changed for any reason, the "item for the pay of a dentist" could be inserted in the academy's yearly congressional appropriation. Saunders had been named the official dentist for the cadets at West Point in 1872 and became the first person officially designated as a dentist in the history of its medical department. He retained his position as post dentist and continued his dental practice as the "Dentist to the Corps of Cadets" at West Point until his death in August 1906.[20,21]

On April 27 the secretary of war submitted Ruger's response to the House Committee on Military Affairs, which, on May 8, decided to reject the bill. Dr AP Merrill, the vice president of the American Academy of Dental Surgery, suggested there had been "some influence brought to bear on the Committee" on behalf of the hospital stewards. However, without the support of West Point officials, the bill was doomed to fail. As an indirect result of Townsend's bill, Dr Thomas Walton, an 1856 graduate of the Baltimore College of Dental Surgery, was appointed to the US Naval Academy with the rank of acting assistant surgeon in 1873. (Discharged on June 30, 1879, Walton served as a contract dentist until 1899. He died the following year.)[22–24]

Continuing Lack of Dental Treatment for Veterans and Active Duty Soldiers

Many veterans with maxillofacial injuries looked to the War Department for continued medical help after the war. However, several were denied treatment because their injuries were not specifically covered under Army Regulations. For example, in September 1870, John Johnston of Penn Run, Pennsylvania, a veteran of Company A, 61st Pennsylvania Volunteers, applied to the surgeon general's office for an "artificial cheek" to repair a wound he received as a 17-year-old at the battle of Spotsylvania Court House. A piece of shell had torn off four inches of his face from his left ear to the corner of his mouth, and his malar bone was broken off at the ear about halfway to his left eye. He wanted an artificial cheek to be made by a "Surgeon Dentist," which would cost $75.[25]

On March 2, 1871, the surgeon general's office informed another veteran, CW Beamendorfer of Lebanon, Pennsylvania, that "commutation" could not be paid for the "loss of the Jaw, or other injuries" that were not specified in the Act of June

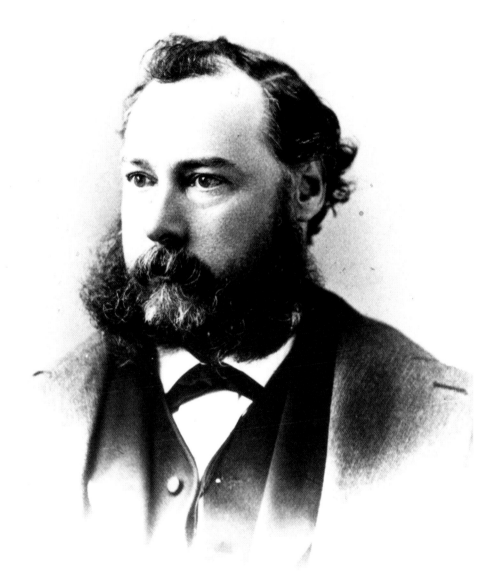

William Saunders, the first person officially designated as a dentist at West Point.
Photograph: Courtesy of US Military Academy Archives, West Point, NY.

17, 1870 (which authorized the surgeon general to furnish artificial limbs to disabled soldiers). In a follow-up letter to Beamendorfer's congressman dated April 1, the surgeon general wrote that the claim for injury to the lower jaw was rejected because there was no "kind of apparatus" available to treat the wound. Nothing of the type had ever been furnished by the government; therefore there was no criterion for judging Beamendorfer's claim. In addition, the surgeon general believed that the acts of June 17 and 30, 1870, were intended to refer to "lesions of the limbs" and other classes of injuries that could be treated by "mechanical appliances."[8] Similarly, on August 7 that year, the surgeon general's office informed John Murphy, a Massachusetts veteran, that his application for an artificial denture was rejected because there was no "appropriation" available from which such "an apparatus" could be funded.[8]

On June 19, 1872, the surgeon general's office told Patrick Fitzpatrick of Hampton, Virginia, a veteran of Company C, 88th New York Volunteers, that the "laws relating to artificial limbs" were not applicable to his injured lower jaw. However, if he would send a description of the "apparatus" he required, the name of the maker, and the cost, his case would be considered. On July 15 Fitzpatrick was notified that he would have to go to the office of Dr CB Davis, a dentist in Philadelphia, for treatment. Davis was to make a denture to "furnish a portion" of the lower jaw for $30, for which the government would pay.[10]

Those on active duty could expect the same limited support for dental matters as veterans. On February 20, 1873, Second Lieutenant George Spencer of the 19th US Infantry stationed at Jackson Barracks, Louisiana, wrote the surgeon general requesting information "concerning the medical treatment of officers and enlisted men of the US Army, for diseases of the teeth." Spencer wanted to know what to do when the attending surgeon was "not competent to give the required treatment in order to preserve the teeth from decay," and if a dentist could be employed "to perform the necessary work" at government expense. On February 26 the surgeon general's office replied that the "government will incur no expense for dental operations."[26]

On October 13, 1874, Dr JS Charles, an Omaha, Nebraska, dentist, wrote to the surgeon general concerning the benefits of dental care for the soldiers on the Western frontier, telling him that "unskilled" surgeons were forced to perform "minor operations of dentistry." On October 17 Joseph Barnes, the Army surgeon general from 1864–1882, replied that the question had been "agitated at intervals for several years but as yet with no practical result." However, he said he would be happy to confer with Dr Charles's congressman on the subject at the upcoming session of Congress.[27,28]

Four years later, things were little improved. On December 17, 1878, the surgeon general's office informed First Lieutenant Valery Havard (1846–1927), an assistant surgeon stationed at Chattanooga, Tennessee, that the Medical Department would not pay for a dental operation required by Corporal John O'Connor of Company A, 18th Infantry Regiment. O'Connor needed an apparatus for "a plug and its support for an alveolus communicating with [the] superior maxilla." The cost was about $50. The surgeon general's office told Havard that the

Medical Department had "no appropriation" from which such expenses could be paid.[29,30]

This situation for the common soldier continued to the last days of the Indian wars. In 1891 Quartermaster-Sergeant Charles Campbell, 7th Cavalry, was shot through the mandible during the engagement at Wounded Knee in December 1890. The bullet shattered the anterior part of the mandible from his right second bicuspid to his left second molar. The initial treatment by the Army surgeons consisted of removing the loose teeth and bony fragments and closing the external lip and cheek wound with sutures. The fracture failed to unite and the fragments of bone sequestrated, leaving the posterior segments freely movable. After 6 weeks, Sergeant Campbell was referred to Dr John Patterson of Kansas City, Missouri, who described his treatment:

> I banded the first lower molar upon the right side and also the first upper molar upon the same side, attaching lugs to the bands for the reception of a screw, and firmly screwed them together. I then placed a jack-screw upon these molars on the palatal side and against the molar on the left side, and forced that side into its correct position, which had been determined by models beforehand. I then banded the upper and lower teeth upon this side as upon the other, and screwed them firmly together.
>
> I then dismissed the patient for ten weeks, the intention being to overcome the growth of cicatricial tissue, which forced the left side against the tongue. I believed the abscesses were caused by the movement of the loose ends upon the soft tissue, and the result proved that this surmise was correct, as they soon healed after the parts were secured firmly to the upper jaw.
>
> At the end of three months the patient returned. He reported himself as very comfortable, save only that he was limited entirely to soft foods. On the removal of the bands the left side, after two or three days, swerved slightly inward and there remained, not quite, but nearly in correct position. I then proceed to make the splint-bridge. . . . It has been worn for six months, and the patient, whom I saw four weeks ago, says he is a new man, and his appearance holds the statement true. He eats solid foods with comfort, and the splint-bridge is a success. I am watching the case as to the growth of new bone where it is entirely gone. He is a young man in good health, and the chances for this are good.[31]

Patterson also commented on the cooperation he had received from the surgeon at Fort Riley, Captain John Van R Hoff, who took care of the external wound of the lip, preventing permanent disfigurement. In his opinion, cooperation between the two professions was in the best interest of the patient and gave the best possible results.[31]

In February 1893 Dr Benjamin Catching of Atlanta urged the readers of the *Southern Dental Journal and Luminary* to lobby their congressmen for a military dental bill. He remarked that since a post was established in Atlanta, he had been besieged by calls from the "ordinary soldier," unable to pay for expensive dental procedures made necessary by the "lack of opportunity" to have the proper routine dental treatment.[32,33]

"No Authority" for the Appointment of Dental Surgeons

On August 6, 1874, at the annual meeting of the ADA in Detroit, Dr Frederick Rehwinkel, a Civil War veteran and the chairman of the ADA's Committee for the Appointment of Dental Surgeons to the Army and Navy, reported that the committee had decided the proposed action to secure the appointment of dental surgeons was "premature." Because Congress was cutting expenses, the timing was poor; therefore, it would be better to let the matter rest for the present. The report was accepted and the committee discharged.[33]

On August 30, 1875, Merrill, the vice president of the American Academy of Dental Surgery, wrote to Surgeon General Barnes concerning the appointment of physician-dentists to the Medical Department. On September 6 the surgeon general replied that there were no legal provisions for authorizing such appointments.[34,35]

That October at a special meeting of the American Academy of Dental Surgery held in New York City, Merrill presented a paper advocating dental surgeons for the services. He argued that the government should not demand "good sound teeth" when recruits entered the service and then fail to provide dental care "to save these valuable organs." He also remarked that General-in-Chief William T Sherman had said he was "'willing to admit the importance of this subject.'" Surgeon General Barnes, although stating that "in the absence of any proper legislation no appointment can be made," acknowledged all the "good influences" upon the health of "skilled Dental Surgery." Merrill also pointed out that the Army physicians were "not as liberal in regard to this question" as those in civilian practice.[4,36]

The same month, at the annual meeting of the Dental Society of the State of Maryland and District of Columbia held in Washington, a committee formed to induce the Army and Navy to collect data on tooth decay and disease reported that it was ready to submit a paper to the surgeons general of the two services. Six members of the society were selected to present the proposal to the government.[37]

On January 24, 1876, at the first session of the 44th Congress, Representative Benjamin Willis of New York, a former colonel of volunteers, introduced a bill (HR 1369) "to provide for the appointment of dental surgeons in the Army and Navy of the United States." Again, the bill was referred to the Committee on Military Affairs and ordered to be printed, but ultimately died.[38] On July 7 the House Committee on Military Affairs reported adversely on the petitions of George Miller and others asking for the passage of a law authorizing the appointment of dental surgeons for the Army, the committee seeing "no reason why the regular Army surgeons cannot render all proper dental service in the Army."[39]

On May 20, 1880, Dr JH Spaulding, a dentist in Fargo, Dakota Territory, applied to the secretary of war for "an *appointment* as *Dental Surgeon*" to the military posts of the upper Missouri and Yellowstone rivers. He wanted the "authority to visit such posts professionally when necessary." If no appointment could be made, he requested a "special permit" for the purpose. The secretary of war referred the matter to the Office of The Surgeon General. On May 27 Surgeon General Barnes replied to the secretary of war:

Since the organization of the Army, it has never been necessary to employ a Dental Surgeon by the gov[ernmen]t for duty with troops and no provision or appropriation has ever been made for such purpose.

Individuals requiring Dental skill prefer to select the person they employ at their own cost and the quasi official endorsement of the applicant by a permit to visit certain posts in his professional capacity would establish a mischievous and troublesome precedent.[40]

On December 28, 1881, the subject was again introduced when Dr Frank Morrison, a dentist in West Chester, Pennsylvania, wrote to his congressman regarding *"employment as dentist* in the regular army." Once more, Barnes asserted that there was "no authority for such appointments" and that no one had ever been "employed in such a capacity."[41,42] Apparently he had forgotten about William Saunders's official work as a dentist at the US Military Academy.

Early in 1882 the *Philadelphia Times* published a colorful editorial, "Soldiers' Teeth," on the merits of a "corps of dentists" for the Army and Navy:

It may be argued that since the old cartridge has been abolished and the infantry have no more biting to do the government has no concern with the teeth of soldiers or sailors. This, however, is a selfish and superficial view. It is well known that a toothless soldier is not apt for half the duty that a well-stocked jaw can render the country. A paternal government cannot afford to close its eyes to the immense advantage to be derived from the sedulous preservation of its soldiers' teeth. A soldier with defective teeth, too, costs the government in doctors' bills, because it has been demonstrated that it requires the full force of an undiseased jaw to masticate the "hard-tack" thoughtfully provided for the military staff of life.

Aching, rotten or hollow teeth break down before the granite strength of this nutriment, and the physical system, responding to the lack of food, disables the soldier to take his place in the ranks. Again, the equipment of each regiment with a dentist will save gun-powder, for it is well known that to alleviate his misery the soldier is prone to fire off his tooth by means of a charge of powder. The picturesque but perilous form of dentistry sometimes blows out the offending tooth and not infrequently the unoffending jaw-bone. Now there are few that will seriously contend that a jaw-less soldier is either a useful or decorative object in garrison or field. Or if the heroic method be not adopted the soldier is apt to fill his mouth with fiery liquids, which, while temporarily assuaging the pain, are apt to end in stealing away the brain by way of the larynx. Nor is the old fashioned "clove" much more comfort, because, as is well known, the clove is the half-way house to the cocktail. Indeed, from whatever point of view this great question may be taken up the need of a dentist in the army is but too plain.[43(pp62–63)]

Dentists in Great Britain were fighting the same battle with the British services. In March 1882 the *British Journal of Dental Science* referred to the *Philadelphia Times* editorial and added that a corps of Army dentists was "a very practical sense of the useful"; a "toothless soldier," it said, was not able to render the same service to his country as one with a "well-stocked jaw." The author went on to say that in the "humorous" *Philadelphia Times* article, the Americans combined "an acute perception of the incongruous with a very practical sense of the useful."[44]

In the spring of 1882 *Medical Record* expressed the general sentiments of the medical profession on the subject. After agreeing that there was an "apparent" need for dental care for the servicemen of both the Army and Navy, the *Record* cited some "practical difficulties":

> We have an army of only twenty thousand men scattered in small garrisons through-out the country. It would hardly be feasible to appoint a dentist for each garrison, and the dental surgeon would have, therefore, to be a rather expensive itinerant. In the navy the difficulty would be still greater. In both branches there would, no doubt, be considerable opposition to admitting dentists to equal rank with medical men. For dentists have no right to call themselves medical or surgical specialist, unless they have gone through the same kind of education and training as that to which the gynecologist, laryngologist, or oculist subjects himself.[45(p94)]

Again, the question of rank for dental surgeons was a barrier; a rivalry existed between physicians and dentists that sometimes outweighed the health of the soldier.

Regardless of editorials or international opinions, the Army surgeon general continued to maintain his position. In 1882 he received several queries regarding the appointment of dentists in the Army. In reply to a letter from Dr JJ Jennelle, a dentist in DuQuoin, Illinois, on March 2, 1882, the surgeon general's office stated that there was "no authority of law under which appointment of Dentists could be made, nor has any one ever been employed in that capacity." On March 20, 1882, the surgeon general's office sent Dr RR Greene, a dentist in Fredonia, New York, the same reply. Saunders's position as the official dentist for the West Point cadets was not mentioned in the letters.[42,46]

George H Perine's Agitation, 1880–1882

In September 1880 Dr George H Perine of New York, former editor of the *New York Dental Journal,* commented in *Dental Cosmos* on the current status of Army dental appointments:

> It strikes us as not a little singular that a movement of such importance has of late received so little notice from the members of our specialty. To those who have given the subject consideration, the necessity of appointments of the character we refer to must be apparent. Sound teeth are among the physical requirements of soldiers and sailors, and certainly no physician or specialist will deny that attention to the preservation of these organs does much towards preserving the health of those in our country's service, and that the evident lack of interest displayed by the government is highly reprehensible. For some years past the establishment of dental chairs in the State medical colleges and the treatment of dentistry as a specialty of medicine have been more or less agitated, and strongly advocated by a large number of the leading members of the profession, and it is doubtful whether any stronger argument can be advanced in favor of such a movement than that contained in this article. A union of dentistry with medicine would be a decided step gained in favor of the appointments herein suggested, in making which the government would incur no additional expense. Doubtless much of the opposition which advocates of the cause have had to

contend with has arisen from the fact that few, if any, of our army and navy surgeons possess a knowledge of dentistry, and that the appointment of physicians practicing our specialty would necessitate a new order of things in this particular direction. At the military stations of the far West, and on board naval training-ships, the services of a dentist are often required, and much suffering is at times experienced for the lack of proper treatment of diseases of the oral cavity. There is no excuse for the indifference displayed by the government in a matter bearing so directly upon the sanitary condition of its servants.[47(p56)]

In September 1881 Perine, who had served as a member of the ADA's Committee on Dentists in the Army during the Civil War, wrote in the *American Journal of Dental Science* that the chief opposition to the appointment of dental surgeons was the prevailing fear among the civilian medical profession that they would displace some of the incumbent medical surgeons. Some argued that this would necessitate the creation of a "dental bureau," increasing the government's expense and resulting in less funding for the Medical Department. In response, Perine advocated the appointment of new candidates (when vacancies occurred) who had graduated from medical colleges where dental surgery was a part of the required curriculum, thus negating the need for a separate bureau.[48]

In the January 1882 issue of *Dental Cosmos*, Perine urged the dental profession to "exert their influence" with their congressmen to secure legislation for dental appointments in the services. He said that currently:

the extraction of teeth appears to be the only remedy resorted to in the service for the relief of aching teeth, and the operation, which is generally performed by an apothecary or hospital steward, is not infrequently attended by unpleasant, if not decidedly distressing results to the patient, for it must be acknowledged that in inexperienced hands the forceps are often productive of serious injury.[49(p56)]

In the meantime, Perine again recommended that candidates be selected on the basis of those "possessing a thorough knowledge of dental surgery." He also noted that servicemen's food was generally of a "coarse quality" and "insufficiently or improperly" cooked, which meant it was harder to digest and required better mastication.[49]

In May 1882 Perine's remarks in *Dental Cosmos* provoked response from Dr WF Hutchinson, one of the small group of preceptor-trained or graduate dentists who served in the US Army as enlisted hospital corpsmen or line soldiers, who was then stationed at Comba, Dakota Territory:

I have been in the army for the past four years, and have done a good deal of dental work, but have met with a great many difficulties; among them the want of a suitable place to perform the work, and the having so many other duties to perform as to preclude the possibility of giving it the necessary time and attention. But, throwing all difficulties aside, I have accomplished much good, especially in my own company, where I can have the men under my care every day. I have impressed on their minds the great necessity of saving the teeth by providing tooth-powders and mouthwashes best suited to each case; distributing Dr. White's little pamphlet, "The Mouth and the Teeth;" filling decayed teeth that would otherwise have to be extracted, etc. The men are all willing to pay for the work, but I think our government should form a special department in the medical department of the army and navy, and provide it with the necessary materials and appliances for the benefit of its soldiers and sailors. Dental surgeons could be appointed or employed as contract assistant surgeons now are in the medical department. The troops stationed on the frontier fare much worse than those close to the cities or towns. They cannot have their operations performed at all, for there are no dentists probably within three or four hundred miles, and consequently an aching or decayed tooth has to be extracted, often by inexperienced hands. It is a want that has long been felt both by the officers and the enlisted men of the army and navy. I propose that the national dental associations make the facts known at their next annual meeting to the Honorable Surgeon-General, and also hope to hear from others on this subject.[50]

In June 1882 Perine wrote in the *Southern Dental Journal* that several state dental societies (Alabama, Georgia, Iowa, Mississippi, Ohio, and Tennessee), the Pacific Coast Dental Society, and certain other dental organizations had already appointed committees to confer with their congressional representatives on the subject of a military dental bill.[51]

The 1881 American Dental Association Meeting

While George Perine continued his efforts to mobilize the dental associations into action, change was also being considered at the ADA meeting in New York City. At the meeting on July 14, 1881, Dr GA Mills told members there was an organized movement among Army officers to petition Congress to appoint Army dental surgeons. He reasoned that if this effort was successful, surely the naval officers would join the movement. Mills offered a resolution supporting the measure, which the ADA adopted.[52]

One of several officers who spoke on the subject, Lieutenant H Whiting of the US Marine Corps said:

I consider the appointment of surgeons who possess a thorough knowledge of dentistry a necessity, and I believe the Government should and will before long take decided steps toward that end. Nowhere is the want of dental treatment experienced more than on board training ships and seagoing vessels (particularly at foreign stations) and in most cases the only remedy resorted to for an aching tooth is the forceps; hence many valuable teeth are sacrificed in the absence of proper dental treatment and other and more serious disorders often follow. From men now in my command that have served in the Army I have learned that the same state of affairs exists at the military posts in the far West. I am fully convinced that much suffering is experienced by soldiers and sailors from the lack of proper treatment of diseases of the teeth. Sound teeth constitutes one of the physical requirements of men entering the service, and it is but right that the Government should bestow upon its servants the care necessary to protect their health. Neither soldiers nor sailors can afford from their limited remuneration, to pay for dental treatment, and it is unjust that a man entering the service with sound teeth should lose them for want of proper care during the term of his enlistment.[48(pp374–375)]

Lieutenant Commander Oscar Heyerman, the executive officer of the receiving ship *Colorado*, agreed, saying, "I am decidedly in favor of the appointment of surgeons in the Navy who possess a knowledge of dentistry. The care of the teeth of sailors is a matter worthy of consideration, and I am greatly in favor of the movement." Major John Janeway, the attending surgeon at Headquarters, Division of the Atlantic, Department of the East, Governor's Island, New York, stated that he had "experienced the necessity of dental services in the Army, and that he had endeavored to supply the deficiency at all times so far as was in his power."[48(p375)] Consensus in favor of military dentists seemed to be everywhere except in the Office of The Surgeon General.

John Sayre Marshall: Advocate for Army Dentistry, 1882

The most important person in the history of the US Army Dental Corps was Dr John Sayre Marshall (1846–1922). In 1882 Marshall entered the fight for dentistry in the Army and did not disengage until his retirement 30 years later. A former Civil War cavalryman from New York, he was a trained dentist, a graduate of Syracuse University's Medical Department (1876), and a dental and oral surgery specialist. In 1882 he moved to Chicago to practice with Dr Walter Webb Allport, a prominent dentist and one of the organizers of the Chicago College of Dental Surgery.[53–60] Marshall was also appointed an instructor of dental and oral surgery on the medical faculty at Northwestern University in Chicago.[56,61–64]

Early in 1882 Marshall began a study of the dental situation in the Army with the intention of making a presentation at the annual meeting of the American Medical Association (AMA) in Saint Paul, Minnesota. He began by writing to a number of prominent military and naval officers to request their views on the need for dental surgeons in their branches of service. Generals Ulysses Grant, William Sherman, Phillip Sheridan, and Winfield Hancock, along with Admiral David Porter, responded unanimously that the Union forces could have used the services of competent dental surgeons during the Civil War. Furthermore, they believed that a continuing need for dental care existed at the frontier forts. Personnel at remote duty stations were forced to travel hundreds of miles by horse-drawn ambulance, often through hostile Indian territory, to receive dental treatment, wasting considerable duty time. Admiral Porter added, "Dental surgeons would be of the greatest benefit to the navy, especially when on long cruises. Had the navy been provided with dentists when I was a youngster I should not now be gumming it."[63]

On April 6, 1882, Marshall wrote to Surgeon General Barnes requesting his written opinion of the "advisability and need of appointing Dentists" to the Army and Navy, provided they were "graduates in Medicine and Surgery." On April 12 the surgeon general informed Marshall that he declined "giving any opinion at present." Two days later, Marshall wrote to Barnes expressing his disappointment, suggesting that perhaps Barnes's "official position" might be "an embarrassment" for him. As a compromise, Marshall requested a list of the "proportion of *dental diseases*" treated by the US Army during the years 1879–1880.[65–67]

On May 4, 1882, the surgeon general's office sent Marshall a listing of the cases of dental diseases reported in the Army from July 1, 1878, to January 30, 1880 (Table 4-1).[68] Accompanying the chart was an acknowledgement of the probable underreporting of actual dental disease cases:

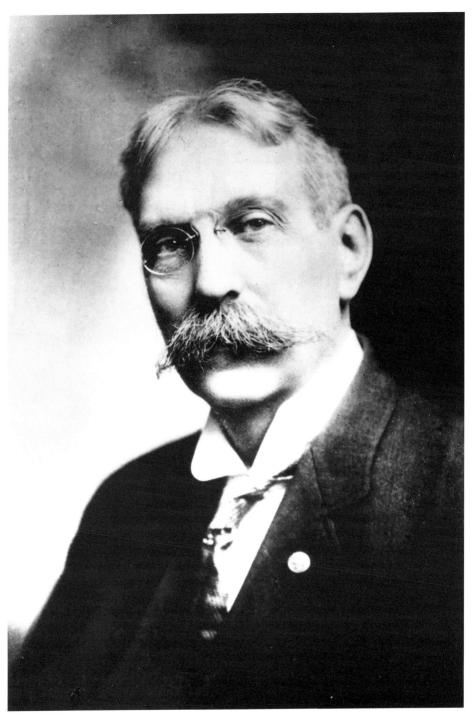

John Marshall, a trained dentist, graduate of Syracuse University's Medical Department, and a dental and oral surgery specialist. Photograph: Courtesy of the National Library of Medicine.

The Statistics, covering this class of cases cannot be relied upon as presenting a true exhibit of the frequency of dental diseases among U.S. Troops, since they do not commonly unfit a soldier for duty, and his name therefore does not often appear upon the monthly reports of sick and wounded from which the above figures are compiled.[68]

On June 7 Marshall used this data in his first detailed report, titled "The Need of Dental Surgeons in the Army and Navy," which he presented to the section on dental and oral surgery at the AMA's annual meeting in Saint Paul.[69] He reminded his audience that the physical requirements for enlistment in government service called for "sound teeth" as a prerequisite, yet once in the service, no dental care was provided. Recognizing the fact that it was no longer necessary for the soldier to bite off his powder cap, he suggested that the sailor still needed good teeth to serve as "an extra pair of hands." He used this illustration: "Many times when reefing topsails in a gale of wind, he is obliged to maintain his position by holding on with his teeth, while his hands are engaged in passing the 'gasket.' The knife, the end of a rope, and many such like things have to be held between the teeth while going aloft."[70]

Marshall also called attention to the fact that the "nature" of the service food required healthy teeth. The food was often dry, hard, and incompletely cooked; he quoted one "old salt" as saying: "The 'hard-tack' furnished by the government was marked B.C. (Before Christ), and the beef was so hard that it made good material from which to carve tobacco-boxes."[70(p493),71] With "diseased teeth," the food was apt to be swallowed before being "thoroughly masticated," which often left troops "unfit for duty" with gastro-intestinal problems.

Recognizing the important role of the surgeon in treating the other parts of the body, Marshall could not understand why diseases of the teeth and jaws were neglected. He said dental caries were "the most common of all diseases" and that few escaped them, including military personnel. Yet the government provided no treatment. The soldiers on the frontier and sailors on long cruises were especially vulnerable. Often "odontalgia" drove the "poor victim" to seek relief by extraction at the hands of a "bungling" hospital steward.[70]

TABLE 4-1

DENTAL DISEASE INCIDENCE IN US ARMY, 1878–1880

	1878–1879		1879–1880	
	White	Colored	White	Colored
Mean strength	21,848	1,964	22,096	2,364
Toothache	52	12	44	17
Dental caries	5	0	7	0
Alveolar abscess	1	0	0	0
Dental abscess	0	0	1	0

Reproduced from: National Archives and Records Administration. Letters Received, 1818–1889. Record Group 112. Captain Benjamin F Pope to Dr Marshall, 4 May 1882. No 2052. Box 124. Entry 12.

Marshall also recalled the great success of Dr James Baxter Bean's interdental splint in treating fractured jaws and gunshot wounds during the Civil War; he argued that dental surgeons would be a valuable asset in treating such injuries in the Army hospitals.[70] At the time, Army and Navy surgeons were opposed to the appointment of dental surgeons, and he concluded that they did not think the problem of dental disease was important enough to justify dental specialists. The 1878–1879 tabulation of dental disease by the Army surgeon general's office showed that of 23,812 US soldiers, there were only 64 toothaches, 5 dental caries, and 1 alveolar abscess, for a total of 70 cases (1 case per 340 soldiers). The 1879–1880 tabulation for 24,460 soldiers listed 61 toothaches, 7 dental caries, and 1 dental abscess, for a total of 69 cases (an average of 1 case per 354 soldiers). Marshall believed that the small number of dental caries was incongruous with the incidence in civilian practice.

The Navy's Bureau of Medicine and Surgery's report on dental disease for 1878 failed to even list dental caries. It reported only 24 cases of odontalgia for the Navy's 7,806 sailors. The Navy chief of the bureau, Commander Philip Wales, told Marshall:

> The Bureau of Medicine and Surgery does not think it advisable, or in the interest of the government to have a separate corps of specially educated dental surgeons. That the necessity does not exist is shown in the reports of the Surgeon-General of the Navy for the years 1879 and 1880, where, in 23,875 cases of disease, there were but 59 of odontalgia and other troubles of the teeth. This very small fraction is due to the fact that in all physical examinations of aspirants for appointment in the navy, persons with defective teeth are rejected.[70(pp495–496)]

Marshall surmised that if these reports were accurate, it would be the dental profession's duty to advise all patients to enter the service to preserve their teeth He concluded that the surgeons obviously "overlooked" dental diseases and considered them not worth mentioning in their reports. Consequently, their superiors were never aware of the problem.[70] To illustrate his point, Marshall quoted a personal letter received from an Army officer on the Western frontier:

> There is, I suppose, among soldiers, as much need of dental surgery as among the same number of men anywhere else; but, as a rule, soldiers are recruited from the lowest walks of life, and are such as pay very little attention to the preservation of their teeth.
>
> Army surgeons are supplied with most complete sets of instruments for *extracting* teeth, and they are kept at every post hospital. The surgeons and hospital stewards usually do all the extracting. Officers and their families, as a rule, so arrange to have all work necessary on their teeth done by their regular dentist when they are East, on leave of absence. . . . Army surgeons never attempt to fill teeth. They merely extract them.[70(p497)]

He also quoted Major General Winfield S Hancock:

> Both officers and men of the military and naval service *need* professional skill in the care of their teeth. Whether the surgeons and their assistants are competent to deal

with their necessities, or to relieve their sufferings, or prevent them until they reach civil assistance, is a question, which I am not prepared to answer. However, I think a fair discussion of this subject before your Medical Society would throw needed light upon it.[70(p498)]

In regard to the Navy, Marshall referred to Admiral Porter's comments in favor of dentists to help sailors properly chew their food and his regret that he had never had the service of a dentist available to him in his younger military days.[70] "If we had had dentists in the navy, I should not have been compelled to live on soft food to-day."[70]

In conclusion, Marshall said that all congressional petitions for a dental service would fail unless the service medical departments endorsed the recommendation. He suggested that the incorporation of dental disease statistics into the regular medical and surgical reports for the services would be the best method of justifying the need for dental surgeons.[70] The subject was discussed by the AMA section members; Dr JL Williams endorsed the paper; Dr DH Goodwillie agreed that Army surgeons should be educated in dental and oral surgery; and Marshall said that the new appointees should have both medical and dental degrees. It was decided that appointees should be able to perform amputations and other surgical procedures that might be necessary on the battlefield.[69]

Dr JB Lawrence wondered how easy it would be to get the Medical Department's endorsement for dental surgeons. From his own Army experience, he knew that any medical complaint "except toothache" would exempt a soldier from guard duty. "I have known of several cases," he said, "where soldiers suffering from severe cases of toothache were obliged to do guard duty, and had their complaints laughed at."[72(pp11–12)] Dr Walter Allport agreed, admitting that the medical officers were "ignorant in regard to the [dental] wants of their men," and recommended that the medical schools be "reformed" to correct this omission in their education. He also cited the previous efforts of Edward Maynard to secure dental appointments in the Army and Navy. But he was optimistic that Surgeon General Barnes would be sympathetic to the cause and offered the following resolution:

> Resolved, That a committee of three be appointed by the Chair for the purpose of considering the subject of appointment of dental surgeons in the army and navy, and that the surgeon-generals of the army and navy, and Dr. E. Maynard, of Washington, be requested to co-operate with this committee.[69]

The resolution was adopted and Allport, Marshall, and Williams were appointed to the committee.[69] On August 18, 1882, Dr Truman Brophy, the secretary of the AMA section on dental and oral surgery, informed the Army surgeon general of the resolution, hoping that Army and Navy surgeons general would lend their support.[73]

The following June at the 1883 AMA meeting in Cleveland, the committee reported that because of a misunderstanding on the part of the "gentleman residing in Washington [Dr Maynard]," who was their line of communication to the surgeons general, nothing had been accomplished. Again, it was recommended that dental disease statistics be incorporated in the medical reports. The committee was extended for another year, but made little progress.[74]

A History of Denistry In the US Army to World War II

Ulysses S Grant's Epithelioma of the Tongue

One of the most prominent 19th Century Army veterans, Ulysses S Grant, could have benefited from a trained corps of dental surgeons in the service, who might have even saved his life. At the recommendation of his physician, Grant consulted Dr Frank Abbott of New York City, a Union veteran, on November 8, 1884. Grant had been suffering for the previous week or so from pain on the right side of his head and face, which his physician attributed to the maxillary right first molar tooth. Barker recommended that it be removed. Upon examining Grant, Abbott found that this tooth was indeed "dead," with an "abscess at the apex of the anterior buccal root." In addition, it was elongated and the roots were covered with tartar. Dr Abbott extracted the tooth and Grant experienced immediate relief from his "neuralgia."[75,76]

On November 14 Grant returned to Abbott's office for a complete oral examination. Abbott found the maxillary right second and third molar teeth next to the extraction site to be elongated (due to missing mandibular opponents), and their roots "thickly coated with a dark brown or black tartar." He advised the immediate removal of these teeth, believing they were a contributing factor to Grant's tongue and throat lesion that had been diagnosed 5 months earlier.[75]

Grant's first cancer symptoms had appeared in June 1884. While eating some fruit, he observed that his "throat was sore," and that peaches, of which he was especially fond, gave him "great trouble." A series of medical referrals followed, which considerably delayed the diagnosis and treatment.[77]

It was not until the fall of 1884 that Grant was first seen by Dr John H Douglas, a highly respected throat specialist, for an "induration" of the tongue. Douglas's clinical examination revealed a well-defined, indurated lesion at the right side of the base of the tongue, which he diagnosed as cancerous. He assured Grant that his case was not hopeless and that he would start "judiciously conservative," non-surgical treatment, including rinsing his mouth and throat with astringent and antiseptic solutions to debride the odorous diseased tissue cells and applying silver nitrate, iodoform powder, and hydrogen peroxide topically to the tongue lesion. He also ordered Grant to stop smoking.[77]

Meanwhile, ulcerations appeared in Grant's mouth, changing his diagnosis to "epithelioma of the tongue and fauces." The base of the tongue on the right side of his mouth was "indurated to a slight extent." The lymph gland under the angle of his right jaw was also affected. The roof of Grant's mouth, at the hard palate line and to the right of the median line, had "three small warty-like excrescences," which showed a "tendency toward cell-proliferation." Grant also suffered from "pain in the right ear." This symptom was treated by a topical application of a 4% solution of cocaine. Cocaine was also administered by injection and iodoform was dusted upon the ulcerations.[78] Grant died on July 23, 1885, at age 64; the cause of his death was listed as "carcinoma of the tongue and tonsil with extension of the tumor into the hypopharynx and larynx."[77]

Some felt that Grant's death in 1885 was due to a disease of dental origin. Abbott, for example, theorized that Grant's broken molar caused the irritation of the base of the tongue, and the condition was aggravated by smoking.[75] The lesion turned cancerous, spreading to the pharynx and lymph glands, and by the time

100

Grant sought treatment, it was too late.[79] In April 1885 the *Independent Practitioner* commented on the case, writing:

> That the oral condition may be, and often is, a prime factor in inducing malignant tumors of the mouth, is a fact that cannot be too quickly and thoroughly comprehended. . . . The case should most certainly be thoroughly investigated from the dental standpoint, that it may prove of greatest benefit to others, for this instance is not at all unique.[80(p210)]

Dental Surgeons, 1886–1890

At the annual meeting of the British Dental Association in London in 1886, Dr George Cunningham, a British crusader for dental health, preventive dentistry, and dentists in the British services (he received the degree of Doctor of Dental Medicine [DDM] from Harvard in 1876), spoke on "Dentistry in its Relation to the State." In his paper, he attacked the lack of dental care in the British services and quoted from a letter of the Army surgeon general on the state of dentistry in the US Army:

> The military academy at West Point has a regular dentist on duty, and it is believed that such is the case at the naval academy at Annapolis. In the army there are several accomplished practical dentists in the corps of hospital stewards, but these are exceptions to the rule. The medical department of the army has tried to arouse interest among medical officers in the matter of the care and treatment of the teeth, by furnishing such instruments as are needed on requisition. The dental cases in the supply list for issue, consist of an extracting case, and a small case for making excavations and temporary fillings. These latter are supplied only to frontier posts, where it is not practical to obtain the services of a dentist. . . . Congress has been appealed to on several occasions to authorise the employment of dentists, but, so far, has taken no definite action. It is probable, however, that, in time, proper provision will be made in this necessary and valuable branch.[81(p12)]

Even though Cunningham presented a more positive picture and admitted that "in time, proper provision will be made in this necessary and valuable branch," the situation regarding dentistry in the Army remained unchanged. On December 29, 1886, Dr Charles Robb, a dentist in Pueblo, Colorado, wrote to the secretary of war asking many of the same questions as Cunningham: were dentists "employed" in the US Army; what were their rank and pay; and what was the procedure for securing an appointment? On January 6, 1887, the surgeon general's office sent Robb the usual reply, saying that the "law makes no provision for the employment of dentists" in the US Army.[82,83]

At the 1887 meeting of the Southern Dental Association at Old Point Comfort, Virginia, Dr William Richards of Knoxville, Tennessee, spoke of the "lamentable condition" of the soldiers' teeth stationed at the adjacent Fort Monroe, Virginia. He said that dentists should not interfere with the work of the physicians, but that the two professions should "cooperate with each other." He urged the association to make an effort to draw the government's attention to this matter.[42,84]

On March 20, 1890, during the first session of the 51st Congress, Congressman Robert Bullock of Florida, a former Confederate brigadier general, introduced

a petition in the House of Representatives from the Florida State Dental Association, requesting that dentists be appointed in the Army and Navy. The petition
was referred to the House Committee on Naval Affairs. On April 7 at the same
session, Senator Matthew Butler from Edgefield, South Carolina, a former Confederate major general, presented a similar petition in the Senate from the same
dental association requesting the establishment of "a bureau of dental surgery"
for the Army and Navy. Again, the document was referred to the Committee on
Military Affairs, but no legislation ever materialized as a result of either proposed bill.[85]

In October 1890 *Dental Headlight* pointed out that if the physicians in the military were as proficient in dentistry as they were in surgery, there would be no need
for dental surgeons. However, this was not the case because they were "proverbi-
ally ignorant" of dentistry.[86] Despite their lack of training, the medical surgeons
stationed at isolated western posts were frequently called upon to perform dental
extractions. Major General William Gorgas (1854–1920), Army surgeon general
from 1914 to 1918, recalled his early days as an Army post surgeon and the use of
the dental key:

> My early professional life for the first twenty years was spent in the west on the
> plains. I had all sorts of work, but a great deal of dentistry fell to my lot, and
> whatever came to hand, I endeavored to turn into the line of tooth extraction. . . .
> I flatter myself that I became exceedingly skillful in this. . . . In my early practice,
> forceps was beginning to be used; I acquired a tolerable degree of skill in the use
> of forceps, but felt absolutely certain I could succeed if I had the key. . . . You put
> the claws of the steel key under the tooth and by revolving the lever got the tooth

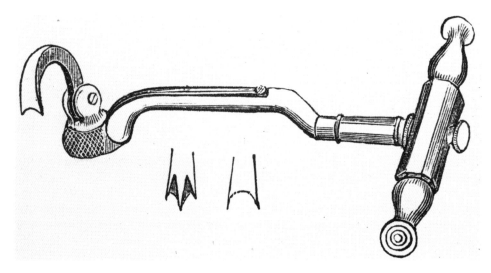

Dental key, circa 1868.
Reproduced from: http://wwwihm.nlm.nih.gov/ihm/images/A/12/377.jpg.
Courtesy of the National Library of Medicine.

out. . . . You always got the tooth, but the trouble was you sometimes got more than one tooth, . . . and frequently you took away a piece of the jaw. But most of my clientele were the Sioux Indians at this time, who had exceedingly firm jawed teeth, and my reputation was increased with the number of teeth I brought out at one extraction, and if I took away a small piece of the jaw I was considered still more skillful.[87]

Comments such as those of Gorgas merely confirmed the quandary in which dentists found themselves when dealing with the Army. On one hand, the Army upheld strict dental requirements for enlistment and reenlistment. On the other hand, it paid no attention to maintaining the dental health of soldiers once they were in the Army. In 1890 Army Surgeon Charles Greenleaf published his latest revised edition of *An Epitome of Tripler's Manual, and Other Publications on the Examination of Recruits*, which was used for many years as a guide for the Army's medical officers assigned recruiting duties. Greenleaf listed the precise dental standards to be met for enlistment or reenlistment in the US Army, but nothing was mentioned about maintaining dental health once in the Army.

"It is deemed impracticable": the 1890s

In 1891 another formal effort to seek federal government support for military dental surgeons was channeled through the ADA's Committee on State Dental Laws and the Appointment of Dentists in the Army and Navy. On August 4, 1891, at the annual meeting in Saratoga Springs, New York, Dr Henry Briss Noble of Washington, DC, reported that he had personally presented the following letter, dated March 27, 1891, to Brigadier General Charles Sutherland, Army surgeon general from 1890 to 1893, and had been cordially received:

The undersigned Committee were appointed by the American Dental Association, at its last meeting, to consider the feasibility of the appointment of dental surgeons in the army and navy.

It is believed that the appointment of dental surgeons in the army and navy would be the means of relieving much suffering and saving the organs of mastication so necessary to health and comfort.

This want is especially felt in our Western military stations by both men and officers far away from any dental surgeon, often requiring them to send members of their families hundreds of miles to get the service of a dentist.

We should be pleased to have your opinion and advice on the above subject.[89(pp20–21)]

On April 13, 1891, Sutherland replied:

I am not in a position to speak as regards the Navy, but so far as the Army is concerned this is a matter which has been considered by the War Department on several occasions. So long as our Army is distributed in small bodies over a vast extent of

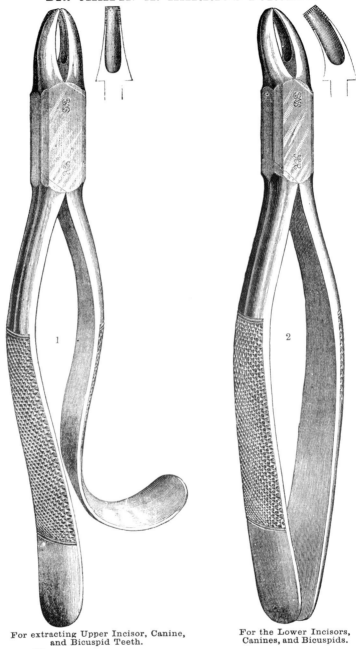

DR. CHAPIN A. HARRIS'S FORCEPS.

For extracting Upper Incisor, Canine, and Bicuspid Teeth.

22

For the Lower Incisors, Canines, and Bicuspids.

Forceps style used in late 1800s and shown in Dental Cosmos *(1878). Designer was reportedly under the supervision of Chapin A Harris. Courtesy of the US Army Medical Department Museum. Borden 017.*

territory and is actually in the field for a considerable part of the year it is deemed impracticable to extend to it the benefits of skilled dental surgery, however desirable this might be on behalf of officers and men. Where troops are massed in garrison, as in a few instances, the military reservation is as a rule in the vicinity of some large city where the services of dental surgeons can be obtained.

I am of the opinion also, that the necessity for special dental service with the troops scattered over the West and South is less needful now than it was some years ago, for increased railroad facilities have brought the most remote posts within a few hours journey of some growing city.[90,91]

Noble sent the same letter to the Navy Surgeon General, JM Browne, who failed to reply. It seemed that the government saw little need for dental care because enlisted personnel served only a short time and could be rejected if they did not pass a preenlistment oral examination.[89]

Dentists in the United States and Britain were not alone in their quest for proper dental care for their armies and navies. On August 17, 1893, at the World's Columbian Dental Congress during the World's Columbian Exposition in Chicago, the Committee to Promote the Appointment of Dental Surgeons in the Armies and Navies of the World (with members from England, Germany, Holland, Denmark, Russia, Switzerland, Italy, Canada, South America, and the United States) met and released a report. Dr M Whilldin Foster, the committee's chairman and dean of the Baltimore College of Dental Surgery from 1894 to 1914, concluded:

That opposition to such appointments came from the surgeons in the army and navy of the United States. The proposition to give the dental surgeon an equal grade with the surgeon was strongly opposed.

It was deemed the better course not to be too urgent at this time, but to send every year a copy of this request to the surgeon-general, to remind him that the effort to place the dental surgeon on an equal grade with the surgeon had not been abandoned.[92]

On September 9, 1893, the new and progressive Army surgeon general (served 1893–1902), Brigadier General George Sternberg (1838–1915), adopted the Medical Department's traditional position, informing Representative John Maddox of Georgia that there was no provision for dentists in the US Army.[93] On September 25, 1894, Richard Doran of Asbury Park, New Jersey, wrote to the War Department for information on military dental surgeons. The surgeon general replied that "no such office existed; the services of a dentist when required being paid for by the officer or enlisted man employing him."[94(p70)]

Despite this opposition to Army dental care, American dentists continued to push the issue at the level of the state and local dental societies. Early in 1897 the Ohio State Dental Society passed a resolution proposing that the government employ dental surgeons for the military. Dr Otto Arnold of Columbus, appointed as its official spokesman, emphasized the incongruity of the government providing soldiers with sanitary quarters, wholesome food, adequate exercise, medical treatment by competent surgeons, and hospitalization when required, yet making no "provision

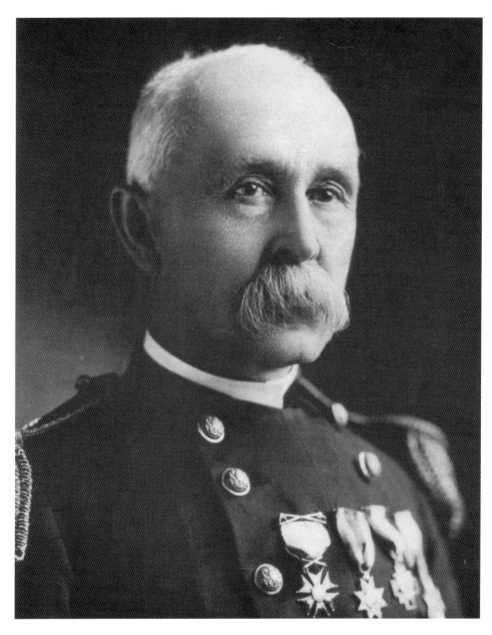

George M Sternberg, surgeon general 1893–1902.
Photograph: Courtesy of the National Museum of Health and Medicine,
Armed Forces Institute of Pathology. NCP 3564.

for his dental organs." He also mentioned that while the recruits' teeth had to pass the entrance physical, "the insidious process of dental caries" was still present and was "no respecter of persons." He deplored the fact that "extraction of the offending teeth" was the only treatment offered and that it was usually performed by hospital stewards, "men wholly without dental training." Arnold also declared that if dentists were on the examining boards, the dental standards of the Army would be elevated merely by their rejection of men with defective teeth. Further, dentists would be invaluable in treating gunshot wounds about the mouth and face.[95,96]

The editor of the *Ohio Dental Journal*, Dr Louis Bethel, urged a "united and organized effort" by the dental profession to secure the needed congressional legislation. *Dental Cosmos* endorsed the desirability of the proposal. Its editor, Edward Kirk, added another "cogent reason for the appointment of dentists in connection with our national defensive service," referring readers to Dr Alton Thompson's article in the same issue on the use of dental records for personal identification; *Dental Cosmos* was one of the first journals to propose forensic dentistry as a reason for commissioning Army dentists. Dr Rodrigues Ottolengui (1861–1937), editor of *Items of Interest: a Monthly Magazine of Dental Art, Science, and Literature*, supported the proposal and thought that the money spent for this service would be better spent than the government funds going to the pensions of Civil War veterans. Dr John Patterson, the editor of the *Western Dental Journal*, who had personal experience treating soldiers, agreed that this "humanitarian" objective should be supported by the entire profession. The measure also received support from England, the *British Journal of Dental Science* expressing its astonishment that the military of both countries could be so "supine" on such an important matter.[97–102]

The editor of the *Pacific Stomatological Gazette*, Dr Frank Platt, took a somewhat different view. He argued that the proposed legislation would be unable to attract "thoroughly competent and well-educated" practitioners because the rank and salary were not comparable to that of medical surgeons. He recommended that the Medical Department's assistant surgeons be required to be "graduates in both medicine and dentistry." This qualification would put the dentists on an equal basis with their medical colleagues. The editor of the *Dental Review*, Dr Alison Harlan, said the "question of rank" would remain the "stumbling block" it had been in the past. It was his opinion that:

> Any rank less than that of second lieutenant or assistant surgeon would not be accepted by our profession. The rank of hospital steward or sergeant would not do for us after having spent three or four years in the study of dental surgery to attain such a position in the army and navy.[103,104]

On April 28, 1897, Murray Acklin, acting hospital steward at Jefferson Barracks, Missouri, wrote to the editor of *Dental Cosmos* in response to the Arnold proposal. He vividly described the soldiers' dental plight from extensive first-hand experience:

> Soldiers cannot always go to a dentist, even though they always have the ready money to pay for their work. Take for instance some of our frontier garrisons, where there is not a dentist located within fifty miles or more of them, and one probably does not

make a visit to the post once in a year; a soldier has an attack of genuine, old-fashioned toothache; it may be a good tooth, one that should not be lost by any means; probably with a few hours' work it could be made nearly as serviceable as ever. But there is no dentist near, and he cannot endure that pain until one comes, probably in six months, possibly longer, so what can the poor fellow do? Nothing but go to the hospital and have it extracted by the steward, and, if the steward is successful in getting it out, the man is relieved of his pain, but he is just one more tooth short; but if it happens to be broken off, and the worst part of it left in the jaw, a condition which very often prevails, the man is worse off than before. In this way thousands of teeth are lost, and eventually there must be many days' service lost to the government, resulting therefrom. Even when soldiers are stationed near cities where dentists are plentiful, they often have a hard time getting work done. The busy dentist must make engagements according to his time, while the soldier, not knowing what duty he may be detailed for, cannot make engagements two days in advance.[105]

On October 27, 1897, at the annual meeting of the sixth, seventh, and eighth district dental societies of New York, Dr CF Bentley of Niagara Falls, New York, read a paper titled "The Care of Army Teeth," and presented a resolution recommending that the various New York dental societies lobby their congressional representatives for dental corps legislation. Bentley emphasized the need for soldiers to have ready access to persons trained and qualified to provide full service dental care. His resolution stressed that no such skilled persons were available in the Army and that the average surgeon could not be expected to have such knowledge. He urged that dental societies throughout New York combine to educate their congressmen on the need and to press for appropriate legislation to give "practicing and competent dentists" military status.[106]

For some years, Bentley had been doing most of the dental work at Fort Niagara. In his experience, he found that the soldiers were "very careless about the care of their teeth, often seeking extraction, but usually having no funds for this purpose." He saw no reason why the government should employ surgeons, veterinarians, and chaplains and not dentists. The Bentley resolution was discussed and passed.[106]

An End to Complacency

Pressure from dental professionals and their sympathizers was mounting to compel the War Department and Army surgeon general to recognize the need for official dental care for the troops. Only extraordinary and unprecedented requirements that could be neither ignored nor avoided could shake the War Department's resolve. These requirements appeared in 1898 when the United States unexpectedly acquired an overseas empire as a result of the war with Spain. A medical officer could no longer advise an ailing soldier with a serious dental problem to seek care from a local civilian dentist, for few of them could be found in such places as Luzon, Mindanao, or Oriente Province in the Philippine Islands, Cuba, or Puerto Rico, where American soldiers were now stationed. In addition, many volunteer soldiers who served and suffered would keep the issue alive upon their return to civilian life and subsequent rise to positions of influence.

References

1. National Archives and Records Administration. Record Group 112. Dr CE Robb to secretary of war, December 29, 1886. Letter. No. 72 (1887), filed with No. 668 (1873). Box 21. Entry 12.

2. National Archives and Records Administration. Record Group 112. Surgeon general's office to Dr Robb, January 6, 1887. No. 72 (1887), filed with No. 668 (1873). Box 21. Entry 12.

3. Perine GH. The necessity of dental appointments in the Army and Navy. *Dental Cosmos*. 1880;22:467–468.

4. Merrill AP. Dental surgery in the Army and Navy. *Mo Dent J*. 1875;7:435–440.

5. Clark FY. The employment of dentists in the Army and Navy. In: *Transactions of the Southern Dental Association*. Cincinnati, Ohio: Wrightson & Co; 1870.

6. Minutes [second annual meeting]. In: *Transactions of the Southern Dental Association*. Cincinnati, Ohio: Wrightson & Co; 1870: 10–12.

7. National Archives and Records Administration. Letter Book No. 18, Military, Jan 3, 1871 to Sept 28, 1872, Surgeon General's Office. Record Group 112. Letters and endorsements sent to medical officers (military letters), Sept 1862–Sept 1872. Entry 7.

8. National Archives and Records Administration. Letter Book No 49, Jan 1, 1871–Dec 15, 1871, Surgeon General's Office. Record Group 112. Letters and endorsements sent, April 1818–Oct 1889. Entry 2.

9. National Archives and Records Administration. Letter Book No. 50, Dec 16, 1871–Dec 31, 1872, Surgeon General's Office. Record Group 112. Letters and endorsements sent, Apr 1818–Oct 1889. Entry 2.

10. National Archives and Records Administration. Letter Book Vol 61, 1881, Surgeon General's Office. Record Group 112. Letters and endorsements sent, April 1818–Oct 1889. Entry 2.

11. Obituary, Dr. Charles Parmele Graham. *Dental Cosmos*. 1904;46:1092.

12. Davenport WF. Obituary, Dr. N. Malon Beckwith. *Dental Cosmos*. 1895;37:160.

13. Obituary, Dr. John Henry Meyer. *Dental Cosmos*. 1919;61:186.

14. Obituary, Dr. Wilbur F. Litch. *Dental Cosmos*. 1913;55:242.

15. Ashburn PM. *A History of the Medical Department of the United States Army*. Boston, Mass: Houghton Mifflin Co; 1929: 108–109.

16. Willey P. *Osteological Analysis of Human Skeletons Excavated From the Custer National Cemetery*. Lincoln, Neb: US Department of the Interior, Midwest Archeological Center, NPS; 1998: i.

17. *Congressional Globe, 42nd Cong, 2nd Sess.* Washington DC: Blair & Rives; 1872: 2072, 3221.

18. National Archives and Records Administration. Correspondence Relating to the Military Academy, 1867–1904. Record Group 94. Colonel Ruger to Secretary Belknap, April 23, 1872. Letter. No. 253. Box 10. Entry 214.

19. National Archives and Records Administration. Superintendent's Letter Book No. 5, Office of the Superintendent. Record Group 404. Letters sent, 1845–1902. Entry 2: 239.

20. Hyson JM Jr. *The United States Military Academy Dental Service: A History, 1825–1920.* West Point, NY: United States Military Academy, United States Army; 1989.

21. National Archives and Records Administration. Letters Sent and Endorsements, 1867–1893. Record Group 404. War Department office, military academy, 1867–1872. Vol 1. Entry 208: 473.

22. Obituary, Dr. T.O. Walton. *Dental Cosmos.* 1901;43: 442.

23. Grady R. The dentist in the United States Navy: an account of the efforts to secure a dental corps. *Dental Cosmos.* 1909;51:601.

24. US Navy. *The Dental Corps of the United States Navy: A Chronology 1912–1962.* Washington, DC: Bureau of Medicine and Surgery, Department of the Navy; 1962: 4–7.

25. National Archives and Records Administration. Record Group 112. John C Johnston to pension office, September 12, 1870. Letter. No. J 53, J 75. Box 49. Entry 12.

26. National Archives and Records Administration. Letter Book No. 51, Jan 1, 1873–Aug 25, 1873, Surgeon General's Office. Record Group 112. Entry 2.

27. National Archives and Records Administration. Record Group 112. JS Charles to surgeon general, October 13, 1874. Letter. No. 3793 (filed with No. 668;1873). Box 21. Entry 12.

28. National Archives and Records Administration. Record Group 112. Surgeon General Barnes to JS Charles, October 17, 1874. Letter. No. 3793 (filed with No. 668:1873). Box 21. Entry 12.

29. National Archives and Records Administration. Letter Book No. 58, Surgeon General's Office, 1878. Entry 2.

30. National Archives and Records Administration. Record Group 112. Office memo, December 20, 1878. No. 5204. Box 75. Entry 12.

31. Patterson JD. Fracture of the lower maxilla by a gunshot wound. Treatment by an interdental splint bridge. *Dental Cosmos.* 1891;33:823–824.

32. Catching BH. Communications. *Southern Dental Journal and Luminary*. 1893;12:83–84.

33. American Dental Association [proceedings, fourteenth annual session]. *Dental Cosmos*. 1874;16:645.

34. National Archives and Records Administration. Record Group 112. Dr Merrill to Surgeon General Barnes, August 30, 1875. Letter. No. 3706 (1875), filed with No. 668 (1873). Box 21. Entry 12.

35. National Archives and Records Administration. Record Group 112. Surgeon General Barnes to Dr Merrill, September 6, 1875. Letter. No. 3706 (1875), filed with No. 668 (1873). Box 21.

36. Merrill AP. Necessity of dentists in the Army and Navy. *Am J Dent Sci*. 1876;9:393.

37. Annual meeting of the Dental Society of the State of Maryland and District of Columbia. *Dental Cosmos*. 1875;17:652–653.

38. *Congressional Record, 44th Cong, 1st Sess*. Vol 4. Washington, DC: Government Printing Office; 1876: 586.

39. US Congress. House. *Dental Surgeons in Army*. 44th Cong, 1st sess, 1876, 743.

40. National Archives and Records Administration. Letter Book No. 16, 1880, Surgeon General's Office. Record Group 112. Entry 6: 147–148.

41. National Archives and Records Administration. Letter Book No. 18, 1882, Surgeon General's Office. Record Group 112. Entry 6.

42. Beecher MP, comp. *Beecher's Dental Directory of the United States*. New York, NY: Beecher & Co; 1888: 49, 123, 156.

43. Soldiers' teeth. *Philadelphia Times*. Quoted in: *Dental Headlight*. 1882;3:62–63.

44. Editorial. *Brit J Dent Sci*. 1882;25:282.

45. Dental surgeons in the Army and Navy. *Medical Record*. Cited in: *Am J Dent Sci*. 1882;16:94.

46. National Archives and Records Administration. Letter Book No. 62, 1882, Surgeon General's Office. Record Group 112. Entry 2; 252, 324.

47. Perine GH. The necessity of dental appointments in the Army and Navy. *Dental Cosmos*. 1880;22:467–468.

48. Dentists for Army and Navy. *Am J Dent Sci*. 1881;15:374–375.

49. Perine GH. Army and Navy dental appointments. *Dental Cosmos*. 1882;24:56.

50. Hutchinson WH. Dentists in the Army and Navy. *Dental Cosmos*. 1882;24:280.

51. Perine GH. Correspondence. *Southern Dental Journal* 1882:184.

52. American Dental Association [proceedings, twenty-first annual session]. *Dental Cosmos*. 1882;24:23,31.

53. National Archives and Records Administration. Compiled Military Service Record. Record Group 94. John Marshall, Second NY Cavalry. Entry 519.

54. National Archives and Records Administration. Record Group 112. Dr Marshall to surgeon general, March 3, 1911. Letter. No. 70760. Box 449. Entry 26.

55. National Archives and Records Administration. Record Group 94. Civil War record, John S Marshall. No. 391988. Box 2730. Entry 25.

56. V[ail] WD. John Sayre Marshall, pioneer Army dental surgeon (1846–1922). *Dental Bulletin Supplement to the Army Medical Bulletin*. 1940;11:111–112.

57. Dyer FH, comp. *A Compendium of the War of the Rebellion*. Vol 2. Dayton, Ohio: Broadfoot Publishing Co, Morningside Press; 1994: 1370–1371.

58. Phisterer F, comp. *New York in the War of the Rebellion 1861 to 1865*. 3rd ed. Albany, NY: James B Lyon; 1912: 51.

59. Crisfield CM, ed and trans. *William Dolphin's Civil War Diary August 15, 1863 through April 4, 1864*. Ossining, NY: Ossining Historical Society; 1991: 113.

60. State of New York. *Annual Report of the Adjutant General of the State of New York for the Year 1863*. Vol 2. Albany, NY: James B Lyon; 1894: 534.

61. A landmark in his profession [Walter Webb Allport, MD, DDS]. *Dent Radiogr Photogr*. 1962;35: 69.

62. Union convention of the fifth, sixth, seventh, and eighth district dental societies of the State of New York [proceedings]. *Dental Cosmos*. 1888;30:920.

63. Koch CRE, ed. *History of Dental Surgery*. Vol 1. Fort Wayne, Ind: National Art Publishing Co; 1910: 138–140, 515.

64. Dummett CO, Dummett LD. *Culture and Education in Dentistry at Northwestern University Dental School (1891–1993)*. Chicago, Ill: Northwestern University Dental School; 1993: 16.

65. National Archives and Records Administration. Record Group 112. Dr Marshall to Surgeon General Barnes, April 6, 1882. Letter. No. 1865: (1882). Box 123. Entry 12.

66. National Archives and Records Administration. Record Group 112. Surgeon General Barnes to Dr Marshall, April 12, 1882. Notation. No. 1865. Box 123. Entry 12.

67. National Archives and Records Administration. Record Group 112. Dr Marshall to Surgeon General Barnes, April 14, 1882. No. 2052. Box 124. Entry 12.

68. National Archives and Records Administration. Record Group 112. Captain Benjamin F Pope to Dr Marshall, May 4, 1882. No. 2052. Box 124. Entry 12.

69. Minutes of the Section on Dental and Oral Surgery. In: *Trans Am Med Assoc*. Vol 33. Philadelphia, Pa: Times Printing House; 1882: 455, 458–459.

70. Marshall JS. The need of dental surgeons in the Army and Navy. In: *Transactions of the American Medical Association*. Vol 33. Philadelphia, Pa: Times Printing House; 1882: 492–498.

71. Mattison RH. *The Army Post on the Northern Plains 1865–1885*. Gering, NE: Oregon Trail Museum Association; 1962: 10–11, 14.

72. Kempton WD. American Medical Association [meeting]. *Dental Jairus*. 1883;4:11–12.

73. National Archives and Records Administration. Record Group 112. Dr Brophy to Surgeon General Crane, August 18, 1882. No. 5557. Box 131. Entry 12.

74. American Medical Association Section on Dental and Oral Surgery [proceedings]. *Dental Cosmos*. 1883;25: 427–428.

75. Abbott F. General Grant's condition. *Independent Practitioner*. 1885;6:218–219.

76. Obituary, Dr Frank Abbott. *Dental Cosmos*. 1897;39:515.

77. Kanterman CB. Ulysses S. Grant's dental dilemmas. *Tic*. 1985;4:5–6.

78. General Grant's condition. *Med Rec*.1885;27:267–268.

79. McPike CL. Army and Navy Dentists. *Pacific Dental Gazette*. 1900;8:151.

80. [Barrett WC]. The case of General Grant. *Independent Practitioner*.1885;6:210.

81. Cunningham G. Dentistry in its relation to the state. *Brit J Dent Sci*. 1887;30:12.

82. National Archives and Records Administration. Record Group 112. Dr CE Robb to secretary of war, December 29, 1886. No 72 (1887), filed with No 668 (1873), Box 21. Entry 12.

83. National Archives and Records Administration. Record Group 112. Surgeon General's Office to Dr Robb, January 6, 1887. No. 72 (1887), filed with No. 668 (1873). Box 21. Entry 12.

84. J MW, comp. Southern Dental Association, Old Point Comfort, Va., nineteenth annual session [proceeding]. Quoted in: *Am J Dent Sci*. 1888;21:392.

85. *Congressional Record, 51st Cong, 1st Sess.* Vol 21. Washington DC: Government Printing Office; 1889: 2452, 3098.

86. Dentists in the Army and Navy. *Dental Headlight.* 1890;11:206.

87. Gorgas WC. Consideration of some of the important changes that have been made in the medical department of the United States Army during the past four years. *J Nat Dent Assoc* 1918;5:1154–1155.

88. Greenleaf CR. *An epitome of tripler's manual, and other publications on the examination of recruits.* Washington, DC: William Ballantyne & Sons; 1890: 41–42.

89. [Noble HB]. Report of committee on state dental laws and the appointment of dentists in the Army and Navy. In: *Transactions of the American Dental Association.* Philadelphia, Pa: The SS White Dental Mfg Co; 1891: 20, 21.

90. National Archives and Records Administration. Record Group 112. American Dental Association Committee to Surgeon General Sutherland, March 27, 1891. Letter. No. 3960 (1891), filed with No. 668 (1873). Box 21. Entry 12.

91. National Archives and Records Administration. Record Group 112. Surgeon General Sutherland to American Dental Association committee, April 13, 1891. Letter. No. 3960 (1891), filed with No. 668 (1873). Box 21. Entry 12.

92. The World's Columbian Dental Congress [proceedings]. *Dental Cosmos.* 1893;35:899.

93. National Archives and Records Administration. Record Group 112. Surgeon General Sternberg to Representative Maddox, September 9, 1893. No. 3960. Box 439. Entry 22.

94. V[ail] WD. Organization day. *Dental Bulletin Supplement to the Army Medical Bulletin.* 1933;4:70.

95. Arnold O. Dental service in the Army. *Ohio Dent J.* 1897;17:145–147.

96. Arnold O. The employment of dentists in the United States Army. *Dental Cosmos.* 1897;39:211–213.

97. [Bethel LP]. Representation in the Army and Navy. *Ohio Dent J.* 1897;17:157–158.

98. [Kirk? EC]. Dentists in the Army and Navy. *Dental Cosmos.* 1897;39:264.

99. Thompson AH. Identification by means of the teeth. *Dental Cosmos.* 1897;39:227–232.

100. [Ottolengui R]. Should dentists enter the Army? *Dent Items Interest.* 1897;19:210.

101. [Patterson JD]. Dentists in the United States Army. *West Dent J.* 1897;11:94–95.

102. Dentists for the United States Army. *Br J Dent Sci.* 1897;40:538.

103.	[Platt F]. Dentists in the Army. *Pacific Stomatological Gazette*. 1897;5:143.

104.	[Harlan? AW]. Dentists in the Army and Navy. *Dent Rev*. 1897;11:135.

105.	Acklin M. Employment of dentists in the United States Army. *Dental Cosmos*. 1897;39:465–466.

106.	Bentley CF. The care of Army teeth. *Dental Cosmos*. 1898;40:307–308.

Chapter V

DENTISTRY ANSWERS THE CALL:
THE SPANISH-AMERICAN WAR, 1898

Introduction

The destruction of the *USS Maine* in the Havana harbor on February 15, 1898, followed by the US declaration of war with Spain on April 25, not only changed the global role of the United States, but also had a dramatic effect on the status of Army dentistry. For the first time, large contingents of US troops had to serve outside the continental limits of the United States without access to qualified civilian dentists. Official reports of the troops' dental discomfort in Cuba, Puerto Rico, and the Philippines during the Spanish-American War and the Philippine-American War (1899–1902) made the War Department and the public aware of the soldiers' need for dental surgeons. This inspired the dental profession to intensify efforts to establish a corps of dental surgeons.

"The Time for Action is Now": Dr John Chapple, January 1898

In January 1898, even before hostilities began, one of the editors of *American Dental Weekly*, Dr John Chapple of Atlanta, Georgia, urged immediate action to promote a dental surgeon measure in pending legislation. Rumors indicated that there were imminent changes in the size and personnel of the Army because of the "small war cloud" that "hung menacingly" over the country. In response to this prediction, Chapple told his readers "the time for action is *now*."[1]

At the 29th annual meeting of the Southern Dental Association in February (its first annual session as a branch of the National Dental Association following its amalgamation with the American Dental Association in 1897) in Saint Augustine, Florida, Chapple offered the following preamble and resolution:

Whereas, The propriety and urgent necessity for the government appointment of dental surgeons to the United States Army and Navy has long been recognized by the dental profession;

And Whereas, This question has been debated so long that, in the opinion of this Association, time for decisive action has arrived: Be it therefore

Resolved, By the Southern Branch of the National Dental Association, that a committee of five be appointed, with instructions to proceed to Washington not later than the first of April next, and urge before the proper authorities the appointment by the government of dental surgeons to the army and navy. Be it further

Resolved, That President [Thomas] Fillebrown, of the National Association, be requested to appoint a similar committee from the other branches of the National Association who will co-operate and act in concert with the committee from this Association.[2(p218)]

The resolution was adopted, and the secretary requested the cooperation of the national body. The association selected a committee (consisting of Drs JA Chapple, B Holly Smith, Mark F Finley, Henry B Noble, and E Beadles) to bring the matter to the attention of Congress.[2]

Dentistry in the Spanish-American War

As in the Civil War, many dentists immediately joined the service when the war with Spain was declared in April 1898, some as line officers or enlisted soldiers and others as members of the Medical Department as hospital stewards or physicians. However, either civilian dentists or unqualified Army surgeons still performed most of the dental work on soldiers. As in the past, some dentists serving in line capacities carried their dental kits with them and performed yeoman service in their spare time, fulfilling the dental needs of the members of their own units. Enlisted soldiers and officers alike underwent a great deal of inconvenience and expense when they required dental attention. Additionally, their absence from their post, garrison, or camp for a considerable time, often many miles away, amounted to considerable lost time to their units.

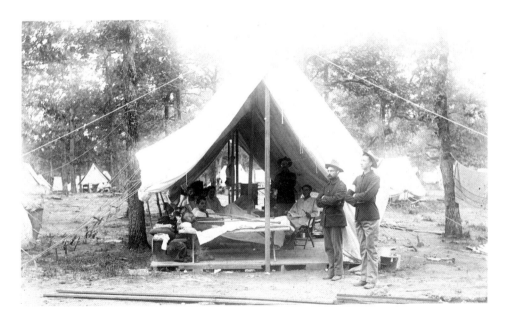

Ward scene with patients and hospital stewards, circa 1898.
Photograph: Courtesy of the US Army Medical Department Museum. Spawar-044.

Despite continued opposition from military medical leaders, the need for dentists to serve the armed forces remained clear, and the nation was equipped to fill this need. In 1898 approximately 25,000 civilian dentists and 8,000 dental assistants were working in the United States, whose population was around 70 million. The prewar US Army of 28,000 soldiers included 177 surgeons and no dentists, yet only 10% of the rejections at the recruiting stations were due to dental causes. According to Dr Williams Donnally (1851–1929) of Washington, "absolutely toothless" recruits were accepted, despite strict official standards, and "artificial teeth" were made for them before their departure for Cuba.[3–5]

William Owen and William Ware:
The Army's First Overseas Dental Infirmary, 1898–1899

As troops and equipment were hastily mobilized for operations in the Caribbean and Philippines, medical officers and their commanders were being compelled to recognize (unofficially) the need for proper dental service. Captain William Otway Owen (1854–1924), an assistant surgeon in the US Army Medical Department, began the process that ultimately established the Army's first dental infirmary in the Philippines. On May 18, 1898, Surgeon General Sternberg recommended that Owen, then on duty at Fort Bayard, New Mexico, be one of the four medical officers ordered to report to Major General Wesley Merritt in San Francisco, California, for duty with the expedition to the Philippine Islands. That same day, the US War Department reassigned Owen to set up the camp hospital in the Richmond district of San Francisco.[6–8]

Within a few days, 160 enlisted hospital corpsmen intended for Philippine duty reported to the camp. This group included two dentists, William Ware (1864–19??) and John Alvin Gibbon (18??–1899), both graduates of the College of Dentistry at the University of California, San Francisco. The two dentists approached Owen, and Ware told him that they had enlisted as hospital corpsmen in the hope of demonstrating that "dentists may be of service to an army." Owen liked the idea and told them to get letters of recommendation from their dean and friends in San Francisco attesting to the validity of their credentials. In a few days, they returned with the necessary papers proving that they were competent graduate dentists.[8–10]

Shortly after his interview with Ware and Gibbon, Owen, now a major, prepared the requisitions for a 1,400-bed hospital for the Philippine expedition. He told Ware and Gibbon to prepare a request for the dental supplies that they would need for a year-long campaign in the Philippines, and to order the instruments and medications that they were "accustomed to use." The surgeon general's office approved the requisition and issued the order.[8,9]

With the arrival of the dental equipment and supplies, Ware began treating Camp Merritt soldiers at the Presidio of San Francisco. When the combat units embarked in August 1898, the two graduate dentists and their full complement of dental equipment and supplies were on their way to the Philippines. Taking advantage of the situation, Ware and Gibbon treated soldiers while en route to Manila.[8]

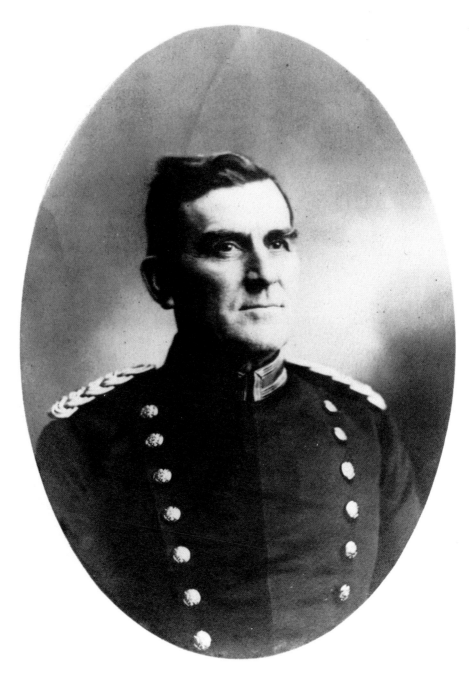

William Otway Owen, an assistant surgeon in the US Army Medical Department
who was ordered to the Philippines in 1898.
Photograph: Courtesy of the National Library of Medicine.

That month, Dr Frank Platt, the editor of the *Pacific Medico-Dental Gazette*, applauded Ware's accomplishment:

> While various attempts have been made throughout the United States to impress upon Congress the necessity for enacting such legislation as would provide for our army an efficient corps of dental surgeons, it has remained for a graduate of the dental department of the University of California to bring this issue to a practical and successful result, at least in so far as our forces now at the Philippines are concerned.
>
> We note with pleasure the fact that Dr. Wm. H. Ware has, with two assistants, Drs. G. F. Ames and J. A. Gibbon, been appointed to serve with General Merritt's army.
>
> To Dr. Ware belongs the credit of having inaugurated the service here, and we earnestly hope this example may be followed at an early date, and that each division of our military service may be given the benefit of skilled dental attendance.
>
> It is of prime importance in considering the physical welfare of man that his teeth should be in such condition as to properly perform the functions for which nature designed them, and we believe it is not carrying this idea too far to say that the efficiency of our army, depending as it does almost entirely upon the physical vigor

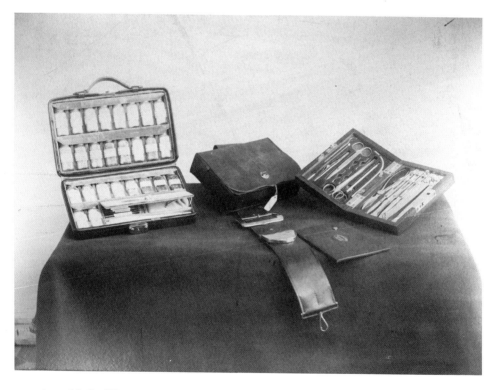

Army Medical Department emergency medicine case and surgeon's field case, circa 1898. Photograph: Courtesy of the US Army Medical Department Museum. Spawar-055.

of its members, depends in turn upon the possession of serviceable and comfortable teeth. That those in authority now recognize this and are turning to the profession for relief is indeed a fact upon which we think we may happily congratulate all dental practitioners.[11]

Shortly after the expedition reached Manila, Gibbon was detailed away from Owen's command. On February 10, 1899, before Owen could have him transferred back, Gibbon was killed in an opening skirmish of the Philippine-American War at Caloocan near Manila. Owen later recalled the incident:

Gibbons [*sic*], instead of being detailed to do work with his dental outfit, like many another poor boy sought the excitement of the battlefield, and one day, returning from the firing-line between the handle-bars of a litter, bringing from the battlefield a wounded officer, Gibbons received a bullet which passed through his heart, and the poor boy died on the field of battle, doing his duty as an upright, honest man. I am sure from the papers and other matters that have come to my attention concerning him that had he been permitted by the Great Master he would have proved himself as faithful to his duty as a dentist as he was in the capacity of litter-bearer on the field of battle.[9,12,13]

Ware remained with Owen's detachment, which established a convalescent hospital for the VIII Corps on the Island of Corregidor in the mouth of Manila Bay. In November or early December 1898, he established the US Army's first semiofficial overseas dental infirmary in 1898. Owen described the historic event:

In one of the old buildings where there was a good light I established Ware as a dental

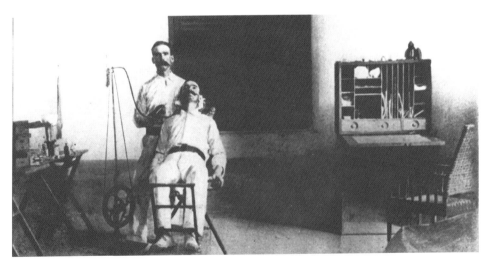

William Ware, one of the initial contract dental surgeons appointed in 1901
and shown here on Corregidor Island in 1898,
was instrumental in establishing dental care for soldiers in the Philippines.
Photograph: Courtesy of the National Archives and Records Administration.

surgeon, and he was kept busy at this work, doing absolutely nothing else but dental work, with one or more assistants to help him keep his room and materials in proper shape, to enable him to do his work as a decent operator should be allowed to do it. It was soon discovered that there was a competent dentist, with proper tools, on duty at the convalescent hospital, and the result was that Ware was kept busy all the time to the limit of his personal capacity to labor—and his capacity was good.[9]

Soldiers from Manila and elsewhere were ordered to Ware's office for dental treatment. There, Ware treated over 300 cases, on which Owen later contended he submitted "the first official reports ever made for purely dental disease."[8] Ware reported on his dental work from his arrival in the Philippines until his discharge on July 11, 1899, writing:

> While it is true that a rigid physical examination is supposed to pass on the qualifications of recruits, it is my unpleasant duty to state that I found the enlisted men almost universally in need of the care of a dental surgeon. The climatic condition, the diet, the exposure, not to mention the water, were in themselves enough, though the physical examination were perfect, to cause the conditions which I found to be almost universal, such as alveolar pyorrhoe [sic], gingivitis, abscesses, etc., familiar to all dental surgeons. In this connection I desire to say that numerous cases were entrusted to my care of fractured jaws, the result of gunshot wounds. These latter cases, as is well known to dental surgeons, require the constant attention and skill of a dental surgeon to restore the natural occlusion for masticating purposes. The surgeons in the army are not prepared nor are they skilled in the science of dentistry to treat successfully such cases.[14]

Owen recalled the case of a young soldier who suffered from a chronic tropical intestinal disease:

> In making the rounds of the hospitals one morning I noticed the condition of his mouth, and sent him to Dr. Ware for treatment. Dr. Ware reported to me that he found nearly every tooth more or less diseased, and many with freely running pus. In three or four weeks the patient's mouth had been placed in fair condition, with the result that the intestinal condition, which had existed for months, ceased, and the man was well without further treatment. In other words, when the pus in the man's mouth was no longer allowed to flow, the intestinal condition was at once cured.[8]

Owen said that Ware worked hard and was "a good man, a good dentist, and a good friend," who rendered "loyal and untiring service." He also later recalled that in early 1899 he had discussed the need for a corps of dentists with Major Charles Boxton (1860–1927), another California volunteer who was a dentist by profession.[15] Owen failed to mention that a third California dentist, Dr GF Ames, served with Ware and Gibbon. Ames and Gibbon were referred to as Ware's "two assistants."[8,9,11]

On March 30, 1899, Dr Luis Lane Dunbar, the dean of the College of Dentistry, University of California, wrote to Surgeon General Sternberg endorsing Ware's appointment as a contract dental surgeon for service in the Philippines and his discharge from his current status as a private in the Hospital Corps. On April 7 the surgeon general's office replied:

Your communication of March 30, 1899 has been received. It relates to the services of Dr. W.H. Ware in caring as a Dental Surgeon for Army patients in Manila, P.I., suggesting his appointment as a contract surgeon for official assignment to such duty. The Surgeon General instructs me to say that there is no authority either in law or regulations for such an appointment. A physical examination of the recruit excludes from service men whose teeth are unsound, while officers have always paid for dental services as they have paid for any other personal service. Treatment by a specialist is authorized in certain cases of "chronic complaints" but dental work has never been regarded as coming within this provision. You will see, therefore, that contract positions for dental work cannot be created without violating established customs.

I should think that there would be a fine field for Dr. Ware in civilian practice in Manila when his connection with the Army is at an end.[16]

Ware was honorably discharged on July 11, 1899, at the Convalescent Hospital, Corregidor Island, Philippine Islands.[10] In 1901 he applied for and was selected to be one of the initial Army contract dentists, serving until his resignation in 1909.

Louis Maus and Jacob Horner: The Army's First Stateside Dental Clinic, 1898–1899

While Owen was preparing his dental clinic in San Francisco, Lieutenant Colonel Louis Maus, chief surgeon on the staff of Major General Fitzhugh Lee's VII Army Corps at Jacksonville, Florida, had a parallel effort underway to organize a dental service for stateside US Army troops. In 1898 Maus organized the hospital service at Camp Cuba Libre, Jacksonville, Florida.[17,18] The entire camp became known for its orderliness and high sanitary standards, which accounted for its low rates of sickness.[19]

Noting the frequency of dental disease among the troops, Maus decided to do something about the problem. Jacob Horner (1864?–19??), an 1898 graduate of the Louisville College of Dentistry, had corresponded with Maus before his enlistment. Upon Horner's arrival, Maus procured $500 worth of dental equipment, rented an office, and put Horner, along with another dentist, John Watts, to work treating the enlisted personnel. Horner agreed to furnish all his own instruments and materials and charge only "the cost of the materials used." He was granted a furlough to return to Indiana to purchase the necessary supplies for his office, and he reportedly spent $600 of his own money on equipment in addition to $17 monthly rent. Maus soon realized that the dentist's talents would be better utilized practicing dentistry than performing the normal steward's duties, and on September 30, 1898, he detailed Horner as "Corps Dentist for the VII Army Corps." On October 1 the commanding officer of Camp Cuba Libre issued a circular announcing that Dr Horner, "Corps Dentist," had established himself in an office in the Hubbard Building at the corner of Forsyth and Main streets in Jacksonville and was "now ready to attend to the teeth of any member of the VII Army Corps. . . . free of cost except for material furnished" (at the time, gold fillings cost from 25 to 50 cents each). On October 30 Maus requested that Private Watts, Horner's assistant, be detailed as an acting hospital steward.[20,21,22]

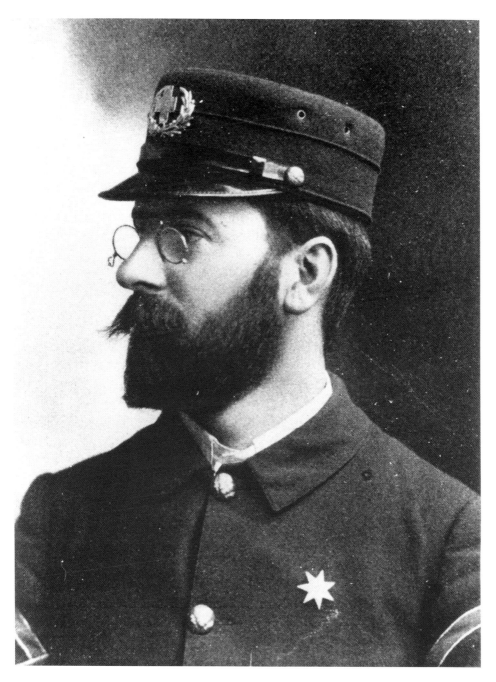

Jacob Horner helped establish the Army's first stateside dental clinic in Florida in 1898.
Photograph: Courtesy of the National Archives and Records Administration.

S. S. WHITE'S
SPECIALTIES IN GOLD.

GLOBE GOLD FOIL.

FOUR VARIETIES:

NON-COHESIVE, or Soft, SEMI-COHESIVE, EXTRA-COHESIVE.

For sale in Numbers 3, 4, 5, 6, 8, 10, 20, 30, 40, 60, 120.

CRYSTALLIZED (Dead Soft).
SURFACE ROUGHENED BY THE KEARSING PROCESS.

Patented December 19th, 1871.   Supplied in Nos. 3, 4, 5, and 6.

GLOBE GOLD FOIL ROLLED.
Prepared with great care, entirely by rolling.
Nos. 30, 40, 60, and 120 kept in stock.

THE QUARTER OF A CENTURY FOIL.
Supplied in Numbers 3, 4, 5, 6, 8, 10.

PACK'S GOLD PELLETS.
TWO VARIETIES.
Patented May 14th, 1872.

SEMI-COHESIVE CRYSTAL GOLD PELLETS
AND
SOFT CRYSTAL GOLD PELLETS.

MEDAL AWARDED AT CENTENNIAL EXHIBITION.

Size 1.   Size 2.   Size 3.   Size 4.

Put up in $\frac{1}{8}$ oz. boxes, Numbers 60 and 120, sizes 1, 2, 3, and 4; also in partitioned boxes containing sizes 1 and 2; sizes 2 and 3; sizes 3 and 4.

We wish to be distinctly understood as affirming that all the varieties of gold which we manufacture are ABSOLUTELY PURE,—no alloy whatever, "slight" or otherwise, is added to produce softness, the required quality being the result of the processes to which they are subjected in the manufacture.

SAMUEL S. WHITE.

16

Advertisement from the 1878 Dental Cosmos *for SS White gold.*
Courtesy of the US Army Medical Department Museum. Borden 002.

From September 30 to December 5, Horner treated 271 patients; inserted 75 gold fillings, 128 amalgam fillings, 35 cement fillings, 33 porcelain crowns, 30 gold crowns, 3 dentures; and performed 28 prophylaxes, 146 extractions, and 108 other treatments. Around November 10 he moved his office to Savannah, Georgia, where the VII Army Corps was transferred, and later to Havana, Cuba, with the corps. From January 1 until April 1, 1899, the two dentists' appointment books were completely full.[20,23]

Maus described what he called the "department of dentistry" in a report to the surgeon general:

> It is almost impossible to realize the great benefit which resulted to the troops from this department, located as they were in the field. Engagements were made as in civil life, and both dentists were kept busy from early morning to late into the night. . . . In my opinion every corps should be provided with a dental department consisting of one chief dentist with the rank of major, three dentists with the rank of captain, and three assistant dentists with the rank of first lieutenant.[24(p87)]

In the July 1899 issue of *Items of Interest*, the editor, Rodrigues Ottolengui, reported on a slightly different plan for a US Army Dental Corps than Maus had proposed. It is unclear whether this plan came before or after the corps dental plan he recommended in his annual report, but Maus's concept provided for one "senior" and two "junior" dentists to be assigned to each of the Army's 15 military departments. The senior dentists would have the rank of captain, and the junior dentists that of lieutenant. The dental surgeons could circulate among the various posts within the command as their services were required. In addition to these 45 dental surgeons, one dental lieutenant colonel and one major would be permanently stationed in Washington. These officers would function in an executive and supervisory capacity rather than in a clinical one. The pay of the dentists would correspond to the pay of mounted officers of the same rank.[20]

Experiences of Dentists Serving with the Troops

Just as during the Civil War, several practicing dentists served as officers of the line in regular, state, and US volunteer units during the Spanish-American War. Many of these dentists often pulled double duty, acting as unofficial unit dentists just as their predecessors had, but they were ill-equipped to undertake the additional duties. Their experiences and observations helped shape dental care for American soldiers in the aftermath of the war with Spain.

Some dentists who also held medical degrees were appointed to serve as surgeons in their respective regiments. Dr Morris Schamberg, for example, served as an acting assistant surgeon. He described his experiences at the Chickamauga encampment and later in Puerto Rico:

> While serving at Chickamauga, many soldiers came to me for the extraction of teeth, and many more could have been relieved had I had proper filling-materials and instruments with me. Nothing tends to bring any condition in the mouth to a crisis as does the life that a soldier leads in the field. Exposed to all kinds of weather, run down

PACK'S GOLD CYLINDERS.

Patented Dec. 19th, 1871, and July 4th, 1876.

THREE VARIETIES.

Manufactured from the Globe Gold Foil, treated according to the Kearsing Patent, December 19th, 1871.

SEMI-COHESIVE CRYSTAL FOIL CYLINDERS,

SOFT CRYSTAL FOIL CYLINDERS, and

SOFT CRYSTAL LOOSE-ROLLED CYLINDERS.

To these we have added two other varieties, made from PLAIN FOIL (*not corrugated*), and distinguished as

PLAIN FOIL SOFT CYLINDERS and

PLAIN FOIL COHESIVE CYLINDERS.

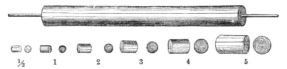

Put up in ⅛ oz. bottles, Nos. ½, 1, 2, 3, 4, 5, and ASSORTED. These Cylinders are loosely wrapped, and can be used, if desired, as Pellets. The manner in which these Cylinders are put up (bottled) is calculated to preserve the gold unimpaired for any length of time.

KEARSING'S GOLD FOIL BLOCKS.

TWO VARIETIES.

Having purchased the patent covering the manufacture* of Kearsing's Blocks and Crystallized or "Surface-roughened" Foil, we offer two varieties, to be known as

Kearsing's Semi-Cohesive Blocks and Kearsing's Soft Blocks,

and made respectively from the Semi-Cohesive and Soft Globe gold foils, treated according to the Kearsing patent of December 19th, 1871.

They are supplied in the following forms and sizes:

Size A.   Size B.   Size C.   Size D.

Put up in ⅛ oz. boxes, Nos. 60 and 120, sizes A, B, C, and D.

If any of our SPECIALTIES are not kept by the dealer in any locality, they will be sent direct from either of our depots, POSTAGE FREE.

The prices of all our varieties of Gold Foil, Pellets, Blocks, and Cylinders, are uniform, as follows:

Price, per ounce... $30.00
"   per ½ ounce... 15.00
"   per ⅛ ounce... 4.00

SAMUEL S. WHITE.

* The patent No. 122,029, of E. G. & L. Kearsing, of December 19th, 1871, for a new and improved process for preparing gold for dental purposes, and for manufacturing gold blocks, belongs to us by purchase.

R. S. Williams, of New York City, has a license under this patent, and is the only other authorized user of this process: all others using the process are hereby notified to discontinue such unauthorized use.   SAMUEL S. WHITE.

6   17

Advertisement from the 1878 Dental Cosmos *for gold cylinders.*
Courtesy of the US Army Medical Department Museum. Borden 003.

This price list from an 1878 edition of Dental Cosmos *lists the cost necessary office supplies, like appointment books.*
Courtesy of the US Army Medical Department Museum. Borden 010.

through fatigue, dependent upon rations which, as a rule, put to a severe test the masticating organs, and non-painstaking as to the hygiene of his mouth by reason of this peculiar life, the soldier proves to be the most needy consultant of the dentist.

During six and one-half months of active service in Porto Rico [*sic*], many cases of interest from a dental stand-point presented themselves to me. Rapidly growing alveolar abscesses were of frequent occurrence, and one case of rather extensive necrosis of the inferior maxilla called for operation. The above-mentioned cases, together with numerous conditions of the mucous membrane which called for treatment, such as ulcerative stomatitis, spongy gums, chancre of the tongue, etc., are proof of the fact that the vicissitudes to which the soldier is subjected render him an easy victim to some of the more serious oral affections.[25]

Dr Herbert Shapard of Austin, Texas, a member of his local militia unit (the Governor's Guard), was mustered into federal service with his company on May 3, 1898. The unit was assigned to the 1st Texas Regiment and was encamped at Mobile, Alabama that June. In July, it moved to Miami for 6 weeks of training. Shapard wrote:

Every day during this period one man or more would come to me and ask me to send after my instruments, as they had dental work to be done. Our Colonel, [Woodford H] Mabry, offered to appoint me regimental dentist (which of course, was an honorary appointment, no provision having been made for such). After due deliberation, I concluded to send after them, and received them at Jacksonville, Florida, about the latter part of August, when I proceeded to open my military dental office in a box house about twelve feet square, which was built for a company commissary. After putting a window sash in the roof, I had a very good office, considering the circumstances. I then proceeded with the aid of a hatchet, saw and pocket knife, to construct a chair out of material consisting of a few pieces of rough one by one and a half and a hard tack box, upholstering it with a piece of red flannel and some moss. This done, I made a table on which to place my instruments. After getting everything in position I was ready for business, although my surroundings were not such as you would expect to find in a regular office. For instance, instead of occupying comfortable rockers while waiting for my services, my patients were expected to sit on a sack of potatoes, or anything that was more convenient, and, instead of such sanitary surroundings as fountain spittoons, etc., patients were expected to expectorate on the floor of mother earth.

My services were in great demand, and besides my regular practice, I was frequently called upon by the surgeons to visit the hospital and treat dental disorders of patients confined therein. I was often awakened from my peaceful slumbers at all hours of the night and requested to get up and treat cases of odontalgia, alveolar abscesses, etc.; in fact, my services were demanded from the colonel down to the company cook, and, during the three months we spent in Cuba, by members of the Second Louisiana, Second South Carolina, and Third Nebraska regiments, and on several occasions by the hospital surgeons themselves. . . . I have had soldiers present themselves to me for treatment whose mouths were in a horrible condition—teeth decayed and filled with decomposed organic matter and food; gums often badly affected with pyorrhea alveolaris, chronic abscesses discharging foul matter into the mouth, this in turn swallowed into the stomach, the thought of which, in itself, is enough to make a man with an iron constitution or a healthy person sick. A great many would tell me that their teeth were in good condition when they enlisted in the army, and it is reasonable to suppose that they were telling the truth, for it is one of the regulations and requirements in order to stand the physical examination to enter the army that their teeth shall be in good order. I knew of several men who were refused admission on account of their teeth not being in proper condition.[26]

Dr Robert Oliver (1868–1937), later one of the three original 1901 examining and supervising dental surgeons and chief of the Dental Corps from 1919 to 1924, had already practiced dentistry for 12 years and served in the Indiana National Guard when he enlisted in the US Volunteers on April 26, 1898. He joined the 27th Battery, Indiana Light Artillery, and during the war served at Chickamauga Park and in Puerto Rico with Major General Nelson Miles's I Corps before being mustered out of service on November 22. With a significant dental and military background, he commented on oral hygiene and the Spanish-American War toothbrush situation:

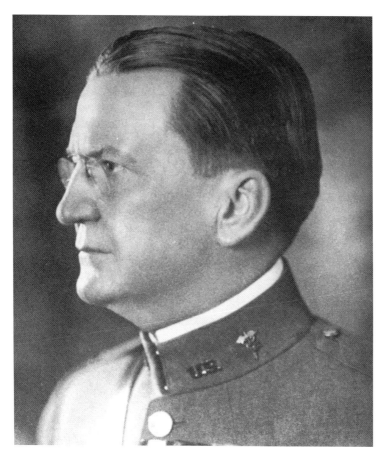

Robert Oliver.
Photograph: Courtesy of the US Army Medical Department Museum. DCC04 Oliver-01.

At that time diligent efforts were put forth, largely by States interested in the welfare of their contingent of volunteers, to supply each soldier with a toothbrush and a small container of dentifrice. This seemed to be the universal idea, but not being under Federal control, there was no plan for furnishing replacement for either toothbrush or dentifrice. The result was that the dentifrice was soon used up. Then the toothbrush alone was used until it began to lose some of its bristles and its efficiency. Through a sort of fad, it became the proper thing to carry the brush by sticking it through the hat band of the campaign hat. I have seen thousands of men marching in the thick dust with toothbrushes sticking through the left side of their hat bands, each brush so filled with earthy particles that at the first rain it was nothing short of a muddy mop. However, the soldier was diligent in the care of this article of his equipment, and retained it through the campaign, but the use for which it was intended was very limited indeed, and not fully productive of beneficial results.[27]

Dr Wilhelm Otto Asseln of Fergus Falls, Minnesota, an 1896 graduate of the Northwestern University Dental School, enlisted as a private in Company F, 14th Minnesota Infantry, in May 1898 and served until mustered out in November.[28] He recalled his Army experience:

Practically all of my professional services while in the Army were "thank you" jobs. I furnished all materials and instruments but the forceps, extractions were always filled; on rare occasions, I would receive twenty-five cents for a particularly difficult

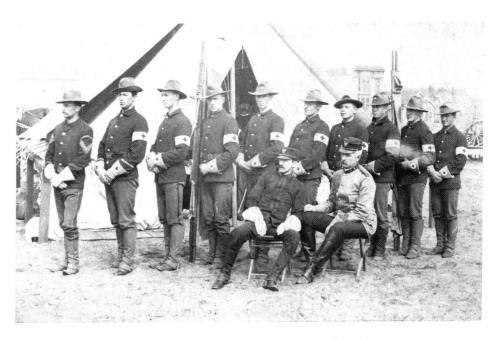

Two Army doctors and 10 hospital corpsmen in front of tent,
Camp Chickamauga, Georgia, circa 1898.
Photograph: Courtesy of the US Army Medical Department Museum. Spawar-047.

filling. I was not in service long before it was known thruout [*sic*] our Army Corps that there was a dentist in the ranks and from that time on, I was frequently called upon, even during the night, to give relief to men suffering from tooth troubles.[21,29]

Years later, he had an opportunity to examine some of his old fillings and found them still giving good service.[21,29]

Dr Homer Croscup, an 1890 graduate of the New York College of Dentistry with a practice in Brooklyn, served as a captain in the 14th Regiment, New York Infantry, US Volunteers, and gave an interesting account of his unofficial work as regimental dental surgeon. After being mustered in with his regiment on May 16, 1898, at Camp Black, Long Island, Croscup moved by rail the next day to Chickamauga. Originally, the regiment was scheduled to sail from New York to Tampa, Florida, but rumors of Spanish gunboats in the area forced them to take the inland route. The nearest town was Chattanooga, Tennessee, 11 miles away, and Croscup soon realized that he would be kept busy in his dual capacity as a company commander and dental surgeon. Among the 1,300 troops in his regiment and the five other regiments in the area (comprising the 1st Division of the III Army Corps), he was the only dentist.[21,30]

Croscup arranged his schedule so he would be at the hospital tent for 1 hour each day, where a line of 20 to 30 soldiers often awaited his arrival. He describes his experiences:

> Of course, extraction, in the majority of cases, was the necessary treatment under the circumstances, but if I had been prepared in the capacity of dental surgeon, nearly all the teeth thus sacrificed could have been saved. In many cases the teeth had been broken by accident; it would have been an easy matter to extirpate the pulps and prepare the teeth for crowning. Many of these accidents occurred in the regular drills and exercises, while serving under the Government and under orders, and the least Uncle Sam could do, would be to give them proper care and treatment.
>
> I remember upon one occasion after a drill in battle formation, extended order, two men came to me suffering from fractured incisors, one having been struck in the mouth with the butt of a rifle, breaking off the right superior central and lateral at the gum margin. From both roots the pulps protruded. I prepared sharp pieces of wood dipped in carbolic acid and forced them into the canals. This is an ancient practice and it came in handily at that time. I have subsequently placed crowns on both roots.
>
> I had many cases from other regiments where the surgeons had made heroic endeavors to extract refractory molars, finally sending them to me to finish up. They, however, could hardly have expected to be successful with the instruments at their command.[30]

Another example of dental service in the Spanish-American War was reported again by Ottolengui, editor of *Items of Interest*. An enlisted soldier in 1st Infantry in Cuba, suffering with a toothache and with no Army dental care available, visited a Cuban dentist, who attempted to extract the tooth but failed to do so successfully. The soldier returned to camp in "great agony" and was found dead the following day from an "overdose of morphine." The officers believed that the soldier had accidentally overdosed trying to relieve his pain, but the enlisted soldiers claimed he had committed suicide to avoid suffering any longer.[20]

As more forces were mobilized, the dental requirements of the growing volunteer force continued to multiply. Private Frank McLin, who spent only 6 months before the war in a dental office, wrote on May 26, 1898, from Camp Thomas, Chickamauga:

> When I return I shall be a full-fledged dentist. I purchased quite a few instruments in St. Paul before I left, together with a package of amalgam and cement, and am making good use of them. I extract from eight to ten teeth each day; am treating toothache and abscess, and I am doing lots of cement and amalgam filling.[31]

On June 14, he wrote: "I don't have as much time to work at dentistry as I should like to, and am going to try and get put on night duty (in hospital). This way I can get a little sleep during the night, and then sleep forenoons and get a tent and work at dentistry in the afternoons."[31]

On August 24, 1898, Colonel [Joseph] Bobletter, 12th Regiment, Minnesota Infantry, also stationed at Camp Thomas, wrote:

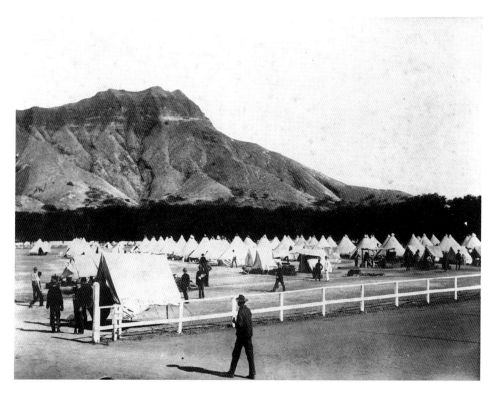

Ward tents associated with Honolulu General Hospital at the base of Diamondhead, 1898. Photograph: Courtesy of the US Army Medical Department Museum. Spawar-035.

The men of my regiment suffer a good deal from tooth trouble. The same occurred during the civil war [*sic*]. Many men suffered and lost valuable teeth, the loss of which no doubt affected their digestion, bowels, and health generally. I believe there should be qualified dentists in the army, say one to each regiment. [31(pp197–198)]

On August 29, 1898, Captain [Walter] Child, a line officer stationed at Lexington, Kentucky, said:

I have noticed several in this camp suffering from toothache. It is an ailment from which a man dislikes to report sick, for if he does he is liable to be compelled to have the tooth extracted by the regimental surgeon, an operation which should not be performed while modern dentistry could so easily prevent it, and one which most of us dread when unskillfully done. In my opinion there should be a dentist with each regiment. It would give us fewer sick men, and hence a much larger fighting force to each company, regiment, brigade, etc. [31]

In September 1898 George Griswold, the former captain of Company H, 12th Regiment, Minnesota Infantry, and an 1889 graduate of the Pennsylvania College of Dental Surgery, underlined the fundamental problem:

On the salary a private gets he cannot afford dentists' bills, and, if he could, he is only allowed to leave camp or garrison duty at long intervals, and feels that his leave is too precious to be spent in a dentist's chair. The result is that his teeth are neglected and decay progresses, until driven by pain he seeks the regimental surgeon, who is unskilled in this specialty, consequently breaks the tooth and mutilates the gum. When his tent-mates have toothache they prefer to stick it out rather than be butchered, and consequently are unfit for duty. How much better it would be if each regiment had its dentist, who, with a capable assistant, could help wonderfully from a physical standpoint to improve the army and naval service of the United States. [31(p198)]

In 1899 Griswold observed that although the average volunteer soldier wanted to take care of his teeth to masticate "Uncle Sam's hard-tack, salt pork, bacon, etc.," he was unable to leave camp long enough to see a dentist, much less pay for dental treatment. As a result of this neglect, he described the following scenario for the soldier eating his rations:

A piece of hard-tack gets into a cavity, crushes through to the nerve, causing him to jump four feet in the air, and yelling like a Comanche Indian, rushes off to the regimental surgeon, who seats him on a camp stool, calmly surveys the offending member, gets two or three grinning hospital stewards to hold the victim, while he produces a pair of antiquated "archaic" weapons that some dealer in surgical instruments has palmed off on him as a universal forceps, grabs the tooth, and, placing his knee on the patient's chest to give him a purchase, gives a long, steady, straight pull that would not bring the tooth in a hundred years, and smash she goes. [32(pp194–195)]

Before sailing for Manila, the surgeon of the 13th Regiment, Minnesota Infantry, Major Reynaldo Fitzgerald, admitted there was "more tooth trouble in my regiment . . . than any other one complaint." [31,33] Once in Manila, Lieutenant LM Bunker of the regiment agreed: "I think that in Manila they could use a few dentists in connection with the army to good advantage. There are a few dentists who enlisted as privates, but to my judgment they are entirely inadequate to the demands."[31]

Major Charles Boxton, an 1883 graduate of the College of Dentistry of the University of California and a practicing dentist in San Francisco, serving as a line officer in the 1st Regiment, California Infantry, in the Philippines, wrote:

> My personal opinion is that the services of our profession are an absolute necessity for the comfort and health of the men. There are three dentists in Manila; one native and two Americans; if one of our men requires attention it takes almost a month's wages. The result is that they neglect the proper care of the oral cavity; their teeth are lost, the gums become diseased; the soldier is then unfit for service and is sent to the hospital, often to become a care on the Government for the balance of his life. I have known of a number of such cases, one man being sent home on account of the loss of teeth.
>
> I have had three different officers come to me for advice. Advice or a little iodin [sic] is the best they can get here at present. Many cases of fever and dysentery are brought about through a deranged condition of the oral cavity. There is no question about that fact, and all fair-minded army surgeons will admit it. All medical men that I have talked to on the subject admit that they cannot handle the work, and that it is very necessary to have dental surgeons in the service for the comfort and general health of the men. In my opinion there should be a dental surgeon with every regiment.[31(p199)]

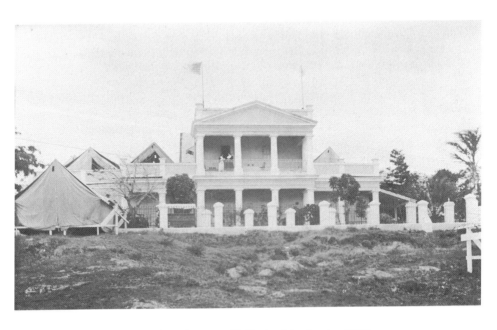

Hospital in Matanzas, Philippine Islands, circa 1898.
Nurse and Catholic nursing sister on balcony.
Photograph: Courtesy of US Army Medical Department Museum. Spawar-054.

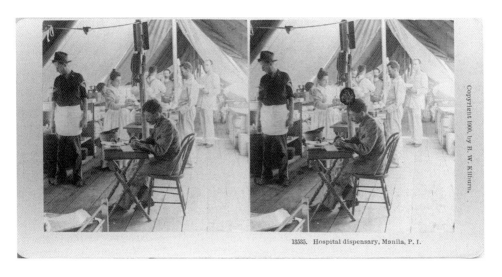

Hospital dispensary, Manila, Philippine Islands, circa 1898.
Photograph: Courtesy of US Army Medical Department Museum. Spawar-038.

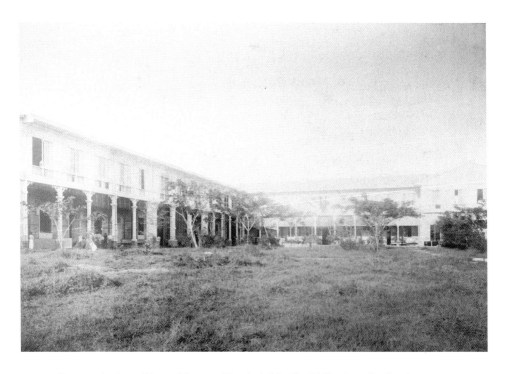

Panoramic view of Second Reserve Hospital, Manila, Philippine Islands, circa 1898.
Photograph: Courtesy of US Army Medical Department Museum. Spawar-049.

Civilian Dentists Shoulder the Burden

When and if they had the time and money, soldiers often visited local civilian dentists for treatment of their dental problems. In some cases, the post or encampment commander made arrangements with local practitioners to visit on a regular basis to treat the soldiers, which saved them time but not money. Dr Benjamin Ford of Chicago, an 1893 graduate of Northwestern University School of Dentistry, visited Fort Sheridan, Illinois, twice a week during 1898 and 1899 to work on the soldiers stationed there. He wrote:

> I have seen recruits come in (particular attention being called to those playing wind instruments) whose teeth were in such bad condition that I formed a support for the lip by molding gutta-percha that they might play their instruments satisfactorily.
>
> The cost of the dental work for these men, charging a very moderate fee, would range from $50 to $100 each, and it would be very hard for them to pay for such services out of a salary of $13 per month.
>
> In the case of some of the men stationed in the west, they were obliged to spend from $10 to $20 to reach the nearest dentist, and I know of one case where a sergeant was sent 200 miles with an escort to be relieved of toothache, and another case of a post quartermaster sergeant who was sent eighty miles by stage to obtain relief.
>
> Very few of the surgeons treat or extract teeth, but they refer the cases to the hospital steward or his assistants.
>
> I know this was true at Ft. Sheridan and I understand that it is true at other posts.
>
> The forceps are not well chosen for this work, and with a poor assortment of instruments and a lack of knowledge upon the part of the extractor, the teeth were frequently so crushed that I found it difficult in many instances to extract the remnants when the patient finally reached me upon the days I was at the post.[21,34(p890)]

In 1898 Dr Charles Stanley of Columbia, South Carolina, was appointed by Captain E[zra?] B Fuller, the mustering officer, to do the emergency dental work needed by the 1st and 2nd South Carolina Volunteer regiments stationed in Columbia before they went into permanent encampment at Chickamauga and Jacksonville. Stanley said:

> I came in professional contact with about two hundred of the officers and men. I extracted between 140 and 150 teeth, most of which were paid for by the government, and the rest were paid for by the men, they not having orders from the surgeons to have the extracting done. For several days after paydays, I devoted all my time to operative work for these soldiers, they paying for the same; and you can well imagine that out of their small salaries, they only had just such work done as required immediate attention.
>
> During my professional relationship with the soldiers, I noticed one case of syphilitic necrosis, two cases of necrosis due to chronic abscessed teeth, six cases of alveolar pyorrhea (none of which had ever received medical attention), three cases of impacted

wisdom teeth with extensive inflammation, and in two cases suppuration. In all of the above cases, I informed the surgeons of the necessity of treatment and what I would have done for the same in my private practice. Out of the 200 men spoken of, there were seven totally incompetent to masticate their food and a number only partly competent to do so.[35(p113)]

The 1st Rhode Island and 2nd Tennessee regiments were also stationed for a while in Columbia. During this short period, Stanley recalls, "I inserted sixty-nine fillings, made five plates, mended three plates and extracted nineteen teeth, all of this work being paid for by the patients. I am sure that the other nine dentists in this city averaged as much work among the men of the Rhode Island and Tennessee Regiments as myself."[35(p113)]

Soldiers who were mustered out after the short war often returned to their civilian homes with serious dental problems. In December 1898 William Whipple of Saint Louis, Missouri, an 1896 graduate of the Missouri Dental College, related his personal experiences treating several returned veterans who had spent the summer at Chickamauga.[15] Their teeth were in "extremely bad condition," and they had "suffered greatly during their camp life with odontalgia." He wrote:

When asked what was done for their relief, they replied "Nothing!" Any one who had trouble with their teeth went to the "Doctor" who pulled them out. One man stated: "A member of my company had toothache and went to have the tooth extracted and the Doctor nearly killed him, so I preferred to suffer rather than submit to such treatment."[36(pp888–889)]

Dr Nicholas Senn on Dental Problems

Lieutenant Colonel Nicholas Senn (1844–1908), a prominent surgeon, professor of surgery, and pathologist on the staff of several medical colleges, was founder of the Association of Military Surgeons in the United States (AMSUS), served as surgeon general of the Illinois National Guard, and was chief surgeon of the US Volunteers during the Spanish-American War. A distinguished Chicago physician, Senn was briefly in charge of surgical work at Camp Wikoff, Long Island, New York, from mid-August until his discharge in mid-September. Camp Wikoff, which was originally intended to be a quarantine and convalescent center for V Corps and other troops returning from the Caribbean with yellow fever or other tropical diseases, exemplified the mismanagement that characterized much of the Army's performance in the war.[37,38] With the focus largely on contagious diseases, little attention was directed to the soldier's dental health.[1]

Two years after his discharge, Senn published his *Medico-Surgical Aspects of the Spanish American War*, in which he recorded his experience with the dental health and habits of soldiers and his own work as a "dentist" during the war:

Of the organs frequently affected among the returning soldiers were the teeth. Patients suffering from carious aching teeth were numerous. In most instances they presented evidence of serious malnutrition following disease and exposure, suppurative alveolitis was less frequent. Infection of many oral cavities showed that teeth had been sadly neglected during the campaign. In Cuba and Porto Rico [sic] I saw occasionally

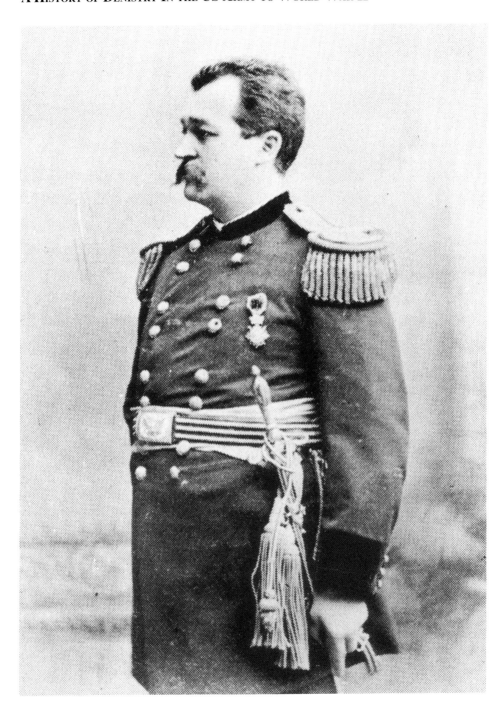

Nicholas Senn.
Photograph: Courtesy of the National Museum of Health and Medicine,
Armed Forces Institute of Pathology. NCP 4104.

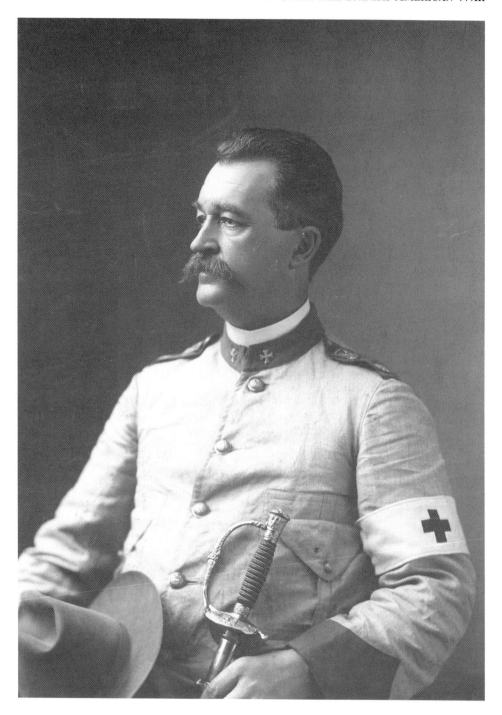

Studio portrait of Lieutenant Colonel Nicholas Senn, MD,
in khaki uniform with Red Cross armband and sword, circa 1898.
Photograph: Courtesy of the US Army Medical Department Museum. Spawar-063.

a soldier with a tooth-brush under the hat band, but I have reason to believe that most of the tooth brushes were either left at home or thrown away on the march, as unnecessary articles of the limited toilet outfit. I did all I could in the way of conservative dentistry by clearing out cavities and packing with cotton saturated with carbolic acid, but in the majority of cases the patients returned and insisted on having the painful tooth extracted. Tooth extraction was a conspicuous and grateful part of the surgery at Camp Wikoff. Hardly a day passed without two or three such operations. A very complete set of tooth forceps furnished by the government did good service in relieving the victims of toothache of their agonizing suffering.[39(pp200–201)]

Senn added his support for dentists in the Army and an important observation on the distribution of dental problems between officers and enlisted soldiers:

Much has been said in favor of attaching a dentist to each regiment to look after the teeth of the men, and the observations made in Camp Wikoff tend to support the propriety of such a much-needed addition to the medical service. It is interesting to know that among these patients there was not a single officer, undoubtedly because the officers were more particular in the care of their teeth than the privates.[40(p171)]

A Clear Need Unseen

The Spanish-American War and opening months of the Philippine-American War clearly indicated a genuine need for dental care for the Army's soldiers. While regular and volunteer officers saw a definite need for dental care in the service, American dentists still needed to convince Congress, the Army surgeon general, and the War Department.

References

1. C[happle] JA. The time for action has arrived. *American Dental Weekly*. 1898;1:217.

2. Foster SW, comp. Minutes of transactions of the southern branch of the National Dental Association, session of 1898. In: *Transactions of the National Dental Association*. Philadelphia, Pa: The SS White Dental Mfg Co; 1899: 218.

3. Wood W, Jr. The necessity of dentists in the Army and Navy. In: *Transactions of the National Dental Association*. Philadelphia, Pa: The SS White Dental Mfg Co, 1900: 202–203.

4. Bentley CF. The care of Army teeth. Cited in: Annual convention of the sixth, seventh, and eighth district dental societies of the state of New York. *Dental Cosmos*. April 1898;40:307.

5. Bennett NG. On the need for the recognition of the assistance of dental surgeons by the war office and admiralty. *J Br Dent Assoc*. 1900;15:607–608.

6. National Archives and Records Administration. Record Group 94. Surgeon General Sternberg to Adjutant General Henry C Corbin, May 18, 1898. Letter. Box 593. Entry 25.

7. National Archives and Records Administration. Record Group 94. Assistant Adjutant General Theodore Schwan to Captain Owen, May 18, 1898. Telegram. No. 81221 (filed with No. 79350). Box 593. Entry 25.

8. Owen W. Establishment of the first dental infirmary in the U.S. Army in the Philippines. *Dental Cosmos*. 1911;53:367–368.

9. Owen W. Pioneer Army dentists in the Philippines. *Dental Cosmos*. 1917;59:728.

10. National Archives and Records Administration. Record Group 112. Application form, William H Ware to surgeon general, March 4, 1901. No. 70437. Box 367. Entry 101.

11. Platt FL. Dentistry in the Army and Navy. *Pacific Medico-Dental Gazette*. 1898;6:442–443.

12. National Archives and Records Administration. Record Group 15. Pension file, Gibbon JA, February 14, 1910. No. 844951.

13. Shore CK, comp. *Montana in the Wars*. Miles City, Mont: Star Printing Co; 1977: 48–51.

14. National Archives and Records Administration. Record Group 112. Dr Ware, November 18, 1899. Box 387. Entry 29.

15. RL Polk & Co. *R.L. Polk & Co.'s Dental Register of the United States 1896–97*. 2nd ed. Detroit, Mich: RL Polk & Co; 1896: 88.

16. National Archives and Records Administration. Record Group 112. Dr LL Dunbar to Surgeon General Sternberg, March 30, 1899. Letter. No. 70437. Box 367. Entry 101.

17. Lee F. *Annual Report of Major General Fitzhugh Lee, Commanding Seventh Army Corps, Camp Cuba Libre, Jacksonville, Fla.* Jacksonville, Fla: Art Printers & Publishers; 1898: 8,13,19.

18. US War Department. *Official Army Register for 1899.* Washington, DC: Government Printing Office; 1899: 23.

19. Wright SH. Medicine in the Florida camps during Spanish–American War: Great controversies. *JFMA.* 1975:21.

20. [Ottolengui R]. Plan for dentists in the Army suggested by Major L.M. Maus, U.S.A. *Dent Items Interest.* 1899;21: 527–528.

21. RL Polk & Co. *R.L. Polk & Co.'s Dental Register of the United States.* 5th ed. Detroit, Mich: RL Polk & Co; 1902: 43, 88, 188, 443.

22. National Archives and Records Administration. Record Group 94. Circular, headquarters, VII Army Corps, Camp Cuba Libre, October 1, 1898. Certificate of disability for discharge, Jacob W Horner, February 10, 1899. Entry 91.

23. National Archives and Records Administration. Record Group 112. Lieutenant Colonel Maus to surgeon general, December 7, 1898. Letter [copy]. Box 387. Entry 29.

24. Lieutenant Colonel Louis M Maus, chief surgeon, VII Corps, to the surgeon general, July 1, 1899. In: *Report of the Surgeon–General of the Army to the Secretary of War for the Fiscal Year ending June 30, 1899.* Washington, DC: Government Printing Office; 1899: 87.

25. Schamberg MI. Army Dentists. *Int Dent J.* 1899;20:356–357.

26. Shapard HH. Dentists in the Army and Navy. *Tex Med J.* 1899;15:81–82.

27. Oliver RT. The rational consideration of oral prophylaxis. *Dental Cosmos.* 1921;63:1118.

28. National Archives and Records Administration. Compiled Military Service Record. Record Group 94. Will O Asseln, Company F, 14th Minnesota Infantry.

29. [Asseln WO]. Letter from patriotic dentist. *J Natl Dent Assoc.* 1918;5:638.

30. Croscup HC. Dentistry in the Army. *Dent Item Interest.* 1899;21:556–557.

31. Leonard L. Dentists in the Army and Navy. In: *Transactions of the National Dental Association* Philadelphia, Pa: The SS White Dental Mfg Co; 1900: 196–197.

32. Griswold G. Dentists in the Army. *Dent Rev.* 1899;13:194–195.

33. Heitman FB. *Historical Register and Dictionary of the United States Army, from its Organization, September 29, 1789, to March 2, 1903.* Vol 2. Washington, DC: Government Printing Office; 1903: 192, 211.

34. The Odontographic Society of Chicago [proceedings]. *Dent Rev.* 1900;15:890.

35. Stanley CC. A few statistical facts, showing the need of dental service in the Army. *Dent Rev.* 1900;14:113.

36. Whipple WL. Dentists are needed in the Army. *Dent Items Interest.* 1898;20:888–889.

37. Cosmas GA. *An Army for Empire: The United States Army in the Spanish–American War.* Columbia, Mont: University of Missouri Press; 1971: 263, 265.

38. Wheeler J. *The Santiago Campaign, 1898.* Port Washington, NY: Kennikat Press; 1971: 207–212.

39. Senn Nicholas. *Medico-Surgical Aspects of the Spanish American War.* Chicago, Ill: American Medical Association Press; 1900: 200–201.

40. Walker WE. Dentists in the Army and Navy. *Dental Registry.* 1899;53:171.

Chapter VI

WISH BECOMES REALITY: DENTAL SURGEONS IN THE ARMY, 1898–1901

Introduction

While dentists served in many capacities in regular and volunteer units from Chickamauga to the Philippines, their civilian colleagues continued to fight for congressional legislation to establish a place for dentists in the US Army. The wartime experiences of dentists in uniform, Army line and medical officers, and enlisted soldiers confirmed the need for professional dentistry in the military. For American dentists and their professional associations and journals, the Spanish-American War initiated a new phase in the long campaign to achieve their goal of dental care for the soldier.

The Mason and Otey Bills

Before the beginning of the war with Spain, Congress tried to get the small frontier army ready, even introducing bills that addressed dental care. On April 16, 1898, at the 55th Congress, Senator Edmund Pettus, a former Confederate brigadier general, submitted an amendment to the proposed civil appropriation bill calling for the appointment of a "dental pathologist" for the Army Medical Museum, and on May 4, 1898, William Mason from Chicago introduced a bill (S 4531) to provide for the appointment of "a dental corps in the United States Army."[1,2]

When the Mason bill was referred to the War Department for remark, Army Surgeon General George Sternberg considered the proposed legislation unwise, saying, "the policy of the Government has always been to make officers and enlisted men responsible for the care of their own teeth."[3(p70)]

Three weeks later, Representative Peter Otey, a former Confederate infantry major from Lynchburg, Virginia, introduced a parallel bill (HR 10508) in the House to establish "a dental corps" in the US Army. The bill provided for an increase in the Medical Corps by the addition of a Dental Corps, "to be composed of one surgeon dentist to each brigade with rank of major, and one surgeon dentist to each regiment with rank of captain, etc." Each dentist had to be a graduate of a reputable dental college and have been in practice full time continuously for the last 5 years. Promotions, pay and allowances, and retirements would be the same as provided in the regulations for the Medical Corps, and all supplies would be furnished in the same manner as for the Medical Corps. The bill was referred to the Committee on Military Affairs. Otey's bill had been written by a friend and constituent, Robert Morgan (1844–1904), another former Confederate infantryman now with a dental practice in Lynchburg.[1,4] Aware of the problem from their own experiences, many influential veterans were beginning to add their voices to the fight for military dental care.

On June 20 the Chicago Dental Society, the Odontographic Society of Chicago, and the Odontological Society of Chicago jointly endorsed a resolution calling for Congress to pass Otey's dental bill. The editor of the *Dental Review*, published in Chicago, also urged its readers to write to their congressmen on the bill's behalf.[5,6]

In July the editor of *Dental Cosmos* and dean of the School of Dental Medicine at the University of Pennsylvania, Dr Edward Kirk (served 1895–1917), commented on the Otey bill:

> As the initial step in securing the desired legislation has been taken, it is important that the bill be modified to such extent as may be necessary to best subserve dental interests in that relation, and that the needful effort to secure its passage by Congress be made at once, so as to avoid the prestige of defeat, which would necessarily impede any subsequent legislative effort in this direction.[2(p593)]

Kirk also referred to the June 20, 1898, appeal of Dr Charles Stanley of Columbia, South Carolina, for all dentists to rally around the bill and pressure their congressmen for its passage. Stanley felt that dental surgery would be a "blessing" to enlisted soldiers.[7]

Also in July, Dr Jonathan Taft, the long-time editor of *Dental Register*, dean of the College of Dental Surgery at the University of Michigan (served 1875–1903), and supporter of Army dental care since the Civil War, called attention to the fact that dentists were employed in hospitals, asylums, and schools; it seemed illogical that their services not be provided to the soldiers and sailors serving the government. He recommended at least one dental surgeon be assigned to each regiment.[8] Despite the groundswell of support from the dental lobby, which was backed by recent military experience, the dental bills failed to get past the Committee on Military Affairs because of the disapproval of the surgeon general and the War Department.

The Dental Journals Press the Issue

The failure of the Otey bill did not deter the dental societies and journals, which continued to press the issue. Dr B Holly Smith of Baltimore, Maryland, a member of the National Dental Association (NDA) who was active in pushing for military dentists, stated in a letter to *Dental Weekly*:

> This abortive effort has, however, made several things plain: (1), that any measure introduced must be an expression of the best thought of the profession; (2), it must receive the unified and enthusiastic support of the same; (3), it must be placed in the hands of an experienced legislator.
>
> When the measure is fairly launched during the next session of Congress, it will then be time for every man to use his personal influence with his representative, for unless we have a large majority of the law-makers prejudiced in favor of such legislation we will still have to reckon with the Surgeon-General.[9(p92)]

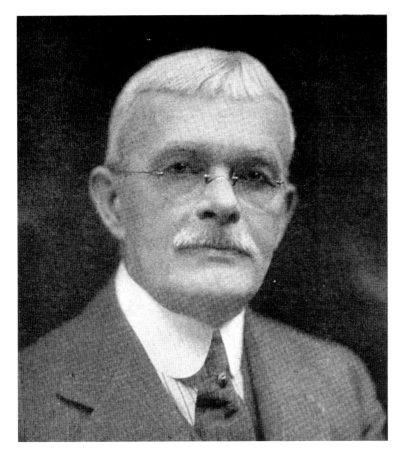

Edward Kirk (1856–1933), the editor of Dental Cosmos.
Photograph: Courtesy of the American Dental Association.

In August 1898 the editor of the *Indiana Dental Journal*, Dr George Hunt, wrote that if Army and Navy dental corps were created, preference should be given to those practitioners who went "to the front" as volunteers: "The dental surgeons who were willing to leave their practice and shoulder a rifle in defense of the country when the call was made for volunteers should have precedence over the stay-at-home contingent in selecting men to fill positions in this corps."[10(p811)]

Hunt also commented on the value of good teeth and on the Army's continuing contradictory position on dental health:

> During the physical examination of the militia recently held, prior to mustering the men into the United States service, a large per cent were rejected on account of defective teeth. The Government wisely believes that good teeth are necessary to the proper mastication of army rations, and if all reports are true, the Government is eminently correct. Proper mastication of rations is essential to proper digestion and assimilation of them and on the correct performance of these latter functions rests the efficiency of the army. An army travels on its belly.

149

> But mark the inconsistency of the methods in vogue at present! The Government en-
> lists men, ordinarily, in the regular army for a period of five years. At present the term
> of enlistment for recruits is the same in the regular army as it is in the volunteer ser-
> vice, namely, the war or two years. During his term of enlistment the recruit is usually
> stationed at points where dental services cannot be obtained, and even if he is quar-
> tered in barracks adjacent to cities or towns, his monthly wages are so small that he
> can ill afford to spare the necessary money for the proper care of his teeth.[10(pp811–812)]

Hunt related his own experiences performing dental work on personnel of the US Army garrison stationed at the Indianapolis Arsenal:

> It was rare when anything but extraction was desired. It must be a pitiful sight to see
> a member of our regular army, one who has gained two or perhaps three stripes for
> his arm, showing ten or fifteen years in the service, chasing a hunk of hardtack or a
> slippery slice of army bacon around his mouth with his tongue and cheeks in an effort
> to anchor it where a lonesome superior second molar may crush it a little bit before
> it slides off of an equally lonesome inferior third molar. And this condition of affairs
> cannot help but obtain if the man is retained in the service.

> To reject a recruit who has already served one or two terms of enlistment on account
> of defective teeth, when the Government is directly responsible for his defects is un-
> just and unworthy of a great nation. If good teeth are a necessity to the raw recruit
> they are equally valuable to the experienced soldier. And the fact that a soldier has
> a set of teeth in good condition at the time of his enlistment does not guarantee that
> they will remain so for several years, unless they receive the surgical attention, which
> they require. The absurdity of the present methods in vogue is amply illustrated by
> this one argument. The Government requires the raw recruit to have a good set of
> teeth because the Government realizes that exposed sensitive dentin, toothache, and
> the loss of teeth result in a soldier of depreciated vitality, a cog in the great army
> machine is defective, and in this the Government is wise. But the Government does
> not recognize the fact that the teeth of the recruit is [sic] just as liable to deterioration
> after enlistment as they were before, and that this deterioration will result in a de-
> fective cog in the mechanism of the machine just as certainly as if it had occurred
> before the recruit was accepted. And in this the Government is not wise. *Quod erat
> demonstrandum* which, freely translated means, that is what we told you in the first
> place.[10(pp812–813)]

The 1898 National Dental Association Meeting

The second annual meeting of the NDA in Omaha, Nebraska, addressed the situation in August 1898, when Charles Butler offered resolutions approving the appointment of dentists to the Army and recommending the creation of an asso-ciation committee to press the issue. Clark Goddard reported that a dental surgeon and two assistants (William Ware, George Ames, and John Gibbon) had already been appointed in Merritt's Corps in California and were about to deploy to the Philippines. After a discussion, the resolutions were referred to the executive com-mittee with instructions to report on the matter before the meeting adjourned.[11]

The NDA executive committee decided that a new committee should have "full control" of the subject of legislation for the employment of dental surgeons in

the Army and Navy and offered a resolution discouraging any "independent action" of state and local societies without the approval of the committee. Close coordination within the NDA was essential to focus its efforts. The association members approved the resolution. Doctors Finley, Donnally, and Butler were appointed
as the new Committee on the Appointment of Dentists to the Army and Navy
(renamed the Committee on Army and Navy Dental Legislation in 1899 and before
World War I merged into the Committee on Legislation). They were instructed to
report on the matter at the next annual meeting.[11] This decision began the NDA's
most pronounced period of active lobbying of Congress and the War and Navy departments. During this time, the NDA strongly encouraged dental legislation that
would introduce dentists into the Army and Navy with commissioned status that
would provide full recognition of their equality with the services' medical officers.
Finley and Donnally remained in the forefront of this struggle for years to come.

The Hull Bill of 1898

On December 7, 1898, Iowa Representative John Hull, the chairman of the
House Committee on Military Affairs, introduced a bill (HR 11022) "for the reorganization of the Army of the United States, and for other purposes." The bill
was referred to the Committee on Military Affairs. On December 20, 10 days after
the formal signing of the Treaty of Paris with Spain that ended the war, the committee reported that "the Army, scattered as it is in remote places, furnishes no
opportunity for the care of the teeth, and the only way this care can be exercised
is for the Government to furnish the skilled dentists to perform the work."[12,13] In
January 1899, while HR 11022 worked its way through the committee, Jonathan
Taft noted that the bill included "a new corps of educated dentists" to be selected
by professional examination.[14]

On January 30 the bill was debated and amended. The rank proposed for dentists was to correspond to the lowest grade of assistant surgeon and the pay and
allowances totaled $1,600 per year. The bill did not provide for dentists' promotion
or increase in pay as it did for medical surgeons, but it did include an amendment
by the House Military Affairs Committee to the Medical Department section for
adding a specific number of dental surgeons to the Army as follows:

> In line 10, section 11, after the word "lieutenant," insert the following: "One hundred
> dentists with rank, pay, and allowances of a first lieutenant, mounted, who shall be grad-
> uates of a dental college and shall pass satisfactory professional examination."[12(p1290)]

James Hay, a representative from Madison, Virginia, offered the following
amendment:

> On page 12, in line 13, after the word "professional," insert the words "competitive,
> and shall be not over 30 years of age." I desire to call the attention of the House to the
> fact that this is an entirely new feature incorporated in the Army bill. It provides for
> a corps of 100 dentists, with the rank of first lieutenant. It does not provide for any
> age limit whatever. It does not provide for any competitive examination, as has been
> heretofore provided for surgeons in the Army.

151

I think in the interest of the service that these dentists ought not to be over 30 years of age. Otherwise you may put in men of 60 years of age. You want men just from college, men who have a college education, men who have some knowledge of dentistry and who can stand a competitive as well as a professional examination, and not a lot of old men with a political pull.[12(p1290)]

Nicholas Cox, a representative from Franklin, Tennessee, submitted a proposition to strike out the entire section providing for the dental surgeons and remarked:

There has never been a corps of this kind in the Army at all, and I want to put myself on record as having been opposed to it in the committee as I am opposed to it here. It does seem to me that we are going absolutely wild about this matter. I can not see any reason for putting 100 lieutenants in the Army as dentists.[12(p1290)]

Representative Hay then offered to change the age limit from 30 to 35, but Cox again moved to strike out the entire section. The Hay amendment was rejected by a vote of 73 to 34, and ultimately the entire dental amendment failed.[12(p1290)]

The Hull bill had originally provided for 500 medical officers for a 100,000-person army, and the committee amendment for 100 dentists was made up on the same basis. When the medical part of the bill came up for discussion in the House in January, the political climate forced the Military Affairs Committee to ask the House to amend every section of the bill. The committee reduced the number of medical officers from 500 to 235 and probably would have reduced the dentists to about 60. Cox, however, led the minority fight in getting the dental amendment totally rejected. Surgeon General George Sternberg continued to withhold support for the bill.[15]

While the committees discussed the bill, the NDA's Committee for the Appointment of Dental Surgeons to the Army and Navy, with Williams Donnally as chairman, had prepared the following substitute for the clause in Hull's bill pertaining to the appointment of Army dental surgeons:

One dental surgeon with rank of colonel, one dental surgeon with rank of lieutenant-colonel, two dental surgeons with rank of major, sixteen dental surgeons with the rank of captain mounted, and seventy-three dental surgeons with the rank of first lieutenant mounted, with right of promotion in the grades named under the rules applicable to the corresponding grades of surgeons and assistant surgeons, all of whom shall be graduates of medical or dental colleges and shall pass a satisfactory professional examination. Provided that dental surgeons appointed as here provided may be transferred to the grade of assistant surgeon by complying with the examination requirements of that grade; and provided further that for all vacancies otherwise occurring in the number of dental surgeons herein provided for there shall be appointed a corresponding number of assistant surgeons, who shall first pass satisfactorily both the examination requirements of that grade and an examination in the special subjects of dental and oral surgery.[16(p188)]

Surgeon General Sternberg replied to Donnally:

I would say that I do not approve of your proposition with reference to dental surgeons. As I have already said to you, I have not been an advocate of the proposition to add to the Medical Corps of the Army the one hundred dentists provided for in

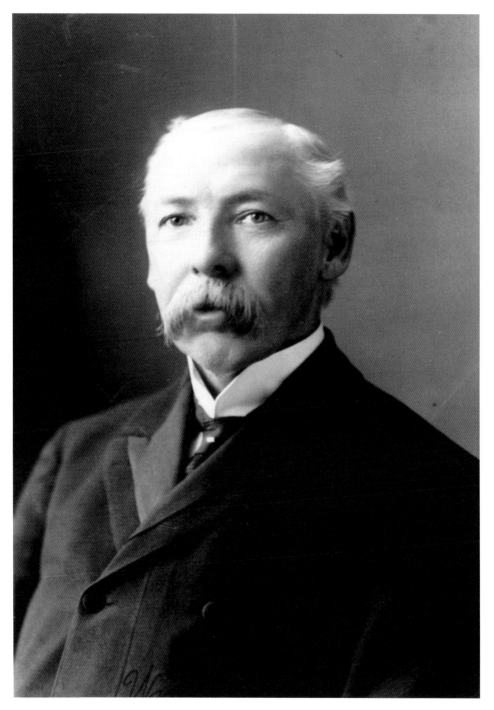

*Williams Donnally, chairman of the National Dental Association's Committee
for the Appointment of Dental Surgeons to the Army and Navy.
Photograph: Courtesy of the American Dental Association.*

the Hull Bill. Moreover, an Army medical officer must serve for five years before he has the rank of Captain; he rarely attains the rank of Major in less than from fifteen to twenty years, the rank of Lieut. Colonel after thirty to thirty-five years service and many of our medical officers have been retired at the age of sixty-four without reaching the rank of Colonel.[3(p71)]

Sternberg also sent a copy of this letter to Hull, the chairman of the House Committee on Military Affairs.[3]

B Holly Smith

By early 1899 approximately 20,000 US troops were in the Philippines, where open fighting was already taking place, but William Ware and George Ames in the Manila area were the only soldiers who could provide affordable dental care (at the time, there was one civilian American dentist in the city, but his rates were high; his charge for the smallest amalgam filling was $10).[17]

The lack of dental care for the soldiers was widely known within the national, state, and local American dental societies, many of which urged their national associations to remedy this situation once and for all. On February 7, 1899, LC Moore of the Detroit Dental Society sent William Walker, president of the Southern Dental Association (now a branch of the NDA) a copy of his society's resolution recom-

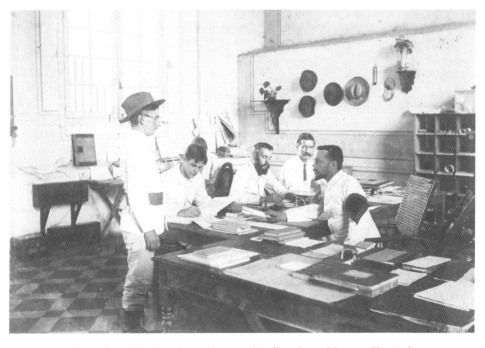

Stewards and clerks in hospital steward's office, Second Reserve Hospital, Manila, Philippine Islands, circa 1898.
Photograph: Courtesy of the US Army Medical Department Museum. Spawar-033.

mending the appointment of dentists to the US Army and Navy. The Southern Dental Association was scheduled to meet in New Orleans within several days and Moore urged Walker to bring the matter up before his association at the "earliest opportunity" because it was "a matter of importance to the profession." Moore believed that if any action from Congress were ever to be expected, dentists had to lobby their congressmen.[18]

At the same meeting, B Holly Smith, an 1881 graduate of the Baltimore College of Dental Surgery and now a member of the Southern Dental Association's Committee on Dentists in the Army and Navy,[19] reported that the committee chairman, John Chapple, had failed to call the committee together or to organize any work during the past year because "he did not think the time propitious for work in this direction; that at a more opportune period he would open negotiations with the powers that be."[19] Smith said that undoubtedly Chapple had "overlooked the great importance of the matter." He urged the society's members to use their personal influence with their congressmen and "beg them to look into the way in which our citizen-soldiers are being neglected." Smith told members "much could be accomplished. The time is right now. Strike while the iron is hot." He assured his listeners that Surgeon General Sternberg, who was a personal friend, thought that there was "no chance" for passage of a dental bill, because all the money was already appropriated for other purposes.[15]

Smith's comments resulted in a round of discussion. Henry JB McKellops, Mexican War veteran and author of the first resolution seeking dentists in the Army, commented that dental surgeon candidates should be trained in both medicine and dentistry. HW Morgan discussed Williams Donnally's work on the NDA's committee, reiterating Donnally's position that every dentist had to appeal to his congressmen. James Crawford contrasted the lack of dentistry for the soldiers at Camp Chickamauga to the care the horses received from the veterinary surgeons:

> Any man who went through one of our military camps, and who saw what I saw at Chickamauga, will have an argument that no man can resist. . . . I saw enough then to convince any one who has enough sense to be a Congressman or a ward politician that it is the duty of the Government of the United States to appoint dental surgeons to the army and navy. . . . There is a very small percentage of horses in the army compared with the number of men, and yet they have veterinary surgeons.[15]

Following the Southern Dental Association meeting in New Orleans, the subject of military dentists became a centerpiece in professional dental journals. The editor of the *Texas Dental Journal*, Dr Josiah Fife, expressed his regrets that so "little effort" had been made, and recommended that such "important a matter" deserved the attention of the entire profession.[20]

In July 1899 Wilbur Litch, editor of *Dental Brief*, wrote in favor of the Hull bill (or any similar measure) that would secure the appointment of dental surgeons for the Army and Navy. He believed that:

> . . . such service, if once properly established, would soon convince the most skeptical of its vast value and importance to the welfare of our soldiers and sailors. If the examinations for appointment are made relatively as severe as those for the present

155

army and navy medical corps, an exceptionally well qualified body of men can be secured, provided, of course, that such inducements as to rank, pay and promotion are offered as they can accept with due regard to their personal and professional dignity; but upon these vital points there must be no compromise and no surrender.[21(pp406–407)]

That same month, Dr LW Sibley of Rochester, New York, supported the need for Army dentists when he observed in *Dental Cosmos*:

At present the Government makes no provision for dental services other than the extraction of teeth. This operation, I am told, is usually performed by the hospital steward, who numbers among his other accomplishments the washing of bottles, doing up of medicines, etc. If the reports of our soldiers returning from Cuba are to be credited, life in the trenches dodging Mauser bullets is a glorious crimson sunset compared to a few minutes with this amateur dentist.[22(p687)]

By way of contrast, he noted: "We are granting to the inmates of some of our prisons the services of a dental surgeon at the expense of the state, and are withholding them from our boys who are to-day fighting under a tropical sun for the honor and dignity of our flag."[22]

In 1898–1899, JJ Ginsti of San Francisco, California, was sent to Manila at the invitation of General Merritt and with Surgeon General Sternberg's approval. Before leaving in July 1899, he examined about 160 soldiers and found that over 80% of them needed dental work. "I went to Manila in the hope of making a report that would induce Congress to act in this matter. . . . Any information or help I

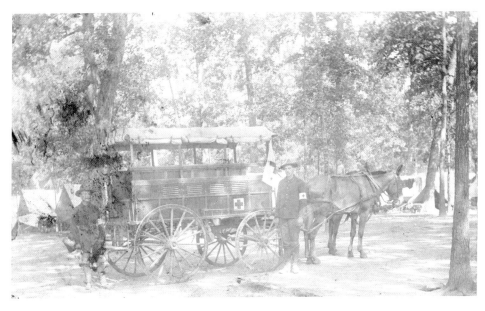

Horse–drawn ambulance, two corpsman standing nearby, Camp Chickamauga, Ga, 1898.
Photograph: Courtesy of US Army Medical Department Museum. Spawar-059.

can give you in that matter I am only too happy to supply, as I consider it one of the most important matters demanding attention in the United States Army at present."[23(p154)]

Dentistry's Dissenting Opinions, 1899

Despite the new sense of urgency, not all dentists agreed on the need for dental surgeons in the Army. William Stark of Kansas City, Missouri, a former major in the 5th Regiment, Missouri Infantry, suggested that the main reason for creating the corps was to provide an opportunity for recent dental graduates to secure "*remunerative* employment" at government expense. He also felt that if the services wanted dental surgeons they would request them of their own accord; forcing dentistry on them seemed to him like "soliciting" (he recommended that the dentists wear a "rampant" forceps as a collar ornament on their uniform blouse). Furthermore, he stated that the Army already looked upon the Medical Department as a "very necessary *evil*," and that a dentist would be considered an "*unmitigated* evil." From "personal experience," he concluded that there would not be enough dental disease to warrant anything besides extractions, the forceps being the "panacea" for the majority of cases. He recommended that dentists enlist as hospital stewards if they wanted an Army career.[24,25]

The editor of the *Western Dental Journal*, Dr John Patterson, wrote that the effort to secure a dental corps was a "useless fight," and that even if dentists were accepted into the Army, "it would not be to the advantage of the dental profession."[26]

In November 1899, at the meeting of the Central Dental Association of Northern New Jersey held in Newark, William Fish, a member of the NDA's Committee for Dentists in the Army and a civilian dentist from Newark, voiced his opposition to the NDA's support of the congressional bill to appoint 100 contract dentists to the Army. He favored a dental corps composed of a lieutenant colonel and a major (purely executive), and one captain and two lieutenants for each of the Army's 15 or 16 geographical departments. He said that to make the corps "effective," its members should be commissioned officers. He argued that it was a recognized fact that Army privates respected only officers: "They respect purely the shoulder straps, nothing more."[27] Craig Work of Ottumwa, Iowa, who had practiced dentistry in the Army as a private, agreed that soldiers would not have as much respect for the dental surgeon if he was not a "commissioned rank officer."[28]

In the *International Dental Journal* that same year, Dr Benjamin Catching of Atlanta admitted that he feared England would have dental surgeons in its army before the United States, yet he agreed that only those with the proper credentials should be chosen, supporting the idea that candidates should have both dental surgery and medical degrees to be eligible for appointment.[29]

The 1899 National Dental Association Meeting

At the annual meeting of the NDA on August 1, 1899, in Niagara Falls, New York, Mark Finley of Washington, DC, read the report of the Committee on the Appointment of Dentists to the Army and Navy. In general, the committee members felt that rather than place the dental profession in an "inferior" position to that of the medical profession, it would be better if no congressional legislation were enacted. The committee felt that this distinction would also extend to the status of the civilian profession. Members believed that those who had entered the Hospital Corps in order to serve as dentists were "detrimental to the attainment" of the objective sought, namely a commissioned dental corps equal in rank to the Medical Corps. The committee concluded that without the support of the surgeon general it was unlikely that any legislation would ever be enacted.[15]

On Donnally's motion, the report was referred to the Committee on the President's Address. This committee did not entirely agree that the association should "work for status only," recommending that the association concentrate on getting dentists into the Army and Navy and then on achieving appropriate status.[15,30]

Despite his favorable view of the Hull bill, in September 1899, Theodore Chupein (1830–1901), a Confederate veteran and the editor of *Dental Office and Laboratory*, worried that 1,000 patients per dental surgeon would be too much for one dentist to handle unless each patient had only a "trifling amount of work to be done." He also thought that the appointed dentists should be selected on their own "professional merits," and not by "political recommendation."[31]

Doctors Fish and Holbrook at Fort Wadsworth

On November 17, 1899, William Fish and Charles WF Holbrook, both civilian dentists from Newark, New Jersey, got permission from the commander of Fort Wadsworth, New York, to conduct a dental examination of the garrison's enlisted personnel. Their examination of 50 soldiers added more justification for a military dental service. They reported that:

Eleven men had what might be called a perfect set of dentures; of these eleven five were new recruits; the balance had been in the service from one to five years. We therefore found 39 men out of 50 in absolute need of dental services. Nine of the thirty-nine men were practically raw recruits, who are supposed to have a perfect set of dentures on entering the service. We found from a very superficial examination the presence of 144 cavities that needed immediate attention; how many more there were that escaped our view no one knows. In many cases where caries existed, the pulps were exposed, and the men complained of toothache to a greater or less degree. Forty teeth had been extracted while in the service. When we take into consideration the present conditions, it is safe to assume that over 50 teeth will have to be removed from those mouths in the next year.[27(p68)]

They also noted that in some instances men had to be relieved while on guard duty because of a toothache; some saying they "needed a dentist more than a doctor."[27]

The Second Otey Bill, 1899

On December 5, 1899, Representative Peter Otey made another attempt in the House of Representatives for Army dental legislation at the 56th Congress. His new bill (HR 972) provided for the appointment of "dental surgeons for service in the United States Army." It was referred to the House Committee on Military Affairs and ordered to be printed.[32,33]

The bill provided authorization for the surgeon general to appoint one contract dental surgeon for every thousand soldiers rather than establish a commissioned dental corps. Those appointed had to be medical or dental college graduates of good character and would have to pass a professional examination. The examination would be conducted and supervised by the first three dental surgeons appointed, who would be selected for their qualifications and compensated an extra $60 a month. Dental college graduates currently serving and satisfactorily performing dental duties could be appointed without examination.[34]

Unlike the Hull bill, Otey's bill proposed that dentists be appointed on a contract basis, under the terms and conditions applicable to Army contract surgeons. Some in the dental profession thought that the position of contract surgeon lacked military dignity and would not command respect. Others argued that the basis of the appointment of dentists in the Army was humanitarian, meant to relieve the sufferings endured by military personnel because of their inability to secure needed dental services; therefore, dentists should be content with the contract basis because rank in the service would not affect the humanitarian character of the work. Also, this plan would be an opportunity for the Army to evaluate the impact of dental surgeons, who would prove valuable and necessary. As a result, better things might come, including the dignity of rank. The Hull bill had aimed higher and lost; the Otey bill's less ambitious approach gave it a good chance of passing. Dentists were urged to write their congressmen in support of the bill. Williams Donnally recommended that they omit "any reflection or even mention of the position" of the surgeon general or War Department in their correspondence.[35]

The Response of the Dental Press in 1900

In January 1900 the editor of *Items of Interest*, Rodrigues Ottolengui, commented on the NDA committee's efforts:

> It will undoubtedly be a disappointment to many who read the bill to note that all that is asked is that contract dentists be authorized, the original and natural desire of our profession being to see dentists established as officers, similarly with the medical corps. The Committee, however, have arduously worked in this cause and are cognizant of so many obstacles in the path of a regular commissioned corps of dentists that they have finally and wisely decided to attempt only that which would not be certain to fail. The defeat of another dental measure would relegate the cause to oblivion for many years, whereas the adoption of the Committee's bill would at least mean the practical trial of the project, with the very possible result that as soon as the usefulness of dentists to the army had been fully felt, much of the present objection would subside and a commissioned dental corps would be more readily attained than now. In such a condition of affairs preference in the appointments would surely be given to those who had well acquitted themselves as contract dentists and who would by then have become familiar with the needs of the soldiers.[33(pp77–78)]

He also urged that all dentists write their congressmen.[33]

In January 1900 *Dental Headlight* stated that it was "the duty of every dentist, both for the love of humanity and his profession, to lend a helping hand." The editor also remarked, "in conversation with a member of the First Tennessee Regiment, recently returned from the Philippines, we learned how badly a dentist was needed, and of the suffering among the soldiers for lack of proper dental treatment."[36]

Also that month, *Dental Digest* commented on the fact that there was both support of and opposition to the proposed dental legislation among the Army surgeons. It quoted the *Brooklyn Eagle* of January 16, which had said that "a prominent army surgeon" was opposed to the idea, claiming, "he thinks that if this bill passes, the government should add tooth-brushes and tooth-powder to the rations. He further says that besides the first cost army dentists would entail on the government there would have to be another outlay for materials." The surgeon reminded readers that Army recruits were not accepted unless their teeth were in good condition and they typically served only 3 years, surely their teeth could not "deteriorate very much in that time." *Dental Digest* thought this statement "so ridiculous" that it did not deserve a reply, and attributed all the opposition to the proposed bill to the "jealousy of army physicians."[37]

On the other hand, *Dental Digest* pointed out that some Army surgeons were strongly in favor of dental legislation. FC Stanton of Chicago, a surgeon in the Illinois state militia and a former acting assistant surgeon, US Army, not only approved of it but also wrote to Otey, commending his efforts. Stanton said:

> This is a matter the importance of which has been gravely underestimated up to the present time. As a surgeon in the volunteer service, I am aware of the frequency with which the services of a dental surgeon are required, and I shall be happy to do anything in my power to further the passage of the bill.[37(p67)]

On the whole, the majority of Army officers, surgeons included, were in favor of the addition of a dental corps to the Medical Department. Most Army officers criticized the bill only because it did not carry rank for the dentists; the objection to giving dental surgeons rank came mainly from members of the medical profession who were not connected with the Army.[38]

The lack of rank was William Fish's main objection to the current Otey bill; he still believed that dentists must be commissioned officers. He added that the association hoped for the appointment of 100 contract dentists. He stuck by his opinion that there should be a lieutenant colonel and a major to handle executive duties and one captain and two lieutenants for each of the Army departments.[27]

In January 1900 the editor of *Dental Cosmos*, Edward Kirk, endorsed the Otey bill while recognizing that the proposed contract status had been criticized in some quarters as "one lacking in military dignity" and "respect." He reminded those taking this view that the main argument for dental surgeons was the "humanitarian motive" and, therefore, rank should not be the important factor for the dental profession's support of the bill. He also pointed out that the Hull bill had aimed higher and had failed as a result. In his view, the Otey bill would be an "entering wedge," after which rank would follow.[39]

The Otey Bill Moves Forward

On January 16, 1900, Surgeon General Sternberg finally endorsed the Otey bill as follows:

> Respectfully returned to the Honorable, the Secretary of War, recommending approval of the bill. The large number of troops in the Philippines, and else where, where the services of competent dentists cannot be secured, makes it desirable that the government should make a reasonable provision for emergency dental work required by officers and enlisted men of the army.[40(p166)]

Sternberg's endorsement, which the secretary of war sent to the Military Affairs Committee, was crucial to the eventual passage of the bill. Now that the Army Medical Department was behind it, it seemed only a matter of time before the bill would become a reality. Sternberg's assent was at least partially the result of the persistent work of Williams Donnally and the NDA Committee on Army and Navy Dental Legislation, which had reached an understanding with Sternberg that the dental surgeons would initially be similar to contract surgeons and later be eligible for commissioned status.[28,41,42] At the 1901 NDA meeting, the committee report confirmed this accommodation:

> There was a distinct understanding with the Surgeon-General that his approval of the terms of the bill was made with the intention of recommending, as soon as authority was granted for the commissioning of Contract Surgeons, that authority would be granted for the commissioning of Contract Dental Surgeons in such numbers as experience in the meantime would warrant. . . . Thus the transition of the corps from the contract to the commissioned status, under restrictions as are suitable to protect the interests of the government and the honor of the profession, was provided in advance.[41(p218)]

On February 28, 1900, the Committee on Military Affairs recommended that the Otey bill (HR 972) be passed with a few minor amendments.[32,43] Representative Hay's report gave the reasons for the committee's approval:

> The necessity for dental surgeons in the Army has been made manifest since the beginning of the Spanish war, and in the light of more recent army service in the Philippine Islands this necessity has been emphasized, and some effective action is believed to be mandatory to accomplish this much-needed end.

> The testimony of army officers of the line, of army surgeons, and the cordial approval of this bill by Surgeon-General Sternberg would be sufficient alone to induce your committee to favorably report the measure, to say nothing of the demands for its passage in the interest of humanity and the health of our soldiers.

> But from almost every State in the Union come to Congress appeals, not from dentists, but from medical men of the highest standing, men of national reputation, expressing their opinion that the measure is one necessary not only for the health of the soldier, but necessary for his efficiency. We would call attention to the fact that Dr. [Nicholas] Senn, of Chicago, a surgeon of world-wide reputation, indorses the

measure. Dr. [Thomas Sargent] Latimer, of Baltimore, of national fame in his profession, heartily approves it. Nearly all members of Congress advocate its passage. . . .

We do not deem it necessary to reproduce in this report the letters of army surgeons, both of the Regular and Volunteer Army; of the distinguished medical men in civil life; of eminent civil officers, and of members of the Senate and House of Representatives. Suffice it to say that all cordially indorsed the proposition of adding dental surgeons to the Army, and in this they were supported by the *New York Herald*, *Nashville American*, *Memphis Appeal*, as well as many journals throughout the country.

Your committee believing that the enactment of this bill into a law will increase the efficiency of the Army and add to the comfort of and retard disease among its rank and file, unanimously recommend its speedy passage.[43]

Also in February, the editor of *Dental Review*, Alison Harlan, reported that the occupation troops in Cuba were "enthusiastic" about having dental surgeons appointed in the Army to treat their dental diseases. Their slender pay made it virtually impossible for them to employ a local dentist. Therefore, they had no recourse but to have their teeth "dug out in the most crude and barbarous way by the regimental surgeon, or more often some amateur butcher," neither of whom had the expertise nor proper instruments for the operation. Frequently, the pa-

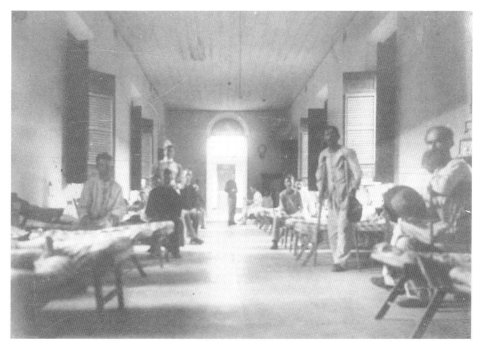

A ward in General Hospital, Santiago de Cuba, 1899.
Photograph: Courtesy of US Army Medical Department Museum. Spawar-002.

tients wound up in the hospital for postoperative care as a result of the "lack of competent dental services."[44]

That same month, James Truman and George Warren, editors of the *International Dental Journal,* agreed that rank was "not of material importance." They also felt that the position of the three supervising dental surgeons was the "weak portion" of the bill. They surmised that it would be difficult to get three competent dentists to serve for the extra $60 a month, and argued that gold, "if used at all," should be reserved for officers, who should pay for the material. Finally, they said that one dentist could not possibly care for a thousand patients; at the rate of seeing six to eight a day, it would take 6 months to see each member of the regiment once.[45]

In March 1900, however, Rodrigues Ottolengui wrote that the prospects were "fair" for congressional approval of the Otey bill. About 200 votes had been pledged in its support in Congress. Some encouragement also came from newspaper reports that Brigadier General Elwell Otis, the Philippines commander, had notified the government that his men were "suffering with their teeth," and that he had requested that dentists should be sent to him. These reports proved to be false, but the Army Medical Department was not as opposed to the dental bill as it had been in the previous year, and Ottolengui thought that the surgeons would pose no obstacle.[46]

Also in March, the majority of Army officers were in favor of the Otey bill, according to Dr Harry Wilson of Chicago. Their only criticism was that it did not carry rank, yet most of this criticism came from the civilian medical profession, not the Army. Wilson took exception to those who said that Surgeon General Sternberg "killed" the Otey bill, whereas he had actually endorsed it in writing to the House Committee on Military Affairs. In its closing, the committee said that passing the bill would "increase the efficiency of the army and add to the comfort of and retard disease" among soldiers. Committee members unanimously recommended its passage.[38]

In April, Ottolengui reported the Otey bill's favorable treatment by the Military Affairs Committee. He also stated that the bill as originally written stipulated that the Army dentist candidates be "graduates of standard medical or dental colleges." The committee amended the bill so that it read "graduates of standard dental colleges" only; Ottolengui thought that the "significance" of this change would be "apparent" and "appreciated" by the dental profession.[47]

That same month, the editor of *Dental Brief,* Wilbur Litch, endorsed the recommendations of Williams Donnally and Robert Oliver of Indianapolis for appointment to the supervising board positions. He stated that Donnally was "a gentleman" who was held in the "highest esteem both personally and professionally by his confreres" in Washington, and had shown "high ability as an organizer" in the effort to secure the passage of the Otey bill. Oliver, he noted, was an oral surgeon, president of the Indiana State Board of Dental Examiners, a faculty member of the Department of Dental Surgery of the University of Indianapolis, Spanish-American War veteran, and known for his "executive ability and powers of organization." The following month, Litch endorsed the recommendation of John Sayre Marshall, citing him as "one of the leading teachers of Oral Surgery and Dental

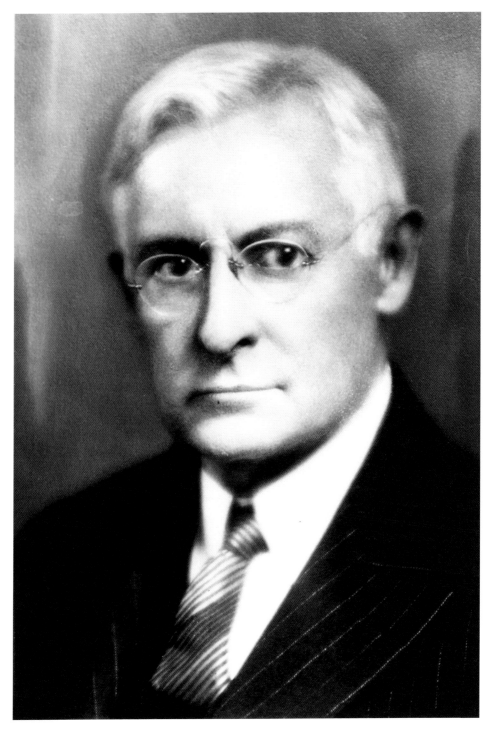

Rodrigues Ottolengui, editor of Items of Interest.
Photograph: Courtesy of the American Dental Association.

Pathology." He noted that Marshall's book, *Injuries and Surgical Diseases of the Face, Mouth and Jaws*, was the standard textbook in nearly all the dental colleges in the United States and Canada, and had even been translated into German.[48]

Dental Office and Laboratory also commented on the new bill:

> A bill for the appointment of dentists to the army was introduced in the last Congress, but failed of passage. The National Dental Association, at its last meeting, appointed a committee who very wisely decided that, in view of the opposition to the project, only the appointment of contract dental surgeons be asked for and not a regularly commissioned dental corps. There is no question of the need of dental surgeons in the army and navy but it is much better to get an entering wedge in this manner than to have the matter again defeated and regulated to the back-ground again for many years as it most surely would be.[34(p91)]

Like many others, the journal urged its readers to write to their congressmen to support the measure.[34]

Also the same month, Dr George Edwin Hunt, the editor of the *Indiana Dental Journal*, added the following remarks in support of the Oliver endorsement:

> Dr. Oliver is peculiarly well qualified by temperament and training to perform the duties attaching to this office. He has powers of organization, executive ability, energy, and brains. His previous military training, while not a necessity, would be an advantage. He has had experience both as a teacher and an examiner, and has acquitted himself with credit and honor in both positions.[49(p535)]

The Otey Bill Stalls

On April 6, 1900, Senator Edmund Pettus of Alabama introduced a companion Senate bill (S 4044) to Otey's House bill to provide for "the appointment of dental surgeons for service in the United States Army." The bill was read twice and referred to the Senate Committee on Military Affairs. On May 17, Pettus, a member of the committee, proposed an amendment, and on June 5, he reintroduced the bill with the amendment recommended by the Military Affairs Committee that limited the number of dentists in the Army to a maximum of 30. The Senate agreed on the amendment, and the bill was read the third time and passed. The next day, the Senate referred the bill to the House Committee on Military Affairs. The Senate then adjourned without taking further action.[32]

At the July 1900 meeting of the NDA at Old Point Comfort, Virginia, B Holly Smith, now the NDA president, commented on the delay of the Otey bill's passage. If the bill reappeared, he recommended Williams Donnally, John Sayre Marshall, and Vines Turner (of Raleigh, North Carolina) be appointed as examining surgeons. He urged the association's Committee on Army and Navy Dental Legislation to continue its efforts to secure passage of the bill. The committee (consisting of Mark F Finley, Charles S Butler, and Williams Donnally) predicted that with the "favor" the measure had already won this session, Congress would pass the dental bill before the close of the next session. The committee was increased to five members and appropriated a maximum of $250 for its work during the coming year.[50–52]

The case of Private Walter Fitzgerald illustrated the continued dental condition of the troops serving in the Philippines in 1900 as Congress and dental associations debated the merits and shortcomings of the Otey Bill. The 23-year-old soldier was one of the first volunteers to reach Manila after Admiral George Dewey's victory in Manila Bay, and had been in the Philippines for 19 months. During his time overseas, Fitzgerald had lost nearly every tooth in his mouth. Tropical fever and the Army diet had affected his gums and caused his teeth to loosen and drop out one by one.[53] Despite many stories like this and more than 2 years of debate and lobbying, as 1900 drew to a close, Congress still had not passed any dental legislation authorizing dental care in the US Army.

The Army Reorganization Bill and the Otey Amendment

The transfer of the Philippines to United States control at the end of the Spanish-American War led to prolonged conflict. A Filipino independence movement, focused on gaining complete sovereignty for the Archipelago, lasted from early 1899 until mid 1902. The confrontation required an unprecedented number of troops, many of whom were federal volunteers who faced expiration of their enlistments early in 1901 despite the continued violence. Mustering out was due to commence in January, but troops could not be withdrawn from at least 400 stations in the Philippines without endangering the safety of those remaining.[54]

As a result of the dangerous situation in the Philippines, a sense of urgency suddenly pervaded Congress on December 3, 1900, when Representative John Hull introduced a bill (HR 12224) for Army reorganization. The Committee on Military Affairs quickly reviewed the bill and a companion Senate bill (S 4300) before referring it to the floor for discussion. On December 6 the Medical Department section (Section 18) of the Senate bill came up for debate in the House. Hull, who had unsuccessfully pushed an Army dental bill in the final session of 1899, presented a letter from Surgeon General Sternberg to the secretary of war lamenting the shortage of medical officers in the Philippines and the inadequacies of the contract surgeons on duty there. Sternberg recommended that 50 of the volunteer surgeons already on duty in the Philippines be commissioned with the rank and pay of major, and 150 of the volunteer assistant surgeons be commissioned with the rank and pay of captain, each for a period of 2 years. It would be much less expensive to the government to retain these officers, who could be mustered out when the emergency was over, than to increase the Medical Corps by adding new permanent officers. James Hay, a representative from Virginia, proposed that this plan be added to Section 18 as an amendment, and the House agreed.[54]

Representative Otey promptly offered an adjustment to the previous amendment of Section 18, which repeated his proposal that a maximum of 30 contract dental surgeons be employed, with a ratio of one for every 1,000 troops. These surgeons, he argued, should be dental college graduates of good moral standing selected by a board of three specially-appointed dentists. The board was to be made up of dentists recommended by the surgeon general and approved by the secretary of war. Dental college graduates currently serving as enlisted soldiers and being used satisfactorily as dentists could be appointed without examination.[54] Otey clarified:

Mr. Chairman, this amendment is the bill which was reported unanimously by the Senate committee, the same bill having been reported by the House committee unanimously on two occasions except that the House bill provided for 1 dentist for every 1,000 men. The Senate changed that to 1 dentist for every 1,000, men but not to exceed 30 in all. I believe every member of this House has been interviewed on this subject, and I have yet to find a single one who has openly opposed it. I have a list of a few of them here which I will give.[54]

Otey listed 50 congressmen, 80 Army officers, and 5 state governors who endorsed the dental amendment before his time on the floor expired. When he had finished, Representative James Slayden of Texas asked, "has the gentleman no way of demonstrating the qualifications of dentists and the necessity for their services without reading the roll of all the public officials in the country?"[54]

Otey did not answer the question but continued:

Now, Mr. Chairman, I do not thrust myself upon the House very often. When I do, I have something to say that is tangible and worth talking about [laughter]. I do not know to what the gentleman from Texas [Slayden] has referred. He reminds me of the Irishman of whom I heard a story. He was eating eggs. The first one he swallowed went down all right; but in swallowing another he heard the sound of a chick as it went down his throat; and then he exclaimed, "Begorrah, you have a swathe voice, but you spake too late [laughter]." I think, sir, that anybody who opposes this bill "spakes" too late. I want gentlemen to come out now and say whether they are going to take care of 3,200,000 teeth, half of which are aching all the time [laughter]. I appeal to gentlemen on this side of the House and on the other side of the House, regardless of recent elections and regardless of political affiliations, to come forward and give the old soldier (that grand old soldier) a chance to get rid of the toothache.

I do not care to occupy further time. I ask for a vote on this question, and I hope every man will stand up or sit down [laughter].[54(p98)]

Hull suggested that the amendment was of such importance that perhaps it should be considered independently of the larger bill. Ultimately, that proved unnecessary and the dental amendment was finally agreed upon, the bill passing the House by a vote of 171 to 133 with all of the House amendments on December 6.[54]

The following January, a *Dental Digest* editorial expressed regret that it was "necessary for dentists to start in the army under such conditions." However, those in high authority felt that if the Dental Corps proved its value, it would become a permanent corps and rank would follow. *Dental Digest* also questioned whether the better qualified, more experienced dentists would be attracted to a service career in view of the insecurity of a 3-year contract with no medical or pension benefits. Furthermore, the journal warned:

Any practitioner who goes into the service with the idea that it is easy will be sadly disappointed, as the work will be very hard, necessitating long hours, and will consist for the most part of extracting, treating and cleaning teeth, inserting amalgam and cement fillings, and perhaps making rubber plates. Some applicants for these positions seem to think they will have electric engines, fountain cuspidors, cabinets, carpets, up-to-date dental chairs, etc. However, the most of our soldiers at present

167

are chasing Filipinos and Boxers, and as the dentists will have to follow the soldiers, an adjustable head-rest or a portable dental chair will be all the office furniture that can be employed, except, of course, where army posts are situated in large cities. . . . From a humanitarian standpoint the bill is beneficial to the army, for even though two or three hundred dentists are needed, thirty will be able to accomplish a great deal. So far, however, as the dental profession is concerned, we regard the measure as an insult rather than an honor. Dentists seem to be viewed by legislators and army officials as on a par with horse doctors, for the appointees are not commissioned, are underpaid, and have little or no control of their own actions. If it were not for the fact that at the present time our soldier boys, who unfortunately can not have any say in this matter, are desperately in need of dental service, we should be glad to see the bill killed in the senate.[55(p65)]

Army Dentists at Last

On January 3, 1901, the Senate began deliberation on the Army bill with the House amendments. On February 1 the bill was signed by the speaker of the House and the president pro tempore. The next day, the president approved and signed the act "to increase the efficiency of the permanent military establishment of the United States." The implementation of this new law was a historic event; a corps of military dental surgeons was officially made a part of the United States Army, a step no other army in the world had taken. Now dental treatment for the common soldier was seen as a government responsibility.[54]

Although the humanitarian cause of dentistry had been served, the profession remained relegated to a second-class status in relation to its medical counterpart because of the lack of commissions for dentists and their status as civilian contract dental surgeons. But that distinction probably did not matter much to Dr Henry JB McKellops, who had first formally proposed the appointment of dentists to the US Army on July 21, 1858, and then fought for the cause for the next 4 decades, because he lived to see his goal achieved before he passed away in April 1901. His obituary in the June issue of *Dental Cosmos* noted, "It is gratifying to know that Dr. McKellops lived to see the accomplishment of his wise suggestion, even after the lapse of forty-two years."[56]

The term "contract surgeon" dated back to the Mexican War, when the number of medical officers in the peacetime Regular Army was inadequate for the expanded wartime army. To meet the need, civilian surgeons were appointed to act in the capacity of regularly commissioned medical officers. These physicians served under contract as "quasi officers," and were referred to by courtesy as "acting assistant surgeon" and by discourtesy as "contract surgeon." During the Civil War, between 5,000 and 6,000 civilian physicians were appointed to the Army, and during the Spanish-American War and Philippine-American War, between 800 and 900 contract surgeons were appointed. In these three wars, the contract surgeons, although never mustered into the Army, wore the uniform and performed all the duties of commissioned medical officers. The contract surgeon's status differed in the following ways: his contract was subject to annulment at any time by the chief medical officer in charge of the department in which he served, with no right to trial or appeal; he was paid less and given fewer allowances than Regular Army assistant surgeons and had no possibility of promotion; he had no sick or disabled pay or right to hospitalization in the Army system; he was not given a pension or retirement benefits unless he was injured in the service, and only then by congressional appropriation; he did not have the right to enter a soldiers' home; and he had no authority to issue orders to enlisted soldiers, even those in the Hospital Corps.[57(pp742–743)] The first contract dental surgeons entered this system of quasimilitary status.

Some years later, John Marshall, who knew the circumstances intimately, explained why the status as contract dental surgeons was necessary at first:

> Although the provisions of this bill were not satisfactory to the profession in general, particularly that section which provided that the dental surgeons should be "employed under contract," it was thought best to strive for its passage in this form rather than cause its defeat by insisting upon a commissioned status for the corps. The main idea at this time was to succeed in establishing a dental corps for the army, that the suffering of our soldiers from dental and oral diseases, at that period so prominently before the country, might be mitigated, and the profession of dentistry recognized as a needful adjunct to that of general medicine and surgery in maintaining the health and physical efficiency of our armies in the field.

> Surgeon General George M. Sternberg was unwilling to recommend to the secretary of war the passage by congress of a bill giving a commissioned status to dental surgeons, as he felt sure that it would not at that time meet with the approval of the military committees of the senate and house of representatives, but he gave assurances that should this bill pass, and the work of the dental surgeons prove to be as beneficial to the services as it was hoped it would, congress would undoubtedly look favorably upon a bill granting commissioned status to the dental corps, and that he would use his best endeavors to secure the passage of such a measure.[28]

The Dental Press: "Better Things in the Future"

The *Dental Review* said it did not desire to comment on the present act, hoping that it would "lead to better things in the future." *Dental Brief* pointed out that contract dental surgeons had "no real military rank," a major disappointment to those who had worked so hard for the dental bill.[58,59]

However, the editor of *Dental Cosmos*, Edward Kirk, applauded the event: "The newly-elected dental corps, as pioneers in their field, will be expected to not only render efficient service, but by the fruits of their labors demonstrate to a large and not uncritical body of observers the rightfulness of the claims of dentistry to a national recognition of its importance in this new relation." Kirk credited the "growth of public appreciation" of dentistry as "one of the common necessities of life" for creating a demand for an Army dental service. The "national recognition" that dentistry received from the act and its significance in advancing the "professional status" of its members would be invaluable to the profession. Kirk concluded:

> The present relation of the dental corps to the government service is that of contract surgeons, and, while the failure to secure the creation of a commissioned corps was cause for disappointment in the minds of many who were actively interested in the matter, there is in the present arrangement ample opportunity afforded for the dental

corps to demonstrate its efficiency, and its future development will determine its status in accordance with its merits. The medical department of the service is fully equipped and organized to the minutest detail, and the official attachment of the dental corps to the medical department is a provision not only natural and eminently wise, but, working as they do for similar ends, it places the dental corps at once upon a basis of the best working efficiency. It is a matter of interest that, while the dental surgeons are classified as "attached to the medical department," the dentist receives his orders from headquarters, not from the army surgeon. The work of each is clearly defined by the army regulations, so that one does not trespass upon the field of the other. It is provided that the dentist and surgeon shall consult upon cases of mutual interest, but under the same ethical professional rules as are maintained in these relations in civil professional life.[60–62]

Foreign dental journals also chided their governments on being behind the times. The *Australian Journal of Dentistry*, for example, recommended that the commonwealth should "keep abreast with the times in the matter of provision of dental service" for its armies and follow the example of the US War Department.[63]

The Dental Examining Board

As soon as the bill became law, the surgeon general named the first three contract dental surgeons who were to compose the dental examining board and serve as supervisory dental surgeons. John Sayre Marshall, the board's chairman, was a widely respected figure in dentistry.[64–71] Also well known was Robert Oliver, who was a veteran of the recent war and prominent in Indiana dental circles.[72,73] However, the third dentist elected to the committee, Robert Morgan, was virtually unknown. An enlisted veteran of the Civil War, Morgan graduated from the Baltimore College of Dental Surgery in 1881 and opened a practice in his native Lynchburg, Virginia.[74,75] In fact, Morgan had drafted the successful versions of dental bill for Representative Otey, who strongly encouraged him to become one of the primary examining dentists. His appointment caused considerable controversy among civilian dentists, but Otey championed Morgan's appointment, saying, "the dentists in the country had not asked for the law. I had not thought of it. It was Dr. R.W. Morgan who suggested it. Then the dentists who had been asleep took it up and did good work to accomplish the results."[76]

Some dental editors, including Kirk of *Dental Cosmos*, Clapp of *Dental Digest*, Litch of *Dental Brief*, and Ottolengui of *Items of Interest*, expressed their regrets that Williams Donnally was not appointed as a member of the examining board, because it was largely through his efforts that this legislation had been passed. Although Surgeon General Sternberg had recommended him, Donnally was not selected because the secretary of war argued that no one who had been "influential" in securing the necessary legislation should "personally profit by the law" (Morgan's role in the legislation was overlooked).[59,60,77–79] This decision left Donnally with considerable ill-will toward Marshall, who was selected in his place, and later caused problems within the NDA.

Dr James Truman, editor of the *International Dental Journal*, commented on the board's composition:

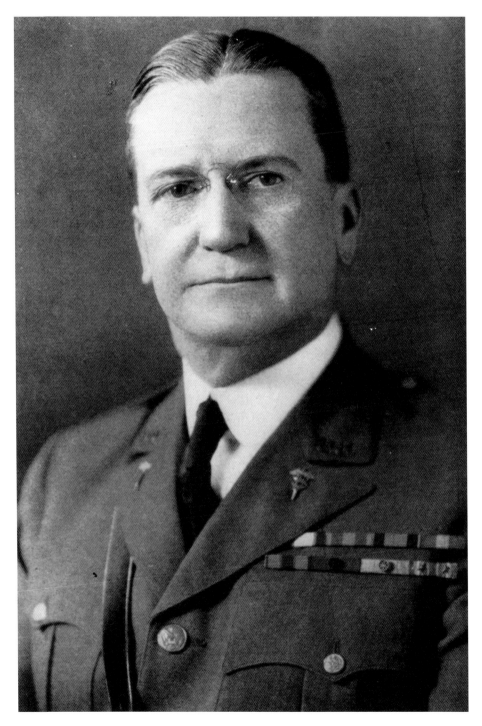

Colonel Robert T Oliver, one of the first three contract dental surgeons chosen to serve on the dental examining board and as a supervisory dental surgeon.
Photograph: Courtesy of Colonel James M Vail.

171

The effort was made throughout the United States to present only the best representative men that could be found willing to accept the chief positions. It was naturally feared that it would be difficult to find that character of men willing to serve on the meager salary provided in the bill. It was well understood that whoever did elect to represent the dental profession in the army, it would be a great pecuniary sacrifice as well as comfort. It was, therefore, something of a surprise that a number of men known to be well qualified, offered their services, and the dentists of the country were not slow to appreciate the fact that this sacrifice was worthy of the men, and, recognizing this, they received cordial endorsement from all sections. It was supposed that the heads of the government appreciated the full measure of responsibility devolving on their selections, and in making these appointments only the highest good of the army would be taken into consideration.

The blow came when it was officially announced that three had been appointed. One man [Marshall] of the three required no endorsement. He was known everywhere as fully equal to all demands; some few knew another [Oliver] by name, but the other [Morgan] was by the writer entirely unknown. This latter appointment cannot be regarded complacently, as it is felt to be entirely at variance with the wishes of the entire dental fraternity that only men well known should fill these important positions.[80(pp391–392)]

Although Truman expressed his satisfaction that Marshall was the board's president and "there is a confidence felt in his ability," he still felt that his selection did not "minimize the disappointment" and "dissipate the unpleasant feeling existing" over Morgan's appointment. He urged the NDA to protest against any future appointments made upon "mere political recommendation." The three men had "a serious responsibility" and would be held to "a strict accountability" by the dental profession. Furthermore, he predicted failure for the corps:

There is no desire to be a prophet of ill-omen in this connection, but it does seem to the writer that the non-success of this experiment is fully assured under present arrangements. The men selected, however able or earnest, cannot fulfill the duties required of them. When this is demonstrated and a demand is made in Congress for the repeal of the act creating contract dental surgeons, let the blame for the failure rest upon Congress, and not upon dentistry, or upon the men who so faithfully worked until the act creating dental surgeons in the army was finally passed.[80(pp393–394)]

Despite his misgivings, he urged the profession's full support of the new service.[81]

The Work of the Dental Examining Board, February–July 1901

Marshall, Oliver, and Morgan began work on February 18, 1901, at 1814 G Street, NW, Washington, DC. The surgeon general instructed the board to plan the format for the examination of the first class of candidates to report the next week, on February 25.[60,82]

In discussions with the examining board, Sternberg told them that many in Congress and the War Department saw contract dental surgeons as "an experiment," but he hoped that they would eventually become permanent and evolve into a commissioned corps. While the board had very carefully selected the best possible dentists to begin the experiment, the surgeon general still reserved the right to select the candidates to be examined by the board. Despite criticism from some in the dental community, Sternberg supported the high standards that the board had set. Marshall believed that dentists would eventually become commissioned and therefore establish permanency in the Army. First, though, they had to prove that they were necessary to the "welfare and efficiency" of the Army. Marshall also thought that any effort to disturb the present status of the dental surgeons during the current session of Congress would be unwise; it was better to wait at least a year for the new dental surgeons to prove themselves. Oliver and Morgan agreed.[83]

The candidates for contract dental surgeons had to be between 24 and 40 years old; graduates of standard medical or dental colleges, trained in all the branches of dentistry; of good moral and professional character (supported by testimonials from well-known professionals); able to pass a rigid physical examination equivalent to that given the candidates for commissioned officer status; and able to pass a thorough professional examination including both theoretical and practical examinations.[84]

On February 25, 1901, the examination of the first eight candidates began. They were examined theoretically and practically in the following subjects and disciplines: anatomy, physiology, histology, physics, chemistry, metallurgy, dental anatomy and physiology, dental materia medica and therapeutics, dental pathology and bacteriology, orthodontics, oral surgery, and operative and prosthetic dentistry. An average score of 75% was required in each subject for the theoretical portion and 85% for the practical. Particular emphasis was placed upon the clinical component. The usual time allotted for the complete examination was 10 to 12 days, but the tests normally ran 2 weeks, with the theoretical followed by the practical. No travel allowances were provided by the government for the candidates' stay in Washington.[84–86]

The candidates were given 2 hours for each subject in the written examinations, with the total written examinations lasting about a week. Elaborate equipment was placed at each candidate's disposal for the practical examination, which was described as follows:

> The practical examination is a thorough test of the candidate as to his manipulative ability. In operative dentistry a patient is assigned to him, and he is required to make an examination of the mouth, recording upon a chart all conditions demanding treatment; and he is graded with reference to the accuracy of his diagnosis and its record. Then follows the removal of deposits; the preparation of cavities both by hand and engine instruments, with a grading upon his instrumentation and technique; the preparation and manipulation of filling-materials, and the insertion of gutta-percha, oxyphosphate, amalgam, and tin fillings; the treatment and filling of root-canals, and preparation of a root for a pivot crown. He is required to show proficiency, and is graded with reference to his ability in the application of the rubber dam, metallic separators, matrices, etc.; his diagnosis, prognosis, and treatment of oral diseases, and the care and sterilization of his instruments and hands. To complete the practical examination in operative dentistry necessitates work at the chair from 9 A.M. until 4 P.M. daily for at least three days, with an intermission of three-quarters of an hour daily for luncheon. In prosthetic work the candidate is examined as to his ability in

173

taking impressions of the mouth, making casts, taking the bite, and adjusting the articulation; the construction of a denture in vulcanite; making dies [sic] and counter-dies from impression to completion; the construction of a swaged plate with metal and vulcanite attachments, and the construction of interdental splints. The swaged plate is to be made from a model of an edentulous jaw carved by the candidate to test his knowledge of the anatomical form of the jaw. The practical examination, including both operative and mechanical practice, consumes about one week, and the candidate is required to attain an average of eighty-five per cent on the total number of practical tests.[62(pp700–701)]

As of March 16, only 2 of 14 candidates successfully passed the board: Seibert Boak (1876–1934) of Martinsburg, West Virginia, a graduate of the National University in Washington, DC; and Clarence Lauderdale (1873–1961) of Naples, New York, a graduate of the University of Buffalo in New York. Both men received appointments as contract dental surgeons and were ordered to report to San Francisco by April 15 to prepare for service in the Philippines.[85]

In his report that day, Marshall expressed the board's general opinion of the candidates:

The board has been disappointed in the professional qualifications of most of the young men who have presented themselves. The examination does not cover any subjects which have not been taught in our best dental schools, and the board believes that the questions submitted have been of a practical nature and eminently fair. It is therefore to be hoped that our colleges will not recommend any young men to come before this board who are not thoroughly well qualified, theoretically and practically, in all of the branches comprising the curriculum of our leading dental schools.[85(p213)]

By July, seven other candidates had successfully passed the examinations for appointment: Franklin F Wing (1876–1942), Montana, Northwestern University Dental School; George L Mason (1871–?), Massachusetts, Boston Dental College; William H Ware (1864–?), California, University of California, Dental Department (who had served as an enlisted dentist in the Philippines in 1898–1899); Hugo C Rietz (1877–?), Wisconsin, Chicago College of Dental Surgery; Ralph W Waddell (1876–?), Ohio, University of Pennsylvania, Dental Department; Jean C Whinnery (1878–1910), Nebraska, University of Pennsylvania, Dental Department; and Frank H Wolven (1878–?), New Jersey, Columbian University Dental Department, Washington, DC.[87]

In addition to those dentists selected by the board in Washington, the February 2 act authorized dental college graduates then serving as enlisted members of the Hospital Corps to be appointed as contract dental surgeons without examination, provided they had been detailed to dental duties for at least a year and had satisfactory performance reports from their commanding officers. Under this provision, five soldiers then serving in the Philippines were released from their enlistments and immediately enrolled as contract dental surgeons: Private Samuel Hussey (University of Michigan College of Dental Surgery, 1897); Private Emmett Craig; Private Alden Carpenter; Acting Hospital Steward Charles Petre; and Private Douglas Foster. After 5 ½ months of continuous service, the dental examining board finally filled its quota. The surgeon general had invited

86 applicants from various states and territories, 70 whom actually appeared to take the examination. The average age of those appointed was about 27 years (the age limit established by the surgeon general was between 24 and 40 years). In general, candidates who had received their dental degrees from 5 to 10 years before failed the theoretical examination, while the recent graduates failed the practical examination (Table 6-1).[88]

Excluding the members of the examining board and those five who were already serving in the Army, the 19 appointees came from 15 states and the District of Columbia: one each from Alabama, California, Iowa, Maryland, Massachusetts, Montana, Nebraska, New Jersey, New York, Ohio, Washington, West Virginia, and Wisconsin; and two each from the District of Columbia, Missouri, and Pennsylvania. The new dentists' assignments reflected the Army's most pressing needs at the time, including orders to the Philippines, Puerto Rico, San Francisco, Kansas, Texas, Illinois, New York, and Virginia.[89]

Although some criticized the difficulty of the board's examinations, in September 1901, Wilbur Litch expressed support for the standards:

> Some exception has been taken to the character of the examinations thus far held. By many the theoretical examination especially has been regarded as unnecessarily severe, indeed in requirement far beyond what can reasonably be demanded of the dental student or practitioner. The subjects embraced in these examinations have, however, been only those found in the curricula of our best schools, and, if a higher standard of attainment in those studies has been demanded than is ordinarily exacted in college examinations, such advanced requirement can hardly be regarded as uncalled for.
>
> It must be remembered that not only were the candidates on trial before the board, but that the board also and those whom they passed will be on trial by the army, the people, and, indeed, the whole civilized world. The success or failure of what must yet be regarded as the experimental organization of the dental corps will be largely

TABLE 6-1

CONTRACT DENTAL SURGEON EXAM STATISTICS

Reasons for Pass/Fail	Number of Candidates (out of 86 invited)
Declined to appear	6
Failed to appear	10
Physically disqualified	8
Fully examined and rejected	3
Failed theoretical examination	7
Withdrew by advice of the examiners (before completion of theoretical examination)	33

Data source: [Litch WF]. Some results of examinations for the Army Dental Corps. *Dental Brief.* 1901;6:551–553.

dependent upon the fitness or unfitness of those selected to inaugurate and carry on its practical work. If they prove thoroughly competent, zealous, and painstaking, possessing not only a high standard of educational fitness, but also practical skill as operators, its success may be regarded as reasonably assured.[88]

Litch later commented that the only real problem with the dental legislation was that far too few dentists had been appointed given the amount of work required.[90]

On July 31 the board completed its assignment after being in session continuously since February 18, and its members were sent to various stations. Marshall's orders to San Francisco included instructions for him to stop in Milwaukee, Wisconsin, to represent the Medical Department of the Army at the NDA meeting in August.[76] The board of examining and supervising dental surgeons was never reconvened.

Fitting Out the New Dental Surgeons

Contract dental surgeons were equipped with a special dental "outfit" especially prepared to meet the requirements of Army practice. Although designed for lightness and portability, it was considered better than what many starting dentists could afford. The portable dental outfit weighed about 450 pounds when cased and was designed to be carried by two horses or mules. It included an Army field desk, two folding chairs, and two folding tables. Canvas covers were provided to protect the cases from rain and moisture.[76] Among the professional items in the outfit were a portable dental chair and a dental engine, packed in separate cases; burs, mandrels, stones, disks, and the like; excavators, chisels, scales, plastic-pluggers, gold-pluggers, rubber dam clamps, clamp forceps, a dam punch, extracting forceps, elevators, a steam sterilizer, and a hand cuspidor. In fact, the kit included all the instruments and adjuncts necessary to perform any operation upon the teeth except crowns, bridges, and artificial dentures. Each outfit contained supplies sufficient for 3 months' service. The smaller instruments and the supplies were packed in two strong cases, arranged with trays and receptacles to hold the contents in place.[91] The general hospitals and other posts designated by the surgeon general were furnished with an additional outfit, which included "a regular office operating chair, Allan bracket, cuspidor, instrument case, extra extracting forceps, and a full laboratory outfit for constructing vulcanite plates, swaged metal plates, interdental splints, crowns, and bridgework."[91]

Establishing Dental Care in the Army

The US Army of the early 20th century ran according to a clearly defined set of regulations that authorized and governed virtually every aspect of daily life. When the House of Representatives passed the Army bill in December 1900, Surgeon General Sternberg realized that it would soon become law, and he subsequently drafted an order establishing the regulations governing the eligibility, appointment, and duties of contract dental surgeons. He forwarded the draft provisions to the adjutant general on December 24 and requested that they be published as soon

176

as the bill passed. This draft, which was modified and amended on March 25, 1901, formed the basis for War Department General Order No. 52.[92–94]

As early as March 21 the War Department began establishing the status, responsibilities, and allowances of potential contract dental surgeons stationed at military posts or in the field. General Orders No. 39 (March 21) and 46 (April 6) authorized contract dental surgeons to make purchases from the quartermaster subsistence stores and to buy "such moderate quantity of mineral oil, lamps, wicks, and chimneys as they may need in the rooms occupied by themselves and their families."[95,96]

On April 17 the War Department issued General Order No. 52, which, in paragraph 1395½, specified the provisions under which contract dental surgeons would operate in the Army. Relying heavily on Sternberg's draft, the four pages of paragraph 1395½ described the qualifications, obligations, assignments, operating procedures, office hours, eligible patients, supplies and equipment, and responsibilities of contract dental surgeons.[94]

Dental surgeons were only authorized to treat "the officers and enlisted men of the Regular and Volunteer Army" during their normal operating hours of 9 AM to 4 PM. Neither the families of officers and soldiers nor civilian employees were eligible for treatment during these office hours; dental surgeons were allowed to provide care for those patients before and after the normal hours, but could not use government-furnished materials on them. The type of work allowed and materials to be used were clearly restricted:

> Emergency work whether for officers or enlisted men should always have precedence. Plate work or restoration of teeth by any method will only be done for those

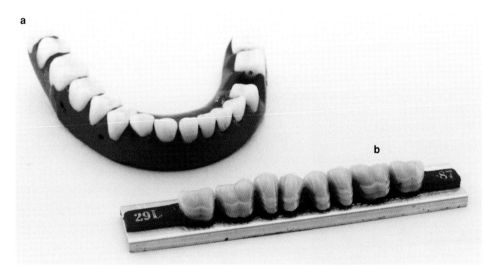

(*a*) *Vulcanite partial denture, circa 1900.* (*b*) *Dentsply Trubyte Teeth, circa 1936.*
Photograph: Courtesy of the National Museum of Health and Medicine,
Armed Forces Institute of Pathology. NCP 3271.

who have lost teeth in the service and in the line of duty. For plate work or filling teeth only the cheaper materials will be supplied, but gold may be used, if the operating dentist sees fit to use it, at the expense of the individual operated upon.[84(pp2–3)]

Each dental surgeon had to keep a record of his work in a bound book, known as the "register of dental operations." Every month, he was required to send a "monthly record of dental operations" to the surgeon general's office. All records were kept permanently as means of identification in case of death or desertion, and for pension claims based upon tooth loss while in the service.[76,91,94]

Several significant differences existed between Sternberg's draft and the final version of Order 52. The draft included information on the uniform of the dental surgeon that was not in General Order No. 52 but was published on April 18 in paragraph 26 of General Order No. 53.[97] According to the regulation, "contract dental surgeons will be permitted to wear the undress and field uniform of an assistant surgeon with the rank of first lieutenant, the straps and ornaments to be in silver instead of gold, and block letters 'D.S.' in silver embroidery to be placed between the bars of the shoulder straps."[98] When General Order No. 52 appeared, it included a lengthy new paragraph that authorized one enlisted soldier, usually detailed from acting hospital stewards or privates of the Hospital Corps, as an assistant for each dental surgeon to help with the instruments and to do other tasks as directed, laying the groundwork for the development of the enlisted dental assistants.[94]

Even as the examining board was still meeting to select the first contract dental surgeons, the Army had already issued the basic regulations that defined their status, duties, uniforms, and medical relations. These details were soon circulating within the American dental community.[99]

"A Department of Military Medical Practice"

At the June 1901 annual meeting of the American Medical Association (AMA) in Saint Paul, the section on stomatology organized a panel on "Military Dental Practice—Its Modifications and Limitations." Commenting on the new dental surgeons' challenges, Dr Henry Hatch of New York recommended that certain types of dental work, like fixed and removable prosthetics, orthodontics, and gold restorations, be completely eliminated from military dental practice because of the extra equipment, time, and expense they required. He also emphasized the value of dental charts and casts for identification purposes, stressing the assistance dental surgeons could give medical surgeons in treating battle casualties.[100]

Dr AH Peck of Chicago then read the remarks of John Marshall, who was still working on examining board matters in Washington. Marshall's paper began with a ringing statement of the importance of what had been done in such a short time:

The passage of the Army Reorganization Bill with its section creating a Corps of Dental Surgeons for the U.S. Army, makes an epoch in the history of modern dental surgery; an epoch which has never had its counterpart before in the history of the world, the influence of which is destined to be far-reaching in its beneficent results, and of great importance in the elevation of our educational and professional standards.[101]

Marshall believed that the creation of a military dental corps was a unique initiative that promised to enhance dentistry's professional status. This was particularly noteworthy, considering that a relatively short amount of time had passed since professional dental education had begun in the 1840s. Since then, the field had grown in prestige and technological sophistication, despite the skepticism of some.[101]

Although many in Congress and the Army viewed the creation of the dental service as an experiment, Marshall saw it as an opportunity for dentists to prove their value and confirm their expertise. He was sure recognition would be forthcoming in the creation of a permanent dental corps with commissioned members. The selection of the first dentists had been thorough and assured quality personnel, a fact that the medical departments of the European armed forces had already noted:

> We have special reason for congratulation also in the fact that the Congress of these United States was the first legislative body in the world to formally recognize the *value* and *need* of the beneficent services of our specialty as a department of military medical practice, and that we have been given an opportunity to prove the wisdom of its action to our country and the world [emphasis in original].[101]

It had been almost exactly 19 years since Marshall had opened his own campaign for Army dentistry with his speech "The Need of Dental Surgeons in the Army and Navy" at a meeting of the same association in the same city.[102]

The Feud between Williams Donnally and John Marshall

As the work of the examining board drew to a close in July 1901, John Marshall wrote to Williams Donnally of the NDA committee to inform him of the board's progress and of their discussions with Surgeon General Sternberg, who had cautioned them not to propose any new dental legislation. On July 29, 1901, Marshall apparently received a rather "extraordinary" reply from Donnally, which took him by "surprise." Marshall could not understand what he had said, done, or written, either in private or public, to "call forth such an epistle," but it was likely connected to Donnally's continuing resentment of not being selected for the examining board. After failing to contact Mark Finley, Marshall went to see Dr HB Noble and together they called on Donnally, but he had already left his office. Marshall then proposed to Donnally that they meet with Finley and Noble to straighten out any misunderstanding that had occurred.[103] In the following years, the Donnally-Marshall cleavage proved damaging to efforts to obtain War Department and congressional approval for the Army Dental Corps.

Laying out the Future

Marshall and Oliver attended the August meeting of the NDA in Milwaukee, Wisconsin, as the official representatives of the Army Medical Department, establishing a pattern of participation and involvement that has continued ever since. In its third annual report, the Committee on Army and Navy Dental Legislation said that its work for the present was concluded, as far as the Army was concerned, with

dangers in our pathway or of the obstacles to be overcome. But I believe that the young men who form the dental corps of the U.S. Army will prove themselves equal to the occasion and bring honor upon the profession to which they belong.[82(p38)]

"The Dental Corps"

After February 1901, John Marshall, Robert Oliver, other contract dental surgeons, and the dental press almost immediately and consistently began using the terms "Corps," "Dental Corps," "Army Dental Corps," "Corps of Dental Surgeons," and even "United States Army Dental Corps" to refer to the 30 civilian contract dental surgeons working for the Medical Department. The Army Reorganization Act of February 2, 1901, established the composition of the Medical Department, including in it medical officers, the Hospital Corps, and the new Nurse Corps, and authorized the surgeon general to employ contract dental surgeons. On March 3, 1911, the Dental Corps was officially authorized in the formal organizational structure and staffing of the Medical Department. Until then, dental surgeons were only referred to as "dental surgeons, as now authorized by law, but never "Army Dental Corps" or "US Army Dental Corps."[105–110]

Marshall's presentation at the NDA meeting in August 1901 used the term "Dental Corps" consistently. On August 30, 1904, at the Fourth International Dental Congress in Saint Louis, Marshall presented a detailed discussion of the selection, functions, and work of the contract dental surgeons in the Army in a paper titled "The United States Army Dental Corps." In addition to the paper's title, one section was called "Plan of Organization of the United States Army Dental Corps." Variations of the term "Dental Corps" were routinely used throughout the dental press in its discussion of contract dental surgeons, in proposed legislation in both houses of Congress, and by the contract dentists themselves in their articles and correspondence. Despite this common use, regulations, correspondence, memoranda, and reports of the US Army and the Medical Department from February 1901 to March 3, 1911, usually used the term "dental surgeons," and only occasionally the terms "Corps of Dental Surgeons" and "Dental Corps."[82,88,90,91,111–114]

Now, if contract dentists proved their value to the Army and Medical Department, they might finally become a commissioned corps. Regardless of the formalities of official Army terminology and organization, what Marshall and many dentists had striven for so ardently since the 1850s at last was a reality, but much hard work remained to be done.

References

1. *Congressional Record, 55th Cong, 2nd Sess.* Vol 31. Washington, DC: Government Printing Office; 1898: 3942, 4561, 5361.

2. [Kirk EC]. Dentists in the Army and Navy. *Dental Cosmos.* 1898;40:593.

3. V[ail] WD. Organization day. *Dental Bulletin Supplement to the Army Medical Bulletin.* 1933;4:70,71.

4. [Ottolengui R]. Dentists in the Army. *Items of Interest.* 1898;20:522.

5. Resolutions adopted by the Odontographic Society, the Chicago Dental Society and the Odontological Society of Chicago. *Dent Rev.* 1898;12:572.

6. [Harlan AW]. Dentists in the Army and Navy. *Dent Rev.* 1898;12:566.

7. Stanley CC. Dentists in the Army and Navy. *Dental Cosmos.* 1898;40:558.

8. [Taft J]. Dentists in the Army. *Dental Register.* 1898;52:345–346.

9. Dentists in the Army and Navy. *Tex Dent J.* 1898;16:92.

10. [Hunt GE]. A failure. *Ind Dent J.* 1898;1:811–813.

11. Walker WE, comp. Minutes of transactions of the National Dental Association, session of 1898. Cited in: *Transactions of the National Dental Association.* Philadelphia Pa: The SS White Dental Mfg Co; 1899: 33, 50–57.

12. *Congressional Record, 55th Cong, 3rd Sess.* Vol 32. Washington, DC: Government Printing Office; 1899: 51, 1253, 1290.

13. US Congress. House. *Reorganization of the Army,* 55th Cong, 3rd Sess, 1898. House Report 1709; pt 1: 2.

14. [Taft J]. Dentists in the Army and Navy. *Dental Register.* 1899;53:46.

15. Finley MF, Butler CS, Donnally W. Report of Committee on the Appointment of Dentists to the Army and Navy. Cited in: *Transactions of the National Dental Association.* Philadelphia, Pa: The SS White Dental Mfg Co; 1900: 12, 56–58, 193, 194.

16. [Kirk EC]. The appointment of dental surgeons in the Army and Navy service of the United States. *Dental Cosmos.* 1899;41:188.

17. Wood W. The necessity of dentists in the Army and Navy. Cited in: *Transactions of the National Dental Association.* Philadelphia, Pa: The SS White Dental Mfg Co; 1900: 205–206.

18. Moore LC. Dentists in the Army and Navy. Cited in: *Transactions of the National Dental Association.* Philadelphia, Pa: The SS White Dental Mfg Co; 1900: 192.

19. RL Polk & Co. *R.L. Polk & Co.'s Dental Register of the United States 1896–97*. 2nd ed. Detroit, Mich: RL Polk & Co; 1896:248.

20. [Fife JG]. Dentists in the Army and Navy. *Tex Dent J*. 1899;17:36–37.

21. [Litch WF]. Army and Navy Dentists. *Dental Brief*. 1899;4:406–407.

22. Sibley LW. The necessity for dental surgeons in the Army and Navy. Cited in: Seventh District Dental Society, State of New York [proceedings]. *Dental Cosmos*. 1899;41:687–688.

23. [Ginsti JJ]. Need of dental services in the Army. *Items of Interest*. 1900;22:154.

24. Stark WT. Dentists in the Army and Navy. *West Dent J*. 1899;13:97–99.

25. Heitman. *Historical Register*. Vol 2. 259.

26. [Patterson JD]. Dentists in the Army and Navy. *West Dent J*. 1899;13:139.

27. Fish WL. Report of committee in relation to dentists in the Army. *Items of Interest*. 1900;22:67–68.

28. Marshall JS. The United States Army Dental Corps. Cited in: *Transactions of the Fourth International Dental Congress*. Vol 1. Philadelphia Pa: The SS White Dental Mfg Co; 1905: 54–55.

29. Catching BH. Army and Navy dental surgery. *Int Dent J*. 1899;20:716,717.

30. National Dental Association [proceedings]. *Dental Cosmos*. 1899;41:916.

31. Chupein TF. Dentists for the Army and Navy. *Dental Office and Laboratory*. 1899;13:142,143.

32. *Congressional Record, 56th Cong, 1st Sess*. Vol 33. Washington, DC: Government Printing Office; 1900.

33. [Ottolengui R]. Dentists in the Army. *Items of Interest*. 1900;22:76–78,218–219.

34. Dentists in the Army, H.R. 972. *Dental Office and Laboratory*. 1900;14:91–92.

35. Donnally W. Army dental surgeons. *Ind Dent J*. 1900;3:103.

36. Dental Surgeons for the Army and Navy. *Dental Headlight*. 1900;21:45.

37. Army dentists. *Dental Digest*. 1900;6:66–67.

38. The Odontographic Society of Chicago [proceedings]. *Dent Rev*. 1900;14:887–888.

39. [Kirk EC]. Dental surgeons in the Army and Navy. *Dental Cosmos*. 1900;42:102–103.

40. Dental surgeons for the Army. *Dental Brief*. 1900;5:166.

41. Donnally W. Report of the Committee on Army and Navy Dental Legislation. Cited in: Transactions of the National Dental Association. *Dental Digest*. 1902:217–218.

42. Finley MF, Butler CS, Donnally W. Report of the Committee on Army and Navy Dental Legislation. Cited in: *Transactions of the National Dental Association*. Philadelphia, Pa: The SS White Dental Mfg Co;1907:20,21.

43. US House. *Dental Surgeons in the United States Army, 56th Cong, 1st Sess, 1900*. House Report 468: 1–3.

44. [Harlan AW]. Dentists for the Army and Navy. *Dent Rev*. 1900;14:162–163.

45. Dentists in the Army. *Int Dent J*. 1900;21:137–138.

46. [Ottolengui R]. Dentists in the Army. *Items of Interest*. 1900;22:218–219.

47. [Ottolengui R]. Dental bills in Congress. *Items of Interest*. 1900;22:306.

48. [Litch WF]. The supervising board of Army dentists. *Dental Brief*. 1900;5:230,289.

49. [Hunt GE]. The supervising board of Army dentists. *Ind Dent J*. 1900;3:535.

50. National Dental Association [proceedings]. *Dental Cosmos*. 1900;42:895,902,903.

51. Finley MF, Butler CS, Donnally W. Report of the Committee on Army and Navy Dental Legislation. Cited in: *Transactions of the National Dental Association*. Philadelphia, Pa: The SS White Dental Mfg Co; 1901: 213–214.

52. National Dental Association [proceedings]. *Dental Cosmos*. 1901;43:72–73.

53. Baldwin AE. Handwriting upon the wall: what does it portray? *Dental Cosmos*. 1900;42:793.

54. *Congressional Record, 56th Cong, 2nd Sess*. Vol 34. Washington, DC: Government Printing Office; 1901.

55. Army reorganization bill as it relates to dentists. *Dental Digest*. 1901;7:62–65.

56. Obituary. Dr. Henry J.B. McKellops. *Dental Cosmos*. 1901;43:702–704.

57. [Litch WF]. 'Contract' Army dentists and surgeons. *Dental Brief*. 1903;8:742–743.

58. [Harlan AW]. The Army reorganization bill. The pressure for dental surgeons as the bill was finally passed. The appointment of examiners. *Dent Rev*. 1901;15:175.

59. [Litch WF]. Dental surgeons in the Army. *Dental Brief*. 1901;6:225,227.

95. US War Department. *General Orders and Circulars, Adjutant General's Office, 1901.* Washington, DC: Government Printing Office. 1902; No. 39, March 21, 1901; par 1280.

96. US War Department. *General Orders and Circulars, Adjutant General's Office, 1901.* Washington, DC: Government Printing Office. 1902; No. 46, April 6, 1901, par 1020.

97. US War Department. Enclosure to letter, Sternberg to the adjutant general, December 24, 1900, 2. *General Orders and Circulars, Adjutant General's Office, 1901.* Washington, DC: Government Printing Office. 1902. No. 77614.

98. US War Department. *General Orders and Circulars, Adjutant General's Office, 1901.* Washington, DC: Government Printing Office. 1902; No. 53, 18, par 26, April 18, 1901.

99. Army Dental Surgeons, rules and regulations. *Dental Brief.* 1901;6:310–311.

100. Hatch HD. Military dental practice: its modifications and limitations. *JAMA.* 1901;37:164–165.

101. Marshall JS. Opening discussion on military dental practice: its modifications and limitations. *JAMA.* 1901;37:165–166.

102. Marshall JS. The need of dental surgeons in the Army and Navy. In: *Transactions of the American Medical Association.*

103. National Archives and Records Administration. Record Group 112. Marshall to Williams Donnally, July 30, 1901. Letter. Entry 311:114.

104. Donnally W. Report of the Committee on Army and Navy Dental Legislation. In: *Transactions of the National Dental Association.* Chicago, Ill: Dental Digest;1901:217–219.

105. *Congressional Record.* Act of Feb. 2, 1901. 56th Cong, 2nd session, Sec 18, 31 Stat 752, Section 1.

106. *Congressional Record.* Army Medical Reorganization Act. Act of April 23, 1908. 61st Cong, 35 Stat 66.

107. The Medical Department. Chap 19. *US War Department, the Military Laws of the United States 1915.* 5th ed. Washington, DC: Government Printing Office; 1917.

108. Office of the Surgeon General. *Manual for the Medical Department.* Washington, DC; Government Printing Office; 1906.

109. National Archives and Records Administration. Record Group 112. John Sayre Marshall to the surgeon general, August 19, 1902. No. 89178. Box 616. Entry 26.

110. National Archives and Records Administration. Record Group 112. John Sayre Marshall to the surgeon general, May 29, 1903. No. 89178. Box 616. Entry 26.

111. Army Dental Corps items. *Dental Cosmos.* 1903;40:983.

112.   Army Dental Corps items. *Dental Cosmos*. 1905;44:543.

113.   The Army Dental Corps. *The Pacific Dental Gazette*. 1904;12:429–432.

114.   Marshall JS. The United States Army Dental Corps. In: *History of Dental Surgery*. Vol 1. Fort Wayne, Ind: National Art Publishing Co; 1910.

Chapter VII

BUILDING THE FOUNDATION: THE EARLY YEARS OF ARMY DENTISTRY, 1901–1904

Introduction

The carefully selected initial group of contract dental surgeons formed the cornerstone for the development of Army dentistry. But until the new dental surgeons actually reached their assigned posts in Cuba, Puerto Rico, the Philippines, and in the United States itself and began to see patients, they could not contribute to the well-being of the soldiers or confirm the wisdom of their service's creation. The new Army dentists learned through trial and error until they and their supervisors became acclimated to the Army and their new duties and gained the confidence and support of the officers and soldiers they served. John Marshall, the senior supervising and examining contract dental surgeon, carried the principal burden of representing the Army's new dental service to the surgeon general, the Medical Department, and the American dental community. Across the Pacific Ocean in the Philippines, Robert Todd Oliver, the second highest ranking dental surgeon, had to build a dental service from scratch for American soldiers heavily engaged in the Philippine Insurrection. The eventual success or failure of Marshall and Oliver in these crucial roles and that of the contract dental surgeons in their daily work would largely determine the future of dentistry in the US Army.

Dentists in the Philippines

The majority of the newly hired contract dental surgeons were to be sent to attend to the more than 60,000 US troops serving in the Philippine Islands. Within days of the passage of the February 2 act, Colonel Charles Greenleaf, Medical Corps, chief surgeon, Division of the Philippines, wrote to the surgeon general about the section of the act that allowed enlisted personnel of the Hospital Corps to be appointed as contract dental surgeons without examination. Such appointments would provide trained dental surgeons in the Philippines much more quickly than would examinations in Washington, but he feared that no members of the Hospital Corps in his division would be eligible because none had been detailed to dental duties continuously for 12 months.[1]

On February 11 the surgeon general wrote to the adjutant general and recommended that Hospital Corps privates Samuel Hussey in Zamboanga, Mindanao, and Emmett Craig in Manila be discharged to accept contracts as dental surgeons. Exactly how this action took place is not clear today, but in April 1901, Craig and

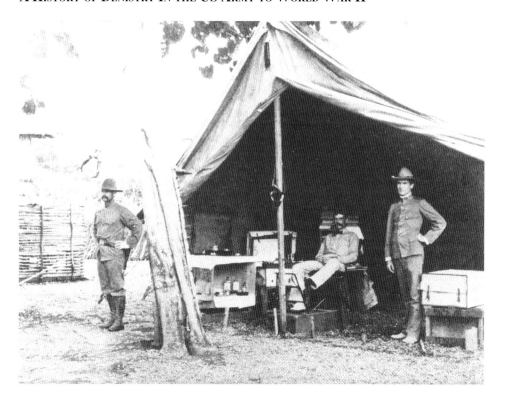

Dental offices under canvas at Camp Weyler, Samar, Philippine Islands, April 1902.
Reproduced from: Dental Cosmos. 1906;48:217.

Hussey were released from their enlistments to sign on as contract dental surgeons without examination, and thus became the first practicing dental surgeons to provide authorized Army dental care to American soldiers.[2,3]

On June 28, 1901, the Army transport carrying William Ware, Ralph Waddell, Hugo Rietz, Seibert Boak, Clarence Lauderdale, and Franklin Wing docked in Manila, which was then under military law. After reporting their arrival to the adjutant general and the surgeon general in Washington, they received orders from the division surgeon that scattered them throughout the various brigades stationed on the islands comprising the Division of the Philippines. In late July, Alden Carpenter, Douglas Foster, and Charles Petre were released from their enlistments to accept contracts as dental surgeons. Jean Whinnery, George Mason, and Frank Stone arrived from the United States on August 17, followed by Frank Wolven and Charles Long on September 6 and 17 respectively. Robert Oliver's arrival in Manila on October 16, 1901, brought the number of contract dental surgeons stationed in the Philippines to 17, over half of the dental surgeons then under contract.[4–6] If the dental surgeons were to quickly establish their credibility and their value to the Army, they had to do it in the Philippines.

While still in Washington on examining board duties in June 1901, Oliver asked

Surgeon General Sternberg for an assignment to the Philippines at the conclusion of the dental board's work. He thought "that the real business of actual supervising would occur in that division, then in a state of war, where a corps organization of dental surgeons would be an absolute necessity. . . ." On August 1, 1901, he received orders to report to Manila as the senior supervising and examining contract dental surgeon, with instructions to "organize and maintain" the dentists according to the needs of the division, which was then heavily engaged in the insurrection. Oliver later recalled that when he reported to the chief surgeon's office, Division of the Philippines, in Manila, the medical officers received him cordially and offered their assistance in organizing dental support.[4]

One immediate problem Oliver faced in Manila was an equipment shortage. Only 10 dentists had been issued the new official Army dental outfits, and even those were only partially complete. The five former hospital corpsmen were still using their own personal dental outfits. One dental surgeon in Laguna Province (probably William Ware) was forced to make do with the small, standard dental case issued to the Medical Department. The dentists moved around the various posts scattered throughout the American-occupied provinces as the dental needs of the

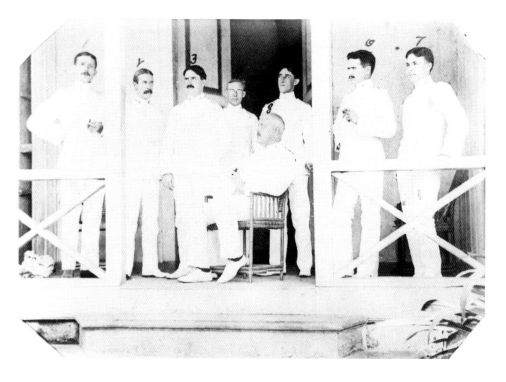

Hospital Operating Staff, Manila, Philippine Islands. From left to right:
1. Dr. Edwards; 2. Dr. Smith; 3. Dr. McAndrews; 4. Dr. Seibert D Boak;
5. Dr. William Waddell; 6. Dr. Keller; 7. Dr. Shook; 8. Major Arthur.
Photograph: Courtesy of Family of Seibert D Boak.

various commands dictated. From the start, they had more work than they could possibly accomplish. Local commanders frequently expected them to complete all necessary dental work in from 5 to 10 days, which Oliver judged to be "utterly impossible." Under such limitations, the dentists barely had sufficient time to provide pain relief, which they termed "emergency treatment," and to do some basic tooth conservation. Virtually every one of the contract dental surgeons assigned to the Philippines commented on the deplorable condition of the soldiers' mouths.[4]

The Philippine Division had more than 140 posts and was divided into the Department of North Philippines (containing the 1st, 2nd, 3rd, and 4th brigades) and the Department of South Philippines (containing the 5th, 6th, and 7th brigades). After his arrival, Oliver reorganized the assignments so the dentists were assigned based on brigade strength (Table 7-1).

There were not enough dental surgeons to assign one to each of the small posts distributed throughout the archipelago. Consequently, dentists were usually based at one of the larger stations in each territory. Using it as their base of operations, they would travel to the smaller posts, spending about 2 weeks at each before moving on. Patients came in from even smaller, adjacent commands for treatment. This itinerant or roving dental service was thought to allow access to more patients than if the patients were required to come in to one central base in each territory.[4]

The itinerant dentists, their assistants, and portable dental outfits usually moved in the mountain districts by pack train under an armed escort to protect them from insurrectionists. Between the various island stations, they traveled aboard native outrigger canoes called "praos." As safety improved, quartermaster wagons, the Manila-Dagupan Railroad, and chartered interisland Army transports were used. The outfit that always traveled with the dentists was packed in four chests and two crates. One crate contained the take-down chair and its equipment. Dental instrument chests contained all the dental supplies as well as operative instruments and appliances, and the dental engine chest held the engine (drill) and its equipment.[4]

TABLE 7-1

NUMBER OF DENTISTS ASSIGNED TO THE DIVISION OF THE PHILIPPINES

Department of North Philippines		Department of South Philippines		Manila	
Brigade	No. of dentists	Brigade	No. of dentists	Brigade	No. of dentists
1st	3	5th	2	N/A	2
2nd	2	6th	1		
3rd	3	7th	2		
4th	2				

Data source: Oliver RT. Three years' service in the Philippines. In: *Transactions of the National Dental Association.* Philadelphia, Pa: The SS White Dental Mfg Co; 1906.

In general, dental surgeons were given an operating room in the various station hospitals that they visited. However, it was not uncommon for them to be assigned space in the office of the quartermaster or even the commanding officer. Sometimes, particularly early in the pacification, their offices were located in various churches, monasteries, and even native shacks that were in close proximity to the hospitals. When no buildings were available, tents were used as operating rooms but proved to be a poor substitute because of lighting problems (direct sunlight was too hot and canvas-diffused light cast false shadows, preventing good visibility into the mouth). The tents were also damp, which caused the dental instruments to rust. Occasionally the dental surgeon was assigned a house to be used as an office and living quarters. At Camp McGrath in Batangas Province, where the 12th Cavalry Regiment was stationed, the commanding officer even had a special dental office built from plans that his dental surgeon submitted. However, this action was the exception rather than the rule.[4]

The dental surgeons soon learned that many dental instruments were not suited to the tropical climate. The first large consignment of supplies and equipment was stored on shelves in a well-ventilated storeroom at the medical supply depot in Manila. After a few weeks, many of the instruments, particularly the delicate root canal broaches, reamers, drills, and the like, were corroded with rust and therefore unusable. To prevent rusting, the larger instruments were wrapped in wax paper, carefully twisted at each end, and the smaller instruments were shipped either dipped in wax or packed in sealed phials.[4]

The contract dental surgeons suffered their first loss in February 1902 with the death of Charles Petre, DDS. After graduating from the Northwestern University Dental School, Chicago, in April 1899, Petre enlisted in the Army on August 9, 1899, as a private for service in the Philippines and was assigned to Company F, 20th US Infantry. Taking his dental instruments with him, he was detailed to the Hospital Corps in September 1899 while en route from San Francisco to Manila. Transferred officially to the Hospital Corps on January 13, 1900, Petre was detailed by "verbal order" of the commanding officer to do dental work for the officers and enlisted soldiers at the military hospital in Aparri, Luzon. On April 21, 1901, he applied to the surgeon general's office for an appointment as a contract dental surgeon, and on July 25 he signed his contract as a dental surgeon. On February 12, 1902, he died of "pyonephrosis intestinal obstruction."[7,8]

Years later, Oliver offered this comment on the Army's oral hygiene and the service that his "little pioneer corps" of dental surgeons rendered during his assignment in the Philippines:

> When the Dental Corps joined the army, during the Philippine Insurrection of 1901, and made its first surveys of the dental conditions, the results were simply appalling. The men had been on active campaign in tropical fields for many months, where no opportunities for dental attention existed. Toothbrushes and dentifrices were not issued regularly, and those of the original issue had long since passed usefulness. The mouths and teeth of these soldiers presented conditions bordering on filth, and in many cases, with resultant pathological lesions. If, at that time, we could have utilized a corps of dental hygienists for the purpose of scaling and cleaning teeth, as a preliminary procedure, the health and welfare of our 60,000 troops in the Philippine Islands would have been greatly improved.[9(p1118)]

a

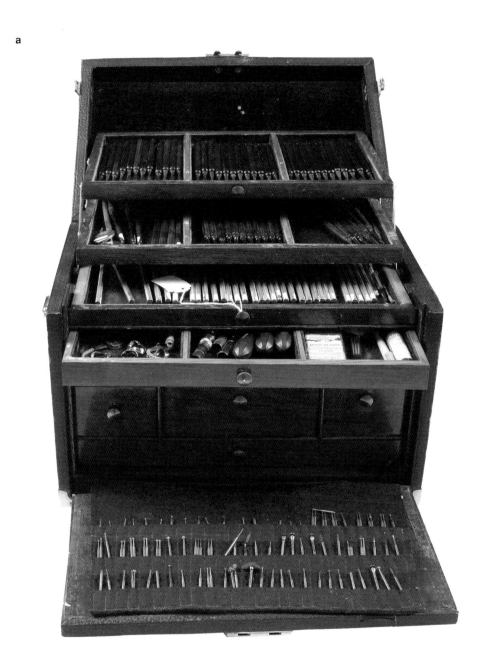

(*a*) Turn of the century dental chest, circa 1901. (*b*) Closed.
(*c*) Removable fabric pouch with space for tools was placed over of the top shelf before closing.
Photograph: Courtesy of US Army Medical Department Museum. Med 7270-1,2,3.

b

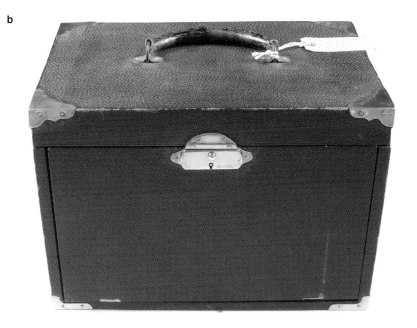

c

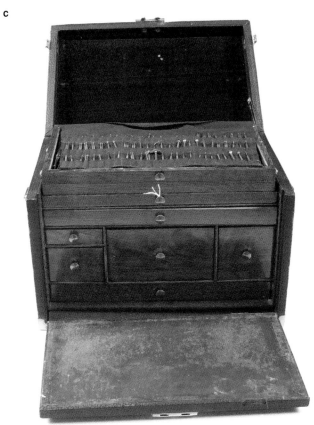

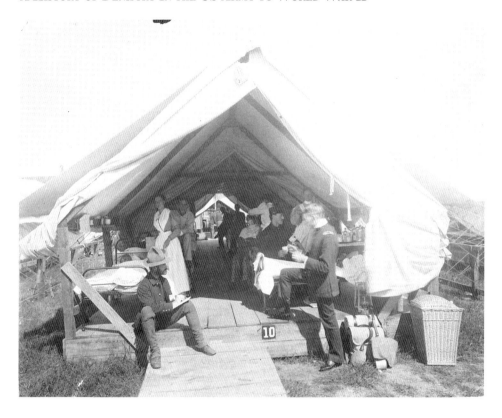

Hospital tent interior showing furnishings and occupants, circa 1898.
Photograph: Courtesy of US Army Medical Department Museum. Spawar-031.

By June 1902 Petre's loss was more than balanced with the arrival of four new dentists from March through May: John McAlister (1872–1935), John Millikin (1876–?), George Casaday (1874–?), and Julien Bernheim (1876–1943; later colonel and Dental Corps chief, 1928–1932), who was selected to fill the vacancy created by Petre's death. When the Philippine Insurrection ended on July 4, 1902, Oliver had 20 dentists at work throughout the islands.[5,10]

In the Field in the Philippines: Boak and Stone

Seibert Boak, the first dentist appointed among the examinees, described his initial Philippine duty assignments on the island of Luzon:

I was ordered to the province of Pampanga, which is about forty miles from Manila on Manila Dagupan R.R. [railroad], and where the finest sugar cane is raised. I arrived just in time for the rainy season, and in my five months' stay there had the experience of going through earthquake, typhoon and flood. Rain! We in the States have never seen a real rain as compared with these, where it rains straight for a month or two at a time. I certainly thought I was going to live to see the deluge reproduced. About the time I got my office fixed up to my satisfaction in one of the above-described nipa shacks of four rooms, a three weeks' rain started in and ended in a typhoon. I had to walk to post headquarters for my meals, and while there eating supper the typhoon started; consequently, we stayed up all night and saw our kitchen blow away. Next morning bright and early I started for my hut through a small river running down the street. The sight of devastation that met my gaze quickened my steps considerably, for the better part of my house was nowhere to be seen. I afterward found all my floatable articles performing aquatic feats in the large pools of water. But with hard work and the assistance of my hospital corps man and muchacho (boy) managed to get the office in shape by 2:00 p.m. So I did all necessary work in the rain until the quartermaster could get a native to fix my roof.[6]

After that experience Boak moved to Zambales Province for 3 months and finally to Tarlac Province. The troops welcomed him wherever he went, and all ranks treated him cordially, though one officer told him, "Your profession is a necessary evil we shall be unable to dispense with after awhile." Unmarried, Boak usually took his meals with the post staff, paying like any visiting officer.[6]

His duty day normally ran from 9 AM to 4 PM. In addition to his cases of equipment, he carried a small reference library provided by the Office of The Surgeon General, which included Burchard's *Pathology*, Marshall's *Oral Surgery*, and the *American Text-book of Operative Dentistry*. The government also provided subscriptions to *Dental Cosmos*, *International Dental Journal*, and *Dental Review*.[6]

Boak found that at least 60% of the personnel he examined had had no dental care other than extractions. Thus, he saw his first mission as overcoming the soldiers' "prejudice against dental treatment." This not only put them on the path to better health, but also conditioned them to seek better dental care once they left the service, benefiting them personally and dentistry in general. The result of better dental care could also be seen in the reduction of gastrointestinal complaints derived from poor oral conditions. Boak encountered many unusual cases that he felt increased his span of knowledge, but serious cases requiring major surgery and prosthetic work had to be referred to the base hospitals at Manila or Cebu because of lack of equipment.[6]

When he received orders to go to a new station, Boak gave advance notice of his arrival to the station commander, who readied an operating room and quarters. Upon arrival, his presence was announced to all commanding officers, who were asked to identify and schedule any of their soldiers who required care. Commanders were also asked to provide a list of all soldiers with syphilis so special precautions could be taken to avert the spread of secondary infection.[6]

With his itinerant deployment, Boak observed that he rarely had time to work a complicated case to satisfactory completion. Often he could only take temporary "emergency treatment" measures and move on. When these failed before his return, he gained an undeserved bad reputation and often caused the patient further discomfort. The remoteness of many posts and the deplorable traveling conditions often meant patients reached the dentist well into the final crisis. The huge volume of work, combined with itinerancy, frequently precluded any follow up, rarely allowing assessment of fully completed treatment. Many soldiers returned to the United States in various stages of dental care, generating some undeserved criticism from military and civilian dentists who took over treatment upon their return.[6]

Boak's first office at San Fernando, about 40 miles north of Manila, was the two-room shack that was destroyed by a typhoon just after he had set up his instruments. In a June 1907 article in *The Dental Register*, he related the many problems he encountered in trying to perform dentistry on the troops:

> Active campaigning, scant water supply, entire time filled with martial duties, constant alertness for the enemy, and in self-preservation, with loss to appear anything but the real fighting machine, this being especially true of the troops stationed in Mindanao and the Sulu archipelago, amongst the Moros, which rendered it almost impossible for a soldier to give even the ordinary care to his person, much less hygienic attention to his mouth. To these conditions add the trouble to secure a soldier after beginning treatment; when sent for he is either out on the firing line, doing guard or old guard fatigue duty, on a scouting expedition, or temporarily attached to some other outfit; or about the time you were in the midst of a month's visit to some command, be ordered away, or the command get field orders; supplies fail to reach you, due to lack of transportation by water or land, leaving you to complete a two months' detail without amalgam, cement, nerve broaches, or other necessary supplies, necessitating the use of mummifying paste, sealed in with cotton and sandarac varnish or gutta percha, where pulps have been extracted. It was often a serious question when out of supplies just what to do to secure permanent relief from pain and suffering, the dental surgeon being thrown on his own resources and ingenuity to accomplish it. A conscientious professional man will not extract except as a last resort, especially if he sees a chance of saving teeth that would otherwise be sacrificed.

> Let me put before you a typical case. I was ordered to go through a battalion of infantry, 450 men in the battalion, in one month, men being brought to the office in squads of twenty under a non-commissioned officer. Upon examining a soldier, find on left side one or two of the superior or inferior molars or bicuspids missing. Right side a molar or a bicuspid, or both, broken down and necrosed, this side bearing the whole stress of mastication. The question is, shall we extract them, leave them in that condition, or begin treatment, knowing the difficulties that will handicap us in the conservative treatment of such cases. If we extract we save our future reputation and take no chances, for if the soldier has trouble, not understanding the conditions or disadvantages we labor under, and has to suffer with no hopes for relief in sight, we get damned for it; for over there it is not a case of getting on a train or boat and in an hour or so get relief, but in most cases it means days. If we make some excuse and put them off, in all probability they will begin to give trouble at a very inopportune time, and a kick is registered by the commanding officer of the company, that a dental surgeon visited that post and left before he finished his work. This being forwarded through military channels, everybody from the C.O. up gets a chance to express their opinion, favorable or otherwise, as the case may be, and in all probability you are called upon to explain why treatment was not furnished in certain cases. If we start in to treat, and when ordered away find root canals are not in condition to fill, we have to place a dressing in the roots, insert cement and trust to nature to do the rest. This also applies to fillings. . . . In the military practice we examine the men as a body and do the required work whether they wish it or not, and the fact of men being ordered to have dental work done, independent of their own desires in the matter is not calculated to secure their co-operation, as general orders require that any soldier unfit for duty, from a cause that is removable by an operation not endangering life, who refuses to be operated upon, will be tried by court-martial and punished.[11(pp289–292)]

Some of the dentists experienced difficult and dangerous field duty. Frank Stone (later colonel and Dental Corps chief, 1934–1938, and the last of the original contract dental surgeons on active duty) was first assigned to Jolo Island and then to Malabang on Mindanao, where active warfare was underway against the Muslim Moros. Carrying his dental equipment on pack mules, he and his assistant accompanied the troops in operations around Lake Lanao. He later stated that his deployment marked "the first time that dental equipment was ever packed and carried in a supply train in actual service in any Army in the world." He frequently came under fire while working on patients in camp. On the march, he moved with the rear guard of the pack train and, because he could not do dental work, its commander used him as a courier to maintain contact with more advanced elements led by Captain (later General of the Armies) John J Pershing. Stone often found himself alone on the trail, sometimes menaced by Moros as he performed his duties. After 2 years of such arduous service, Stone was not in good health and was happy to get orders for duty at the hospital in Manila. Unfortunately, his field service left him so ill with amoebic dysentery that he left Manila on October 10, 1903 headed back to the US Army General Hospital at the Presidio of San Francisco as a patient rather than a practitioner. Stone was subsequently stationed there until 1906.[5,12]

Marshall at the Presidio of San Francisco

While Oliver was still on his way to Manila, Marshall arrived at the Presidio of San Francisco to find himself faced with a major organizational problem. Apparently some misunderstanding had arisen about whether Surgeon General Sternberg intended to assign Marshall to the post of the Presidio or to the US Army General Hospital, Presidio of San Francisco, Department of California. On September 2, 1901, Lieutenant Colonel (later Colonel and Brigadier General) Alfred Girard (1841–1914), Medical Corps, the hospital's commanding officer, telegraphed the surgeon general's office asking where Marshall was to be assigned. The ambiguous answer came back that Marshall was assigned to duty at the post, but that he could work at the hospital and at other posts in the Department of California under temporary assignments.[13,14]

Marshall was unhappy with this arrangement. On September 6 he wrote to Colonel William Forwood, the acting surgeon general, while Sternberg was in the Philippines, telling him that before leaving Washington Sternberg had directed that Marshall would be stationed at the general hospital, where he would have "greater opportunities for professional service and study than any other station in the country." Although his dental outfit had arrived, as of September 6 Marshall had not been assigned either an office or quarters. It seemed that there was a shortage of quarters for officers and that the post hospital was overcrowded. Girard, too, had expected him to be stationed at the hospital, not the post. On September 12 Forwood informed Marshall that although he personally favored assigning him to the hospital, the orders that Sternberg had left before his departure were that he should be assigned to the post.[15,16]

Upon his return to Washington, Sternberg telegraphed Marshall on October 11,

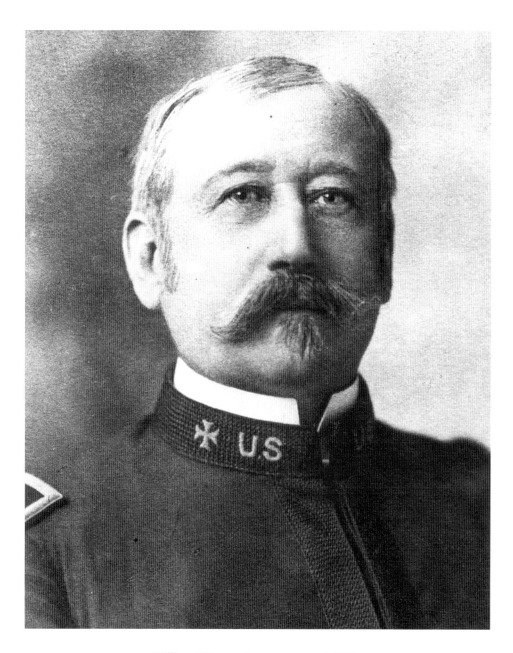

William H Forwood, surgeon general, 1902.
Photograph: Courtesy of the National Museum of Health and Medicine,
Armed Forces Institute of Pathology. NCP 3565.

asking whether he still preferred to be assigned to the general hospital. The next day, Marshall replied that although the current arrangements were "satisfactory," he still preferred to be assigned to the general hospital as soon as quarters were available there. Currently, he had quarters at the post with a one-room office at the hospital administration building, thanks to Girard. The situation at the Presidio was such that unless the quartermaster general built him an office building (which was unlikely to happen), no space was available. At the general hospital, room would become available as soon as the new officers' ward was completed. Marshall thought he needed at least three rooms, one for an office and waiting room, one for an operating room, and one for a laboratory and extracting room. The surgeon general directed Girard to provide the rooms that were accordingly furnished for dental operations. Marshall remained assigned to the post of the Presidio, but physically worked in the Presidio General Hospital until late July 1905.[17–22]

In addition to better accommodations, Marshall soon found that being in the Presidio General Hospital put him at the center of Medical Department activities at the Presidio and Department of California. Because of its mission in support of American forces deploying to and returning from the Philippines, the Presidio General Hospital was the largest and most important Army facility. As such, its commanders were carefully selected, and included Lieutenant Colonel George Torney (1850–1913), who took over in March 1904 and commanded it until he was chosen in November 1908 to succeed O'Reilly as Army surgeon general. Working for 4 years with Torney provided some advantages to Marshall in his dealings with the surgeon general's office after January 1909.[23]

New Contract Dental Surgeons Join the Army

Although the original dental examining board never reconvened and was officially dissolved on March 9, 1905, the three examining and supervising dental surgeons, John Marshall, Robert Oliver, and Robert Morgan (replaced in late 1901 by John Hess), were constantly called upon to examine candidates for their physical and professional fitness to be offered contracts as dental surgeons.[21,24,25] After Oliver reached the Philippines, he examined three enlisted soldiers for appointments as contract dental surgeons in late 1901, but found none to be qualified.[5] In February 1902 John Hess examined and passed Frank McDermott, who never served after accepting his contract.[26–28] From November 4, 1901, through July 5, 1902, Marshall handled the bulk of the examinations, which, he informed the surgeon general, "have been conducted with the same degree of care and thoroughness, as were those conducted by the full board during its sessions in Washington, D.C."[21] He examined 13 candidates at the Presidio and passed eight to fill existing vacancies or to be added to a list of eligible dentists who could be offered contracts should a vacancy occur.[21,29,30] The final three of the original 30 authorized contract dental surgeon positions were filled by candidates examined and passed by John Marshall: Alexander Bacon on November 25, 1901, who was ordered to Cuba to replace Robert Morgan; John McAlister, Jr (1872–1935) on January 23, 1902, who was assigned to the Philippines, where he arrived on March 10; and George Casaday (1874–?) on February 3, 1902, who was ordered to the Philippines, where he arrived on April 21.[31]

On February 17, 1902, Marshall examined and passed John Millikin (1876–?), who signed his contract on March 3 and replaced Hess, who had taken Morgan's position. The next two candidates Marshall examined eventually became chiefs of the Dental Corps: Julien Bernheim (who signed a contract on April 9 and was ordered to the Philippines to replace the recently deceased Charles Petre) on March 22, 1902; and Rex Rhoades (1875–1959), on July 5, 1902. Rhoades (later colonel) accepted his contract on November 10, 1902, and was the only two-time Dental Corps chief, serving before and after Bernheim from 1924 to 1928 and from 1932 to 1934. A sufficient pool of eligible candidates now existed, so no further examinations were held. When Bacon's contract was annulled in late June 1903, William Hammond replaced him. When some of the initial dental surgeons left the service upon expiration of their contracts in 1904, George Stallman replaced William Fisher on July 21, 1904, and George Gunckel replaced George Decker on August 6, 1904.[31]

American Forces in Cuba and Puerto Rico and Morgan's Replacement

As soon as contract dental surgeons were authorized, Army leaders in Cuba began pressing to have some assigned. In May 1901 Colonel Frank Baldwin, commanding the 7th Cavalry and garrison at Columbia Barracks in Havana, urged that at least one dentist be sent to his post. Lieutenant Colonel Valery Havard, the Army of Occupation's chief surgeon, and Major General (later Lieutenant General) Leonard Wood, its commander, both enthusiastically supported the request. They observed that the number of troops in Cuba justified the assignment of at least two dentists, one based at each end of the island and roving to provide support to other garrisons. Morgan and Dr George Decker were assigned in August 1901.[32–35] Shortly afterward Morgan became ill, and on October 31, 1901, Havard, now chief surgeon, Department of Cuba, reported his condition "serious" and recommended that he be granted immediate leave and be returned to the United States.[36,37]

Morgan left Cuba on November 3 on a month's sick leave, which the surgeon general subsequently extended to 2 months. Sternberg determined that Morgan was too sick to return to duty and that his contract would be annulled for physical disability, which it was on February 3, 1902.[37] On November 29, after learning more fully of Morgan's problems, Sternberg asked Marshall to recommend a replacement from among the current dental surgeons. On December 6 Marshall identified doctors Edwin Tignor, Robert Updyke, and John Hess as the best candidates to replace Morgan, but recommended Tignor as "the best qualified man in the Corps for this position." However, Sternberg selected John Hess (1870–1932) as the third supervising and examining dental surgeon, which Marshall later agreed was "a wise selection." The surgeon general instructed Marshall to give Hess "such instructions as you may think necessary regarding these examinations, the preparation of reports thereof, and other matters your experience may dictate," so that Hess would be uniform with Marshall and Oliver in his examinations and reports.[37–41]

Morgan's replacement in Cuba was Alexander Bacon, whom John Marshall had examined and passed and who accepted a contract on November 25, 1901. Bacon was assigned to Cuba and served there until April 30 the following year.[42]

Dr Hugo Voorhies reported for duty in Puerto Rico after passing his examinations

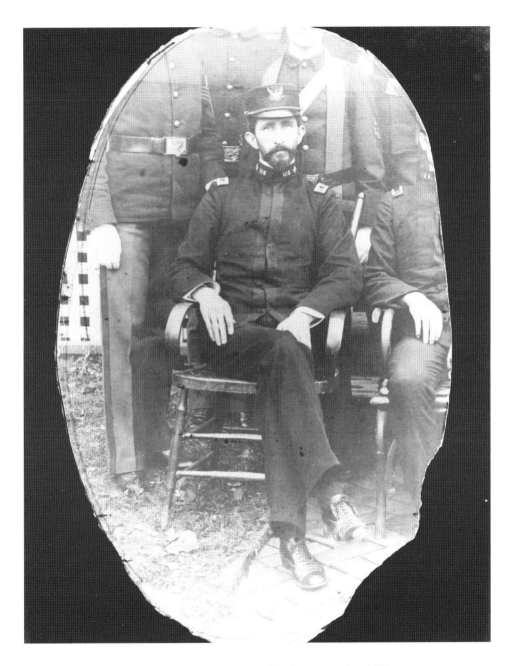

Edwin P Tignor as a contract dental surgeon, circa 1901.
Photograph: Courtesy of Lorraine Tignor.

and being hired in 1901. Although warned that military officers would receive him "very abruptly and formally," he later commented in an article in *The Dental Forum* that "on reporting, Col. Buchanan, Commanding Officer, and Capt. Blunt, Adjutant General of Porto Rico, greeted me with: 'Doctor, we are glad to see you;' 'been expecting you,' 'needing you,' and many other pleasing remarks which I was glad to hear."[43] He was courteously received wherever he went, and at the Officers' Club "some of them immediately proceeded to tell me about this tooth and that they wanted me to look after, so I began to feel, for the first time, a little at home and something of a fixture."[43] During his months on the island before transferring to Fort Porter, New York, in December 1902, Voorhies found very poor dental health among the soldiers but he reported that his work appreciably helped to change their dental hygiene habits:

> As to the nature of the work, there is considerable extracting, owing to the poor condition of the men's teeth, who have been in the service for some time, and who had not or did not save sufficient means to have their teeth attended to and are beyond redemption. The officers, as well as the enlisted men, highly appreciate the dental services rendered, and often remark what a great benefit it is to them. . . . We clean a good many teeth and do work for soldiers who never before received treatment of any kind. We instruct them in regard to caring for their teeth, and see that they furnish themselves with tooth brushes.[43(p176)]

While he noted that in Puerto Rico and later assignments the soldiers at every level seemed to genuinely appreciate his arrival as he rode his circuit, he also commented that "no doubt my departure was as equally enjoyable to them."[44] The beneficiaries of dental care immediately sensed the value of the new contract dental surgeon, even if they still retained much of their fear of dental treatment.

Voorhies's "The Care of the Teeth"

While in Puerto Rico, Voorhies had grown deeply concerned about the dental health of the soldiers he was treating. This concern prompted him to prepare an article titled "The Care of the Teeth" in English and Spanish, which he submitted to the chief surgeon of the Department of the East on May 29, 1902, and recommended for distribution to officers and enlisted soldiers on the island. In his article, one of the first preventive dentistry tracts prepared in the Army, he outlined the fundamentals of dental and oral health and laid out a basic concept that has guided much of preventive dentistry: "Precaution in youth is prevention in maturity: habits formed in childhood are practiced throughout life. If you properly care for your teeth in early life, you will not be apt to neglect them in after years." He recommended "a good tooth brush with bristles long enough to penetrate well the space between the teeth, have them stiff but not too stiff . . .," brushing after rising and every meal and before retiring at night, regular flossing, occasional use of mouth washes, removal of tartar deposits on the teeth, care of the gums, and visits to the dentist for examinations every 6 months. In his article, Voorhies concluded that "one person in a hundred have good teeth, ninety-nine in a hundred could have good teeth with proper attention." Although Voorhies's tract was written in

1902, it reads as if it were recently released by the American Dental Association.[45]

Brigadier General William Forwood (1838–1915), who succeeded Sternberg and served as Army surgeon general from June 8 to September 7, 1902, promptly sent Voorhies's proposed circular to John Marshall for comment on June 12. On June 23 Marshall replied that it was a good idea to place information on dental care and prevention of caries and oral diseases "in the hands of the Officers and enlisted men of the Army. . . ."[46,47] He went on:

> I believe if the enlisted men could be taught the value of oral hygiene, dental caries and the diseases which result from it would be much less prevalent than they are at present, while gastric and intestinal diseases, which are so common in camp life, might be greatly lessened.[47]

Marshall thought that "if a few simple rules upon the hygiene of the teeth and mouth, expressed in cogent language, were printed and distributed to each command sufficient in quantity to reach the enlisted men, that this would be sufficient to call proper attention to the subject."[47]

On July 1 Forwood returned Voorhies's article and asked Marshall "to prepare suitable rules for the care of the teeth and hygiene of the mouth, to be embodied in a circular for distribution among the officers and enlisted men of the Army." Marshall returned the requested information to the surgeon general's office on July 16.[48,49] Forwood retired on September 7 and Robert O'Reilly (1845–1912), who had been the chief surgeon of the Department of California at the Presidio of San Francisco since June 1902, became the surgeon general (1902–1909). A few days later, O'Reilly told Voorhies that his proposed article on dental hygiene was "duly considered." However, "it was not deemed advisable to publish it in circular form."[50] There is no indication that the Voorhies circular ever appeared, but Marshall's work was just begun and would resurface in September 1903, soon after he presented his paper at the NDA meeting in late July.

John Marshall's 1902 Report on the Presidio's Dental Service

All of the contract dental surgeons, especially John Marshall, spent endless hours writing about their status and work for dental journals and speaking at national, state, and local dental societies whenever and wherever they could. A good example of this was Marshall's speech in June 1902 at the annual meeting of the California State Dental Association at San Francisco, where he spoke about the first year of the dental service at the Presidio of San Francisco. *Dental Cosmos* reported as follows on Marshall's talk:

> The necessity of dental surgeons in the army is very great. In the last nine months at the Presidio 3452 sittings were given and between five and six thousand operations performed. Three chairs are in continual service from 9 A.M. to 4 P.M., with an hour's intermission at noon for lunch. A great many diseases are encountered that are peculiar to the tropical climates, and inflammatory conditions of the mouth that the speaker has not seen before are apparent in the mouths of the returning soldiers from the Philippines. There is an ulcerated condition of the gums and the oral

mucous membrane, beginning at the festoons, sweeping in both directions following the gum line and traversing the entire mouth. The teeth become loosened, but there is no other evidence of scorbutic symptoms. Most cases have a great deal of salivary calculus, and, in treating these lesions of the mouth, dysentery and diarrhea are cured in a few weeks that without treating the oral cavity would have required care for months.[51(p1072)]

Marshall then described the Presidio dental clinic's personnel:

I have with me in my office four hospital corps men. One of them is a graduate of the Toronto Dental College. The other man has had one year in college, and I learned afterwards that he had about five years in some of these cheap John offices as an operator. I have another man who acts as clerk and keeps the records, and a fourth man who assists me individually at my chair. There are three chairs going all the time from 9 o'clock in the morning until 4 o'clock in the afternoon, with an hour or an hour and a quarter intermission. We are doing every day just as much work as it is possible for three men to do. I had an idea that there would be a time when the work would let up but we are just as busy to-day as we were when we first started in. I could keep five men busy at the Presidio. We have something like 5,000 troops all told, that is, in camp, in quarters and in the hospital. More than that, all the outlying posts in this department come to the Presidio for their dental care. So I do not expect we shall ever find the time when we shall have a let up in the amount of work we have to do.[52(p530)]

John Marshall's Official Reports on the Work of the Dental Surgeons, 1901–1903

As the senior supervising and examining contract dental surgeon, John Marshall was responsible for reporting officially to the surgeon general on the annual activities of all of the dental surgeons in the Army. He also reported widely to the dental community through the dental press and journals, such as *Dental Cosmos* and *Dental Review*, and spoke often at national, state, and local dental societies to keep dentists fully informed on what the Army dentists were doing. Despite the problems noted by the dentists in overseas positions, in a letter published in the February 1902 *Dental Review*, Marshall assessed the overall situation for Army dentistry as favorable. The support of the retiring Surgeon General George Sternberg, who "has given the dental corps every facility for its work" and "gave his hearty approval to all that we asked for," was largely responsible for this situation. Already commonly referred to among themselves and in the dental press as the "Dental Corps of the Army" or more simply the "Army Dental Corps," the contract dental surgeons were now deployed throughout the Army, hard at work, beginning to change dental hygiene habits, and were generally well received (Table 7-2).[53–55]

Marshall's official reports for 1902 and 1903, actually covering calendar years 1901 and 1902, provide a more detailed look at the work of the dental surgeons, the dental health of the US Army of the time, and some of the major issues with which the dental surgeons dealt. Since 1818 the Army surgeon general had compiled a detailed report on the annual activities of the Medical Department that was submitted to the secretary of war and published as the "Annual Report of The Surgeon General." On August 19, 1902, after tediously collecting as much data as he

TABLE 7-2

THE 1902 ROSTER OF CONTRACT DENTAL SURGEONS, US ARMY

Examining and Supervising Dental Surgeons	Location
John S Marshall	San Francisco, California
Robert T Oliver	Manila, Philippine Islands
John H Hess	West Point, New York
Contract Dental Surgeons	
George M Decker	Havana, Cuba
Alexander P Bacon	Havana, Cuba
Hugh G Voorhies	San Juan, Puerto Rico
Robert P Updike	Fort Leavenworth, Kansas
Edwin P Tignor	Fort Riley, Kansas
William C Fisher	Fort Sheridan, Illinois
Ord M Sorber	Fort Sam Houston, Texas
William H Chambers	Fort Monroe, Virginia
John D Millikin	Philippine Islands
Julien R Bernheim	Philippine Islands
Emmett J Craig	Philippine Islands
Samuel W Hussey	Philippine Islands
Clarence E Lauderdale	Philippine Islands
Seibert D Boak	Philippine Islands
Franklin F Wing	Philippine Islands
George L Mason	Philippine Islands
Hugo C Rietz	Philippine Islands
William H Ware	Philippine Islands
Ralph W Waddell	Philippine Islands
Jean C Whinnery	Philippine Islands
Frank H Wolven	Philippine Islands
Frank P Stone	Philippine Islands
Douglas E Foster	Philippine Islands
Alden Carpenter	Philippine Islands
Charles J Long	Philippine Islands
John A McAlister	Philippine Islands
George H Casaday	Philippine Islands

Data source: Roster of dental surgeons, US Army. *Dental Cosmos*.1902;44:402.

could from the dental surgeons (the returns from the Philippines were incomplete), Marshall submitted his initial report summarizing the selection, assignment, and work of the initial contract dental surgeons. Delays in shipping and receiving equipment and supplies, especially in the Philippines, he noted, had prevented some of the dentists from being fully operational until late in 1901.[56]

Marshall reported that in less than a year in 1901, the dental surgeons had seen 9,148 patients—9,125 regulars (2,872 in the United States, 5,174 in the Philippines, and 1,079 in Cuba and Puerto Rico), and 23 volunteers (7 in the United States and 16 in the Philippines), but again noted that the Philippine reports were incomplete and the numbers there would likely be higher. Dental procedures performed on these patients included treating 8,408 teeth with caries, of which 7,035 teeth were filled and 2,072 extracted. The large number of extractions was due to severe dental caries found among soldiers in Cuba, Puerto Rico, and the Philippines. The dental surgeons were instructed to conserve all teeth that could be made healthy with treatment to minimize their loss. Marshall noted that dental caries seemed to be more active after the soldiers had been in the tropical climate for several months. The exact cause for this was not then clear, but Marshall believed that it was a combination of poor dental care during active operations, the effect of the tropical climate, and food and dietary changes.[56] He concluded:

> . . . pyorrhea alveolaris and inflammatory and ulcerative conditions of the gums and oral mucous membrane are very prevalent among officers and enlisted men who have served, or are serving in the tropics. These conditions are more noticeable in those who have been in the Philippines for a considerable period, and in those who have suffered from certain forms of illness. These conditions seem to be largely due in the former to the enervating and debilitating effects of the hot climate etc., and in the latter to such wasting diseases as gastritis, diarrhea, dysentery and the continued fevers.[56(p4)]

TABLE 7-3

DENTAL CARE IN THE US ARMY, CALENDAR YEARS 1901–1902

	No. of Cases	
	1901 (partial year)	1902 (full year)
Cases of dental caries	8,408	31,092
Fillings (all types)	7,035	24,652
Extractions	2,072	6,043
Patients	9,148	16,161
Total operations	13,498	49,483

Data sources: (1) Office of the Surgeon General. *Annual Report of the Surgeon General.* Washington, DC: OTSG; 1902: 18–24. (2) Office of the Surgeon General. *Annual Report of the Surgeon General.* Washington, DC: OTSG;1903: 20–29.

Marshall's reports for 1902 and 1903 contain the first detailed accounts of the dental health of the US Army at the time. Though much had been written in previous years, the details only became clear when the dental surgeons actually began their daily work with the soldiers (Table 7-3). Perhaps more significant in reinforcing Marshall's conclusions are the statistics when broken down by geographic area for calendar year 1902, the first full year of dental operations (Table 7-4). But Marshall's report often read more like an advertising pamphlet for the dental surgeons and the establishment of a permanent dental corps:

> The service of the dental corps have been highly appreciated by the officers and enlisted men of the regular and volunteer armies and have proved very satisfactory to the Medical Department, because they have been able to relieve a great amount of acute suffering, and to conserve a large number of teeth and restore them to a healthy condition, thus almost immediately returning to duty many cases that were previously carried for days upon the company sick-report. This has resulted in greatly reducing the loss of valuable time to the service, incident to diseases of the mouth, teeth and jaws, and relieving and hastening the cure of such gastric and intestinal disorders as were due to defective mastication, and infective and suppurative conditions of the teeth and oral cavity. . . . The cost of maintaining the dental corps is small when compared with the relief from suffering obtained and the greater efficiency of the officers and men, who have received the services of the dental surgeons. Good teeth are an essential factor in maintaining the general health of our troops and consequently of their efficiency, and on account of the increasing prevalence of dental caries and the abnormal condition growing out of the disease the dental surgeon has become a necessity to the army. Early provision should therefore be made for the establishment of a permanent corps of dental surgeons attached to the Medical Department.[56(p6)]

TABLE 7-4

DENTAL CARE IN THE US ARMY BY STATION, 1902

	No. of Cases			
	United States	Philippines	Cuba and Puerto Rico	Total
Cases of dental caries	11,206	18,626	1,260	31,092
Fillings (all types)	9,310	14,468	874	24,652
Extractions	2,017	3,632	394	6,043
Patients	6,940	8,153	1,068	16,161
Total operations	18,971	28,115	2,897	49,483

Data source: Office of the Surgeon General. *Annual Report of the Surgeon General*. Washington, DC: OTSG; 1903: 20–27.

Marshall's report was printed in the 1902 annual report largely as he submitted it, his editorializing included. His report of July 2, 1903, contained as much opinion as did his earlier report, but this time Major (later Brigadier General) Walter Mc-Caw, Medical Corps, who edited the annual compilations in the surgeon general's office, used a generous red pencil. Marshall's more opinionated comments never appeared in the printed 1903 annual report, which was more statistical and factual. When finally printed, a new paragraph, probably written by McCaw, was inserted in the report, stating:

> The foregoing interesting tabulations, with professional comments, have been ably prepared for this report by Dr. John S. Marshall, contract examining and supervising dental surgeon, U.S. Army. The work of the contract dental surgeons has been of a high order and deserves commendation. Reports from experienced officers of the Army indicate that appreciation of the faithful and efficient services of the army dentist is steadily growing among officers and men.[57–59]

What Marshall actually submitted in his report was as follows:

> In the report of 1901 attention was called to the value of dental surgeons, from the economic standpoint, and the statement was made that "the cost of maintaining the Corps of Dental Surgeons was small when compared with the relief from suffering obtained, and the greater efficiency of the officers and enlisted men who had received the services of the Dental Surgeons." It may be added that the financial saving to the government will be very considerable in the future by preventing the loss to the service of the officers, enlisted men and nurses, by reason of incapacity for duty incident to dental diseases and their sequelae, and also to the probable future reduction in the number of claims for pensions, by preventing the loss of the teeth from disease while in the service. . . . The Dental Surgeons have therefore become an indispensable adjunct to the Medical Department of the Army, and it is recommended that suitable legislation be enacted to place them on a permanent basis in the service.[60]

The surgeon general's office would not allow such explicit lobbying for a dental corps to be published in its official report to the secretary of war, especially when the dental associations were lobbying for the creation of a commissioned corps to replace the contract dental surgeons and the secretary opposed it.

In collecting the data from his fellow dental surgeons for these annual reports, Marshall noted serious shortcomings in the system of recording and reporting dental operations. On September 12, 1903, he wrote to the surgeon general of the importance of the numerical reports. He wanted a structured system of accurate reports using a more detailed form and wanted all the reports to come to him:

> Reports of this character to be of scientific value must be correct and it goes without saying that there has never been in the history of the profession any method of gathering and tabulating statistics upon these subjects, which cover so large a number of cases and with such completeness of details as do those of the Corps of Dental Surgeons, U.S.A. . . . These statistics are bound to be quoted, discussed and written about a great deal in the future by dental authors and on this account they should be made as accurate as possible.[61]

It took more than a year for Marshall to finally bring the surgeon general's office around to his views on the inadequacies of its proposed register of dental operations and to accept his suggested form for standardized reporting.[62,63] Accurate and complete data collection on dental operations was an important tool in patient care and in demonstrating the value of the dental surgeons' work to improving the health of the Army in an era that prized the powers and benefits of modern science and research. Marshall placed emphasis on this aspect of his work because it could contribute significantly to winning the argument for commissioned status.

John Marshall and the 1903 Annual Meeting of the National Dental Association

In June 1903 politics surfaced when the president of the National Dental Association (NDA), Dr LG Noel of Nashville, Tennessee, wrote to the surgeon general requesting that Marshall not be appointed as the Army's delegate to the association's annual meeting in Asheville, North Carolina. Apparently Mark Finley, the chairman of the association's Committee on Army and Navy Dental Legislation, did not want Marshall to attend, going so far as to call on O'Reilly in person to express his opposition to Marshall's attendance. Noel stated that although he did not desire to make this incident "an open fight" with Marshall or "stir up trouble" among the dental surgeons, he wanted to "stop his coming." He hinted that Marshall had caused "trouble" 2 years earlier at the 1901 Milwaukee meeting. Noel contended that the entire committee, as well as the chairman of the executive committee, Dr JD Patterson, and three of its other members, were also opposed to Marshall.[64–66] The other most influential member of the Army and Navy committee was Williams Donnally, who had originally desired Marshall's position on the dental board for himself and had been at odds with him since 1901. On July 6, 1903, the surgeon general's office informed Marshall that the secretary of war, "after careful consideration of the matter," thought it not "practicable" to designate him as the Army's delegate.[67]

Not only did Marshall show up in Asheville, however, but he also presented an important paper on preventive dentistry and the oral diseases peculiar to the troops in the Philippines. Because the Presidio was the primary reception center for soldiers either embarking or disembarking for service in the Pacific theater, Marshall was stationed at the ideal location to evaluate the troops returning from the Philippines. The surgeon general's report for the year ending June 30, 1903, showed that dental diseases were 18.27% higher among the troops serving in the Philippines than those stationed in the states. Periodontal disease was especially high. The disease called "sprue," a chronic inflammation of the alimentary canal, also caused sore mouth.[68]

Marshall was a keen observer of the soldiers' medical and dental conditions and began to focus on the poor hygienic conditions of the soldiers' mouths. Soon he came to connect soldiers with chronic diarrhea and dysentery with ulcerated conditions of their gums and mucous membranes. "These cases of intestinal disease often make exceedingly slow progress towards convalescence," he noted, "some of them remaining in the hospital month after month with little permanent improvement." He wrote:

In a conversation with Colonel A.C. Girard, who was at that time in command of the hospital, I suggested that there might be some important relationship existing between chronicity of the disease and unhygienic condition of the mouth, and that is was not improbable that in some of these cases the unclean condition of the oral cavity was a source of secondary infection. He therefore issued an order directing that all obstinate cases of these diseases be sent to me for examination and treatment of any abnormal oral conditions that might be present. In some of the most obstinate cases I found the mouth and teeth in very unclean condition, the gums inflamed and turgid, the oral mucous membrane inflamed, and in some of the worst cases the mucous follicles were enlarged, forming vesicles which later ruptured, leaving small ulcerated patches, which in the course of twenty-four hours were covered with a curdy white pellicle.[68(p556)]

Marshall began treating these cases by spraying patients' mouths with a 25% solution of hydrozone, painting their gums with an iodine and aconite mixture, and touching the ulcerated patches with a 10% solution of silver nitrate. Within 10 days, the mouth symptoms were cured, "and almost immediately thereafter the general condition of the patient began to improve, and many after a few weeks more were discharged as convalescent." Marshall concluded: "This I think proves the fact that in those cases in which rapid improvement in the general condition of the patient followed the cleansing of the teeth and the treatment of the mouth, the chronicity of the disease was due to constant reinfection from the unhygienic condition of the oral cavity."[68(pp556–557)]

Already a strong proponent of preventive dentistry and of the dental hygiene movement of the era, Marshall's medical background also led him to believe that many illnesses began in the mouth:

The menace to the general health through an unclean mouth and diseased teeth is by no means even approximately appreciated either by the medical and dental professions or the laity, as is evidenced by the fact that very few physicians take into account the influence of diseases of the mouth and teeth upon the general health when examining a patient for some obscure disease of the general system. . . . Many cases of what have appeared to be due to malarial influences or bad plumbing have been traced to an unclean or diseased condition of the teeth and mouth, while numerous cases of gastric and intestinal affections have been traced to the same source.[68(pp559–560)]

After 2 years of treating soldiers, Marshall knew from first-hand experience that soldiers neglected the care of their teeth and mouths despite the repeated admonitions of Army surgeons and dental surgeons to keep their teeth and mouths clean, use toothbrushes, and rinse their mouths after meals. The general public was no less guilty than the American soldiers in their poor oral and dental hygiene habits. Marshall believed that the dental surgeon had to educate both the public and the soldier. He noted "if we do not teach this in season and out of season we are not performing our duty to our patients nor fulfilling our obligations to the state."[68(p560)]

Marshall's approach to get his point across began in his office in the Presidio General Hospital, where he placed large cards that read "Clean teeth do not decay" and "Do not ask the dental surgeon to treat your teeth until after you have brushed them." These helped get the message to his patients, who showed marked improvement after some months and visits. "I have been greatly pleased with the good impression that this information and suggestion has had upon men, for after the first or second visit there is a marked change in the appearance of their teeth," he noted. "These men also spread the information among their fellows, and I can already see a marked change in the care given to the teeth by the men of the whole garrison."[68(pp560–561)]

Marshall's Proposed Circular and the Soldier's Handbook

On September 14, 1903, following close on the heels of his NDA paper at Asheville, Marshall wrote to Surgeon General O'Reilly about the need for a circular on the "Hygiene of the Teeth and Mouth" that should be issued "to the Army for its instruction in the care of the teeth and mouth and as a prophylactic measure against dental and oral disease." He told O'Reilly that he had originally prepared the circular at Surgeon General Forwood's request in July 1902, but apparently his draft was lost during the change of command to Robert O'Reilly. Marshall continued:

> I have therefore deemed it my duty as the senior officer of the dental corps to call attention to the fact that much of the suffering experienced by our own troops through diseases of the teeth and the mouth could be prevented by the employment of such hygienic methods, as are recommended in this circular. . . . My experiences in military dental surgery during the past two and a half years has proved to me that there is a very general lack of information upon the part of the enlisted men of the army, of the means which they can employ to prevent dental caries and other diseases of the mouth. Good teeth are so important to the comfort and health of the individual, and consequently to the efficiency of an army, that the question of the preservation of these organs becomes an important one from the military standpoint.[69]

Like Voorhies's proposed circular of the previous year, Marshall's covered all the main points of good dental care and explained how dental caries and diseases of the teeth and mouth occurred and how to prevent them. He recommended proper methods of caring for the teeth and mouth, including brushing, use of tooth powders "to keep the teeth clean and bright," rinsing the mouth after meals, flossing, and antiseptic mouth "lotions." "It may be stated, therefore," he said, "as a general fact, that clean teeth do not decay."[69]

Unlike Voorhies's 1902 proposal, Marshall's circular eventually produced some positive results, although no known circular from the surgeon general's office ever appeared. On January 18, 1904, Marshall sent a pamphlet on "Hygiene of the Teeth" to the surgeon general with a recommendation that it be included in the next edition of *The Soldier's Handbook* that every soldier in the Army was issued. On April 16, 1904, the adjutant general informed Marshall that the surgeon general had forwarded two paragraphs to be considered for inclusion in the next edition.[70] The proposed paragraphs encapsulated much of what Marshall desired for educating the soldiers:

> A soldier should care for his teeth because their damage or loss will result in improper chewing of food and thus in various diseases of the digestive system. Decay, which is the commonest disease of the teeth, is caused by allowing particles of food to remain on and between them. These should be removed by thorough brushing. It is well to use a good tooth powder once or twice daily.

a

REDUCTION IN PRICES.

Glass Jars and Bottles for Tooth Powders,

WITH SPOON ATTACHMENT.

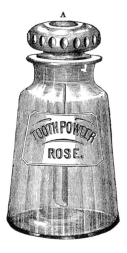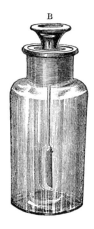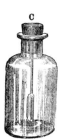

To save purchasers the inconvenience and annoyance of filling small boxes from the cans, we have adopted the above forms of jars and bottles with the spoon attachment, by which the desired quantity of powder can be taken out without spilling or wasting.

"A" is a ground stoppered jar, holding about two pounds of powder, with a neat glass label, "Tooth Powder—Rose," or "Tooth Powder—Wintergreen." These are very convenient for filling small boxes for *office sales.*

" B " is a ground stoppered bottle, holding one pound, and " C " one-quarter pound tooth powder. These are intended for *family use.*

The glass stoppers of "A" and "B" are made hollow, so as to contain the cork into which the spoon is fastened.

" C " has an ordinary cork, with spoon attached.

PRICES.

"A," Empty Jar... $1.25
" B," " One-Pound Bottle... 35
" C," " Quarter-Pound Bottle... 20

41

(a) In the late 1800s, tooth powders were kept in jars like these ones advertised in an 1878 issue of Dental Cosmos.

b

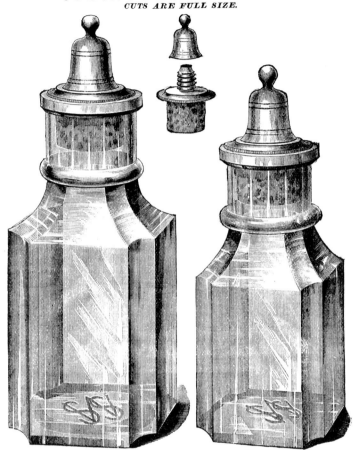

REDUCTION IN PRICES.
TOOTH-POWDER BOTTLES.
CUTS ARE FULL SIZE.

No. 1, Large.   No. 2, Small.

These bottles are made of flint glass. The mouths being wide, permit their being easily filled, the tapering necks allowing the powder to flow readily, without choking up, as is the case with most patterns now in the market.

The tightly-fitting corks with screw tops are advantages which are fully explained by the cuts. The cut showing the construction of the cap is half actual size.

This convenient manner of keeping tooth powder meets with general favor, avoiding waste, and the bottle can be readily carried when traveling. The fragrance of the powder is retained, and several may use from the same bottle with propriety.

No. 1. (Large)......................................per doz. $1.50.   Each 15 cents.
"   2. (Small)........................... ....   "   1.25.   "   12   "
"   1. Filled with our No. 1 Tooth Powder...   "   4.50.   "   40   "
"   2.   "   "   "   "   "   "   ...   "   3.25.   "   30   "

NOTE.—These bottles can also be supplied, *on order*, with the same cap, adapted for mouth washes, at same rates as above.

42

(continued). (b) Notice the SS White logo on the bottom of each bottle. Courtesy of US Army Medical Department Museum. Borden 020, 021.

In order that decay of the teeth may be detected before serious damage has occurred, a contract dental surgeon should be consulted at frequent intervals. Toothache indicates that the deeper parts of the teeth have become diseased and a soldier should not, therefore, wait until the teeth ache to consult a dentist, as by that time destruction may be so great as to much increase the severity of the dental operations needed or even to make impossible any effective repair.[70]

The next and subsequent editions of *The Soldier's Handbook* included these exact words in the section titled "Take Care of Your Health."[71] After some initial struggles, Marshall was beginning to make some headway in his campaign to improve oral and dental hygiene in the Army.

O'Reilly's Agenda and Continuing Problems with Contract Status

Throughout his tenure as surgeon general, O'Reilly focused his energies most heavily on correcting problems in the Medical Department that the Dodge Commission had identified in its investigation of the military performance in the Spanish-American War. In addition, he was especially determined to undo the deficiencies in the numbers and grades of commissioned medical officers that the Army reorganization of February 2, 1901, had imposed, forcing the use of what O'Reilly called in his last annual report of 1908 "the objectionable device of employing civilian physicians under contract. . . ."[72] O'Reilly tried annually to correct this problem, even submitting his own bill "to increase the efficiency and enlarge the Medical Department" in 1903 and 1904, but had little success in Congress until 1908.[73,74]

On Christmas Eve 1903, O'Reilly, who had now been the Army surgeon general since September 1902, submitted his draft bill to Chief of Staff Lieutenant General Adna Chaffee, and wrote that "In my opinion certain grave defects exist in the present organization of the Medical Department, which interfere with its efficiency in time of peace and its successful expansion in time of war." In his attached detailed memorandum, O'Reilly enumerated the most serious defects as inadequate numbers of commissioned medical officers, the lack of sufficient pay and promotion opportunities to attract young physicians, and "no satisfactory means of expansion to meet war conditions and special needs in time of peace (epidemics, 'little wars', etc.)." Heretofore, the only means of expansion was the use of contract surgeons "to supplement insufficient commission personnel," but O'Reilly had finally reached the conclusion that this "has always been wasteful and unsatisfactory, and has now become absolutely impractical because of the recent decision that the contract surgeon not being an officer obedience to his orders cannot be enforced even in the case of enlisted men of the Hospital Corps."[75]

The decision that prompted O'Reilly's action occurred in April 1903, when the Army judge advocate general ruled that contract surgeons had no authority to issue orders to any enlisted personnel, including those in the Hospital Corps. The same rule applied to contract dental surgeons. Early in 1903, the chief surgeon, Department of Luzon, had prepared a circular authorizing contract surgeons to assume command of posts or detachments when, "by the exigencies of the service," no commanding officer was present and the command reverted to a noncommissioned officer. Brigadier General George W Davis, the commander of the Philippine

Division, then requested that legislation be enacted to confer "military rank upon contract and dental surgeons." However, in April 1903, Judge Advocate General Brigadier General George B Davis, disagreed, arguing that contract surgeons were employed "to treat the sick" and contract dental surgeons were employed "to care for the teeth" of enlisted soldiers, and not to "exercise military command." Since the establishment of the Hospital Corps in 1887, the contract surgeon's position had become an "anomalous one." The Act of July 16, 1892 (27 Stat 175), had discontinued their employment, but the acts of May 12, 1898, and February 2, 1901, again authorized their appointment out of necessity. Davis recommended that Army legislation be directed towards replacing them by an increase in the size of the regular medical establishment, something that O'Reilly ardently but unsuccessfully sought.[76]

O'Reilly's lengthy memorandum of December 24, 1903, reported that the Medical Department had 200 contract surgeons and 320 commissioned medical officers. He believed that the February 2 act had seriously harmed the Medical Department by limiting the number of medical officers and replacing them with contract surgeons—he now wanted commissioned officers to replace the contractors and the contract system eliminated. He estimated that 450 regular medical officers would be sufficient for the Army's peacetime needs. Since the Spanish-American War, there had been 1,604 contract medical surgeons appointed and 1,512 discharged, the average number in service at any given time was 347. Considering the cost of transporting these contract surgeons home, often across the Pacific, and the cost of sending new surgeons to replace them, it was an expensive proposition for the government. Also, other factors to be considered were their ignorance of military duties and administration, loss of property by inexperience, and errors in record keeping for pension cases. With all these negatives, "the contract surgeon will be found to be by no means an economical substitute for officers of higher ranks and pay and of experience."[76]

While the contractors themselves faced a number of problems, O'Reilly believed that the system was dysfunctional and needed to be replaced:

> The uncertainty of his tenure of office, the lack of dignity and authority inherent to his status as a civilian in a military organization, his ungracious title, and the uniform which he is now compelled to wear which has been carefully stripped of all insignia of official rank, all are productive of discontent and tend to drive out the able and energetic while they are accepted by the sluggish and unambitious. The tendency of the system is therefore to the survival of the unfit and incapable. Finally the recent decision of the War Department that contract doctors cannot command enlisted men even of the Hospital Corps . . . has made a longer retention of the system impracticable.[76]

John Marshall was no less opposed to contract status for the dental surgeons than O'Reilly was to it for surgeons. To Marshall, the contract status was a temporary expedient that allowed an Army dental service of some sort to be established and that had to be replaced with a commissioned "Dental Corps" for dentists to receive professional and personal recognition. To O'Reilly, contract surgeons robbed the Medical Department of the uniformed physicians he needed to maintain the Army's health and would remain "the objectionable device of employing civilian physicians under contract. . . ." In exchanges with O'Reilly in November 1903 to January 1904, Marshall advanced arguments about the long-run negative effects of contract status on the Army's dental surgeons that differed very little from those that O'Reilly put forth in his memorandum for more commissioned medical officers.[77–80]

Contract Status and the "DS" Uniform

In a paper on his initial 3 years in the Philippines (from October 1901 to October 1904) that he presented at the NDA annual meeting in July 1905, Robert Oliver attacked the entire contract status of the dental surgeons:

> The present status of the contract dental surgeon is continually a source of humiliation and degradation to all, and to those more sensitive men who have occupied social positions at their homes equal to the best in their several communities it is of course keenly felt.[4(p70)]

While Oliver despised contract status, he saved some of his most critical comments for another issue that possibly irritated the contract dental surgeons the most—their uniforms. Oliver pointed out that dentist's uniforms themselves implied a separate, second-class status. On December 31, 1902, the adjutant general's office prescribed a change in uniform, whereby no full-dress uniform was authorized for contract dental surgeons. Their dress, service, and white uniforms were to conform to those of medical officers, but without the shoulder straps of a first lieutenant that they had formerly worn. Collar ornaments for dress and white uniforms were to be silver block letters "DS" in place of the coat-of-arms of the United States, and the collar ornament on their service uniform was to be dull bronze letters "DS."[4,81]

On September 6, 1904, while still in the Philippines, Oliver had had enough of the "DS" uniform and wrote to the military secretary, outlining his complaints and requesting changes and a return to the previous uniform:

> The wearing of an officer's uniform, in contradistinction to the hybrid one now prescribed, would tend to elevate the official station, the social standing, and the self-respect of Dental Surgeons, more nearly commensurate with the dignity of their profession and their standing as gentlemen; and would stimulate them to exert their best efforts and highest attainments toward the betterment of the Army Dental Service; would give them justifiable pride in the new specialty of the Army Dental practice, and would, altogether create a spirit of contentment and satisfaction to the individual membership of the Corps, without which any organization has its limitations of efficiency.[82]

Oliver's request was forwarded to the War Department and on to the general staff, surgeon general, and quartermaster general for comment. The surgeon general's office replied on October 26 that contract surgeons and dental surgeons:

> . . . should either not be required to wear uniform or should be given one which would clearly indicate that they have the relative status of commissioned officers. This the present uniform does not do. The uniform formerly worn by these men was believed to be satisfactory. Of course, it is understood that the wearing of shoulder straps will not confer to Contract Dental Surgeons the authority to command.[83]

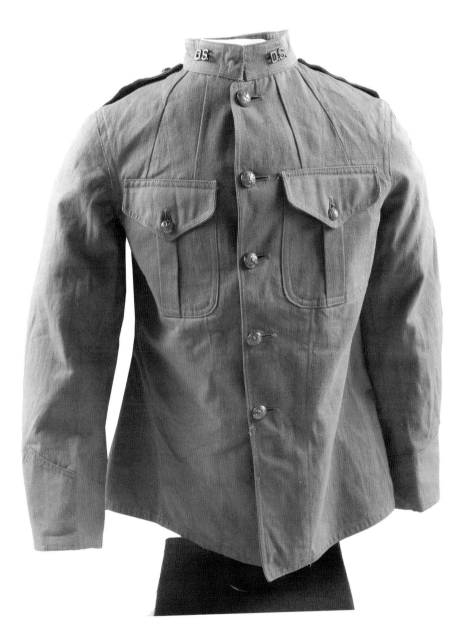

Early Dental Service uniform, circa 1902.
Photograph: Courtesy of US Army Medical Department Museum. Med7271-1.

Lieutenant Colonel James Kerr, acting chief of the general staff's 1st Division, made an exhaustive study of Oliver's complaint and responded with a five-page memorandum report on November 15, 1904. He concluded:

> It is not believed that the wearing of shoulder straps by dental surgeons will cause enlisted men to show them more respect, or elevate their official status, social standing, etc. Enlisted men are required by orders and regulations to salute dental surgeons and to pay them proper respect, and their official status and social standing do not depend on whether or not they wear shoulder straps. . . . The uniform as now prescribed is considered by Dental Surgeon Oliver to be a hybrid one, but it is not considered that it will be any less hybrid by adding to it a hybrid shoulder strap such as he desires. The objectives to the present uniform of dental surgeons are not deemed well founded. It is, therefore, recommended that no change be made in it.[84]

On November 22 Chief of Staff Chaffee approved no change. Three days later, the military secretary's office informed the commanding general, Philippines Division, that "no change be made in the present uniform of Contract Dental Surgeons."[85]

By the time that the War Department response reached the Philippines, Oliver was already in the United States and on his way to his next assignment at West Point. In a paper presented at the July 1905 NDA meeting (and included in the NDA's *Transactions* in 1906), he continued his attack. When in the blue uniform, he noted, the uninformed might presume the dental surgeons were liveried servants. While wearing the other two uniforms, the dentist looked like an enlisted hospital corpsman and sometimes was ordered about as one until his status was clarified. Finally, Oliver pointed out that because dentists were not authorized dress uniforms, they were excluded automatically from all formal events and formations. Oliver believed that such treatment in the short run adversely affected their management and discipline, and in the long run would affect recruiting and retainment of dentists of high quality.[4] He wrote:

> It seems a great injustice to educated professional men who have spent years in acquiring a technical and scientific knowledge of their specialty and who have qualified before a competent examining board before entering the service, to be so meanly uniformed as to be indistinguishable from ordinary soldiers. . . . You may all say that there is no disgrace in the wearing of civilian clothing as above stated, which is quite true; but at any army post where one is supposed to be an officer, or at least a quasi-officer, and is strenuously struggling to maintain even that status, I must say that to appear different from all the rest places a dental surgeon in a more or less humiliating position and indicates to him that he is one of the army only through sufferance.[4(pp70–71)]

In 1903, after 2 years of service, Dr Hugh Voorhies reported that the "DS" insignia signified "Don't Shoot," which may have reflected the attitude of some of the line officers and enlisted soldiers toward the new dental surgeons and their role in the Army.[43] While an unimportant minor detail to the War Department and many line officers, the dental surgeons saw the matter of "DS" uniforms as a major irritant that lessened their authority and hard-won social standing as professionals.

BUILDING THE FOUNDATION: THE EARLY YEARS OF ARMY DENTISTRY

Dr Hussey: Itinerant Dentist in the Department of Dakota

After returning from the Philippines in April 1903, Dr Samuel Hussey was assigned to duty with John Marshall at the Department of California before departing for the Department of Dakota on August 1, 1903. His 1903–1904 report indicated the type of dentistry performed by a contract dental surgeon working as an itinerant dentist in a geographical department. He recalled:

> The dental service rendered in the Department of Dakota, from August 12th, 1903, to June 30th, 1904, has been almost entirely of an emergency character.
>
> My first tour of duty from August 12th to September 18th, 1903, I visited all the posts in the Department [10 posts in Minnesota, North and South Dakota, Wyoming, and Montana] for the purpose of examining the teeth of all the officers and enlisted men and perform[ed] operations only that required immediate attention, and upon arrival at Ft. Snelling, I reported to the Department Commander the probable length of time required to complete the necessary dental work at each post.
>
> After remaining on duty at Ft. Snelling, Minn., from September 18th to November 30th, 1903, I was sent out on the second tour of duty to visit all the posts in the Department and perform all the necessary dental work.
>
> On this tour my services were very largely extractions, restorations by permanent fillings of gold, amalgam and oxy-phosphate, removing of salivary deposits, and treatment of abscesses and other ordinary diseased condition of the teeth and gums.
>
> The hours for Sundays and holidays have been found necessary for the relief of the suffering in new cases and redressing of cases already under treatment.
>
> The office hours have been the greater part of the time from 8:30 A.M. to 5:00 P.M., except during the short days of the winter, when the light was not quite sufficient.
>
> Total number of patients treated, 815, as follows: Officers, regular, 55; Enlisted men, 674; Retired soldiers, 1; General prisoners, 3; Civilian attaches, male, 16; Civilian attaches, female, 66. Total number of sittings, 2,200; Total number of sittings per each working day, 9; Average number of sittings per patient, 3; Average length of time required for completing treatment of each patient, one hour and twenty minutes.
>
> The force of dental surgeons in the Department of Dakota, is still inadequate to meet the demands of all classes of operations, e.g., it has been impossible for the present dental surgeon to perform restorations by artificial dentures, except while stationed at Ft. Snelling, Minn., because it is impracticable to carry an extensive laboratory equipment on tours of duty while visiting posts from two weeks to two months and the greater demand requires treatment and filling of such a nature as has been mentioned above, therefore the laboratory outfit has been lying idle at Fort Snelling, Minn., for several months.[86(pp578–580)]

The majority of dentists generally seemed satisfied while performing under demanding conditions, even as their status continued to be argued in the War and Medical departments and in Congress.

Dentists in the Field

Army dentists worked hard in the field but were often frustrated in their attempts to instill new habits of dental hygiene among their patients. In November 1903 *Dental Cosmos* quoted the *Army and Navy Journal* on one significant problem:

> The dental surgeons are experiencing considerable difficulty in getting enlisted men in the army to properly attend to their teeth. A proposition is now under consideration by the medical department of the army to have the dental surgeons give lectures to the enlisted men under their charge on the urgent necessity for the care and preservation of the teeth.[87]

At the Fourth International Dental Congress in Saint Louis, Marshall commented on many aspects of dental practice in the Army. Even though the government only provided tin and plastics for filling materials, he noted that dentists could use gold at the patient's expense. In fact, in some cases the Army furnished the necessary instruments for gold work. Then, too, the dental surgeon was furnished with an enlisted Hospital Corps assistant to help him with the work. Marshall pointed out that the dentist's first mission was to alleviate suffering and to stop further decay. Consequently, much of his work must be a stopgap until the patient could get permanent treatment at a general hospital. Within these constraints, Marshall believed the dentists were performing well. Those located at the hospitals had all the facilities necessary to perform any kind of work required. At major posts dentists could expand their skills through the treatment of families, gaining experience in pediatrics and orthodontics, as well as in jaw work. In fact, in the absence of a surgeon, dentists were authorized to perform any medical procedure for which they were competent. Marshall thought that expanding experience would mandate changes that he was sure would occur in due course.[88]

Despite such positive views in 1904, contract dental surgeon Ord Sorber (1867–1922), who served at Fort Sam Houston, Texas (1901–1904) and then the Philippines (1904–1907) before resigning to pursue private practice, commented in *Dental Brief* on his inability to take advantage of the provisions for deriving additional income from the patients who were not entitled to "free service":

> As authorized by law and specified by regulations only officers and enlisted men are entitled to free service, but persons not entitled to free service may be operated upon before nine o'clock A.M. or after four P.M.; provided the dentist's services are not required by those entitled to them. This is to enable us to add to our income if we so desire, but it has not been of any use to me, because the amount of work required by those entitled to free service has been far greater than I could possibly perform, only about one-third of the work required having been performed, though it was by no means confined to prescribed hours. It soon became apparent that if the regulations were to be obeyed all thought of outside work must be given up.[89(p252)]

He emphasized the problem with the backlog of work:

> The amount of dental work in demand is enormous. If I may judge of the state of affairs in the rest of the army by the conditions found in that part of it stationed in the Department of Texas, it will require at least three times the present number of dentists

to properly care for even the urgent cases. The number of men newly enlisted each year would alone be sufficient to keep us all busy.[89(p254)]

Sorber cited the advantages of a military dental practice, such as relatively few bills to collect from patients and few problem patients. But then he listed as the disadvantages: the uncertainty of a contract renewal, no possibility of increasing one's income, inadequate dental facilities at the majority of posts, constant change of station, lack of opportunity to perform the finer types of dentistry, cost of uniforms and living expenses in remote places, necessity for using equipment not suited to one's preference, and the constant pressure from persons not entitled to "free service" to induce violations of the regulations governing dental treatment.[89]

His conclusion was not favorable to a military dental career:

The Inspector-General's Department has taken testimony regarding the desirability of making the service permanent, and in course of time it may be made a commissioned service, but to the writer this appears to be a very remote possibility, in view of the proverbial slowness with which such matters move. But should it come to pass, the service will still fall far short of being a desirable birth [*sic*] for a capable man.

In conclusion, I would suggest that, in view of the attainments necessary to pass the examination, any one who can successfully take it is well able to command a much larger income in private practice in any of the larger towns or cities.[89(pp254–255)]

On the other hand, contract dental surgeon Charles Long, who had served in the Philippines since 1901, expressed his satisfaction with the service when writing to Brigadier General William Dougherty, formerly in the Philippines but now assigned to Fort Jay, New York:

I have been in the Islands now, two years and nine months, and although Staff Officers are supposed to complete their tour here in three years, I doubt whether or not we will be relieved on time, as there are not enough men in our Department in the States to relieve us all out here; however, I am in good health and stationed here in Manila I enjoy myself very much, so I am not particularly anxious to go home.[90]

Dentists in the Philippines: 1902–1904

The changed operational situation in the Philippines and the end of most active military operations also altered the dentist's work pattern as the number of troops decreased and numerous smaller posts were consolidated. The postinsurrection reorganization of the Philippines into Luzon, Visayas, and Mindanao resulted in fewer posts and soldiers. After the peace declaration on July 4, 1902, the number of Army posts was decreased from about 140 to less than 50 by October 1904. In 1903 dental surgeons were assigned to only the larger stations and patients came to them from the surrounding small posts according to a previously arranged appointment schedule determined by the dental surgeon and the commanding officer.[4(p47)]

By June 1902 McAlister, Craig, Wolven, Rietz, Ware, Wing, Carpenter, and Foster were assigned to Luzon; Mason, Bernheim, Lauderdale, Whinney, and Millikin

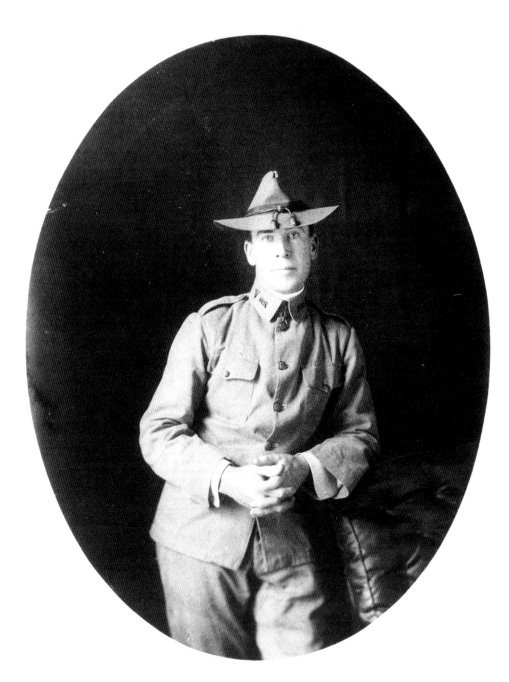

Charles J Long, contact dental surgeon who had served in the Philippines.
Photograph: Courtesy of National Archives and Records Administration.

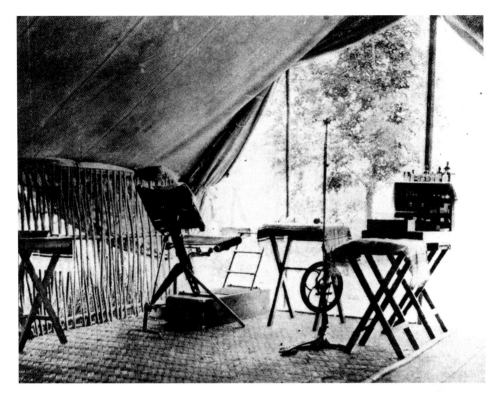

Portable dental outfit set up in dental office at Camp Stotsenberg, Luzon, June 1903.
Reproduced from: Dental Cosmos. *1906;48:217.*

were assigned to Visayas (which included Dental Base Station No. 2); Boak, Hussey, Stone, and Casaday were assigned to Mindanao (which included Dental Base Station No. 3); Waddell and Long were at Dental Base Station No. 1 in Manila; and Robert Oliver was assigned to the chief surgeon's office.[10]

Base stations were one of Oliver's innovations where prosthetic cases could be treated, because it was impossible for itinerant dental surgeons to carry the laboratory equipment needed to perform this type of dentistry. The first station, Dental Base Station No. 1, was opened at the First Reserve Hospital in Manila in early March 1902. All of the prosthetic cases from the Department of North Philippines were sent there for treatment. Dental Base Station No. 2 was established for the Department of South Philippines at its headquarters in Cebu. In October 1902, with the reorganization of the Philippine Division into the three departments of Luzon, the Visayas, and Mindanao, the base station at Cebu was transferred to Iloilo, the headquarters of the new Department of the Visayas. A new station, Dental Base Station No. 3, was opened at Zamboango for the Department of Mindanao. All oral surgery cases were referred to Oliver in Manila.[10]

In Oliver's system, the base stations were home stations where dentists spent anywhere from 2 to 10 months a year. The rest of the year they rotated among smaller stations where soldiers from outlaying posts could meet them for examination

227

and treatment.[10] John Millikin's schedule for 1903 illustrates how the system worked and how time-consuming the constant moving, shipping, setting up, breaking down, and packing up must have been (Table 7-5). Millikin's home station was Catbalogan, Samar, and Hospital Corps Private Patrick Curley served as Millikin's person in charge of property and "as a guard for same during this time."[91]

All of the changes in stationing and reduction in troops in 1902 and 1903 also meant that fewer dental surgeons were required. Strength dropped steadily from a high of 20 in June 1902, to 18 in June 1903, and then 17 in 1904, before Oliver's return to the United States in October. However, the surgeon general's office fixed an official authorized level of 14 dental surgeons in April 1904. Oliver complained in his final report that this number was insufficient to provide dental care, given the time the dental surgeons lost in moving from post to post. He insisted that at least 17 surgeons were still required.[5] He went on to say:

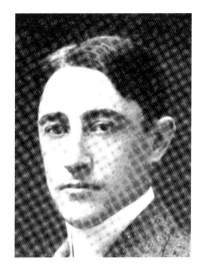

Dentist RW Waddell, who served in the Philippines, pictured here in 1918.
Reproduced from: JASMUS. 1919;3:14.

> This unfortunate condition of affairs is much to be regretted, as it is considered only fair that every soldier should have an equal opportunity of having his teeth filled and saved, especially when he is detailed for duty at remote stations in this division where it is absolutely impossible for him to obtain dental treatment from civilian dentists, even at his own expense.[5(p3)]

As the dentists settled into their work, the need for each of them to have two enlisted assistants became increasingly evident. In his 1903 report to the surgeon general, Oliver envisioned one soldier "working as an operating assistant at the chair" and also responsible for the care, sterilization and preservation of the instruments and materials. The other assistant should be trained in maintaining dental records and reports, as well as in supply procedures. He estimated that the extra time given the dentist as a result of this help would at least double the number of patients who could be cared for. The dental assistant was at the dental surgeon's disposal "at all times" and accompanied him on his circuit, although carried on the hospital's muster rolls.[5,92]

The turnover in dental surgeons was heavy in 1903 with Hussey, Craig, Carpenter, and Foster all returning to the United States for reassignment and Stone being evacuated with illness, and no new arrivals to replace them. The situation in 1904 was even worse because the 3-year contracts expired and Ware, Waddell, Rietz, Boak, Lauderdale, Wing, Whinnery, Wolven, Mason, Long, and Oliver were all scheduled to depart. To offset some of the departures, four new dental surgeons arrived in the Philippines for duty in 1904: Rex Rhoades, WG Hammond (contract annulled January 1911), GE Stallman, and GI Gunckel.[5]

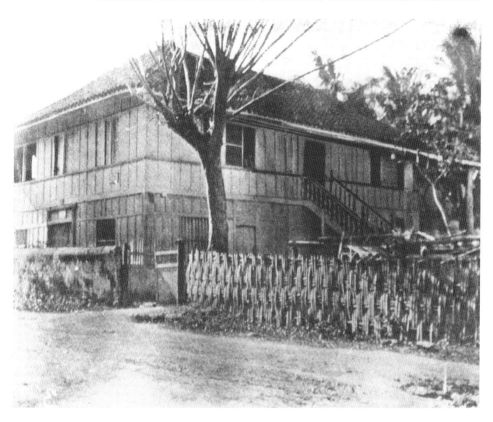

Exterior view of the office at Cebu, Philippine Islands, May 1902.
Reproduced from: Dental Cosmos. 1906:48;213.

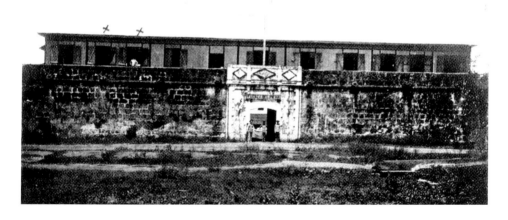

Exterior view of the office at Zamboanga, Mindanao, Philippine Islands, May 1902.
Reproduced from: Dental Cosmos. 1906:48;215.

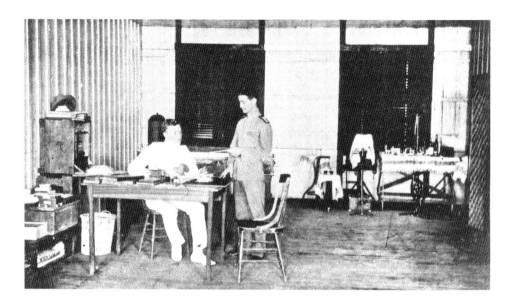

Interior view of the office at Zamboanga, Mindanao, May 1902.
Reproduced from: Dental Cosmos. *1906:48;213.*

TABLE 7-5

JOHN D MILLIKIN ITINERANT SCHEDULE, 1903

Location	Duration
Catbalogan, Samar (substation: Gandara River)	2 months
Calbayog, Samar	3 months
Laguan, Samar (substation: Catubig)	2 months
Borongan, Samar	2 weeks
Guinan, Samar	2 weeks
Basey, Samar	1 month
Santa Rita, Samar	1 month
Binatic, Samar	2 weeks
Daram, Daram Island	2 weeks

Data source: National Archives and Records Administration. Record Group 94. Order No. 44, W.S. Scott, captain, acting assistant adjutant general, Division of Philippines, to John D. Millikin, 5 January 1903. Letter. No 472628. Box 3319. Entry 25.

To make personnel matters even worse, after stalling for nearly a year, in February 1904 Oliver was ordered to Peking, China, for temporary duty with the US Legation Guard. Upon his arrival on April 21, he was informed that all the officers and enlisted soldiers of Company B, 9th Infantry, required dental treatment. There had not been a dental surgeon assigned previously, and the two local civilian Chinese and Japanese dentists lacked professional ability. Examination of the command showed that over 96% of the 142-person garrison was in need of immediate dental treatment. Several had been temporarily relieved from duty and placed on sick leave because of dental and oral disease, which could not be treated by the hospital medical staff. Oliver did not return to the Philippines until August 1, 1904.[5,93,94]

While in the Philippines, Oliver compiled and submitted two extensive reports covering the work of the dental surgeons for fiscal year 1902 (July 1, 1902, to June 30, 1903) and for the entire period from April 1901 to October 1904. He later revised these reports to prepare a major presentation for the NDA's annual meeting in late July 1905, and they were subsequently published in *Transactions of the National Dental Association* as "Three Years' Service in the Philippines" (Table 7-6). In them, he reported on the work accomplished by the dental surgeons in the Philippines, who were "an honor to our noble profession, as they certainly create the world's record of dental service, for never before has there been an equal number of dental surgeons banded together in one organization working toward a common end."[4,5,10]

Oliver's pointed comments on the oral and dental condition of the soldiers in the Philippines revealed an abysmal situation:

> Judging from the kind of cases first presented it could be easily seen that the vast majority of soldiers had never known what dental attention was, as the neglected condition of their mouths and teeth indicated beyond all doubt that the individual paid very little or no attention to the welfare of these important organs. When we consider that there were probably sixty thousand troops in the Philippines at the time, a majority of whom had been on duty in the tropics about two years with no possibility at hand of obtaining dental treatment from civilians or otherwise, and with the manifold effects of the tropics, character of food, and continuous active service against a wary foe, which prevented even the ordinary care to their personal toilet, it can be imagined what condition the mouths of these men presented.[4(p60)]

TABLE 7-6

SELECTED DENTAL SERVICES IN THE PHILIPPINES, MAY 1, 1901 TO SEPTEMBER 30, 1904

Total Cases	Cases of Dental Caries	Operations	Fillings (all types)	Extractions	Patients
75,587	55,567	82,562	41,061	12,844	30,262

Data sources: (1) Oliver RT. Three years' service in the Philippines. In: *Transactions of the National Dental Association*. Philadelphia, Pa: The SS White Dental Mfg Co; 1906. (2) National Archives and Records Administration. Record Group 112. Robert T. Oliver to surgeon general, USA (through channels), [April 1901–October 1904], 15 October 1904. Report. No 89178. Box 616. Entry 26.

Severe campaigning conditions contributed to poor oral and dental health, allowing soldiers little time for personal hygiene. Few appeared to make any serious efforts to clean their teeth even when out of the field and in permanent installations. Serious dental problems affected 80% to 90% of the soldiers.[4] Oliver commented:

> This neglect, often accompanied by the direct local effects and indirect systematic effects of poorly cooked food upon the oral tissues, together with a general loss of tone due to fatigue and the rigorous tropical climate, were prominent etiologic factors in the foregoing pathological conditions mentioned.[4]

Oliver disagreed with previous observations about the effect of tropical climates upon teeth and gums. He believed that "the tropical effects were only incidental and can be traced to a general loss of tone in the individual and the consequent lessening of nutritive activity."[4]

Located as they were thousands of miles from San Francisco and New York meant that supplies of dental equipment and materials were often inadequate or entirely lacking. In his 1904 report, Oliver noted that this situation largely arose from the delay in receiving supplies following approval of annual requisitions: "The last annual requisition was forwarded February 25, 1904, and supplies did not begin to arrive until June, 1904, and then only in small part, with additions coming September 10, and a large part yet to arrive."

Oliver wanted semiannual requisitions to prevent shortages. In addition, he wanted the medical supply officer in New York to notify Manila when requisitioned items could not be issued. Oliver would then have the opportunity to purchase the items locally, "instead of having to wait several months to see if said articles would arrive in the next consignment of goods."[5]

In his report on 1902 and 1903, Oliver commented extensively on the need to reorganize what he called the "Dental Corps, U.S.A":

> . . . giving it an official status in the permanent establishment. . . . The new organization should contemplate the establishment of four grades (one file only for the highest), with the rank, privileges, emoluments, etc., equal to that of the corresponding grades of the Medical Department.[10]

He went on:

> This reorganization would be of untold benefit to the Corps in the future, as it would be a means of attracting the very best professional talent from the better class of young practitioners, would assure the future for the Corps members by giving them rank and pay commensurate with the dignity of their profession, their status as professional men and more nearly in proportion to the value of their services as specialists. It would also be a stimulus for them to render their best services to the Government and would greatly assist in maintaining a high degree of efficiency and "Esprit de Corps," without which any branch of the service deteriorates. At the present time the Corps enjoys the distinction of having a first class reputation and a high degree of professional talent. This on account of the established high standard for qualification demanded by the Examining Board and upon the high class of professional men who were admitted to the Corps, all of whom joined with the expectation of finally becom-

ing a part of the permanent establishment of the Army, thereby obtaining an assured and honorable position during active life, with ample provisions for the future. A majority of these men now on duty in the Division of the Philippines are beginning to manifest a spirit of unrest and discontent at the present status, and it is extremely doubtful if many of the better class remain long in the Corps with a contact status which, if allowed to remain in force, will result in getting only such a class of men as will be attracted to and satisfied with a status of inferiority and degradation. . . .[10]

Oliver largely repeated these comments, with some slight changes, in his overall report for the period 1901 to 1904.

On October 25, 1904, Colonel Joseph Girard, chief surgeon of the Philippines Division, agreed with Oliver's recommendation that 17 dental surgeons be assigned to the Philippines, as well as with his assessment of the growing importance of dental care in the Army:

In this connection the undersigned respectfully invites attention to the fact that since the addition of Dentists to the Medical Department of the Army, their services have been demanded by an enormous, ever-growing proportion, reaching, perhaps 90 per cent, of the rank and file. That is the case not only in the Philippines, where the climate is supposed, whether correctly or not, to induce dental caries, but in the home garrisons just as well. As the majority of the men is made up of young soldiers in their first enlistments, the conclusion is unavoidable that the diseased condition of their teeth cannot, in most cases, be due to the exposure or hardships connected with the military service, but must have existed at the time of their enlistment. The calls for Dentists from the various Army posts, both in the United States and the Philippines, are now so frequent and urgent, that, if it is contemplated to properly repair every recruit's jaws and keep them thereafter in good working condition, the number of Army Dentists must be greatly increased, more than doubled, certainly, for it is patently insufficient at present.[95]

When he came to Oliver's views on dental reorganization, Girard's opinions stiffened significantly and probably reflected the sentiments of most of his physician colleagues in the Medical Department:

With regard to the recommendation for a reorganization of the so styled "Dental Corps, U.S.A." (See page 7), the undersigned desires to enter his emphatic disapproval of any such expression, and of all measures or efforts tending to give Army Dentists a separate standing in the Army by establishment of an independent hierarchy of grades, whether outside of the Medical Department or within and in connection with that Department itself, in the latter case, a sort of "imperium in imperio" subversive of military discipline by the division of authority, and wholly contrary to the interests of the service. The care of soldiers' teeth, considered by itself, is undoubtedly a serious matter, and should be sedulously provided for, but, when looked as from the broad point of view of the Sanitary Service of the Army, it assumes much more modest proportions, and becomes simply an incident and a subordinate subject among a multitude of far more important questions; the tendency, evident in this report, to unduly magnify the import of Dentistry in the Army by the establishment of a special, and prospectively independent hierarchy of grades, the erection of Dental Hospitals, etc., etc., can be characterized only as extremely mischievous, totally unnecessary, and wasteful of public funds. The Medical Department of the Army should be one and indivisible, constituting but one Corps under a single head and with but one line of grades, all, including dental and other assistants, subordinate to one another according to rank and deriving their faculties from the same fountain head of authority.[95]

Despite this view, Girard fully understood the problems of professional status and standing that the contract dental surgeons faced and clearly believed that this situation required action to correct:

> While expressing himself thus strongly on this special subject, the undersigned is quite disposed to advocate granting military commissions to Dental Surgeons; he is of the opinion that the system of employing professional men in the Army, on a quasi military footing as Contract Surgeons and Contract Dental Surgeons is radically wrong, as long as those men are expected to associate on equal terms with military officers. Their present position is ambiguous, humiliating and unsatisfactory in every way. Either let them be and remain civilians pure and simple, and stand on their own merit, or confer upon them military commissions which, by placing them on a level with their associates, will safeguard their self-respect and secure to them the regard which they are legally entitled to from officers and enlisted men.[95]

There is no record of how Oliver's report or Girard's endorsement were received at the surgeon general's office in late 1904.

A Foundation for Army Dentistry

These early years of Army dentistry were filled with significant accomplishments and profound disappointments for contract dental surgeons. With John Marshall and Robert Oliver leading the way, a few dentists achieved much in the Army. The work of the dental surgeons in the United States and especially in the Philippines had revealed the wretched state of the Army's oral and dental health beyond any doubt. In their work, dentists were contributing to the overall readiness of the Army by reducing the number of soldiers who were absent from their units or lost altogether to the Army due to oral or dental diseases.

Despite the legislative setbacks, much was accomplished during these early years of Army dentistry, proving the contentions of those who had argued for so long that the Army and American soldiers deserved the excellent dental care that American dentistry could provide and would be better for it. Firm foundations for future development were established, even if they appeared to be somewhat shaky to many at the time.

References

1. National Archives and Records Administration. Record Group 112. Colonel Charles R Greenleaf, chief surgeon, Division of the Philippines, to the surgeon general. Letter. No. 80254. Box 539. Entry 26.

2. National Archives and Records Administration. Record Group 112. Sternberg, surgeon general, to adjutant general, February 11, 1901. Letter. No. 78774. Box 519. Entry 26.

3. National Archives and Records Administration. Record Group 94. Personnel folders for Emmett J Craig and Samuel W Hussey. Entry 91.

4. Oliver RT. Three years' service in the Philippines. In: *Transactions of the National Dental Association*. Philadelphia, Pa: The SS White Dental Mfg Co; 1906.

5. National Archives and Records Administration. Record Group 112. Robert T Oliver to surgeon general, USA (through channels) [April 1901–October 1904], October 15, 1904. Report. No. 89178. Box 616. Entry 26.

6. Boak SD. Army dental surgeon and his work in the Philippines. *Dental Register*. 1903;57:301–308.

7. National Archives and Records Administration. Record Group 112. Index, First Lieutenant George A Skinner, hospital commander, to letter of Charles A Petre to chief surgeon, Division of the Philippines, April 23, 1901. No. 75469. Box 357. Entry 101.

8. National Archives and Records Administration. Record Group 112. Major General Adna R Chaffee to Adjutant General, February 14, 1902. Cablegram. No. 75469. Box 496. Entry 26.

9. Oliver RT. The rational consideration of oral prophylaxis. *Dental Cosmos*. 1921;63:1118.

10. National Archives and Records Administration. Record Group 112. Robert T Oliver to surgeon general [July 1, 1902–June 30, 1903], June 30, 1903, 1. Report. No. 89178. Box 616. Entry 26.

11. Boak SD. Dental Army service in the Philippines. *Dental Register*. 1907;61:289–292.

12. Stone FP. Personal experiences in the Army Dental Corps. *Wash Univ Dent J*. 1937;3:121–125.

13. National Archives and Records Administration. Record Group 112. Lieutenant Colonel Girard to surgeon general's office, September 2, 1901. Telegram. No. 70760. Box 449. Entry 26.

14. National Archives and Records Administration. Record Group 112. Surgeon general's office to Girard, September 3, 1901. Letter. No. 70760. Box 449. Entry 26.

15. National Archives and Records Administration. Record Group 112. Marshall to Colonel William H Forwood, September 6, 1901. Letter. No. 70760.

16. National Archives and Records Administration. Record Group 112. Forwood to Marshall, September 12, 1901. Letter. No. 70760.

17. National Archives and Records Administration. Record Group 112. Sternberg to Marshall, October 11, 1901. Telegram. No. 70760.

18. National Archives and Records Administration. Record Group 112. Marshall to Sternberg, October 12, 1901. Telegram. No. 70760.

19. National Archives and Records Administration. Record Group 112. Marshall to the surgeon general, June 1, 1903. Letter. No 70760.

20. National Archives and Records Administration. Record Group 112. John S Marshall to the surgeon general, June 1, 1903. Personal service report [September 1, 1901–June 30, 1902]. Letter. No. 70760. Box 449. Entry 26.

21. National Archives and Records Administration. Record Group 94. War Department Special order no. 168, July 22, 1905. No. 391988. Box 2730. Entry 25.

22. Biographical files of Brigadier Generals AC Girard and George Torney. Biographical Files, Research Collection, Office of Medical History, OTSG/MEDCOM, Falls Church, Va.

23. National Archives and Records Administration. Record Group 112. O'Reilly to Marshall, Oliver, and Hess, March 9, 1905. Orders no. 79325. Box 527. Entry 26.

24. National Archives and Records Administration. Record Group 112. Correspondence with Marshall and Hess pertaining to dental examinations in 1902 and 1904. No. 79325. Box 527. Entry 26.

25. National Archives and Records Administration. Record Group 112. Frank E McDermott. Case files. No. 82082. Box 352. Entry 101.

26. National Archives and Records Administration. Record Group 112. General correspondence. No. 82082. Box 557. Entry 26.

27. National Archives and Records Administration. Record Group 94. Document file. No. 424245. Box 2961. Entry 25.

28. National Archives and Records Administration. Record Group 112. John S Marshall to surgeon general, July 5, 1903. Personal service report [July 1, 1902–June 30, 1903]. Letter. No. 70760.

29. National Archives and Records Administration. Record Group 112. John S Marshall to surgeon general, July 25, 1904. Personal service report [July 1, 1903–June 30, 1904]. Letter. No. 70760.

30. Dental Corps Biographical Files. Research collection. Office of Medical History, OTSG/MEDCOM, Falls Church, Va.

31. National Archives and Records Administration. Record Group 112. FA Baldwin to adjutant general (through channels), May 8, 1901. Letter with index. No. 78773. Box 519. Entry 26.

32. National Archives and Records Administration. Record Group 112. Havard May 9, 1901. Letter. No. 78773. Box 519. Entry 26.

33. National Archives and Records Administration. Record Group 112. Wood May 10, 1901. Letter. No. 78773. Box 519. Entry 26.

34. National Archives and Records Administration. Record Group 112. Ward to Wood August 22, 1901. Telegram. No. 78773. Box 519. Entry 26.

35. National Archives and Records Administration. Record Group 15. Major Valery Havard, chief surgeon, Department of Cuba, Havana, October 31, 1901, pension file. Letter. Certificate No. 584073.

36. V[ail] WD. Organization of the Dental Corps. *Dental Bulletin Supplement to the Army Medical Bulletin*. 1933;4:172.

37. National Archives and Records Administration. Record Group 112. Sternberg, surgeon general, to Marshall, November 29, 1901. Letter. No. 70760. Box 449. Entry 26.

38. National Archives and Records Administration. Record Group 112. Marshall to Sternberg, December 6, 1901. Letter. No. 70760. Box 449. Entry 26.

39. National Archives and Records Administration. Record Group 112. Sternberg to Marshall, January 4, 1902. Letter. No 70760. Box 449. Entry 26.

40. National Archives and Records Administration. Record Group 112. Marshall to surgeon general, January 12, 1901. Letter. No. 70760. Box 449. Entry 26.

41. Personnel files on Alexander P Bacon. Research Collections. Office of Medical History, OTSG/MEDCOM, Falls Church, Va.

42. Voorhies HG. Dentistry in the service. *The Dental Forum*. 1903;1:176–179.

43. Voorhies HG. Dentistry as practiced in the U.S. Army. *Dental Brief*. 1910;15:619.

44. National Archives and Records Administration. Record Group 112. HG Voorhies to chief surgeon, Deptartment of the East, May 29, 1902. Letter with enclosure; The care of the teeth. No. 70417. Box 97. Entry 25.

45. National Archives and Records Administration. Record Group 112. Second endorsement, WH Forwood, surgeon general, to Marshall, June 12, 1902, to letter, Voorhies to chief surgeon, Department of the East, May 29, 1902. Letter. No. 70417.

46. National Archives and Records Administration. Record Group 112. Third endorsement, Marshall to surgeon general, June 23, 1920, to letter, Voorhies to chief surgeon, Department of the East, May 29, 1902. No. 70417.

47. National Archives and Records Administration. Record Group 112. Fourth endorsement, Forwood to Marshall, July 1, 1902, to letter, Voorhies to chief surgeon, Department of the East, May 29, 1902. Letter. No. 70417.

48. National Archives and Records Administration. Record Group 112. Fifth endorsement, Marshall to surgeon general, July 16, 1902, to letter, Voorhies to chief surgeon, Department of the East, May 29, 1902. Letter. No. 70417.

49. National Archives and Records Administration. Record Group 112. June 30, 1902, and first endorsement, O'Reilly through chief surgeon, Department of the East, to Voorhies, September 12, 1902. Memo. No. 70417.

50. Roller OP. California State Dental Association [proceedings]. *Dental Cosmos.* 1902;44:1072.

51. Marshall JS. Work done at Fort Presidio by the Dental Corps. *Pacific Gazette.* Quoted in: *Dental Register.* 1902;56:530.

52. Marshall JS. The Dental Corps of the Army. *Dent Rev.* 1902;16:171.

53. Roster of dental surgeons, U.S. Army. *Dental Cosmos.* 1902;44:402.

54. Army Dental Corps. *Dental Cosmos.* 1902;44:1100.

55. National Archives and Records Administration. Record Group 112. Contract dental surgeons. Report, enclosure to letter, John S Marshall to the surgeon general, August 19, 1902. No. 89178. Box 616. Entry 26.

56. National Archives and Records Administration. Record Group 112. Contract dental surgeons. Report, enclosure to letter, John S Marshall to the surgeon general, July 2, 1903. No. 89178. Box 616. Entry 26.

57. National Archives and Records Administration. Record Group 112. Walter D McCaw, surgeon general's office, to John S Marshall, July 8, 1903. Letter. No. 89178. Box 616. Entry 26.

58. Office of The Surgeon General. *Annual Report of the Surgeon General, 1903.* Washington, DC: Government Printing Office; 1903: 30.

59. National Archives and Records Administration. Record Group 112. Contract dental surgeons [July 2, 1902]. 21.

60. National Archives and Records Administration. Record Group 112. Marshall to surgeon general, September 12, 1903. Letter. No. 89178.

61. National Archives and Records Administration. Record Group 112. Marshall to surgeon general, October 31, 1904. Letter. No. 89178.

62. National Archives and Records Administration. Record Group 112. Major Charles F Mason, surgeon general's office, to Marshall, December 16, 1904. Letter. No. 89178.

63. National Archives and Records Administration. Record Group 112. Dr Noel to surgeon general, June 14, 1903. Letter. No. 70760.

64. National Archives and Records Administration. Record Group 112. Dr Finley to surgeon general, June 14, 1903. Letter. No. 70760.

65. National Archives and Records Administration. Record Group 112. Dr Finley to surgeon general, June 17, 1903. Letter. No. 70760.

66. National Archives and Records Administration. Record Group 112. Surgeon general's office to John Marshall, July 6, 1903. Letter. No. 70760.

67. Marshall JS. Certain abnormal oral manifestations peculiar to tropical and sub tropical climates, as manifested among the American troops in the Philippine Islands. *Dental Digest*. 1904;10:551–561.

68. National Archives and Records Administration. Record Group 112. Marshall to the surgeon general, September 14, 1903. Letter with enclosure; Marshall, hygiene of the teeth and mouth. No. 70417. Box 446. Entry 26.

69. National Archives and Records Administration. Record Group 112. WP Evans, assistant adjutant general, to chief surgeon, Department of California, April 16, 1904. Letter with enclosure; Memorandum for soldier's hand book. No. 105637. Box 709. Entry 26.

70. *The Soldier's Handbook for use in the Army of the United States*. Washington, DC: Government Printing Office; 1908: 80.

71. Ashburn PM. *A History of the Medical Department of the United States Army*. Boston, Mass: Hougton Mifflin Co; 1929: 285–290.

72. National Archives and Records Administration. Record Group 165. General staff folder, medical department efficiency bill, 1904. Box 19. Entry 3.

73. Gillett, MC. *The Army Medical Department, 1775—1818*. Vol 3. Washington, DC: Center of Military History, United States Army; 1981: 320–322.

74. National Archives and Records Administration. Record Group 165. O'Reilly to the chief of staff, December 24, 1903. Letter with enclosure; Memorandum to accompany a bill to increase the efficiency of the Medical Corps, U.S. Army. General staff folder, Medical Department Efficiency Bill, 1904.

75. National Archives and Records Administration. Record Group 165. Contract surgeons: eligibility of, to command troops. Judge Advocate Davis to adjutant general, April 8, 1903, Appendix IV to memorandum, enclosure to letter, O'Reilly to the chief of staff, December 24, 1903.

76. National Archives and Records Administration. Record Group 112. John S Marshall to Surgeon General O'Reilly, November 30, 1903. Letter. No. 70760.

77. National Archives and Records Administration. Record Group 112. Surgeon general to Marshall, December 12, 1903. Letter. No. 70760.

78. National Archives and Records Administration. Record Group 112. Marshall to surgeon general, January 2, 1904. Letter. No. 70760.

79. National Archives and Records Administration. Record Group 112. Surgeon general to Marshall, January 4, 1904. Letter. No. 70760.

80. US War Department. General orders no. 132. In: *General Orders and Circulars, Adjutant General's Office, 1902*. Washington, DC: Government Printing Office; 1903: paragraphs 58–59.

81. National Archives and Records Administration. Record Group 94. Robert T Oliver to the military secretary, September 6, 1904. Letter. No. 407861. Box 2837.

82. National Archives and Records Administration. Record Group 94. Fourth endorsement, CL Heizman, acting surgeon general, to quartermaster general, October 26, 1904. No. 407861.

83. National Archives and Records Administration. Record Group 94. Lieutenant Colonel James T Kerr, acting chief, 1st Division, general staff, November 15, 1904. Memorandum report. No. 407861.

84. National Archives and Records Administration. Record Group 94. HP McCain, assistant adjutant general, to commanding general, Philippines Division, November 25, 1904. Letter. No. 407861.

85. Hussey SW. The life of an Army dentist. *Dental Register*. 1905;59:578–580.

86. The Army Dental Corps. *Army & Navy Journal*. Cited in: *Dental Cosmos*. 1903;45:902.

87. Marshall JS. The United States Army Dental Corps. Cited in: *Transactions of the Fourth International Dental Congress*. Ed. Kirk E. Philadelphia, Pa: Press of the Dental Cosmos; 1904: 48–49.

88. Sorber OM. The United States Army Dental Service. *Dental Brief*. Cited in: *Pacific Dental Gazette*. 1904;12:252–255.

89. National Archives and Records Administration. Record Group 112. Long to Brigadier General William E Dougherty, June 5, 1904. Letter. No. 106047. Box 712. Entry 26.

90. National Archives and Records Administration. Record Group 94. Order No. 44, WS Scott, captain, acting assistant adjutant general, Division of Philippines, to John D Millikin, January 5, 1903. Letter. No. 472628. Box 3319. Entry 25.

91. National Archives and Records Administration. Record Group 112. War Department Circular No. 33, July 1905. Box 54. Entry 26.

92. National Archives and Records Administration. Record Group 94. Robert T Oliver, China service, 1903–1904. No. 516526. Box 3596. Entry 25.

93. V[ail] WD. The Dental Corps. *Dental Bulletin Supplement to the Army Medical Bulletin.* 1934;5:158–160.

94. National Archives and Records Administration. First endorsement, Colonel JB Girard, chief surgeon, Philippines Division, to report, Oliver, April 1901–October 1904.

Chapter VIII

THE DRIVE STALLS: CONTINUING EFFORTS TO CREATE A COMMISSIONED DENTAL CORPS, 1901–1904

Introduction

While the new contract dental surgeons labored to establish their credibility with the soldiers in the field, the National Dental Association (NDA) and the dental press continued its drive for legislation that would create a commissioned corps of dentists in the Army. John Marshall played an increasingly prominent role in this process from inside the Army Medical Department and War Department beginning in October 1902, while continuing his daily dental practice and supervising the overall work of the dental surgeons. Whether or not the NDA and the American dental community ever achieved the goal for which they so ardently continued to agitate—a commissioned corps of military dentists within the Army Medical Department—depended as much on the success or failure of John Marshall and his colleagues in their daily work as it did on the efforts of the dental lobbyists.

Secretary Root Trumps Efforts to Gain New Legislation

On April 24, 1902, Alabama Senator Edmund Pettus, a veteran of the Mexican War and former Confederate brigadier general instrumental in promoting previous dental bills, submitted a bill (S 5420) to "reorganize the corps of dental surgeons attached to the Medical Department of the Army." The bill proposed a ratio of one dentist per 1,000 troops, a ratio that had become a fixture in legislative efforts. More importantly though, it proposed that dentists be appointed into the Army in grades comparable to the Medical Corps and that the contract dental surgeons presently on duty fill the initial appointments; he wanted dentists to be full commissioned members of the Medical Department on a career track. Tennessee Representative Walter Brownlow submitted a similar bill (HR 79) to the House the next day.[1,2]

Surgeon General Sternberg had already promised the NDA that he would accept a transition from contract dental surgeons to commissioned status while the February 1901 act was still under discussion, so he readily gave his personal endorsement to these bills on April 29, 1902, and recommended that dentists be made commissioned officers, just as physicians were:

> The dental surgeons appointed in accordance with the act of February 2, 1901, are rendering excellent service, and their services are highly appreciated by the officers

a

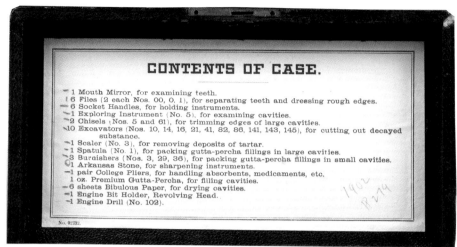

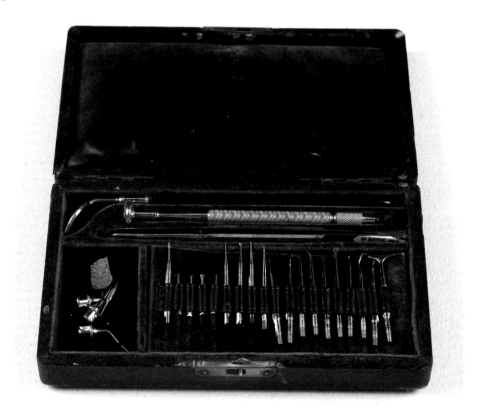

and enlisted men of the army. A larger number could be utilized to good advantage; and the permanent retention of dental surgeons as part of the military establishment will, in my opinion, be in the interest of the service.[3,4]

Despite Sternberg's endorsement, on May 3, 1902, Secretary of War Elihu Root wrote to the chairman of the House Committee on Military Affairs opposing the

c

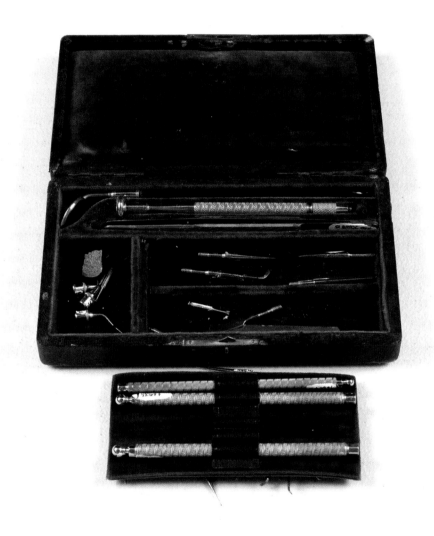

(*a*) *A smaller version of a portable dental case, possibly for field use.*
(*b*) *Inventory of smaller portable chest was attached to the inside of the lid.*
(*c*) *Open, with removable storage pouches taken out.*
Photograph: Courtesy of the US Army Medical Department Museum. Med7268-1,2,3.

bill. In his opinion, the contract dentists were needed only while large numbers of troops served in the Philippines, and he hoped that was a temporary situation. He also considered dentistry "not military in character" and wanted to avoid creating more noncombatant officers. Furthermore, Root believed that the original dental law needed more time to be assessed in actual practice before making changes.[5,6]

In a June 1902 editorial, Dr Wilbur Litch, editor of *Dental Brief*, rebutted Root's position, saying the bill was a "measure of simple justice" to those members of the dental profession serving as Army dental surgeons. Despite the surgeon general's recommendation, Root's opposition was critical to the bill's failure to pass in Congress. The struggle for commissioned status continued for 9 more years.[7]

At the meeting of the NDA in Niagara Falls, New York, in late July 1902, Mark Finley, Williams Donnally, Charles Butler, and Gordon White of the Committee on Army and Navy Dental Legislation expressed their disappointment over the bill's failure and singled out Secretary of War Root as the main cause:

> This bill received the approval of Surgeon General George M. Sternberg, in accordance with his purpose formed two and a half years ago, and at the time expressed to your committee. . . . The Secretary of War promptly and vigorously disapproved the commissioning of dental surgeons, for the alleged reason that their duties are in no sense military. In this connection we digress to mention that of the first two dentists sent to the Philippines with General Merritt's Army one was killed in battle soon after his arrival [John Gibbon], and some of the contract dental surgeons are constantly exposed to the dangers of war and of the military service. There are members of both the Senate and House Military Committees who will continue to favor commissioning dental surgeons notwithstanding the disapproval of the Secretary of War.[8(p274)]

The committee again laid out the three, often-stated, fundamental objectives pertaining to dental legislation for the Army that were set out in the NDA meetings of 1899 and 1901 and had guided its efforts with Congress, the War Department, and the surgeon general:

> *First.* That there may be secured to the officers, men, and boys in the U.S. military service the benefit of the services of educated, ethical, and efficient corps of dental surgeons.
>
> *Second.* That the value of dentistry to the general health, comfort, longevity and efficiency of the military man may be more universally recognized.
>
> *Third.* That the educational value of the dental college course, the importance of the function of the Doctor of Dental Surgery, and the civil status of the dental profession should be conceded as sufficient to entitle the military dental surgeon to equality with other professions in certain grades, pay, and allowances.[8(p273)]

To the committee, this was a serious matter of professional recognition and pride as well as service to the nation and soldier. The committee went on:

> As has been fully explained heretofore, the status secured through the efforts of this Committee for the army dental surgeon was acceptable because he entered the service on the "terms and conditions" applicable to more than two-thirds of the medical

officers in the Army, because the War Department had by regulations so adapted the contract system that the contract surgeon was at no social, professional or official disadvantage, and for the further important reason that the contract system adopted by Congress at the beginning of the Spanish War afforded the only available means to commissioned positions for either surgeons or dental surgeons. However, nothing else than commissioned rank for army officers can be altogether satisfactory to the professions they represent, or to the military service.[8]

For more than a year, the committee continued to work quietly with the Army and Navy surgeons general and Congress to remedy the major problems of an Army bill. However, for the first time in the 4 years since its establishment in 1898, the Committee on Army and Navy Dental Legislation did not file a meaningful report at the 1903 NDA meeting. This did not mean that their lobbying had ceased; it had just taken other directions. Three years later, Williams Donnally noted in his report to the NDA meeting—which is probably the best overall summary of the committee's intimate involvement in the legislative process from 1898 through 1906—that in 1902 and 1903 the committee had turned its attention "to oppose all recommendations for the establishment of a contract dental corps for the navy." By an understanding with the Navy surgeon general, after April 1902 the committee adopted the approach that the Army and Navy bills would be "identical in proposed grades of rank and corps organization, and for the same reason the earlier passage of the Army dental bill was more urgently attempted" because the adoption of either Army or Navy bill "would immediately become a precedent for the adoption of the other."[9(pp21–23)]

At the NDA's annual meeting in late July, 1903, in Asheville, North Carolina, the committee reported that "the prospect of securing a satisfactory commissioned rank for the Military Dental Surgeon is favorable" but did not go into details of its continuing efforts on Capitol Hill.[10] The report concluded "that an educated and efficient dental service, representative of the attainments of the profession, cannot be maintained without a commissioned personnel is practically conceded, and nothing less will be accepted by your Committee or your true friends in Congress."[10]

John Marshall and the Surgeon General

As the senior supervising dental surgeon and president of the examining board, John Sayre Marshall played the most critical role in the development of Army dentistry during its formative years. His stature in the American dental profession provided him with contacts and credibility that were almost unmatched at the time. From the very first, he was the principal spokesperson for the dental surgeons within the profession and Army and his interactions with the surgeons general he served shaped Army dentistry. While no documents available today shed any real light on the personal relationship of Surgeon General O'Reilly and Marshall, the two men appear to have known each other at the Presidio of San Francisco when O'Reilly served as chief surgeon of the Department of California from June through August 1902. The volume of correspondence between the men testifies that they had a significant interaction during O'Reilly's time as surgeon general. Regardless of their personal relationship, Marshall's

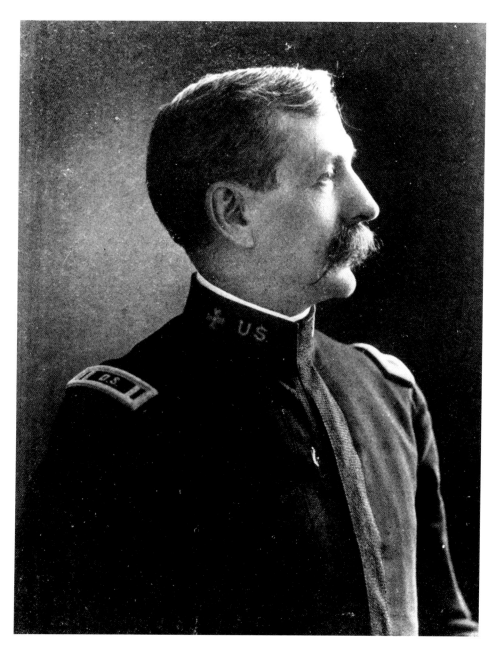

*John S Marshall, senior supervising dental surgeon and president of the examining board,
played a critical role in the development of Army dentistry during its formative years.
Photograph: Courtesy of the American Dental Association.*

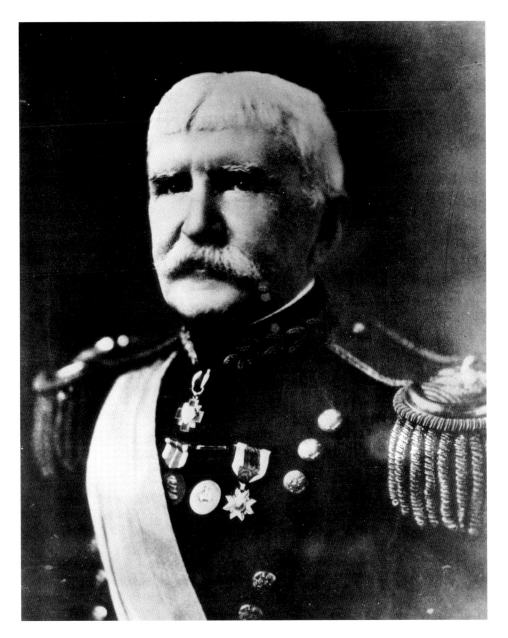

Robert M O'Reilly, surgeon general 1902–1909.
Photograph: Courtesy of the National Museum of Health and Medicine,
Armed Forces Institute of Pathology. NCP 3566.

position as a practicing dentist in the field during these years and the lack of an official dental presence in the Office of The Surgeon General in Washington seriously hampered his ability to influence the policies and decisions pertaining to dental matters.

The difficulties facing the Army's dentists as contract dental surgeons, the details of establishing a functioning dental service, and the need for legislation to create a commissioned corps of dentists formed major themes in John Marshall's correspondence with O'Reilly. While not taking any discernible role in the 1902 legislation struggle, Marshall began his personal dialogue on dental legislation with the new surgeon general on October 14, 1902, with a letter and attached draft of a bill to provide commissioned rank for the officers of a "Corps of Dental Surgeons."[11] The proposed bill for the reorganization of the contract dental service into a commissioned corps was titled, "Bill for the Organization of a Corps of Dental Surgeons to be attached to the Medical Department of the U.S. Army and under the direction of the Surgeon General," and read as follows:

> Be it enacted by the Senate and House of Representatives of the United States of America in Congress assembled.
>
> *Sec. 1.* There is hereby created a corps of dental surgeons to be under the direction of the Surgeon General of the Army and whose duty shall be to give dental treatment and services to those now entitled or who may hereafter be entitled to treatment and services of the medical corps of the army and to perform such other duties as may from time to time be directed or authorized by the Secretary of War.
>
> *Sec. 2.* The corps shall consist of three (3) Dental Surgeons, each with the rank, pay and allowances of Major, six (6) assistant dental surgeons, each with the rank, pay and allowances of Captain, mounted, and twenty-one (21) dental surgeons, each with the rank, pay and allowances of first lieutenant, mounted.
>
> *Sec. 3.* The President, by and with the advice and consent of the Senate, may first appoint the three dental surgeons with the rank of major, provided for by this act, from the contract dental surgeons now in the service who have demonstrated their mental, moral and professional fitness therefore.
>
> *Sec. 4.* Vacancies created by this act or which may hereafter occur shall be filled by appointment by the President, by and with the advice and consent of the Senate, of candidates from civil life who must be citizens of the United States between 24 and 30 years of age, of good moral character, graduates of standard medical or dental colleges, and thoroughly trained in all the departments of dental surgery, of unquestioned professional repute, and who shall be required to pass the usual physical examinations and such professional examinations as the Secretary of War may prescribe, which examination will consist, among others, of the subjects that comprise the curricula of the standard dental colleges of the United States, and tests of skill and proficiency in all the practical departments of dental surgery, provided that those contract dental surgeons now in the service who have demonstrated their mental, moral and professional fitness may be appointed assistant dental surgeons.

Sec. 5. Promotions in the corps of dental surgeons, as prescribed in Sec. 2 of this act, shall be by seniority, provided, that all promotions shall be subject to such examinations and regulations as the President may direct, and provided further that service as contract dental surgeon shall be computed as commissioned service.

Sec. 6. That in time of war or when war is imminent the President may, by and with the advice and consent of the Senate, appoint volunteer dental surgeons with the rank, pay and allowances of first Lieutenant, mounted, provided that the total number of dental surgeons shall not exceed one to each 2000 enlisted men in the regular volunteer forces.[11]

In his letter, Marshall enumerated the reasons why a reorganization of the corps was necessary:

- Dental diseases were as prevalent among the officers and enlisted soldiers of the US Army as they were in the civilian population and even more so among the troops serving in Cuba, the Philippines, and Alaska.
- "Serviceable" teeth were essential to maintaining the "general Health" and "highest efficiency" of an army serving in the field, especially in the tropics.
- It would be advantageous from an economic standpoint for the government to provide dental surgeons to treat the dental diseases that caused loss of duty time.
- The dental service had passed the "experimental stage" and proved its "great value" to the Army. Therefore, it should be continued as a "permanent service."
- The "contract system" currently in vogue was not "adequate to the requirements of a permanent service."[11]

Marshall argued that dental surgeons had demonstrated their worthiness of commissioned rank with the right to promotions and retirement benefits. After laying out his arguments for a commissioned corps, he concluded:

I would, therefore, most respectfully solicit your consideration of the merits of the case, and your suggestions upon the various features of the measure as presented, with the hope that you will see the propriety and advisability of recommending to the Secretary of War the passage by Congress at its next session of this or some other measure which in your judgment might seem more desirable.[11]

On October 23 O'Reilly acknowledged receipt of Marshall's proposal.[12] Nothing more was heard about his proposed bill until more than a year later, when Marshall again wrote to O'Reilly to take up his invitation "to be free in suggesting for your consideration such matters as seemed to me to be of importance for the well being and efficiency of the Dental Corps." Thus, Marshall began a series of exchanges with O'Reilly on the need for a commissioned dental corps at the very time that O'Reilly himself was working on his own bill to eliminate contract surgeons and enlarge the number of medical officers. Marshall stressed that a "change in status" of the Dental Corps was of "vital importance" to its numbers, who had appealed to him as their senior dental surgeon to broach the subject to the surgeon general. Many of the best young dentists were "getting uneasy and more or less dissatisfied" with their "status and future prospects." Several were considering leaving the service. If they were assured that the dental surgeons would be placed on a commissioned basis with prospects of promotion, their services could be retained. Marshall reminded O'Reilly that placing the dental surgeons on commissioned status would actually save the government money. A first lieutenant's pay was less than the contractors were receiving. Marshall believed that the current dental surgeons would trade the slight pay difference (they would lose $200 a year) for "improved status" and therefore remain in the service.[13]

Marshall recommended that his October 23, 1902, proposal for new dental legislation be substituted for the bill (HR 79) that Walter Brownlow of Tennessee had introduced in Congress on November 9, 1903. Marshall expressed the hope that legislation would be passed during the upcoming congressional session to place "the corps in the honorable position to which they aspire and to which the learning and the high standing of their profession entitles them to occupy."[13,14]

On December 12 the surgeon general informed Marshall that although he understood that "rank and commission" would be "desirable" and "important" to the dental surgeons, he failed to see how the government would benefit from the change to a commissioned corps. He reasoned as follows:

- Dental surgeons were employed for a "special line of work," which did not necessitate their accompanying the troops into the field where they would be obliged to command and discipline enlisted soldiers. Therefore, he failed to see why they needed commissioned rank and how it would improve the dental service.
- If dental surgeons were commissioned as first lieutenants, their pay would be less than that of contract dentists. They would stand to lose $200 per year. A more effective solution would be for the contract dentists to keep their present status or receive a pay increase in exchange for their services.
- As commissioned officers, the dental surgeons' entire time would be "at the disposal" of the government, thereby preventing the after-duty hours private work they were able to perform under the current arrangement (under Army Regulation [AR] 1584).
- The Brownlow bill was prepared by someone "not conversant with the service," and its discussion, in the surgeon general's opinion, was therefore not worth the time. As for Marshall's own bill, O'Reilly wondered about the nature of the "other duties" to be authorized by the secretary of war to which Marshall referred.[15]

On January 2, 1904, Marshall sent a lengthy and detailed reply to the surgeon general, pointing out the following:

- While it was true that dental surgeons were engaged in a "special line of work," there were other commissioned officers in the Army, such as paymasters and chaplains, who held rank but did not normally command troops in the field. Dental surgeons were normally assigned an enlisted soldier from the Hospital Corps who served as an assistant (under AR 1581). At base and general hospitals, sometimes two or more assistants were under the "command and discipline" of a dental surgeon. In the Philippine Islands, dental surgeons did accompany the troops in the field; the dental outfit used by contract dentists was designed specifically for that purpose. Duty "under arms" at isolated posts where night attacks often occurred was common.

- The problem with the contract system was not one of pay, but one of status. Military rank, which would render the service more attractive, was the main desire of the dental surgeons. A dentist with a university degree felt that he should be accorded commissioned status like his medical colleagues and other professionals in the service. The dental surgeons had the same responsibilities as officers, but not the rank; under Army law at the time, dental surgeons were not authorized to issue orders to their enlisted assistants or even their patients. Therefore, the majority of the contract dentists preferred to hold the rank of first lieutenant and accept the pay difference ($133.33 per month, rather than the $150 they were receiving).
- As for AR 1584, the majority of dental surgeons felt that the same rules for professional service should apply to the Dental Corps as to the Medical Corps. Fees for work excluded by the government could be collected by the dental surgeons and turned over to the proper authority.
- The "other duties" to which Marshall referred in his bill were included to provide for nonprofessional duties, such as court martial boards, and could be omitted.[16]

Marshall concluded:

Finally, I would respectfully suggest that the importance of the work of the dental corps and its general acceptability to the Army, justifies giving them a status that will further contribute to their efficiency while the members of the Dental Corps, individually and collectively, have fully demonstrated their professional ability, proficiency and faithfulness to the service, and, are, therefore, in my judgment, worthy of the honorable status to which they aspire.[16]

After receiving Marshall's detailed report, O'Reilly said that "the proposition to confer rank and military status on Contract Dental Surgeons has been received, and will have, as it merits, attentive consideration." (It is interesting to note in these exchanges that whereas Marshall invariably referred to the "Dental Corps" or "corps," O'Reilly always used the terms "contract dental surgeons" or "dental surgeons.") The surgeon general told Marshall that he remained unconvinced of the need to commission the dental surgeons, "But I am open to conviction."[17]

On January 13, 1904, Marshall replied and reminded O'Reilly that the $200 in pay that the contract dentist would lose would be more than compensated for by his gain: commutation of quarters, right to forage, disability or age retirement with pension and "self respect." Forage rights would allow the dentists to keep a horse for "outdoor exercise," which would benefit their health because they worked in a "cramped" position while operating. Commissioned rank would also allow the dental surgeons to inspect themselves and conduct examinations for promotion. The "glamour of the quasi military position" was wearing off for the younger men, and something had to be done to improve their morale. Again, the surgeon general's office filed Marshall's "additional arguments" for "future consideration," but no action was taken, despite the fact that the foreign tours of some of the contractors stationed in the Philippines had already exceeded 2 years.[18,19,20]

The Brownlow Bill (HR 79): Proposed Reorganization of the Dental Surgeons, 1903–1904

The O'Reilly-Marshall exchange played out at the same time that the original 1901 dental surgeons' 3-year contracts were expiring. After February 1904 and the failed legislative effort of 1902, efforts to enact new dental legislation were renewed. On November 9, 1903, at the first session of the 58th Congress, Representative Brownlow introduced in the House another new bill (HR 79) "to reorganize the corps of dental surgeons attached to the Medical Department of the Army." This bill was essentially the same as the 1902 bill and it was quickly referred to the Committee on Military Affairs.[14,21,22]

On March 25, 1904, the Odontological Society of Cincinnati sent a petition to the new secretary of war, William Taft, recommending the passage of the pending bill. It cited the upcoming expiration of the 3-year contracts of the original contract dental surgeons and the desirability of retaining their services. The letter was passed to Surgeon General O'Reilly for review and comment.[23]

On April 15, O'Reilly returned the correspondence and informed the Army chief of staff that he did not believe HR 79 was needed and suggested that a new bill be prepared. O'Reilly's comments were critical and frequently referred to as the Medical Department's official position on Dental Corps legislation throughout his years as surgeon general. He told the chief of staff the following:

> In considering the Bill (H.R. 79) organizing a dental corps composed of officers of various grades and with military rank, this office has hitherto taken the position that rank was not needed to further the proper performance of the duty devolving on a dental surgeon whose functions are strictly limited to the care &c. of the teeth of officers and enlisted men of the Army. Assurances are, however, given from credible and responsible sources that the possession of rank would result in giving better service than can be procured under the present contract system. This being the case, I have the honor to recommend that a Bill be drawn to accomplish this purpose and that it be submitted to Congress for legislative action. The Bills referred to–which are now in Committee–are defective and should not pass.
>
> In my opinion, the Bill to be proposed should contain provisions to the following effect:
>
> 1. Prescribing age limit and professional qualifications. 2. Providing examining boards to determine physical fitness (a board of medical officers) and a dental board (to consist of one dental surgeon now in the military service, to be designated by the Secre-

tary of War, and two dental surgeons nominated to the Secretary of War by the President of the American Dental Association, who while so serving should be properly compensated) and without the recommendation of these two boards no one shall be appointed. 3. No more than five original appointments shall have the same date of commission. On being commissioned they shall be entitled Dental Surgeons and shall rank as First Lieutenants. After five years service, those holding this grade who shall have passed a satisfactory physical and professional examination shall rank as Captain, and after an additional 10 years service, shall, subject to a similar examination, rank as Major. The pay and allowances of Dental Surgeons shall be the same as those of a First Lieutenant. But their right to command should be absolutely limited to the Dental Surgeons and such enlisted men as may be detailed for duty with them, so as to prevent them from assuming command of hospitals. 4. The whole number of Dental Surgeons should not exceed thirty of whom three shall have the rank of Major, five the rank of Captain and twenty-two the rank of First Lieutenant.[25]

One of the "credible and responsible sources" that influenced O'Reilly's position on commissioned rank versus contract status must have been John Marshall, who repeatedly attacked the contract system. However, items 1 through 4 of O'Reilly's letter became the main points of discussion and disagreement between the War Department and the surgeon general on one hand, and Marshall and the Army's dental surgeons, the NDA's Committee on Army and Navy Dental Legislation, and the dental profession and press on the other.

On April 21, 1904, Senator Pettus sent a note to Surgeon General O'Reilly and attached a copy of HR 79. He told O'Reilly that the Senate Committee on Military Affairs was considering the bill, and "I most respectfully ask your opinion of this bill; and also your opinion as to the best mode of providing the Services of Dental Surgeons for the Army & the number needed." O'Reilly responded, saying that day that he thought

the bill mentioned you should not pass because it is very carelessly and loosely drawn (for instance there is no such rank known in the Medical Department of the Army as "Passed Assistant Surgeon")[a Navy rank]. There is no proper provision for examinations; there is no limit on age at admission (which might result in the appointment of men to the highest proposed rank and their retirement for age under the general law after a very short service).[9,25,26]

O'Reilly noted that the number of dental surgeons "while not excessive, appears to be sufficient." He referred the senator to his April 15 letter to the chief of staff, which stated his position on the actions necessary to correct the deficiencies in the current bill:

I have written and forwarded for the action of the Secretary of War certain suggestions in regard to legislation for the Dental Surgeons. These suggestions, if adopted, will substantially meet what I understand is the main point desired by the American Dental Association, that is, permanent tenure of office with proper rank, to be increased on length of service proportionate to that in the Medical Department of the Army.[26,27]

Two years later, Williams Donnally provided some additional perspective on what had occurred:

> The War department declined making a report on dental bills offered after April 1902, and the Military Committees refrained from consideration of these bills because they were not reported on by the War department. Your committee, with a view to creating a sentiment in favor of the bills, used all the support at its command with both the War department and the Military Committees, until finally we induced these committees to make simultaneous special requests for a report on H.R. 79, and on the corresponding Senate bill. In response to a request of the Military Committee for a report, H.R. 79 was reported upon unfavorably by the Surgeon-general under the date of April 15, 1904, and unfavorably by the general staff (a body composed of about thirty selected army officers), unfavorably by the chief of staff, General Chaffee, unfavorably by Secretary Taft, and returned to the Senate and House military committees.[9]

The main points of contention became age limitations, distribution of rank, time in grade for promotion, pay and allowances, composition of the examining board, and the physical and professional reexamination of those contract dental surgeons already serving. After the April 15 memo, Donnally's committee began discussions with Surgeon General O'Reilly and his staff:

> with a view of reaching an agreement whereby the Surgeon-general would, at a later suitable time, affirm his approval of every detail of the terms of a bill to be drawn and presented to Congress by your Committee along the lines of his recommendations of April 15, 1904, but the terms to be more favorable in several respects, especially with reference to the special recognition to be accorded those already in the contract service.[9]

As these negotiations dragged along on a new draft bill, Senator Pettus submitted another bill (S 5906) to the Senate Committee on Military Affairs on December 12, 1904, "to reorganize the corps of dental surgeons attached to the Medical Department of the Army."[29–31] The general staff referred the new Senate bill to the surgeon general for review and comment. On December 17, O'Reilly responded by returning both S 5906 and HR 79 and inviting attention again to his April 15 letter. He recommended some changes that limited commissions to those now in service who had rendered "satisfactory service" for 3 or more years and met all other qualifications of the law, "were within the age limit required by regulations at the time their original contracts were signed," and passed the standard physical examination for commissioning.[32] Clearly, such an age limit did not favor retaining the most experienced of the contract dental surgeons, including Marshall, Oliver, and Hess, and Donnally's committee continued to debate these critical points with the surgeon general.[9]

Growing Army Support for New Dental Legislation

In addition to the dental community, significant support for a substantive dental bill also came from many of the Army's line officers, who increasingly understood the value that dental surgeons added to maintaining soldiers' health and overall unit readiness. By the fall of 1903 some Army department commanders and surgeons believed that experience to date indicated a need for more dental surgeons and better

operating rooms at the various posts. In his annual report for 1903, Major General
John Bates, commanding the Department of the Lakes, described the department's
dental service, which was typical of all stateside dental activities:

> One contract dental surgeon is on duty in this Department, who, during the year
> visited each post, and to the best of his ability extended his service to the officers and
> enlisted men thereat. He treated 1,966 cases. The work performed has been largely
> of an emergency character owing to the lack of facilities for laboratory work at most
> stations. Application was made for the assignment of an additional dentist to duty in
> this Department, as the work was thought greater than one could properly perform.
> It was the intention to recommend the establishment of a dental office at a central
> point in the Department, where one dentist could attend to operative and prosthetic
> dentistry and make one annual or semi-annual visits to all stations. It was believed
> this arrangement would place the dental service on a more satisfactory footing in this
> department. *No other dental surgeon was available for this detail, and the one at present on
> duty continues to make periodical visits to the various stations until such time as it may be
> practicable to obtain the assignment of another to this department.*[33]

On May 20, 1904, Colonel Marion Maus, the commander of the 20th Infantry
Regiment, wrote from his headquarters at Malate Barracks, Manila:

> I have the honor to invite your attention to the importance of dentists in the army, es-
> pecially at remote stations in order that officers and enlisted men have proper dental
> attention.
>
> While in command at Camp Marahui, Mindanao, certain officers including myself,
> and a number of enlisted men suffered very much from want of such service; later,
> however, a dentist was provided and great relief and benefit were realized.
>
> There are times when the services of a dentist are as necessary as that of the Army
> Surgeon. From my experience in the service, including all posts of the United States
> and Dependencies, I can testify to the importance of this branch of the service, and to
> much suffering from the want of it.
>
> It would, perhaps, be desirable to have Dental Surgeons assigned to certain regiments
> in the same way as Chaplains.
>
> The Dental Surgeons that I have known are experienced and excellent men. I would
> strongly urge that their position be made permanent, the number increased and that
> they be given rank equal to that of Assistant Surgeons, they being in their profession,
> fully as important. It is certain that first class Dental Surgeons cannot be kept in the
> service unless they are offered sufficient inducements.
>
> In this climate teeth rapidly decay and disease appears to attack the mouth more
> rapidly than in the States, although in remote districts in the United States the Dental
> Surgeon is fully as necessary.
>
> I strongly urge legislation making a permanent Corps of Dental Surgeons in number
> suited to the demands of the service, with permanent rank and pay.[34]

Despite Maus's strong endorsement, the medical officers in the Philippine command took a different view. On May 25, 1904, the chief surgeon at headquarters, Department of Luzon, Manila, Colonel John Hall, disapproved Maus's recommendation, stating "the present system seems sufficient." On May 27 the chief surgeon's office, headquarters, Philippine Division, concurred, stating, "the present system of dental service appears to be satisfactory, and so far as known in this office no difficulty has been experienced in securing competent dentists under it." Major General (later Lieutenant General and Chief of Staff, 1910–1914) Leonard Wood, himself a former medical officer, then the commanding general for the Department of Mindanao, agreed with his medical officers that "the present system is satisfactory."[35,36]

On June 20, 1904, Major (later Lieutenant General and Chief of Staff) Hugh Scott, 14th Cavalry Regiment, commanding the post at Jolo, Jolo Island, Philippines, added his support for military dentists in a letter (through military channels) to the military secretary:

> I have the honor to invite your attention to the great importance of and the vast benefit derived from the services of a Dental Surgeon at this post.
>
> The Post is about 600 miles from Manila where it would be necessary for officers and enlisted men and members of their families to go for dental treatment but for the presence in the post of a Dental Surgeon. The necessity to travel this long distance and use of the infrequent transportation available here, would often occasion great hardship and inconvenience and would sometimes keep an officer away from his duties for a whole month.
>
> There are a number of Posts in the Philippine Islands and even in the United States where similar conditions would hold and to which the same remarks would apply.
>
> I recommend legislation making a permanent Corps of Dental Surgeons with permanent rank and pay and sufficient in number to meet the demands of the service.[37]

However, the division's chief surgeon, Colonel Hall, once again disagreed and endorsed Scott's letter on July 16, 1904:

> It does not seem to follow that the present system of furnishing dental service should be changed, and new legislation be called for, because the small post of Jolo may find it convenient to have a permanent dental surgeon. The present system is found to work well enough. All that is needed is to make the supply more commensurate with the demand.[38]

On November 2 Lieutenant Colonel George Chase, the commander of the 12th Cavalry Regiment stationed at Camp McGrath, Batangas, endorsed the legislation (through military channels) for dental commissioned status:

> I have the honor to recommend that such action may be taken by constituted authority as may be deemed advisable, leading to the establishment of a corps of dental surgeons with commissioned officers as its members. There are at present not enough contract dental surgeons to meet the demands of the service. The 12th Cavalry, now under my command, has no dental surgeon on duty with it and has not had since July 1, 1904. The officers and men of the regiment are continually asking

for authority to go to Manila for dental treatment, thus depriving the government of their services and entailing upon them a considerable expense. My experience with troops in the past in isolated places with no means at all of dental treatment, and especially now in the Philippines, teaches me that the care of the teeth is as essential to the health and efficiency of troops as is the care of other portions of the body, in short a man with bad teeth is almost sure to have bad general health in addition to great discomfort. The present system of employing dental surgeons is an excellent step in the right direction. I am convinced that a trained commissioned corps of dental surgeons would be a great improvement upon the present system and would be an economical measure.[39]

Colonel Joseph Girard, chief surgeon of the Philippines Division, endorsed Chase's letter on November 15, 1904:

My views upon the subject of this communication have been expressed at length in an endorsement to the Report of Supervising Dental Surgeon R.T. Oliver to the Surgeon General, on his being relieved from duty in this Division [see Chapter VII, The Philippines, 1902–1904]. I stated therein that practically ninety per cent of the present rank and file of the Army, whether in the Philippines or in the United States, were, judging from my experience, in need of dental treatment, and that considering the short period of service of the majority, they must have been afflicted with bad teeth before enlistment; that in consequence, either dentists enough should be provided to repair and put in sound condition the jaws of every newly enlisted recruit, before he joins his command, or else, stringent orders must be issued to recruiting officers and examining surgeons to reject every applicant with unsound teeth; under the latter provision, I am convinced that the present number of Dentists allowed by law is sufficient for all legitimate purposes; in the other case, at least twice and probably three times the legal number will be required. I see no good reason why Dental Surgeons should not be commissioned, although I decidedly object to the creation of a so called "Corps" which I consider totally unnecessary.[40]

The dental surgeons also drew stateside support from the line. On July 19, 1904, Colonel Ralph Hoyt, the commander of the 25th Infantry Regiment stationed at Fort Niobrara, Nebraska, endorsed the dental corps bill (through military channels):

I have the honor to recommend that Dental Surgeons be added to the Commissioned force of the Army the same as other permanent Officers, and that the claims of the Contract Dental Surgeons now in the service be given prior consideration for appointment.

The service of Dental Surgeons with the Army in the Insular possessions and at frontier stations in the United States in relieving suffering has demonstrated the necessity of providing for its continuance on a permanent basis. It is believed that they should be assigned permanently to regiments that are located at stations away from cities and that their promotion to additional grades should be in proportion to the advance of officers of like grades and duties in the line with which they serve.[41]

On July 22 Department of the Missouri Chief Surgeon Colonel Charles Byrne concurred: "According to my observation in two military departments, the number of contract dental surgeons is not sufficient to do the amount of dental work which is necessary for the comfort and health of the soldiers of the Army."[42]

Support from Civilian Dentists

In addition to Army line officers, dental colleges and numerous dental societies sent in petitions to the War Department in support of new legislation. On May 14, 1904, the faculty of the dental department of the University of California signed a petition recommending that Congress pass legislation creating a commissioned dental corps. The dean, Harry Carlton, forwarded the petition on May 27 to the secretary of war. On June 24, the faculty of the Indiana Dental College likewise petitioned Congress in favor of a commissioned dental corps.[43,44] Many dental societies joined the effort to persuade Congress and the War Department to enact legislation creating a commissioned dental corps with grades from first lieutenant to lieutenant colonel. From June to December 1904 20 major dental societies, including the state societies from California, New Jersey, Wisconsin, and Utah, wrote to Secretary of War Taft, the surgeon general, or their senators and representatives expressing their wholehearted support for a commissioned Army dental corps.[45–47] The American Medical Association's section on stomatology showed its support when, on July 13, it sent Taft the petition adopted at the June AMA meeting in Atlantic City, New Jersey.

To all of these, the War Department responded promptly and politely. The response to the California State Dental Association on June 1, 1904, summed up the War Department's position: "by direction of the Chief of Staff, that this recommendation will be held in view for consideration of the Secretary of War in case further legislation on the subject shall be recommended by the Department."[48–50]

Williams Donnally's Reports of 1904

In June 1904 Williams Donnally, the chairman of the International Committee on the Promotion of the Appointment of Dentists to the Armies and Navies of the World and long-time member of the NDA's Committee on Army and Navy Dental Legislation, reported that the "unsupplied requisitions" of Army department commanders and post surgeons for more dental surgeons not only proved the necessity for an increase in the size of the Dental Corps, but also the "value" of the corps and the need for its commissioning. The committee requested that dentists contribute papers on the subject to be presented at the Fourth International Dental Congress to be held in Saint Louis August 29 through September 3 in conjunction with the NDA's eighth annual meeting. Donnally also noted that "the present Surgeon General has only recently encouraged the committee of the National Dental Association to expect his official endorsement of our contention for commissioned rank for military dental surgeons."[51,52] Unfortunately, Donnally was incorrect on this point.

On September 2, 1904, at the International Dental Congress, Donnally read the report of the international committee and offered two resolutions. First, he suggested that the world's military organizations provide dental care; and second, that an international committee, consisting of one representative from each country, be appointed to lobby for the same. The dental congress passed the resolutions.[53]

CONTINUING EFFORTS TO CREATE A COMMISSIONED DENTAL CORPS

John Marshall at the Fourth International Dental Congress

The Fourth International Dental Congress and the NDA annual meeting in Saint Louis were ideal platforms for John Marshall to describe the development of Army dentistry since February 1901. His paper, presented August 30, 1904, was titled "The United States Army Dental Corps," which perhaps expressed his dreams for the future rather than the realities of the present Army organization.[54] Combined with his annual reports and his paper from the 1903 NDA annual meeting, his report provided another clear picture of the inadequate dental health of the Army in the early years of Army dentistry.

According to Marshall, statistics for the Army showed that dental diseases were:

> . . . as prevalent among the officers and enlisted men of our army as among individuals in civil life . . . while among the troops who have served in tropical and semi-tropical climates these diseases are much more prevalent. Dental diseases affected 42.85% of troops who served only in the United States, but the numbers rose to 61.12% of those serving in the Philippine Islands and 64.02% for the troops who served in Cuba and Porto Rico [sic].

> The records of my office at the General Hospital, Presidio of San Francisco, show that from October 1, 1901, to July 1, 1904, 4533 cases have been examined and treated for dental and oral diseases, and, out of this number only one person has been found who was absolutely free from dental caries; this was a young lieutenant just graduated from West Point military academy.[54]

Two of Marshall's assistants had examined two infantry regiments recently returned from the Philippines and found 87.62% (632 out of 711) of the soldiers in one regiment and 93.46% (744 out of 765) in the other required immediate dental treatment. Troops in the first regiment had 2,280 dental caries and required 321 extractions, while in the second unit soldiers had 3,565 dental caries and required 197 extractions.[54]

After providing a detailed account of dental disease and work done since 1901, Marshall compared the Army's dental health to that of the British and German armies and discussed the dental diseases that adversely affected the soldier's oral wellbeing and efficiency. He then described what he called the "Plan of Organization of the United States Army Dental Corps," merely reviewing the Medical Department's current policies and procedures governing the contract dental surgeons, along with their official status (which he noted was "a somewhat anomalous one"), examination and selection of candidates, and pay and allowances. He outlined the duties and responsibilities of the dental surgeons, their equipment, their conditions of employment, operating procedures, and reporting system.[54]

Concluding his presentation, Marshall said:

> From the foregoing it will be seen that the War Department, through recommendations of the Surgeon-general, has provided for the care and treatment of the dental and oral diseases of the army in as thorough and as scientific a manner as is possible

under the exigencies of military life and movements. Experience, however, may make it necessary to institute certain changes and modifications in the present system of service, and when such action is proved to be essential to the welfare of the army and an increased efficiency of the corps there is no doubt that the proper authorities will immediately institute such changes and modifications.[54(pp48–49)]

Marshall's presentation elicited heated discussion on the current status of dentists in the Army and Navy. Among those who spoke was Williams Donnally. After outlining what the NDA committee had accomplished since 1898, he noted that its work was instrumental in crafting the bills now under consideration in Congress that would provide commissioned rank to both Army and Navy dental surgeons.[54] Donnally said:

As members of the committee of the National Dental Association, Dr. Finley and I are authorized to say to this Fourth International Dental Congress that an agreement has been reached by which the War and Navy departments concede the committee's contention for commissioned rank for military and naval dental surgeons, and, if the arrangement is not defeated by antagonistic influences, it is confidently expected that this committee will, in cooperation with those departments, secure reasonably satisfactory legislation by Congress at its next session. . . . the battle has been waged for years, and now that an agreement has been reached on the essential claim of the profession—commissioned rank—there can be no doubt that the military and naval committees of Congress, always favorable to our contention, will accord us at all that the War and Navy departments concede.[54(pp50-51)]

The same day, at a concurrent meeting of the NDA, the Committee on Army and Navy Dental Legislation reported "progress" in the quest for commissioned status. In light of Donnally's ongoing negotiations with Surgeon General O'Reilly to resolve the many differences outlined in O'Reilly's April 15 letter to the chief of staff, this was apparently an accurate appraisal.[9]

Considering the American and international audience, Marshall's paper was probably the most important presentation to that time on the status and significance of dentistry in the US Army. Certainly, it was the clearest overall exposition so far on the roles, responsibilities, and challenges of the contract dental surgeons and on the dental health of the US Army. It was a critical, if still little-known, milestone in the history of the evolution of the US Army Dental Corps that ranks along with his paper before the NDA meeting in August 1901.

Marshall's Draft Bill, December 1904

On December 16, 1904, Marshall, still stationed at the Presidio of San Francisco, once again sent his proposed "Bill to increase the efficiency of the Army" to the military secretary through the surgeon general. The bill provided for reorganization of the current dental surgeons into a commissioned corps. Identical to his October 23, 1902, proposal to Surgeon General O'Reilly except for some minor wording and an allocation ratio of one dental surgeon per 1,000 enlisted soldiers (rather than the previous one for 2,000 soldiers), this bill incorporated the changes in "status and organization" that Marshall thought were necessary for a more "economic administration" of the dental surgeons and about which he commented in Saint Louis in late August.[55]

Marshall accompanied his proposed bill with a lengthy memorandum justifying the creation of a permanent commissioned dental corps, which drew heavily from his thoughts in his earlier exchanges with O'Reilly. He maintained his corps' strength at still only 30. In his memo, he cited the positive performance of the contract dental surgeons and the subsequent reduction in sick time lost and concurrent improvement in the overall health of the force. The need to attract high quality dentists to support the Army mandated an improvement in dentists' status and chances for career advancement. Furthermore, in Marshall's view, dentists had to have the necessary authority over subordinates and patients to effectively carry out their duties. He did not feel that the change from contract to commissioned status would have much effect on costs. On December 23 O'Reilly forwarded Marshall's proposed bill and memorandum to the military secretary, "inviting attention to [his] letter of April 15th, addressed to the Chief of Staff, in which [his] views are expressed in regard to the organization of the Dental Corps." Marshall's proposal and O'Reilly's letter were forwarded to the chief of staff on the 27th.[56,57] O'Reilly's own bill (S 4838; HR 13998) was also before Congress for consideration, carrying the approval of the secretary of war.[58]

The Drive is Stalled

By the end of 1904, nearly 4 years after the Act of February 2, 1901, the NDA's efforts to gain congressional legislation to create an Army dental corps had stalled against the opposition of the War Department and Surgeon General O'Reilly. Even though John Marshall had become increasingly involved in discussing new dental legislation with O'Reilly, he had made little or no progress. The progress toward what most American dentists, dental associations, and the dental press believed to be the promised commissioned "Dental Corps" had not been as swift, or apparently as certain, as it had seemed it would be back in 1901. More years of struggle lay ahead.

References

1. *Congressional Record, 57th Cong, 1st Sess*. Vol 35. Washington, DC: Government Printing Office; 1092.

2. Bills before the Senate, Fifty-Seventh Congress. *Int Dent J*. 1902;23:456–457.

3. National Archives and Records Administration. Record Group 112. Endorsement, Surgeon General Sternberg to secretary of war, April 29, 1902. No. 106047. Entry 26.

4. San Francisco Dental Association [proceedings]. *Pacific Dental Gazette*. 1909;17:136.

5. National Archives and Records Administration. Record Group 94. Endorsement, Root to chairman, House Committee on Military Affairs, May 3, 1902. No. 432377. Box 3017. Entry 25.

6. National Archives and Records Administration. Record Group 94. Adjutant general's office, May 1, 1902. Letter. No. 432377. Box 3017. Entry 25.

7. [Litch WF]. Commissioned status for Army and Navy dental surgeons. *Dental Brief*. 1902;7:336.

8. Finley M, Donnally W, Butler CS, White G. Report of Committee on Army and Navy Dental Legislation. In: *Transactions of the National Dental Association*. Chicago, Ill: Dental Digest Press; 1903.

9. Finley M, Donnally W, Butler CS, White G. Report of Committee on Army and Navy Dental Legislation. In: *Transactions of the National Dental Association*. Chicago, Ill: Dental Digest Press; 1906.

10. Finley M, Donnally W, Butler CS, White G. Report of Committee on Army and Navy Dental Legislation. In: *Transactions of the National Dental Association*. Chicago, Ill: Dental Digest Press; 1904.

11. National Archives and Records Administration. Record Group 112. John S Marshall to the surgeon general, October 14, 1902. Letter with enclosure; An act to increase the efficiency of the Army. No. 70760. Box 449. Entry 26.

12. National Archives and Records Administration. Record Group 112. Surgeon General O'Reilly to Marshall, October 23, 1902. Letter. No. 70760. Box 449. Entry 26.

13. National Archives and Records Administration. Record Group 112. John S Marshall to Surgeon General O'Reilly, November 30, 1903. Letter. No. 70760. Box 449. Entry 26.

14. *Congressional Record, 58th Congress, 1st Sess*. Vol 37. Washington, DC: Government Printing Office; 1903.

15. National Archives and Records Administration. Record Group 112. Surgeon general to Marshall, December 12, 1903. Letter. No. 70760.

16. National Archives and Records Administration. Record Group 112. Marshall to surgeon general, January 2, 1904. Letter. No. 70760.

17. National Archives and Records Administration. Record Group 112. Surgeon general to Marshall, January 4, 1904. Letter. No. 70760.

18. National Archives and Records Administration. Record Group 112. Marshall to surgeon general, January 13, 1904. Letter. No. 70760.

19. National Archives and Records Administration. Record Group 112. Surgeon general to Marshall, January 21, 1904. Letter. No. 70760.

20. National Archives and Records Administration. Record Group 112. Marshall to surgeon general, December 4, 1903. Letter. No. 70760.

21. National Archives and Records Administration. Record Group 112. US Congress, House. HR 79. 58th Cong, 1st Sess, November 9, 1903. No. 106047. Box 712. Entry 26.

22. Army Dental Corps items. *Dental Cosmos*. 1903;45:1009.

23. National Archives and Records Administration. Record Group 112. Petition, Odontological Society of Cincinnati to Secretary of War Taft, March 25, 1904. No. 106047. Box 712. Entry 26.

24. National Archives and Records Administration. Record Group 112. Surgeon General O'Reilly to chief of staff, April 15, 1904. Letter. No. 106047. Box 712. Entry 26.

26. National Archives and Records Administration. Record Group 112. Surgeon General O'Reilly to Senator Pettus, April 21, 1904. No. 106047. Box 712. Entry 26.

27. National Archives and Records Administration. Record Group 112. Senator EW Pettus, to Surgeon General O'Reilly, nd. Letter with enclosure; HR 79. No. 106047. Box 712. Entry 26.

28. National Archives and Records Administration. Record Group 112. O'Reilly to Pettus, April 21, 1904. Letter. No. 106047. Box 712. Entry 26.

29. *Congressional Record, 58th Cong, 3rd Sess*. Vol 39. Washington, DC: Government Printing Office; 1905.

30. National Archives and Records Administration. Record Group 94. US Congress, Senate. Bill 5906. 58th Cong, 3rd Sess, December 12, 1904. Letter. No. 524625. Box 3645. Entry 25.

31. Bills before Congress. *Dental Cosmos*. 1905;47:163.

32. National Archives and Records Administration. Record Group 94. Endorsement, surgeon general to secretary of war, December 17, 1904. No. 524625. Box 3645. Entry 25.

33. National Archives and Records Administration. Record Group 112. Extract from annual report, Major General Bates, Department of the Lakes, 1903. No. 106047. Box 712. Entry 26.

34. National Archives and Records Administration. Record Group 112. Colonel Maus to military secretary, May 20, 1904. Letter. No. 106047. Box 712. Entry 26.

35. National Archives and Records Administration. Record Group 112. Endorsement, chief surgeon, headquarters, Department of Luzon, May 25, 1904, chief surgeon's office, headquarters, Philippine Division, June 2, 1904. No. 106047. Box 712. Entry 26.

36. National Archives and Records Administration. Record Group 112. Endorsement, Major General Wood, headquarters, Department of Mindanao, June 16, 1904. No. 106047. Box 712. Entry 26.

37. National Archives and Records Administration. Record Group 112. Major Scott to military secretary, June 20, 1904. No. 106047. Box 712. Entry 26.

38. National Archives and Records Administration. Record Group 112. Endorsement, Colonel Hall to adjutant general, Philippine Division, July 16, 1904. No. 106047. Box 712. Entry 26.

39. National Archives and Records Administration. Record Group 112. Lieutenant Colonel Chase to military secretary, November 2, 1904. Letter. No. 106047. Box 712. Entry 26.

40. National Archives and Records Administration. Record Group 112. Endorsement, Colonel Girard, chief surgeon, Philippine Division, November 15, 1904. No. 106047. Box 712. Entry 26.

41. National Archives and Records Administration. Record Group 112. Colonel Hoyt to military secretary, July 19, 1904. Letter. No.106047. Box 712. Entry 26.

42. National Archives and Records Administration. Record Group 112. Endorsement, Colonel Byrne, chief surgeon, Department of Missouri, July 22, 1904. No. 106047. Box 712. Entry 26.

43. National Archives and Records Administration. Record Group 112. Dr Harry P Carlton, dean, dental department, University of California, to secretary of war, May 14, 27, 1904. Letter and petition. No. 106047. Box 712. Entry 26.

44. National Archives and Records Administration. Record Group 112. George E Hunt, dean, Indiana Dental College, to secretary of war, June 24, 1904. Letter and petition. No. 106047. Box 712. Entry 26.

45. National Archives and Records Administration. Record Group 112. Letters and petitions, various dental societies to secretary of war, various dates [June–December 1904]. No. 106047. Box 712. Entry 26.

46. Peck CD. Resolution on appointment of dentists to Army and Navy. *Dental Summary*. 1904;24:659–660.

47.   The Army Dental Corps resolution. *Pacific Dental Gazette.* 1904;12.

48.   National Archives and Records Administration. Record Group 94. Section on stomatology, American Medical Association, to secretary of war Taft, July 13, 1904. Petition. No. 524625. Box 3645. Entry 25.

49.   National Archives and Records Administration. Record Group 94. JS Pettit, assistant adjutant general, to CL Goddard, and others, California State Dental Association, June 1, 1904. No. 529913. Box 3645. Entry 25.

50.   National Archives and Records Administration. Record Group 94. HP McCain, assistant adjutant general, to Eugene S Talbot, MD, July 19, 1904. Letter. No. 902272. In: No. 524625. Box 3645. Entry 25.

51.   [Donnally W]. Address of the Committee on the Promotion of the Appointment of Dentists to the Armies and Navies of the World. (*Dental Register*). Quoted in: *Pacific Dental Gazette.* 1904;12:500–501.

52.   Donnally W, White G, Brown AJ. Address of the Committee on the Promotion of the Appointment of Dentist[s] to the Armies and Navies of the World. *Dental Register.* 1904;58:315.

53.   Donnally W. Report of the Committee on the Promotion of the Appointment of Dentists to the Armies and Navies of the World. In: *Transactions of the Fourth International Dental Congress.* Vol 1. Philadelphia, Pa: The SS White Dental Mfg Co;1905:57,60.

54.   Marshall. The United States Army Dental Corps. In: *Transactions of the Fourth International Dental Congress.* Philadelphia, Pa: The SS White Dental Mfg Co; 1904: 39–56.

55.   National Archives and Records Administration. Record Group 112. Marshall to military secretary, December 16, 1904. Letter [and proposed bill]. No. 106047. Box 712. Entry 26.

56.   National Archives and Records Administration. Record Group 112. John S Marshall, examining and supervising dental surgeon, US Army, to military secretary, December 16, 1904. Memo. No. 106047. Box 712. Entry 26.

57.   National Archives and Records Administration. Record Group 112. Endorsement, Surgeon General O'Reilly to military secretary, December 23, 1904. No. 106047. Box 712.

58.   National Archives and Records Administration. Record Group 94. Lieutenant Colonel James T Kerr, acting chief, 1st Division, general staff, January 5, 1905. Memorandum report. No. 24625. Box 3645. Entry 25.

Chapter IX

THE STRUGGLE FOR A COMMISSIONED CORPS CONTINUES, 1905–1908

Introduction

During their first 4 years of service, contract dental surgeons had demonstrated their importance to improving both the health of the American soldier and the Army's overall readiness. Yet they seemed to many about as far away as ever from their goal of complete professional recognition: commissioned status in a US Army Dental Corps that was equal to its colleagues within the Army Medical Department. The dental surgeons and their supporters in the National Dental Association (NDA) and American dental community believed that Surgeon General George Sternberg had agreed to commissioned status. Now his successor, Brigadier General Robert O'Reilly, distanced himself from Sternberg's position as he fought for a major reorganization of the Medical Department that would relieve the shortage of medical officers left after the Act of February 2, 1901. Moreover, the War Department general staff, created in the major Army reorganization of 1903 as the primary advisor to the secretary of war and chief of staff in all matters of planning, organization, and operations, had set itself solidly against the establishment of a commissioned dental corps of any sort. The dental community entered 1905 with two bills (S 5906 and HR 79) under consideration in Congress, as well as John Marshall's draft bill under study in the War Department general staff. But before anything could happen, the American dental community had to repair some of its own fences as personal rivalries and disunity emerged as major obstacles to a united political "dental" front.

The General Staff Report

On January 5, 1905, Lieutenant Colonel James Kerr of the War Department general staff submitted his report on legislation Senator Pettus (S 5906) and Representative Brownlow (HR 79) had introduced and that John Marshall had forwarded in December 1904. The report also covered the general Medical Department bill that Surgeon General O'Reilly had sponsored (S 4838; HR 13,998). Kerr called attention to two "crucial" considerations that had to be determined. First, Kerr questioned whether or not the dental surgeons were performing satisfactory service under the present contract system. Second, if they were, he questioned why it was necessary to commission them in order to maintain this efficiency.[1]

Drawing upon John Marshall's memorandum, Kerr answered the first question in the affirmative—it appeared from the experience of the years 1902 through 1904 that the dental surgeons were "efficient" and their service was "highly satisfactory." The second question was more difficult to answer because the necessary data was lacking. Although in his memorandum of December 16, 1904, Marshall had said that commissioned status was necessary to attract the "better class" of dental surgeons, Kerr thought that actual experience showed that a "very good" representation of the dental profession had been recruited under the contract system, including Marshall himself. Also, retention did not seem like much of a problem because most of the dentists had remained in the service. As far as cost savings and increasing the work load, Kerr did not agree with Marshall's argument to maintain the number of dentists at 30:

> although he asserts that the dental surgeons have never been able to perform more than from thirty to fifty per cent of the dental work required at the posts where they have been stationed. . . . It is difficult to understand how thirty contract dental surgeons, who, in time of peace, are able to perform only from 30 to 50 per cent of the work expected of them, would, if made commissioned officers, be able to perform 100 per cent of such work."[1(pp5–6)]

It seemed to make more sense to Kerr to increase the number of dental surgeons rather than commission them. He asserted:

> It is not apparent why a dentist, employed in connection with the Army, should have rank and the right to command men. . . . The work required of dentists in the Army is essentially the same as that performed by dentists in civil practice. . . . His work, valuable as it is, is not of a distinctly military character, such as performed by Majors, Captains and Lieutenants, and it, therefore, seems not only unnecessary, but inappropriate, to give the dentist the rank and title of a military officer.[1(pp6–7)]

Major General George Gillespie, the assistant chief of staff, approved Kerr's report on January 9, 1905, and agreed that the dental surgeons did not require rank to perform their duties because they had "no occasion to exercise command, and it is best that they should not."[2] He also drew attention to the fact that they wore an undress uniform. On January 10 Lieutenant General Adna Chaffee, the chief of staff, forwarded the memorandum to Secretary of War Taft. He concurred with the findings of his staff and recommended that "no change be made in the existing law."[3] Further:

> The nature of their employment is such as not to necessitate or justify the exercise of command. There appears no necessity to constitute them commissioned officers of the Army. It does not seem to the Chief of Staff as at all probable that the commissioned status would tend to efficiency; on the contrary, he believes that efficiency will be best maintained under the contract system. By this system inefficiency may be quickly remedied by annulment of contract and employment of efficient in lieu of inefficient men.[3]

The dental surgeons themselves did not remain on the sidelines during this discussion. Robert Oliver and SD Boak met with Secretary of War Taft on January 11, 1905, to support the current bills for a dental corps. Boak followed up the

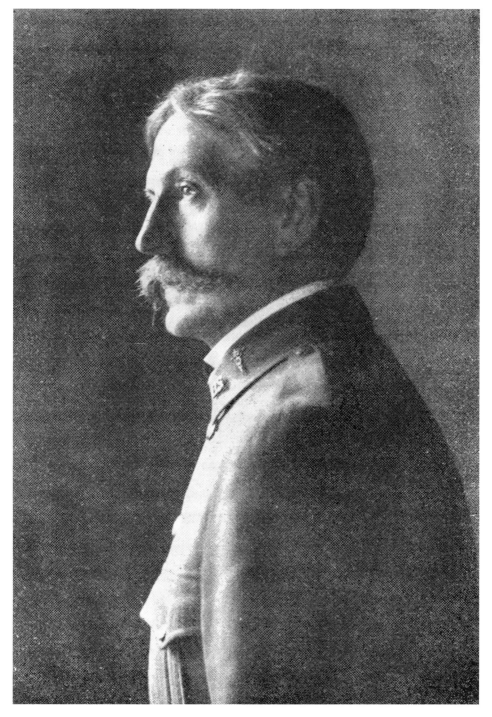

John S Marshall, 1907.
Reproduced from: Items of Interest. *29;1907: 5.*

SUPERIOR FRENCH TOOTH BRUSHES.

MADE EXPRESSLY FOR OUR SALES.

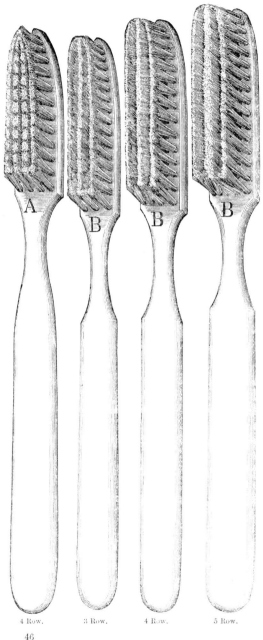

These brushes are made expressly for our sales, and are of the best French manufacture. Waxed backs.

This style of brush has received the approval of many of the most intelligent practitioners. The arrangement of the bristles is such as to allow their entrance between the teeth, and into depressions and irregular spaces, thus insuring greater cleanliness than can be secured by a flat-faced brush.

A is pointed, as shown in cut, 4 rows.

B is less pointed, and in three sizes, 3, 4, and 5 rows.

PRICES.

" A " 4 row, per doz. $3.00
" B " 3   "   "   2.30
" B " 4   "   "   3.00
" B " 5   "   "   3.80

Having a demand for a smaller size brush of the " A " pattern, for children's use, we have recently added them to our stock; they are made with three rows of bristles, of a soft grade; the bristle portion is one and a half inches in length.
Price, per dozen.........$2.30

SAMUEL S. WHITE.

4 Row.   3 Row.   4 Row.   5 Row.

46

*A precursor to Dr Rhein's 1884 toothbrush design,
pictured here in an 1878 issue of* Dental Cosmos.
Courtesy of US Army Medical Department Museum. Borden 007.

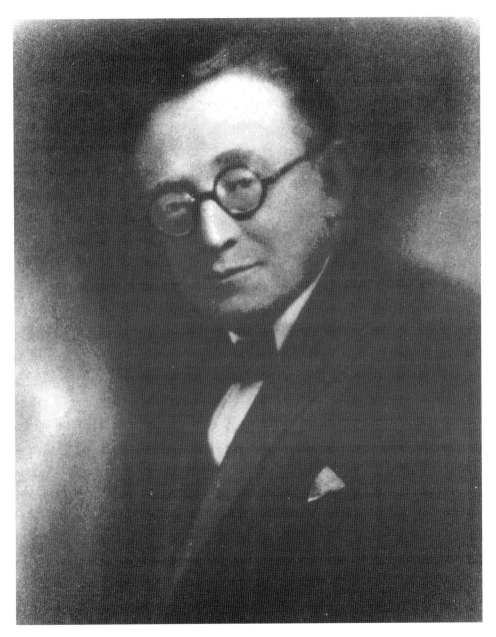

Doctor Meyer L Rhein, a civilian dentist, developed and patented an early toothbrush.
Photograph: Courtesy of the National Library of Medicine.

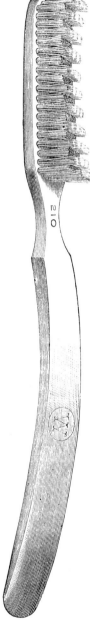

TOOTH BRUSH No. 210.

Suggestion of Dr. G. W. Adams.

Dr. Adams claims that by the curvatures of the handle every part of the mouth can be reached. The cut of the bristles facilitates their penetration between the teeth. The handle being tapered, forms a scoop for conveying powder to the mouth, thus avoiding the wetting and spoiling of that left in the box.

These are made of the best stock, the bristles being wired in and the backs waxed.

Price..per doz. $4.00

SAMUEL S. WHITE.

CASE-MAKING DEPARTMENT.

We have recently completed the fitting up in our manufactory of a department devoted to the making of Operating and all other kinds of Dental Cases, in wood and leather. This department being now under our immediate supervision, we can

GUARANTEE THE WORKMANSHIP

of every article. Estimates furnished on application. Parties ordering cases or asking estimates will please give particular description of the dimensions, style of case, quality and color of lining, etc. When instruments or appliances are desired to be fitted in a case, it will be necessary to send them to us.

SAMUEL S. WHITE.

EXAMINATION BLANKS.

These neat and convenient blanks are greatly appreciated by all who use them. They are 5⅜ inches long by 3½ inches wide. On one side of each slip is a cut of the full upper and lower set of teeth, together with the deciduous set. The other side is ruled for memorandum accounts.

Put up in tablets each containing 50 blanks. Price per tablet, 50 cents.

Samples sent on application.

Dentists may have their own name and address printed on each blank without extra charge by ordering six or more tablets at one time.

SAMUEL S. WHITE.

48

Several toothbrush designs were on the market prior to Dr Rhein's, and many were advertised in this 1878 issue of Dental Cosmos. Courtesy of US Army Medical Department Museum. Borden 009.

care. The surgeon general agreed with Greely and directed the Department of the Columbia to arrange for an annual visit by a dentist. The department surgeon, Lieutenant Colonel Rudolph Ebert, pointed out that the extended travel to and around Alaska consumed about 7 months, meaning the rest of the department would be left without a dentist for over half the year. He suggested that the units be brought up to full dental health prior to their rotations into and out of Alaska every 2 years. The alternate year visits would then be sufficient to deal with crises. Greely still urged that annual visits be considered, although he agreed that the only interim measures possible were intensive predeployment care and authorization of special payments to civilian dentists in Alaska in the event of emergencies. The majority of the officers serving in Alaska endorsed the need for more dental surgeons in the command.[13]

Despite the shortcomings that Greely and Millikin identified, dental surgeons were actually making notable achievements under difficult conditions. Dr Meyer Rhein offered the following critique and endorsement of Army dental care after his 1905 visit to John Marshall's dental office at the Presidio:

> There is nothing the dentists of America can feel prouder of than the Army Dental Service as I saw it at San Francisco under the direction of Dr. John S. Marshall . . . , and I only wish I could get the committees of congress and of the senate having these matters in charge to see what Dr. Marshall has done, not only in the fitting up of the different offices that he has there for the accommodation of his patients; not only in the wonderful system of supplies and dental instruments by which the U.S. Army Dental Surgeon can travel with his corps or division and carry his entire office paraphernalia with him, but also the remarkable methods of registration of work which makes an absolutely enduring record of everything that has been done. I never for a moment imagined that so much work could be accomplished by the dental surgeons who have been appointed in the army as I saw there. And this, gentlemen, is entirely due to the work of one man, Dr. John S. Marshall, who gave up a lucrative practice in Chicago to accept the position he now occupies for a paltry salary of twenty-five hundred dollars a year. No man ever made himself a martyr to a worthy cause more than Dr. Marshall has in this respect, and, because of what he has done, his name is bound to live forever in the annals of American dentistry. Dr. Marshall has not the rank that he should have, nevertheless he is treated as an equal by many who rank above him and by the head of the Medical Staff there, and anyone who knows the conditions in an army post concerning rank will appreciate what this means, and no words that I can utter can speak louder for the value of his services than does this one fact.[14(pp902–903)]

John Marshall's Work at the Presidio

In July 1905 John Marshall was officially relieved from duty at the Presidio of San Francisco's post and transferred to duty at its general hospital, where he assumed his duties on August 1. He had a graduate dentist, Private Burdette Conway, serving under him. Conway had enlisted in the Army hoping for the opportunity to take the examination to be a dental surgeon. However, there were no examinations scheduled for some time. The only thing that Marshall could do for this "valuable" man was to recommend that he be promoted to sergeant.[15–19]

In August 1905 Marshall adopted a new card system for dental patients to replace the old register of dental operations. The cards were color coded: white for infantry, yellow for cavalry, red for artillery, blue for Staff Corps, and gray for military dependents and civilian employees. This change allowed for an instant record that had not existed in the old system, in which all the operations were listed in a day book and then transferred under the patient's name to a register at the end of the month. The cards were made out in duplicate so that one set could be kept at the post and the other sent in to the surgeon general's office.[19]

The same month, Marshall recommended to the surgeon general that dental surgeons and their enlisted assistants be instructed to wear the "regulation white, washable, blouse" while on duty in the operating room and laboratory; he and his staff wore the blouse in the interest of "personal appearance, cleanliness, and the most approved principles of hygiene and sanitation," but some dental surgeons wore their woolen blouses while treating patients. Marshall felt that this practice was:

> . . . contrary to all correct surgical principles, and cannot but be detrimental to the best interests of any patient who is being operated upon for a dental or oral disease having a break in the continuity of the soft tissues or which necessitates any surgical procedure upon these tissues. Surgical cleanliness is as important in the treatment of diseases affecting the teeth and oral tissues as in any other department of surgery.[20]

The surgeon general replied that the recommendation would be considered for insertion in the next revision of the Medical Department's manual.[20,21]

On November 23, 1905, Surgeon General O'Reilly wrote to Lieutenant Colonel George Torney, commander of the Presidio General Hospital, concerning the "constant complaint" that there were not enough dentists to perform the Army's dental work. He wanted to know if the two dentists assigned to his hospital were sufficient to handle the load. He was also curious if they spent "a great deal of their time" treating the families of officers and doing "outside practice." He emphasized that the paragraphs of the Army Regulations that described the dental surgeons' duties (1425 and 1426) should be strictly complied with. He was also aware that some complaints had been made against members of the Dental Corps for overcharging the enlisted personnel for gold work.[22]

Torney referred the matter to Marshall, who provided a report on December 17. Replying through Torney, Marshall stated that his annual report for 1902 showed that he was "overwhelmed with work" and that three dentists could have been kept "constantly busy." No patients not connected with the Army had ever received treatment in his office. In addition, he had used his own supplies when treating those not entitled to free treatment under Army Regulations. Marshall pointed out that he had the additional duty of examining the applicants for appointments as dental surgeons. He was forced to conduct these examinations in his office operating room while he was treating patients. During the practical examination, he was obliged to have the candidates operate at a chair placed next to his own so that he could inspect the various stages of their work. Thus, his own chair work was "very arduous," but the "necessity of the situation called for this sacrifice." The workload required Sunday and holiday office hours to keep up with the backlog. Longer weekday hours had frequently been necessary in the "interests of suffering humanity." Therefore, he simply never had the "time or inclination" to do any "outside practice."[23]

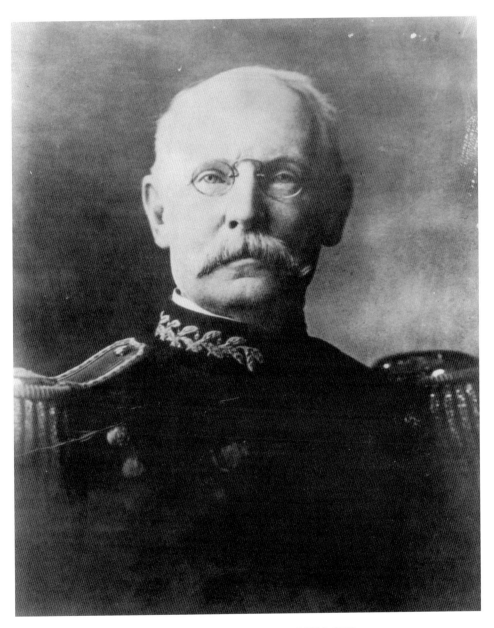

George H Torney, surgeon general 1909–1913.
Photograph: Courtesy of the National Museum of Health and Medicine,
Armed Forces Institute of Pathology. NCP 3567.

As for as the subject of gold, Marshall pointed out that the surgeon general established the charges for gold work in 1901. The fees for gold foil restorations had been set at $1 minimum and $2 maximum both for officers and enlisted personnel. These fees barely covered the cost, considering the natural waste and loss of material incident to this type of filling. The fees for gold crown and bridgework had never been officially established. Marshall had arbitrarily set a fee range of $5 to $10 for crowns, based on a figure that was half the civilian fee. This arrangement had proven satisfactory in all but one case, where the officer-patient thought he had been "overcharged" on a fee of $34 for 4 crowns. Marshall said that during the fiscal year ending June 30, 1905, his department had treated 382 officers (about 10.32% of the entire commissioned strength of the Army) and 1,465 enlisted soldiers (about 2.61 % of the Army). He expressed doubt that this record was duplicated at any other Army station.[23]

In his December 22 endorsement, Torney disagreed that the dental surgeons were overworked or needed additional help. He reported that "the services of the senior dental surgeon [Marshall] at this hospital are given almost exclusively to the officers of the Army and the members of their families, while those of the junior [Frank Stone] and his enlisted assistants are rendered to the enlisted men." In addition, Torney raised the issues of gold fillings and of allowing the dentists to charge for work done on officers and enlisted soldiers during nonduty hours. Torney said:

> The statement made by Dr. Marshall on page 26 of his report relative to the scale of charges for gold fillings, and on page 28 relative to crowns and bridge work, seems reasonable, but the principle is wrong, as I do not think that an enlisted man should be compelled to pay for any service rendered him by an officer. Holding this opinion, and also the belief that plastic gold is not essential for the preservation of defective teeth in the human subject, and, further, that the materials issued to the dentists by the Medical Department of the Army are equally as applicable and as efficient as gold when utilized as fillings for cavities in teeth, and, also, in prosthetic dentistry, I recommend that in their practice in the cases of enlisted men the dentists of the Army be required by order to use these materials exclusively, and further that they be prohibited from accepting from such patients any remuneration whatever, either for additional expensive materials or for services rendered. It is believed that such requirement would protect the enlisted men against extortion, which has undoubtedly occurred in some instances in the past, and would remove the cause for much complaint against the dental surgeons.[24]

On January 19, 1906, O'Reilly replied to Torney, thanking him for the report and agreeing with his conclusion that additional dental surgeons were not needed. However, the surgeon general was not pleased with the information that Marshall was "given almost exclusively" to the officers and their families:

> I desire . . . to state that the law authorizing the employment of dental surgeons provides that their work shall be confined to the treatment of officers and enlisted men of the regular and volunteer army. The Regulations also provide that dental surgeons shall operate between the hours of 9 a.m. and 4 p.m. upon those officers and enlisted men who are entitled to their services. During the last four years so many reports have come to this office that the dental surgeons at the Presidio Hospital were working from early morning to late at night (Sundays included) that I desire hereafter their

work during the hours prescribed by regulations shall be confined to treating those who are entitled to their services. The families of officers and civilian employees are not under the law entitled to dental treatment.[25]

O'Reilly told Torney that the issue of limiting the dental surgeons to use of Medical Department materials for treating enlisted soldiers would be addressed soon.[25]

Marshall's work at the Presidio General Hospital was sharply interrupted on April 18, 1906, when the great San Francisco earthquake struck, followed by disastrous fire. Marshall's dental office, including his electric panel switchboard, dental cabinet, and many instruments, sustained considerable damage. The fire also destroyed his personal Army records. After the disaster, Marshall served as the sanitary inspector of the refugee camp at Point Lobos. His duties included building latrines and supervising the sanitary and hygiene conditions in the camp. Marshall was issued emergency drugs, instruments, and supplies for treating the refugees at Fort Mason.[26–30]

Major Febiger's Report and Questions of Dental Care

Serious issues with current Army Regulations governing dental care and dissatisfaction with the contract system were not limited to medical officers and dental surgeons. On February 27, 1906, Major Lea Febiger, assistant inspector general at headquarters, Pacific Division, in San Francisco, California, filed a critical report on the dental service that reflected its limitations. Febiger declared that on the whole he was satisfied with the performance of the contract dentists and praised them as "competent, energetic and attentive to their duties." However, he noted that "certain apparent abuses, prejudicial to the accepted army standards," had to be corrected. The inspector said the "commercial idea" was too prominent. For example, using gold restorations on soldiers who could not afford them, then dunning their pay for reimbursement or requiring payment in advance of treatment. There was a chance that some "unscrupulous" dentists would take advantage of the soldiers through "unfair dealing." The dental surgeons were in an "anomalous" position contrary to normal Army policy when they were forced to be involved in financial transactions for "personal service" rendered to enlisted soldiers. Because dentists' prospects lacked promotions and pay raises under the existing system, Febiger believed there was a temptation to "make hay" from their "outside practice" at the expense of official time. If dentists were commissioned, these problems would disappear, giving them "dignity" and ending the disparity allowing them to charge officers' and soldiers' families for some services when contract surgeons could not. Also, dental supplies could be issued and accounted for in the same way as medicine, solving another potential problem. Febiger concluded by observing that regulatory office hours were not being observed. He urged that dentists be allowed to do more than just "temporary or emergency" work because "permanent" work on dependents would improve the dental surgeons' skills in the "finer and more difficult operations of their craft."[31]

On April 10 O'Reilly responded to Febiger's report. He explained that the only reason he had recommended rank for dental surgeons was that he was assured by "creditable sources" (probably the NDA, Donnally, and Marshall) that rank would get a "better class" of dentists into the service. However, he did not believe that rank was necessary for this purpose. He rejected the idea of increasing the dental supply table to include the "finer" materials for the more "elaborate" dental work. He also recommended that dental surgeons confine their use of materials on enlisted soldiers to the free materials furnished by the government, unless the patient had the ready money for gold. He stressed that Army Regulations be strictly enforced to prohibit work during the regular office hours on other than free patients. He disapproved of the recommendation that dental surgeons be required to treat the families of Army personnel.[32]

The War Department responded quickly to this matter and on April 30, 1906, issued Circular No. 26, which required contract dental surgeons to use the dental materials that the Medical Department furnished when operating on enlisted soldiers, unless the soldier had "funds in hand" to pay for the "finer materials." A week later the military secretary sent letters to the various Army departments informing them that the secretary of war directed that paragraph 1426 of the Army Regulations be "strictly enforced." This was the paragraph that fixed the dental surgeons' hours from 9 AM to 4 PM and prohibited them from "operating on those not entitled to free service during these hours." Any failure to comply with this paragraph would be cause for contract annulment.[33,34]

Febiger's report raised another question on the exact extent of dental entitlements. Earlier, responding to a request to refer patients to a local civilian dentist, the surgeon general's office opined that the small number of dental surgeons authorized in the 1901 legislation implied lawmakers presumed outside care would still be required. The surgeon general assumed the dentists would have to give priority to isolated posts where civilian counterparts were not available. The new dental surgeons were assigned to departments with the understanding they would rove within them as circumstances dictated. The Medical Department reasoned that far greater numbers of dentists would have to be authorized before full dental care could be granted to all military personnel and their families. It did not believe that such care was guaranteed in the same way medical treatment was. Ultimately, military personnel were responsible for their own dental care if they did not have access to an Army dentist, and dental work was guaranteed only in cases of duty trauma, such as a gunshot wounds. Even if an Army dentist was available, specialized work such as "artificial plates," which could not be produced with government materials, were the patient's financial responsibility.[35–39]

New Dental Bills

In December 1905 Representative Brownlow and Senator Pettus submitted modified versions of their earlier, unpassed bills to upgrade the status of dentists in the Army.[40] Both bills (HR 31 and S 2355) again called for commissioning dentists, creating "a corps of dental surgeons" to be attached to the Army Medical Department, and giving priority for admission to the present contract dentists. Pettus's bill also proposed maintaining the corps strength at 30 dentists at all times.[41–43]

On February 1, 1906, the Senate Committee on Military Affairs reported favorably on the Pettus bill (S 2355) and recommended that it be passed without any amendments. The committee said that the "injustice of the treatment of dental surgeons" in the Army and Navy of the United States had been "a matter of serious consideration" in Congress for several years. For the past 9 years, the Army surgeons general had recommended "the organization of a dental corps on the lines suggested by this bill." Many prominent Army officers had testified to the "great importance" of the dental surgeons' work.[40,44]

The committee also reported that there should be no difference in rank between medical and dental surgeons because in the universities and colleges of the United States they were "educated alike." The committee pointed out that:

> Senators who have served in any Army of the United States know what importance is attached and should be attached to military rank. Chaplains have military rank, and they should have it. Quartermasters have military rank, and it ought to be given to them. Commissaries have military rank, and they need it. Physicians have military rank, and they also need it. Quartermasters and commissaries require, to fit them for their office, a business education and not the years of learning which is necessary to qualify a man for one of the learned professions. Your committee are of the opinion that great injustice has been done by the law of the land in reference to dental surgeons. They are not even entitled by the customs of the Army to associate with commissioned officers, though they may be admitted as a matter of courtesy, and they should have a right to such association. By the customs of the Army dental surgeons, though they have no right to associate with commissioned officers, would not be allowed by such commissioned officers to habitually associate with the rank and file, for if they did so they would lose caste.[44(p3)]

The committee concluded that rank would make the contract dental surgeons "more efficient." The next day the bill was announced as next in order but was allowed to "go over" because of an inattentive Senate. On February 2 the bill was announced as the next business in order on the Senate calendar. Pettus asked that it be favorably considered, saying:

> Bills on the line of this one have been approved by every Surgeon-General of the Army for the last nine years. The bill has had the unanimous sanction of the Committee on Military Affairs, so far as I have heard. I will say that this is one of the most modest bills that I have seen introduced in the Senate. The whole idea in the bill is to give rank to the men of this learned profession in the Army, and it is very modest rank at that.[40,44]

The following day Senator Eugene Hale of Maine, who had been absent from the previous meeting due to illness, requested that the dental bill be reconsidered and restored to the calendar. His main objection to the bill was that it increased the expenses of the War Department. Unfortunately, Pettus was absent that day and the bill was ordered restored to the calendar.[44]

The same day, February 6, Dr Rodrigues Ottolengui of *Items of Interest* wrote to the surgeon general about Pettus's bill. He was concerned with a section of the bill that provided:

> That the Surgeon General of the Army is hereby authorized to organize a board of three examiners to conduct the professional examinations herein provided for, two of whom shall be civilians whose qualifications are certified by the executive council

of the National Dental Association and whose proper compensation shall be determined by the Surgeon General, and the third examiner shall be selected by the Surgeon General from the contract dental surgeons eligible under the provisions of this Act for appointment to the dental corps.[95]

Ottolengui interpreted this provision to mean that the executive council of the NDA would control the appointment of dental surgeons in the Army, as it would have the "power to appoint the majority of the board of examiners." Also, he feared that this bill would "throw out of the service" Marshall and Oliver.[45] On February 10 the surgeon general's office replied that O'Reilly would "oppose any attempt to exclude" the current examining and supervising dental surgeons (Marshall and Oliver). However, he approved of the composition of the board as stated with the two civilian members. Later, if this plan proved unsuccessful, it could be changed.[46]

On February 9 O'Reilly sent the chairman of the Senate Committee on Military Affairs a copy of his report on the bill. Under the proposed reorganization, the surgeon general's office estimated that the cost of the 30-person commissioned dental corps, allowing for 3 captains and 27 first lieutenants, would be close to $52,850 for 1907. After 10 years the cost for 4 majors, 10 captains, and 16 first lieutenants would be just over $70,073. If the corps was increased to 60 dentists, the cost of 3 captains and 57 first lieutenants was estimated to be about $100,850 for 1907, and around $135,755 after 10 years for 7 majors, 18 captains, and 36 first lieutenants.[47]

On March 29 Pettus asked that the bill be reconsidered. After some debate, it was placed back on the calendar on April 13, and debate on the bill resumed on April 23.[40] Senator Hale led the opposition to the bill, arguing that it was unneeded, as there were no dental corps in the armies and navies of Great Britain, France, or Germany. He looked at it as "a movement" to increase the size of the Army. Senator Henry Cabot Lodge of Massachusetts recommended that the controversial section of the bill be amended. He moved that the examiners all be military appointed by the surgeon general. Pettus had no objection to the amendment, and the revised section now read:

That the Surgeon-General of the Army is hereby authorized to organize a board of three examiners to conduct the professional examinations herein prescribed, one of whom shall be a surgeon in the Army, and two of whom shall be selected by the Surgeon-General from the contract dental surgeons eligible under the provisions of this act to appointment to the dental corps.[40]

Hale agreed that this was "a very fitting and proper amendment" and an improvement on the bill. The amended bill was read three times, reported without further amendment, and passed the Senate on April 23, 1906.[40] It was referred to the House Committee on Military Affairs on April 25. Three days later, the committee referred the bill back to the House Committee of the Whole House on the State of the Union.

Some amendments were recommended in the accompanying report that the Committee on Military Affairs submitted with the bill. For example, the number of dentists was not to exceed 45. Before commissioning, candidates were to have served at least 1 year as contract dental surgeons. The initial dental examining board was changed back to include two civilians nominated by the NDA and one contract dental surgeon selected by the surgeon general. Other modifications included pay calculations for contract dentists who became commissioned and waivers of examination for those already in service. The bill also specified grade distribution among the 45 dentists.[40,48]

The report included additional endorsements for the bill and for military dentistry. Brigadier General Frederick Grant, Department of Texas, stated:

While the comparatively recent beginning of dental service in the Army makes the matter still one of an experimental nature only, opportunity has already been offered for sufficient observation to warrant the conclusion, not only that the dental surgeons should be indefinitely continued, but largely increased, in order to meet the full demands of the service. . . .

In my opinion, after careful investigation, the principal needs of the service, with respect to dental surgeons, are: First, more dental surgeons; second, a suitable operating room at each post; third, some positive and practicable methods compelling enlisted men to give proper attention to personal care of the teeth. I believe that there should be three dental surgeons assigned to this department, if possible, but not less than two under any circumstances.[48]

In his testimony to the Senate military committee, Major William Owen, the Army surgeon who had established the Army's first dental office in the Philippines, stated:

For seven years I have been giving especial attention to the diseases of the mouth and teeth because of their influence on the general health. During the time in which I was in charge of Corregidor hospital about three hundred soldiers, more or less disabled by dental disorders, were under treatment. I recall one case in particular, a diarrheal trouble of several months' standing, which resisted treatment until placed under the care of a dentist, whose treatment, directed to the mouth alone, effected a cure and the restoration of the soldier to active duty in two weeks. There were fifteen or twenty similar cases, known as pyorrhea of the sockets of the teeth, with pus bathing the teeth, mixing with food, and entering therewith the alimentary tract. Neglected, such cases cause a pensionable disability.[48]

Brigadier General George Randall, the commander of the Department of Luzon in 1904, reported:

There are not enough dental surgeons in the department for the work required. The recommendation for an increased number is approved. In this connection I invite attention to the excellent results obtained in the health and comfort of men from the work of dental surgeons, and it is recommended that they be given permanent positions and commissioned rank in the Medical Department.[48]

The report concluded with the following statement:

While the Military Committee, in recommending the passage of the bill, have been guided by a purpose to meet an urgent need of the Army on sound business principles, it is nevertheless gratifying to your committee to incidentally accord a small measure of recognition to a profession whose members have contributed much to the public weal and to suffering mankind everywhere.[48]

Reorganization of the Dental Corps

Meanwhile, hearings were held concurrently in the House Committee on Military Affairs on Brownlow's modified bill, now numbered HR 9737. It covered the same ground as before, proposing a commissioned corps of dental surgeons be added to the Medical Department. It differed primarily in proposing the strength of the corps be premised on one dentist for every 1,000 troops.[49]

In a hearing before the House Committee on Military Affairs on March 13, 1906, Surgeon General O'Reilly said he thought an exception should be made in the bill for the three examining and supervising dental surgeons (Marshall, Oliver, and Hess) to permit them to be commissioned without examination. The NDA proposed an amendment to cover this situation and O'Reilly approved. It read:

> That dental surgeons attached to the Medical Department of the Army at the time of the passage of this act may be eligible to appointment, three of them to the rank of captain and the others to the rank of first lieutenant, subject, in each case in which the Surgeon-General may deem such further test of qualification necessary, to any or every part of the requirement herein prescribed for original appointments.[49]

Williams Donnally, also at the hearing, argued that the subject of placing a limit of 45 on the number of dental surgeons to be appointed was covered by an amendment recommended by the Senate version of the bill. The estimated cost of the 45 dental surgeons under the bill was $75,639.[49] University presidents, deans, and professors from the following schools also appeared to testify to the worthiness of commissioned status for their dental graduates: George Washington University, Philadelphia Dental College, Georgetown University, University of Michigan, Harvard University, University of Pennsylvania, and Columbian University.[49]

The Dental Press:
Reaction to S 2355

In an editorial in the March 1906 issue of *Items of Interest*, Rodrigues Ottolengui criticized the proposed civilian "Board of Control," for the Dental Corps. He wrote that it was inappropriate for civilians with no military experience or sense of Army Regulations to select the professionals who were to practice Army dentistry. He also noted that as the bill was currently worded, neither Marshall nor Oliver would be eligible to be appointed to the board or appointed to captaincies. Neither man had been required to pass an entrance examination under the 1901 dental act, but in order to make captain, they would have to pass an examination before a board, two of whose members were to be chosen by the executive council of the NDA. Only then could they be appointed to the examining board.[50]

In the March 1906 issue of the *Dental Register*, Editor Nelville Hoff agreed with Ottolengui's assessment of the Pettus bill and urged changes. His recommendation was to appoint one of the Army dental surgeons to the rank of major, appoint

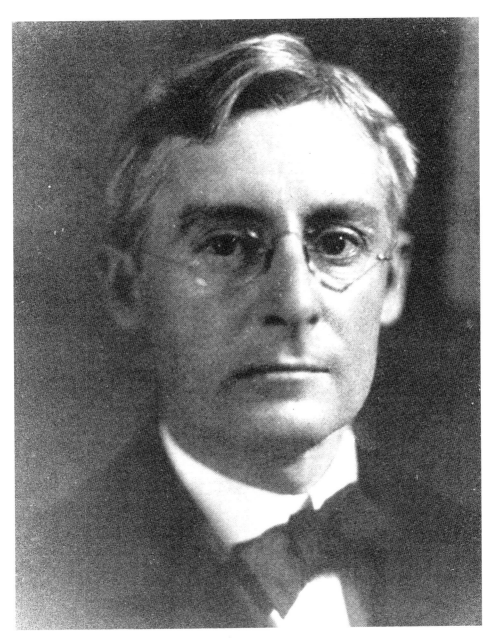

Rodrigues Ottolengui, editor of Items of Interest, *often used his journal to express his opinions about military dentistry. Photograph: Courtesy of the National Library of Medicine.*

a Navy dental surgeon of similar rank, and appoint three civilian dentists—one from the NDA, one from the National Board of Dental Examiners, and one from the National Association of Dental Faculties—to a five-person examining board. This board could then certify all candidates for both the Army and Navy dental corps.[51]

Dr John Patterson, the editor of the *Western Dental Journal*, also took exception to the civilian majority composition of the board. In particular, he objected to the requirement that those selected be "certified" by the executive council of the NDA and not by the association itself. The council had originally been set up to expedite business matters and keep such discussion out of the association's general sessions. At no time was it intended that the council be given the authority to select "men for a public national service."[52]

Dr CN Johnson, the editor of *Dental Review*, concurred with Ottolengui that it would be difficult to support any legislation that would cause any "humiliation" to Marshall and Oliver in view of the sacrifice of their "private interests" in 1901 to accept contracts as Army dental surgeons.[53] On May 3, 1906, Ottolengui again called the surgeon general to task regarding the status of Marshall and Oliver in S 2355 as amended by the House Committee on Military Affairs. In Section 2, lines 5 and 6, the clause "and who are within said age limit at the time their original contracts were signed may be eligible," seemed to preclude their appointment. The surgeon general's office responded that as the bill had not yet received the endorsement of the War Department, it was inappropriate for the surgeon general to intervene at the present time.[54,55]

Perhaps inspired by Ottolengui's appeal, on May 9, 1906, Surgeon General O'Reilly addressed the problem of the overage dental surgeons to Representative John AT Hull, the chairman of the House Committee on Military Affairs. Under the House bill, seven current contract dental surgeons would be barred from appointment to the commissioned corps; namely, Marshall, Oliver, Hess, Sorber, Stallman, Voorhies, and Ware. O'Reilly recommended that "a more liberal age limit be inserted" in Section 2. At the time these men signed their contracts, the age requirement was between 24 and 40 years.[56] The following day, Hull replied that he saw a "good reason" for admitting the men who were between 24 and 40 when they entered the service, but thought that including Marshall, who was near the age of retirement, would "require a very wide latitude."[57]

On May 19, 1906, John Marshall sent a letter to the military secretary expressing his concern for the provisions that would exclude the commissioning of 10 of the current contract dental surgeons (including himself). He pointed out that the three examining and supervising dental surgeons had given up large lucrative practices in order to assist the surgeon general in 1901. At that time, they were assured that if and when the corps would be commissioned, they would be retained and commissioned. If the House-amended bill were to pass, these men would be dismissed from the service without a pension. Marshall thought this scenario a "great injustice" to those who had contributed so much to Army dental care. He recommended that the age amendment be removed from the bill.[58]

On July 13, 1906, another of the supervising dental surgeons, John Hess, then stationed at the Department of California (San Francisco), wrote to the surgeon general concerning S 2355. After thanking him for supporting the commissioning of dentists, Hess said during his 5 years as a contract dentist his status had been an "embarrassment" and he was certain that without commissions, the quality of applicants was bound to decline. According to Hess, the hope for commissions was the magnet keeping quality dentists in the present service. He urged that the age limit be reconsidered to include those who had come in under the 1901 conditions; otherwise a large body of expertise would be lost and those effected would suffer an injustice. He supported the surgeon general's desire that a board of both civilian and military dentists select dentists for the corps and that Army surgeons be excluded from this board.[59] On July 20 the surgeon general's office replied that O'Reilly had addressed the age limit status with Representative Hull and was in favor of a more "liberal age limit" being inserted in Section 2 of the bill.[60]

On September 4 Williams Donnally recommended that all of the seven Army contract dental surgeons who would be considered overage under the Pettus bill stick together for their collective common good and that the entire dental profession support their retention if the bill passed.[61]

The editor of *Dental Summary*, LP Bethel, pointed out that the pending Army medical bill would eliminate the status of contract medical surgeons, leaving the dental surgeons as the only group still as contract personnel or "Mex" officers. He urged all members of the dental profession to support S 2355 and H 9737.[62]

On December 4, 1906, Secretary of War William Taft requested legislation to add an additional dental surgeon so that another dentist could be assigned to duty at West Point to replace William Saunders, who had passed away in August after 48 years as the academy's dentist. It was not until an act of March 2, 1907, that Congress finally authorized the requested increase in the number of contract dental surgeons by one to a total of 31, so that a second dentist could be assigned to the US Military Academy. However, 1906 ended with no new dental legislation being passed.[63–65]

The Cuban Pacification, 1906–1909

When the United States returned to Cuba from June 1906 to April 1909, demand for dental support renewed concurrently with the assignment of troops to what was then called the Army of Cuban Pacification (AOCP). In December 1906 the commanding officer of the 28th Infantry stationed at Matanzas, Colonel Owen Sweet, sent an urgent request asking for dental support from AOCP headquarters. He was personally suffering from painful "abscesses in three back teeth" and reported that 60 of his soldiers needed dental care. Headquarters told him that no dentists were available, but he was not authorized to employ a civilian dentist. The only dentist in the command, Alden Carpenter, was on circuit and would eventually reach Matanzas. Sweet argued that, according to the regulations, he was entitled to dental and medical care, especially when his condition impaired his ability to perform his duties. He asked again for the authority to employ a civilian dentist despite the expense to himself, saying it was inappropriate and would be even more expensive if he had to go on leave to the United States for treatment. Headquarters responded again that he could not hire a civilian and gave him the encouraging news that a second dentist (Seibert Boak, back from the Philippines) was scheduled to arrive soon.[66–68]

Boak and Carpenter tried without success to meet the needs of the command in 1907. Although all agreed a third dentist was needed, they remained the only

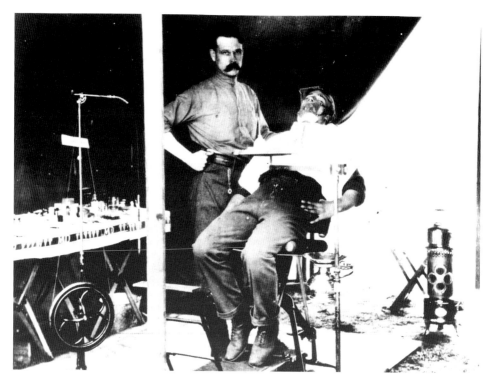

Dental office in Camp Columbia, Cuba.
Photograph: Courtesy of the National Museum of Health and Medicine.

dentists assigned until the command closed; Carpenter returned to the United States in January 1909 and Boak followed in March. In the meantime, the two men had so much to do that they were working themselves to the point of exhaustion. Because demand was so great, neither could be granted leave to recuperate. Their problem was made worse by the unexpected need to give support to the 1st Provisional Marine Regiment. Its plight surfaced in a letter from one of its commanders requesting dental help because his troops were insufficiently paid to resort to local civilians who were "very indifferent and exceedingly expensive." Although the Marines were not technically entitled to Army dental care, they were a working part of the AOCP, so dental treatment was authorized as a courtesy and a necessity. Soldiers and Marines with severe dental problems were recommended by their unit surgeons to be transferred to the field hospital in Havana. Their cases included jaw injuries, severe infections, and broken dental plates. There, the dentist not on circuit did what he could for them. The large number of absences generated by this practice represented considerable lost duty time. This became such a concern that the AOCP commander, Major General Thomas Barry, directed all requests for dental care at the hospital be sent to him for review before orders were issued, saying "this dental business can be run into the ground." As it turned out, the requests were an accurate reflection of the needs of the command and served as further evidence of the heavy workload carried by the two dentists prior to the command's withdrawal. Their assignment to a temporary unit meant that dental service had had to be curtailed elsewhere in the Army and no one considered the implications for any further joint service deployments.[69–71]

The Dental Surgeons in 1907

Once the situation in the Philippines had stabilized at 14 dental surgeons after 1904, the remaining 16 were distributed throughout the United States. Because two of the 16 contract dental surgeons assigned to the US military departments were required to provide dental care for the AOCP, the stateside surgeons were spread even thinner. As of April 1, 1907, the 31 contract dental surgeons were stationed as follows:

- Philippines Division: 14.
- Department of the East: 1.
- Department of the Gulf: 1.
- Department of the Lakes: 1.
- Department of Dakota: 1.
- Department of the Missouri: 2.
- Department of the Colorado: 1.
- Department of Texas: 1.
- Department of California: 2.
- Department of the Columbia: 1.
- Army of Cuban Pacification: 2.
- Fort Slocum, New York: 1.
- Columbus Barracks, Ohio: 1.
- US Military Academy, West Point, New York: 2.

There was no fixed period for the dental surgeons' duty at the various posts. Rather, the dental needs of the posts determined their itineraries. With only a few exceptions (such as West Point) the dental surgeon's duty station was considered to be the department and not an individual post.[72]

Meanwhile, demands for additional dental surgeons came in from various post commanders. The continuing problems in the Pacific Northwest were especially noteworthy. When Inspector General Colonel John Chamberlain visited Alaska in 1907, Dental Surgeon Jean Whinnery urged the assignment of at least one more dentist to the Department of the Columbia (despite Greely's efforts of 1905, there was still only one dentist for the vast area). As such, only minimal dental care could be provided, mostly emergency. Whinnery said that during the period from January 20, 1905, to June 7, 1907, he had rendered 4,653 operations and treatments in 25 different locations. Despite that, he had met only the minimal needs of the command, compelling many soldiers to seek civilian care. Chamberlain agreed that at least one more dentist was desirable. The problem persisted the next year. Whinnery was away from Vancouver Barracks, Washington, his home base, for the full 12 months, serving posts throughout the department. This meant that the 1,500 soldiers at the barracks had not gotten military dental care for a total of 22 consecutive months.[73–75]

On November 18, 1907, Major General Greely, now the commander of the Department of the Columbia, reported from his headquarters at Vancouver Barracks that 94 enlisted soldiers (mostly recruits) of the 14th Infantry Regiment, destined for the Philippines, were awaiting dental work. Another 200 recruits were expected to arrive shortly, compounding the need for more dentists. If another dental surgeon could not be assigned for temporary duty, Greely requested permission to hire a civilian dentist. He felt that it was a shame to send his troops overseas with defective teeth.[76] The next day, Surgeon General O'Reilly advised the adjutant general that no dental surgeon was available to send to Vancouver Barracks. He suggested that some of the work might be performed either at the recruiting depots where there were dental surgeons or in the Philippines, where 11 contract dental surgeons were stationed. On November 21 the adjutant general notified Greely of the surgeon general's decision.[77,78]

The Uniform Issue

Dr Robert Oliver had long insisted that dentist's uniforms themselves implied a separate, second-class status. In 1907 the question of shoulder straps for contract dental surgeons, contract surgeons, and veterinarians resurfaced. On December 9, 1907, Jean Whinnery, dental surgeon, EW Bayley, contract surgeon, and Daniel Le-May, veterinarian, all stationed at Vancouver Barracks, Washington, complained that the absence of shoulder straps on their uniforms was "exceedingly humiliating and insulting to one's self respect." They recommended that they should wear "plain silver" shoulder straps and that this change would "exact proper respect and obedience" from their enlisted personnel. The commanding general, Greely, concurred. When the correspondence reached the surgeon general's office, the acting surgeon general, Colonel Valery Havard, responded favorably:

> It is the opinion of this office that contract surgeons and contract dental surgeons should either not be required to wear a uniform, or should be given one which would clearly indicate that they have a relative status of commissioned officers. This the present uniform does not do. The uniform formerly worn by these men was supposed to be satisfactory. Of course it is understood that the wearing of shoulder straps will not confer to contract dental surgeons the authority to command.[79]

However, Major General William Duvall, the assistant to the chief of staff, did not agree that any change in the contract doctors' uniform was necessary. He emphatically stated:

> Paragraphs 62, 63 and 64, General Orders No. 169, War Department, c.s., prescribe a uniform for Contract Surgeons, Dental Surgeons and Veterinarians, which it is thought is sufficiently distinctive to prevent mistakes as to the official status of the wearer. It is believed the shoulder strap should be worn by commissioned officers of the Army only.[79]

The year ended with no change in any aspect of the dentists' status, despite substantial efforts by Congress and some members of the Army.

Continuing Issues with Army Regulations Governing Dental Care

Although Surgeon General O'Reilly had attempted to fix shortcomings in the Army Regulations governing dental care during 1906, he had not completely succeeded. On November 20, 1906, the surgeon general's office wrote to all of the chief surgeons of the geographical departments about "numerous complaints of the inadequacy of the dental services." He directed them to investigate and report on their departments, especially with reference to paragraphs 1426 and 1428, Army Regulations, which fixed office hours from 9 AM to 4 PM and limited dental work during those hours only to those entitled to free service.[80]

On December 7 Colonel Clarence Heizmann, chief surgeon of the Department of California, replied that John Marshall reported compliance with the applicable paragraphs with some exceptions, such as treating Army nurses in transit to and from the Philippines, emergency cases "as an act of common humanity," and only treating families of soldiers outside office hours.[81] Also in December, George Torney wrote to the surgeon general about paragraphs 1426 and 1428, Army Regulations. He recommended the following changes:

> *1426.* Dental surgeons will operate between the hours of 9 a.m. and 4 p.m. upon those officers and enlisted men who are entitled to their services. They may not operate upon others, not entitled to free service, before and after these hours, when their services are not required by those entitled to them, but material issued to them by the Government will only be used in operations upon officers and enlisted men of the Army. Emergency work, whether for officers or enlisted men, shall, at all times, have precedence over those not entitled to free service, without regard to the hours of duty.

> *1428.* For plate work or for filling of teeth only the materials supplied by the Government will be used, and dental surgeons are forbidden to enter into any financial agreement with enlisted men involving an obligation for payment for silver, platinum, or gold used for filling cavities in teeth, for the construction of bridge work, for the fitting of crowns, or the making of artificial dentures.[82]

Then he reminded O'Reilly that he had written about this matter in December 1905 and repeated his previous words (see "John Marshall's Work at the Presidio"):

> . . . in order that I may emphasise [*sic*] the expression of my opinion regarding the necessity for prohibiting Contract Dental Surgeons from entering into any financial agreement with enlisted men of the Army for the payment for work performed or materials furnished, as such transactions are detrimental to the interests of the service in as much as they are the cause of dissatisfaction and are productive of disputes which should never be allowed to occur.[82]

On April 16, 1908, John Millikin, the dental surgeon for the Department of the Lakes at Fort Sheridan, Illinois, wrote to the surgeon general about the use of gold, platinum, and porcelain for fillings, crowns, and bridges and those entitled to his services. He acknowledged that "there is much dissatisfaction in the Army about the charges made by Army dental surgeons for dental gold work and for work done for officers' families." He noted that civilian practitioners were often not nearby and were too expensive when it came to permanent dental work, which "cannot be done without the use of gold, platinum and porcelain." His use of these materials was fairly infrequent, for he had done only 415 operations with gold, platinum and porcelain out of over 11,000. He recommended that a scale of charges be published so that everyone knew what they were, and "in this way regulate all charges by dental surgeons and eliminate much trouble and dissatisfaction." Millikin addressed the problem of free dental care for families and how much trouble it had caused him in his practice, saying:

> There is no practical way to allow officers' families treatment free during regular office hours as it would take up too much time, that should be given to the officers and men. A dental surgeon refusing to do the officers' dental work for officers' families, is in as much disfavor as the one over charging for his work. Not withstanding A.R. 1426 most officers, and especially their families, think officers' families are entitled to free dental treatment at any hour, this often leads to much trouble and loss of time explaining why they are not entitled to free dental treatment and not during regular office hours.[83]

On May 15, 1908, in addition to returning Millikin's letter, O'Reilly recommended to the adjutant general that paragraphs 1426 and 1428, Army Regulations, be amended as Torney had suggested in December 1907.[84,85] O'Reilly explained:

EXHIBIT 9-2

JOHN D MILLIKIN

John D Millikin graduated from the University of Pennsylvania's School of Dentistry in 1898. John Marshall examined and accepted him as a contract dental surgeon in February 1902, after which Millikin was assigned to the Philippines, where he worked from March 1902 to May 1905. He later served at Fort Leavenworth from 1905 to 1908, then returned to the Philippines until 1911. In November 1911 he was found physically unfit for commissioned service in the Dental Corps, probably due to his service in the Philippines, and his contract was annulled on March 4, 1912. He moved to San Francisco and later rose to civilian distinction. He always remained very supportive of Army dentistry and was deeply involved in the Association of Military Dental Surgeons of the United States. He served on the General Medical Board of the Council of National Defense from 1917 to 1919 and also served 10 years as a lieutenant colonel in the Dental Reserve Corps.

Data source: National Archives and Records Administration. Record Group 112. John D Millikin to surgeon general's office, 1 May 1905, with indices. Letter. No 105637. Box 709. Entry 26.

The Medical Department furnishes the necessary material to enable dental surgeons to do good work for officers and enlisted men of the Army except in special cases, but under paragraph 1428, A.R., gold and the more expensive materials may be employed if the operating dentist sees fit to use them at the expense of the individual operated upon. This is not believed to be good policy, as the arrangement has led to many misunderstandings; moreover it is believed to be detrimental to the best interests of the service for dental surgeons to enter into financial agreements with enlisted men of the Army for payment for work performed or materials furnished.[85]

On May 21 Major General Duvall, the assistant to the chief of staff, approved O'Reilly's recommendations with some changes in paragraph 1428 to make it clear that enlisted soldiers would only use government furnished materials "and no other." Any "financial agreements with enlisted men" for silver, platinum, or porcelain dental work were strictly forbidden. Duvall did not agree with any of Millikin's recommendations, and his letter was filed "without further action."[86]

On August 12, 1908, the War Department published General Order No. 128 with new paragraphs 1418 and 1420, which amended the former paragraphs 1426 and 1428. Limitations on those entitled to free dental service and the type of materials to be used were put into place, along with a prohibition on financial arrangements between dental surgeons and enlisted soldiers as outlined above.[87] Despite the Army Regulations, these issues were not resolved and continued to be a major source of trouble for dental surgeons over the next several years.[88–91]

In a letter to the editor in the December 1908 issue of *Dental Cosmos*, an anonymous writer, "XYZ," complained about the new paragraphs of the Army Regulations, writing:

Enlisted men will not go to a dentist who is authorized to do only certain kinds of work, and who can use only certain kinds of material, any more than they would in civil life to a physician who was allowed to use only two kinds of medicine. The success of this corps depends upon the confidence of the enlisted men, and nothing could more completely have aroused resentment and refusal to receive treatment than the limitations recently placed upon the dental surgeon and the treatment that enlisted men may receive. . . . This order will work untold hardship on the men stationed in the Philippines, Cuba, and Alaska, where civilian dentists are few and their prices beyond the reach of the enlisted men. In the Philippines, outside of Manila there are no dentists, so men going on foreign service for two years, with a dentist visiting a post every four to six months, means the wholesale loss of front teeth. . . . Under the provisions of this order, crown and bridge work cannot be done, consequently many teeth that can be saved and made useful will have to be extracted. . . .

In closing, I would like to state that the dental surgeons, most of whom have industriously endeavored to maintain a status that would reflect credit on their corps and the profession at large, feel that regulations like the inclosed [sic] one are a reflection on their decency and self-respect, and a reflection on the profession at large as scientific men.[92(p1443)]

This issue soon resurfaced, and, just as "XYZ" had predicted, it happened in the Philippines.

The Pettus Bill: S 2355
"What has Become of It?"

Considerable recrimination and discussion followed the failure to produce satisfactory dental legislation. In January 1907 Rodrigues Ottolengui urged the dental profession to encourage its congressmen to vote for the Pettus bill without the House amendments. If the House amendments were added, he feared the two bills would not be passed before the present Congress adjourned and dental legislation would have to start over again the next session. Ottolengui also wrote to Secretary of War Taft, requesting his support for the bill. Ottolengui believed that although neither the Senate nor the House bills were perfect, the establishment of a commissioned dental corps was the most important point; "faults" in the new law could be taken care of later.[93,94]

The Pettus bill did not even get the full approval of the NDA's Committee on Army and Navy Dental Legislation. It influenced the House Military Affairs Committee to change provisions that were not acceptable to the majority of the dental profession. The bill was reported favorably in the House and recommended for passage, but failed to pass by the end of the session and died with the 59th Congress.[95,96] On July 27, 1907, Senator Edmund Pettus of Alabama, an ardent supporter of Army dentistry since 1898, passed away and left a major gap in the ranks of congressional support for a commissioned dental corps.[97]

In the November 1907 issue of *Dental Cosmos*, Edward Kirk published an editorial titled "What Has Become of It?" He referred to the fact that over the past few years, committees had been formed, meetings held, money spent, bills introduced and lobbied in Congress, and still there was no commissioned permanent dental corps. He criticized the efforts of the NDA's committee charged with working on an acceptable dental bill.[98]

On November 12, 1907, B Holly Smith, the chairman of the NDA's 1907 legislative committee, replied that some positive steps had been taken, despite the failure to pass the dental bill. "Friends" had been made in Congress, and, after all, the medical bill to eliminate contract surgeons had fared no better, despite the support of the medical profession. The two primary reasons for the defeat of previous dental bills, he argued, were the dental profession's failure to unite behind the legislative committee's efforts and independent attempts to seek alternative measures. Ultimately, he felt "outsiders" had perhaps caused the whole affair to drag on.[99]

On December 10, 1907, Ottolengui expressed his dissatisfaction with Smith's remarks on the "organized band of knockers and kickers" opposing the legislative committee's efforts. As a member of the legislative committee, Ottolengui professed to be one of the "organizers" of that band. He explained that his opposition to the original Army dental bill was not because of any "personal animosity" toward Williams Donnally. Nor did his opposition to the current bill have anything to do with any "personal friendship" with Marshall and Oliver. Instead, he insisted his break with Donnally had been precipitated by Donnally's willingness to accept contract status for Army dental surgeons; in Ottolengui's opinion, nothing less than "an officered corps" should have been accepted. Regarding Marshall and Oliver, Ottolengui said he did not know Marshall except by reputation, and had met

Oliver only once or twice. Nevertheless, he was not in favor of any Army dental bill that would exclude these two men or would place the "patronage" of the dental appointments in the control of a "small body of civilians"; Marshall and Oliver had earned their right to serve in the commissioned corps and supporting any bill that would exclude them would be a "disgrace" to the dental profession.[100]

On December 16 Meyer Rhein stated that the real problem was not outside the legislative committee, but was in the committee itself. Donnally, it seemed, was strongly biased against Marshall, who was the senior supervisory dental surgeon. When this information came out at the 1906 Atlanta meeting, a "tacit gentleman's agreement" was reached that Donnally and Finley, who had served since the committee's establishment in 1898, should no longer serve on the legislative committee. B Holly Smith also had similar feelings toward Marshall. Rhein regarded Marshall as a "strictly honest man" who had no time for politics. He also criticized the fact that the dental committee was trying to pass legislation through Democratic members of a Republican House, when it was a political axiom that no important legislation was ever passed by Congress when introduced by a minority member. This fact, he felt, demonstrated the "unfitness" of the men serving on the dental committee.[100]

Smith reminded Rhein that it was members of the minority party, Representative Otey in the House and Senator Pettus in the Senate, who had secured the passage of the 1901 dental bill. Smith also stated that the NDA's legislative committee had indeed worked very hard to secure legislation that would include the commissioning of the two overage members of the corps, Marshall and Oliver. In fact, the original bill drafted by the committee had included a provision for all the members of the current Dental Corps. The age limit issue had been raised by a member of the House Military Affairs Committee. Once introduced, Representative Hull, the chairman of that committee, announced that he would not allow the bill to be reported if it provided for Marshall's commissioning. He argued that Marshall was almost 60 years old and would be able to retire in about 2 years on three quarters pay. The surgeon general agreed with Representative Hull and said he would not support the bill's passage. He stated he would, however, favor a private bill to promote Marshall in view of his excellent service. With this dilemma facing them, the committee had no choice but to carry on rather than jeopardize the legislation. At the surgeon general's suggestion, a clause was added providing for the civilian examiners. This loophole could allow Marshall a place on the board.[101]

On November 25, 1907, William Fisher, a former 1901 contract dental surgeon who had left the Army in 1904, added his support to those critical of the NDA's efforts to secure legislation for a commissioned dental corps. Fisher argued that when he entered the service in 1901, he was assured that before his 3-year contract was up, Congress and the Army would recognize the necessity for commissioned dental surgeons. The congressional term of the winter of 1903 to 1904, just prior to the expiration of the contracts of the original 1901 dental surgeons, was the key time to press the issue before Congress. The legislative committee had missed this "golden opportunity." In 1904 Fisher had resigned from the Army, "disgusted with the manner in which the National Dental Association was looking after the interests of those who had done much toward the advancement of the profession within the government service, and, thoroughly dissatisfied with the contract status." Others, too, had left for similar reasons. Following a visit to some friends in the War Department in 1906, Fisher said he reached three conclusions:

> First, that the committee on army and navy affairs from the National Dental Association was most certainly doing no effective work. Secondly, that there was an underlying obstinate and effective opposition from the medical department of the army as represented within the office of the Surgeon-general. Thirdly (and this from my three years' experience), that there was not any opposition from so much as five per cent of the "line" and other "staff" officers.[102]

In his opinion, only the combined efforts of all state and local dental societies and the entire dental profession would produce a successful legislation.[102]

John Marshall in the Philippines

In October 1907 Surgeon General O'Reilly contemplated sending John Marshall to the Philippines for duty to replace John Hess, who was ill. The surgeon general kept one of the three examining and supervisory dental surgeons in the Philippines due to the large number of dental surgeons there and their work load. Hess had switched places with Oliver, with Oliver going to West Point and Hess to Manila in January 1905. On October 17 O'Reilly postponed the reassignment because Hess's return date was indefinite and he wanted Marshall to hold an exami-

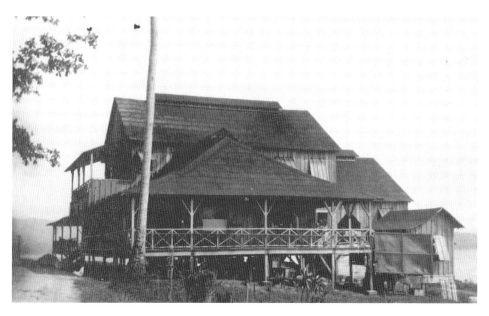

Post Hospital, Camp Bumpus, Tacloban, Leyte, Philippine Islands, April 1907.
Photograph: Courtesy of National Archives and Records Administration.

nation of candidates in December. After the examinations were completed in January 1908, Marshall was granted a leave of absence and traveled to Chicago.[103–107]

While in Chicago, Marshall attended a meeting of the Chicago Odontographic Society on January 21, 1908 (Exhibit 9-3).[108] Before he commented on the night's paper, Marshall spoke briefly of his work as the senior Army dental surgeon:

> My position has been a somewhat peculiar one—an unique one, I may say—one that no other man up to this time has ever occupied. I have been placed, as it were, in the limelight where I could be criticized and have been criticized sometimes most unmercifully, but criticism hurts no man if he takes it in the right spirit, and I have tried to take the criticism which has come to me in that spirit. It has not made me sour, because some people rip me up the back; I am as happy as I ever was, and keep on in the same old way trying to do my duty as I understand it. I could not expect to please everybody, and I never try to please everybody. I have tried to do my duty as I have understood it, always keeping in mind the best interests of army dental surgery and the honor of our profession.[109]

Finally, on February 1, 1908, Surgeon General O'Reilly recommended that Marshall be ordered to duty in the Philippines on the Army transport sailing on about March 5. Marshall received his orders on February 4, 1908, and left San Francisco on board the transport *Thomas* bound for Manila. He did not return until July 1910.[110–114] The senior spokesman for the Army's contract dental surgeons was very remote from the legislative efforts in Washington to authorize a commissioned corps.

From his work at the Presidio with soldiers returning from the Philippines, Marshall already knew of the poor oral and dental hygiene of the troops serving in that tropical environment. On October 24 Marshall recommended to the chief surgeon of the Philippines Division, Colonel John Van R Hoff, that the following procedures be implemented:

EXHIBIT 9-3

THE CHICAGO ODONTOGRAPHIC SOCIETY MEETING, JANUARY 21, 1908

Among the Chicago dental luminaries in attendance that evening was Dr William HP Logan (1872–1943), then dean and chief of oral surgery at the Chicago College of Dental Surgery (Loyola University of Chicago). Logan was called to active duty in World War I and served as the first chief of the dental division in the Office of The Surgeon General from 1917 to 1919.

Data source: Biographical File of Colonel William HP Logan. Biographical Files, Research Collections, Office of Medical History; OTSG, US Army. Falls Church, Virginia.

(1) Dental surgeons should avail themselves of every opportunity to instruct the enlisted men in the care of their teeth by lectures and demonstrations.

(2) Enlisted men should be required to "thoroughly brush their teeth at least once daily" and the non-commissioned officers or squad leaders be responsible to see that they complied.

(3) Regular inspection of the mouth by the company or detachment commander be mandatory, just like the inspection of the enlisted men's feet.[115]

On the same day, Marshall forwarded his detailed "Report on the Need for Dental Prophylaxis in the United States Army" to the surgeon general through Colonel Hoff. The report renewed his previous attempts to convince the surgeon general and Army to adopt "some efficient means of preventing, in a measure at least, the appalling ravages" of dental and oral diseases:

Good teeth, or at least serviceable teeth, are very necessary as a means of maintaining the general health, & consequently the highest efficiency of any army, particularly when campaigning in the tropics, where conditions of the climate & necessary changes in the food and the habits of life are so enervating & debilitating to the general system. . . . Resistance to disease under these conditions is greatly lessened & the individual is consequently predisposed to certain classes of diseases among which are dental caries, pulpitis, pericementitis, dento-alveolar abscess, pyorrhea, alveolaris, necrosis of the jaws, inflammatory & ulcerative conditions of the gums, of the oral mucus membrane, the throat & the tongue.[116(p1)]

Marshall recited information from the annual reports of the surgeon general on the continuing poor oral and dental health of soldiers in the Philippines compared with those in the United States. He again recommended "the great need of adopting vigorous measures" among the soldiers to enhance oral and dental hygiene and prevent dental caries:

This, I believe, may be accomplished by educating the soldiers through lectures & demonstrations given upon dental hygiene & sanitation by the dental surgeons at the post schools, & by requiring soldiers to thoroughly brush their teeth at least once each day. . . . To gain the greatest benefit however, from this cleansing it should be done after each meal. . . . A good tooth brush & pure water are all that is really necessary for the removal of fermentable material from the teeth & mouth. Many enlisted men do not carry a tooth brush in their kit & never cleanse their teeth in any way; while some of them have such filthy, disgusting looking mouths when they report to the dental surgeon for treatment that they need to visit a scavenger before it is safe for the dental surgeon to operate or to make an examination of their mouths. The infections from an unclean mouth are very virulent & exceedingly dangerous to one inoculated with them, & as a consequence the dental surgeon must be constantly on his guard to prevent such infection of his hands.[116(pp8–9)]

Then Marshall laid out his recommendations as noted in Hoff's letter. As with many of Marshall's previous efforts to prompt action, on December 1, 1908, the surgeon general's office thanked him for his report and commented that it would be given "due consideration."[116,117]

300

The Bulkeley Dental Bill: "The Iron is Hot"

On January 14, 1908, at the beginning of the first session of 60th Congress Senator Morgan G Bulkeley (1837–1922) of Connecticut, a Union Civil War veteran, took up where Pettus had left off and introduced the same dental bill that had passed the Senate 2 years earlier as an amendment to the Army medical bill (S 1424) but that had died with the termination of the 59th Congress. The Senate Military Affairs Committee opposed attaching the dental bill to the medical bill and recommended that Bulkeley report his dental amendment as a separate bill.[95,118,119]

On January 27 Bulkeley submitted a report from the Committee on Military Affairs, accompanied by his bill (S 4432) "to reorganize the corps of dental surgeons attached to the Medical Department of the Army." The committee had recommended that the bill be passed. The bill again proposed creating a commissioned dental corps with a strength premised on one dentist per 1,000 troops. Appointees were to be between 22 and 30 years old and subjected to physical and professional standards satisfactory to the surgeon general. A professional examining board of an Army surgeon and two contract dental surgeons, all appointed by the surgeon general, would determine qualifications. Contract dental surgeons currently serving with "satisfactory" reports and entrance examinations could be commissioned without further examination. Dentists could be promoted up to the rank of major. The mix of lieutenants, captains, and majors was set in a series of ratios to each other, while the maximum number of dentists in the Army was set at 30.[118,120–122]

On January 28 the bill was read again at Bulkeley's request just at the close of the morning hour. The next day it was read the third time and passed the Senate. The following day, January 30, it was referred to the House Committee on Military Affairs, which in turn referred it to the War Department for comment. Chief of Staff Major General J Franklin Bell sent it to Surgeon General O'Reilly for his opinion.[96,118]

In the February 1908 issue of *Items of Interest*, Ottolengui pointed out that if a dental bill (such as S 2355 or HR 9737) passed with the civilian board clause (Section 4), then the Army dental appointments would be more or less under the control of the council of the NDA. At the time, the council had seven members, therefore four members constituted a majority.[123] In the February 1908 edition of *Dental Digest*, the editor, Dr George Clapp, urged his readers that their professional duty, "individually and collectively," was to use all "honorable means at their command" to get their congressmen to support the passage of the dental reorganization bill.[124]

Contract Dental Surgeon George Casaday asked the surgeon general if it would be permissible for the dental surgeons as a group to retain an attorney to represent them in the current dental legislation, because the majority of the dental surgeons approved the measure. In addition, he wanted to know if the surgeon general approved of a dental board with two civilian members and one dental surgeon or a board with one medical surgeon and two dental surgeons.[125] On February 17 the surgeon general's office replied that the employment of an attorney to "influence legislation" was a violation of Army Regulations. Regarding the constitution of the board, the surgeon general could not comment because the bill had not yet been referred to his office for discussion.[126]

In March Edward Kirk wrote that Bulkeley's bill had gone farther toward enactment than any previous bill. He urged the dental profession, using Clapp's phrase, to unite "collectively and individually" to secure its passage into law.[127] CN Johnson, editor of *Dental Review*, also favored the current bill, as long as it included the "older members of the corps." He thought the political situation was "ripe" for the bill's passage, writing: "The iron is hot. Will not the profession mold it into shape by a few vigorous strokes?"[95] Wilbur Litch, editor of *Dental Brief*, added to the momentum by telling his readers that the current bill seemed to "embody all that could reasonably be expected" at the time.[128] Ottolengui even supported the new bill and printed the names and Washington addresses of all the members of the House Committee on Military Affairs in *Items of Interest* so that they would "receive about ten thousand letters from dentists." The Indiana and Illinois dental societies also contacted Secretary Taft in support of the pending dental bill.[119,129,130]

Another important factor working against the dental bill was the American Medical Association (AMA). In December 1907 the dental bill got little support from the medical profession because the House of Delegates of the AMA favored keeping dental legislation in abeyance until after the general medical bill for the reorganization of the Medical Department was passed. It was reportedly killed by an Army surgeon who was a delegate.[131-133]

Although his own reorganization bill was on the verge of success, on April 1, 1908, Surgeon General O'Reilly rendered his opinion on Bulkeley's dental bill to the chief of staff:

> The enclosed bill in my opinion is defective and should not be passed in its present shape. I recommend that this matter be referred to the General Staff for their careful consideration.
>
> Whatever may be the advantage of organizing a corps of commissioned dental surgeons I think it extremely important that any steps in that direction should be taken with a full knowledge of what may be expected if such a bill becomes a law. If Congress gives its approval to a corps of dental surgeons, such an act will simply announce that the government assumes the dental care and treatment of all persons who are now entitled to medical care and treatment. The conclusion that must be drawn from this announcement is that a sufficient number of commissioned dental surgeons must be provided to give this treatment, or the department must be supplied with means to procure the necessary treatment from civilian sources, just as is now done by the Medical Department for medical treatment. With the present dental corps this would entail the expenditure of thousands of dollars annually.
>
> I think it only fair to make this frank statement, as I do not desire to, in any way, be the means of securing the War Department's approval to a bill that would ultimately entail great additional expense to the government without doing my part in presenting all the facts necessary for the intelligent consideration of the measure.[134]

Major General Bell, the chief of staff, concurred with this opinion, and the bill went back to the House committee where it remained.[95,135]

A Fractious Dental Lobby Presses On

On April 9, 1908, Williams Donnally, the chairman of the Committee on Army Dental Legislation of the NDA, wrote to Secretary of War Taft regarding the Bulkeley bill. He pointed out that virtually everyone acknowledged the need for a dental service of some sort in the Army. It was the status of those providing the service that was the source of contention, he argued; what happened to the approximately 30 contract practitioners was not really what was at stake:

> Your denial of the equity of the claim of the dental profession for a limited measure of the social, professional and official advantages of the grades of rank accorded all other professions represented in the military service (which claim is recognized in repeated Acts of the Senate and in H.R. Military Committee Report No. 3642, 59th Congress) would not only wound the pride of the members of the profession who have taken their degrees in the universities and colleges of the states, thousands of whom are practicing in this and every civilized country under the most favorable social and professional advantages, but would, especially if it should avail to arrest the legislative progress of the Act of the Senate, turn many of the more discriminating and ambitious young men from the dental to other professions.[136]

In conclusion, Donnally argued that formal dental education was American in origin and continued to set the global standards. Dentistry had reached a level of complexity similar to any other medical specialty, and its members deserved the Army's acknowledgment of their skills and education. Not commissioning its dentists implied a "dishonor [to] the profession with a continuance of a discreditable and humiliating military relation." He urged Taft's support for the law.[136]

Surgeon General O'Reilly's long-sought bill to "increase the efficiency of the Medical Department of the U.S. Army" finally passed Congress and was signed into law on April 23, 1908. It provided for a medical corps, medical reserve corps, hospital corps, nurse corps, and "the dental surgeons, as now authorized by law."[5,137] The Medical Reserve Corps, the first such reserve organization of any kind in the history of the US Army, replaced the former contract surgeons. The passage of this act prompted Meyer Rhein, a member of the Committee on Medical Legislation and the National Legislative Council of the AMA, to write to O'Reilly expressing his continuing disappointment in the surgeon general's lack of support for a "commissioned dental corps."[138]

On May 27 the surgeon general replied to Rhein, saying that he still held the same viewpoint on dental legislation that he had expressed to the chief of staff on April 15, 1904. Because the general staff, the chief of staff, and the secretary of war disapproved his opinions, he told Rhein he did not care to make any further statements until the War Department announced a "definite policy" regarding dental legislation.[139]

In May 1908 an unidentified medical officer, reportedly "very close to the S.G.O.," stated that the attempts to attach the dental bill to the Medical Department bill without consulting the surgeon general's office was the crux of the problem. Apparently O'Reilly was "very hot about it" and believed that he had been "ignored," prompting him to endorse S 4432. In general, O'Reilly was "friendly" to the dental surgeons' cause, but the surgeon general's office and the general staff could not be ignored.[140]

On June 3, 1908, the dental lobby received some very good news. With the Medical Reorganization Act, the AMA's House of Delegates passed a resolution authorizing its Committee on Legislation to support "such bills as meet the approval of the War Department."[131–133] The House of Delegates also endorsed the proposed dental legislation, saying:

> The House of Delegates of the American Medical Association, recognizing the great importance of the services of the dental corps of both the army and navy, and appreciating the importance of placing both on a commissioned basis, authorizes the Committee on Medical Legislation to assist in securing the passage of such bills as meet the approval of the War Department or the chief of the Bureau of Medicine and Surgery of the Navy Department.[132,141]

Coming from an organization that represented 80,000 physicians, this support was indeed welcome.[132]

In September an unidentified contract dental surgeon wrote to the NDA's executive council that Donnally and Finley had not only been "antagonistic" to the surgeon general's office and the general staff, but had "ignored" them for the past 6 years. According to the source, Army dental surgeons had lost confidence in Donnally's and Finley's abilities to secure new legislation. The author suggested that Rodrigues Ottolengui, WW Walker, and ML Rhein would be better suited for the committee.[142]

Another unidentified contract dental surgeon stated that Donnally's committee had "done more harm than good"; it had altogether failed to consult the Army dental surgeons on the issue. This source blamed the committee for constructing bills without consulting Marshall and Oliver, who had done more for Army dentistry than the entire profession combined. He believed that this slight was not accidental. The sentiment among the contract dental surgeons was that Donnally and Finley should be removed from the committee.[143] The ill-feelings that existed between Donnally and Marshall, which dated back at least to 1901, had adversely affected the struggle for acceptable legislation since then.

Still another contract dental surgeon called for Donnally's resignation, arguing that the dental surgeons should not suffer simply because Donnally was doing his "best." He thought that "two fractions" were now working for dental legislation, which meant that nothing was being accomplished.[144]

At the Northeastern Dental Association meeting in Hartford, Connecticut, in October 1908, Senator Bulkeley commented on his bill, saying that "apparent jealousy among the dentists themselves" had obstructed the bill's passage, and the only way to assure the dental law's passage was to have a "united effort" from the part of the dental profession. The question of rank alone would prevent action on the bill unless the dentists stopped quibbling about it. "Nothing," he said, "would add more to the comfort of the soldiers than skilled dental surgeons," and he hoped that he would see the bill's passage during his term in the Senate.[99]

On October 20, 1908, Donnally declined reappointment as chairman of the NDA's Committee on Army and Navy Dental Legislation. He had been either the committee's secretary or chairman for the past 10 years, except from 1906 to 1907, when Doctors Ottolengui, Sanger, and Smith constituted the committee. He cited financial loss, "mental and physical strain," and interference with "personal, social, and family interests" as his reasons for resigning and offered to donate $500 to any fund that the executive council set up to support the pending Army bill.[99]

On November 26, 1908, Donnally wrote to Surgeon General O'Reilly defending his position and contradicting statements made that he had "antagonized" the surgeon general and "completely ignored" his office in the NDA committee's attempts to secure the passage of the dental bill. He attributed these remarks to the dental profession's "mischief-making, muck-raking insurgents."[145] On December 16, 1908, O'Reilly replied that the dental surgeons had a perfect right to express their opinions; he was not responsible for their views. He also absolved Donnally of any responsibility for the Bulkeley amendment.[146]

Growing Discontent among the Dental Surgeons

With all that had transpired in Congress, the Medical Department, and the NDA in recent years, a number of contract dentists began to show growing disenchantment with their status. In November 1908 Dr Ord Sorber, a former contract dental surgeon who had left the service in 1907 after 6 years to pursue a civilian career, painted a less than flattering picture of Army dentistry. He criticized the lack of security in the contract system as well as his "relative rank." The latter meant that even the most junior Army officers bumped him from bunks on Army transports and from government housing. The lack of a commission meant he got neither foreign service pay nor longevity increases. He confronted an ever expanding workload with no prospect of it decreasing, though he was pressured to provide more and more services. He found his working environments marginal, whether in Arkansas or the Philippines, in part because of climate, but also because of the inadequate clinic space provided. Substantial paperwork and inadequate or inappropriate supplies made it even harder to maintain professional standards. "Your correspondent expended about five hundred and fifty dollars of his own funds on office equipment and supplies in the effort to keep things going and finally asked for the annulment of his contract," Sorber wrote.[147]

In the December 1908 issue of *Dental Cosmos*, Edward Kirk pointed out that the contract system was both unsatisfactory from a "professional standpoint" and from the "standpoint of the relationship of the corps to the line." He regarded the contract system as merely "an entering wedge" that would eventually give dentistry the "status and recognition" to which it was entitled. The path toward commissioned status had been a "long and devious" one, "strewn with the wrecks of personal ambitions and personal friendships." He called for a "concerted effort" from the profession.[99]

In December 1908 Dr Raymond Ingalls, a contract dental surgeon wrote a letter to the editor of *Dental Cosmos*, stating that the recently passed medical bills that gave contractors a reserve commission had left contract dentists in an insulting and anomalous situation. In a practical sense, it meant that there would be increasing pay disparities between dentists and the rest of the Medical Department. The notoriously rigorous entrance examinations for dentists meant that the Army hired some of the best practitioners in the profession and then relegated them

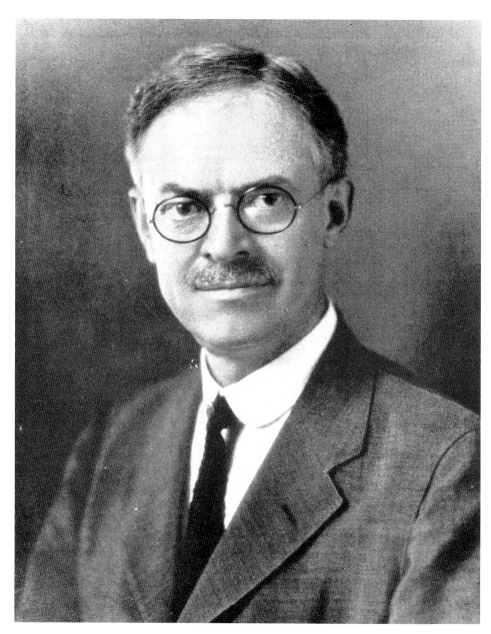

Ord Sorber, a contract dental surgeon from 1901–1907,
spoke out about the rank problems with the system.
Photograph: Courtesy of the National Library of Medicine.

to second-class status. Ingalls believed this sent the wrong signals to the Army and society in general and to the dental profession in particular that could lead to a reduction in the quality of future dental applicants. He argued that granting commissions would make up for many other shortcomings, writing: "Our present status makes us servants of the Army; rank would put us in the Army." In his opinion, achieving successful legislation for Army dentists required extensively educating Congress and gaining consistent support from every dentist and dental organization in the country.[99]

Despite their disappointment, however, Army dentists were increasingly appreciated by their beneficiaries. For example, on November 11, 1908, Major General John Weston, commander of the Philippines Division, endorsed a commissioned status for the Dental Corps in a letter to Major General Fred Ainsworth, the Army's powerful adjutant general:

> I write to invite your attention to the anomalous condition of the Dental Corps, and to ask that you, so familiar with organization and legislation, have it put upon a commissioned basis in the Army. The Corps is really a good one, is of material benefit to the Army, is doing good work here and elsewhere, is deserving and should be classed with other professions in the line of the Army, and is so recommended.[148]

Surgeon General O'Reilly's Final Position

As he prepared to end his second term as Army Surgeon General, O'Reilly addressed the pending dental legislation after discussing it with his successor, George Torney. On December 16, 1908, O'Reilly sent a lengthy memorandum to Chief of Staff J Franklin Bell. After his appointment as surgeon general in September 1902, he had initially favored commissioned status for contract dental surgeons. However, his first and overriding priority was to correct the "injustice" that the Army Reorganization Act of February 2, 1901, had done to the Medical Corps. Now that this situation had been remedied by the April 1908 act, it was time to discuss the commissioning of dentists in the Army. In April 1904, when Brownlow's HR 79 was under consideration in Congress, O'Reilly had said that rank was not necessary to the "proper performance" of the dental surgeon. However, "creditable and responsible sources [the NDA committee and perhaps John Marshall]" had convinced him that rank would greatly improve the dental service. Therefore, he had recommended that legislation be drawn up to provide commissioned status for the dental surgeons. Now, late in 1908, O'Reilly leaned again toward his earlier opinion that rank was not necessary. Finally, he had realized that there were "fractions" among the dental profession, which seriously eroded his earlier confidence in the credibility of the NDA. He broke his arguments down to the following conclusions:

- Good dental care could be provided by contract dental surgeons at less expense than a commissioned dental corps.
- It was doubtful that the dental associations would be satisfied with the rank that would be given dental surgeons if legislation were enacted. They

would probably continue to lobby for higher rank and perhaps block the passage of Army legislation, particularly that pertaining to the Medical Department.

- The commissioning of dentists was "wholly without precedence" in the Army. No corps had ever been created in the Army that had "no distinctly military relations and duties." Any "competent" dentist could perform his duties effectively without prior military training.

- Dentistry was "generally held in the medical profession as a minor and mechanical specialty of the medical sciences." Commissioning dentists would "cheapen" the commission in the Medical Corps, especially the Medical Reserve Corps. It could also lead to the pharmacists, veterinarians, and even the architects in the quartermaster department demanding commissions.

Ultimately, O'Reilly recommended that dental surgeons not be commissioned.[149]

The Chief of Staff's Position Changes

On November 24, before O'Reilly had even prepared his final comments, J Franklin Bell, the War Department chief of staff, wrote him a note and forwarded a copy of Bulkeley's bill. He explained that he had met Dr Emory Bryant, President Theodore Roosevelt's personal dentist, at the president's home at Oyster Bay, Long Island, New York. They had discussed the bill, a copy of which Bryant later left at the chief of staff's office. However, Bell told Bryant that he "could not recognize him as a representative of the Dental Surgeons, and he asked me whom I would recognize as authorized to speak for the Dental Surgeons." Bell recommended John Marshall. Bryant asked if he could invite Marshall to write to him about the dental bill, and Bell agreed. However, no letter from Marshall to Bell has yet been found.[150]

On December 22, after receiving O'Reilly's December memorandum, Bell wrote a memo to the Second Section general staff, detailing his thoughts about the dental bill. He noted that he had sided with O'Reilly and opposed the Bulkeley bill the previous April because of the impending action on the Medical Reorganization Bill. However, his action did "not indicate any opposition to the bill by the Chief of Staff."[152] Writing in the third person, Bell explained:

> In the judgment of the Chief of Staff there is just as much reason why dental surgeons should have rank as that any other surgeon should, and he believes that both dental surgeons and veterinary surgeons should have rank. It will certainly be the only way to settle the question so that the dental and veterinary corps can get what they are entitled to.[151]

Bell considered the Bulkeley bill "entirely reasonable." He was not bothered that the bill would create several positions for majors:

> The fact that it will confer the rank of major on a few who have served only ten years is no reason why they should be deprived of all rank. It would be quite reasonable to raise the limit of service necessary to attain the rank of major to a greater length of

time, if the Second Section considers it advisable. A certain number might be given the rank of major, for instance, after fifteen years' service, and thereafter depend upon rising to that rank by promotion to vacancies, or any equitable arrangement giving to them what may be conceded to veterinary surgeons, and approximately what is conceded to surgeons of the medical corps would seem proper for dental surgeons.[151]

In the fall of 1908 Bell solicited the views of the Army dental surgeons. He said that while the Medical Department was against giving rank to dentists, the "General Staff was not to be dictated to by the Medical Department." He did not favor doing anything to benefit the Army dental surgeons or the dental profession at large. However, he would approve a bill for commissioning the Army dental surgeons if it could be shown that the dental service could be improved with the whole Army as the beneficiary. In his annual report, dated December 26, 1908, Bell wrote: "The bill [S 4432] now before Congress for the dental surgeons should be passed." At last some progress was apparently made in gaining the War Department's support for a commissioned corps, even if the surgeon general was now openly opposed.

Progress toward Commissioned Status

The years from 1904 to 1908 marked steady progress for dental surgeons in their work on the Army's oral and dental health. They had also made some headway in improving the dental habits of officers and soldiers. As a result, commanders increasingly valued the contributions that the dental surgeons made to the readiness of their soldiers and units. Although Chief of Staff J Franklin Bell adopted a more favorable position toward dental legislation, no real progress toward commissioned status had been achieved. In 1909 a new president and a new surgeon general had the opportunity to change this dismal record.

References

1. National Archives and Records Administration. Record Group 94. Memorandum report [on dental surgeons], Kerr, January 5, 1905. No. 524625: 3–7.

2. National Archives and Records Administration. Record Group 94. Endorsement to Kerr report, January 5, 1905, Major General Gillespie, assistant chief of staff, January 9, 1905, to Lieutenant General Chaffee, chief of staff. No. 524625.

3. National Archives and Records Administration. Record Group 94. Endorsement to Gillespie, Lieutenant General Chaffee, chief of staff, to secretary of war, January 10, 1905. No. 524625.

4. National Archives and Records Administration. Record Group 112. SD Boak to Mr Carpenter, secretary to WH Taft, January 13, 1905. Letter. No. 106047. Box 712. Entry 26.

5. Gillett MC. *The Army Medical Department, 1775-1818*. Vol 3. Washington, DC: Center of Military History, United States Army; 1981: 321.

6. National Archives and Records Administration. Record Group 112. Assistant secretary of war to Donnally, January 25, 1905. Letter. No. 106047.

7. National Archives and Records Administration. Record Group 112. Various dental societies to secretary of war [January–July 1905]. Letters and Petitions. No. 106047.

8. National Archives and Records Administration. Record Group 112. Donnally to secretary of war, January 12, 1905. Letter. No. 106047.

9. National Archives and Records Administration. Record Group 112. Assistant secretary of war to Donnally, January 25, 1905. No. 106047.

10. [Hoff NS]. The Army dentist. *Dental Register*. 1905;59:544–545.

11. Motley WE. *History of the American Dental Hygienists' Association 1923–1982*. Chicago, Ill: American Dental Hygienists' Association; 1986: 9.

12. National Archives and Records Administration. Record Group 112. John D Millikin to surgeon general's office, May 1, 1905. Letter with indices. No. 105637. Box 709. Entry 26.

13. National Archives and Records Administration. Record Group 84. Brigadier General Greely to military secretary, October 20, 1905. Letter. No. 524625.

14. Rhein ML. Recollections of the Portland Congress. *Items of Interest*. 1905;27:902–903.

15. National Archives and Records Administration. Record Group 94. Surgeon general's office to military secretary, 20 July 1905. Letter. No. 70760.

16. National Archives and Records Administration. Record Group 94. Special orders no. 168, par 2, War Department, July 22, 1905. No. 391988. Box 2730. Entry 25.

17. National Archives and Records Administration. Record Group 112. Marshall to military secretary, August 1, 1905. Letter. Entry 357.

18. National Archives and Records Administration. Record Group 112. Marshall to commanding officer, USA General Hospital, Presidio of San Francisco, August 29, 1905, 24, 27. Letter. Entry 357.

19. National Archives and Records Administration. Record Group 112. Marshall to surgeon general, November 9, 1905, 32–33. Letter. Entry 357.

20. National Archives and Records Administration. Record Group 94. Marshall to surgeon general, August 21, 1905. Letter. No. 70760.

21. National Archives and Records Administration. Record Group 94. Surgeon general's office to Marshall, September 21, 1905. Letter. No. 70760.

22. National Archives and Records Administration. Record Group 112. Surgeon General O'Reilly to commanding officer, US Army General Hospital, Presidio of San Francisco, 23 November 1905. Letter. No. 77614. Box 509. Entry 26.

23. National Archives and Records Administration. Record Group 112. Marshall to commanding officer, US Army General Hospital, Presidio, 17 December 1905. Letter. No. 77614.

24. National Archives and Records Administration. Record Group 112. Endorsement, Lieutenant Colonel Torney, December 22, 1905, to Marshall to commanding officer, US Army Hospital, Presidio. No. 77614.

25. National Archives and Records Administration. Record Group 112. Surgeon general to Lieutenant Colonel Torney, January 19, 1906. No. 77614.

26. National Archives and Records Administration. Record Group 112. Dr Marshall to Shutts, Walters & Co, Surgical Instruments & Appliances, May 17, 1906. Entry 357.

27. National Archives and Records Administration. Record Group 112. Dr Marshall to surgeon general, May 23, 1906. Entry 357.

28. National Archives and Records Administration. Record Group 112. Dr Marshall to commanding officer, Presidio of San Francisco, May 28, June 4, 1906. Entry 357.

29. National Archives and Records Administration. Record Group 112. Dr Marshall to chief surgeon, Presidio of San Francisco, June 18, 1906. Entry 357.

30. National Archives and Records Administration. Record Group 112. Dr Marshall to adjutant general, May 16, 1907. Entry 357.

31. National Archives and Records Administration. Record Group 94. Major Febiger to military secretary, February 27, 1906. Letter. No. 524625. Box 3645. Entry 25.

32. National Archives and Records Administration. Record Group 94. Endorsement, Surgeon General O'Reilly to military secretary, April 10, 1906. No. 524625. Box 3645. Entry 25.

33. US War Department. *General Orders and Circulars, Adjutant General's Office.* Washington, DC: Government Printing Office; April 30, 1906: No. 26.

34. National Archives and Records Administration. Record Group 94. Military secretary to commanding generals, Atlantic, Northern, Southwestern, Pacific, and Philippines Divisions, May 8, 1906. Letter. No. 524625. Box 3645. Entry 25.

35. National Archives and Records Administration. Record Group 112. To chief surgeon, Department of California, August 23, 1902. Letter. No. 77614-I. Box 509. Entry 26.

36. National Archives and Records Administration. Record Group 112. Reply from chief surgeon, Department of California, September 2, 1902. No. 77614-I. Box 509. Entry 26.

37. National Archives and Records Administration. Record Group 112. Sixth endorsement to inquiry to military secretary. Dentist employment, Dr AC Senecal, December 9, 1905. No. 108929. Box 151. Entry 25.

38. National Archives and Records Administration. Record Group 112. Fifth endorsement, May 18, 1906 to inquiry RO Lexington, KY, April 21, 1906. No. 108929. Box 151. Entry 25.

39. National Archives and Records Administration. Record Group 112. Comment A, fifth endorsement, November 16, 1916 to inquiry regarding Private Alex De Villers from commanding officer, Walter Reed General Hospital, June 15, 1916. No. 108929. Box 151. Entry 25.

40. *Congressional Record, 59th Cong, 1st Sess.* Vol. 40. Washington, DC: Government Printing Office; 1906.

41. National Archives and Records Administration. Record Group 94. HR 31, 59th Cong, 1st Sess, December 4, 1905. Bill. No. 524625. Box 3645. Entry 25.

42. National Archives and Records Administration. Record Group 112. S 2355, 59th Cong, 1st Sess, December 20, 1905. Bill. No. 106047. Box 712. Entry 26.

43. Two bills which are up before Congress: 59th Congress, first session. S. 2355. *Items of Interest.* 1906;28:230–231.

44. US Congress. Senate Reports (Public). 59th Cong, 1st Sess. Vol 1. Washington, DC: Government Printing Office; 1906. S report 585, 1–3.

45. National Archives and Records Administration. Record Group 112. Dr Ottolengui to surgeon general, February 6, 1906. Letter. No. 106047.

46. National Archives and Records Administration. Record Group 112. Surgeon general's office to Dr Ottolengui, February 10, 1906. Letter. No. 106047.

47. National Archives and Records Administration. Record Group 112. Surgeon general's office to chairman, Senate Committee on Military Affairs, February 9, 1906. Report. No. 106047.

48. US Congress. House Reports (Public). 59th Cong, 1st Sess. Vol 2. Washington, DC: Government Printing Office, 1906. H report no. 3642. 1–2.

49. National Archives and Records Administration. Record Group 112. Hearing before the House of Representatives Committee on Military Affairs having under consideration a bill (H.R. 9737) to reorganize the corps of dental surgeons attached to the Medical Department of the Army. March 13, 1906. No. 106047.

50. Ottolengui R. The minor details' in the Army and Navy Dental Corps bills, at present advocated by the Legislation Committee of the National Dental Association. *Items of Interest.* 1906;28:209–212.

51. [Hoff NS]. Army and Navy dental bills. *Dental Register.* 1906;60:109–111.

52. Patterson JD. The Army and Navy dental bills. *Items of Interest.* 1906;28:361–363.

53. [Johnson CN]. Army and Navy legislation. *Dent Rev.* 1906;20:514.

54. National Archives and Records Administration. Record Group 112. Dr Ottolengui to surgeon general, May 3, 1906. Letter. No. 106047.

55. National Archives and Records Administration. Record Group 112. Surgeon general's office to Dr Ottolengui, May 5, 1906. Letter. No. 106047.

56. National Archives and Records Administration. Record Group 112. Surgeon General O'Reilly to Representative Hull, May 9, 1906. Letter. No. 106047.

57. National Archives and Records Administration. Record Group 112. Representative Hull to Surgeon General O'Reilly, May 10, 1906. Letter. No. 106047.

58. National Archives and Records Administration. Record Group 94. Dr Marshall to military secretary, May 19, 1906. Letter. No. 524625.

59. National Archives and Records Administration. Record Group 112. Dr Hess to Surgeon General O'Reilly, July 13, 1906. Letter. No. 106047.

60. National Archives and Records Administration. Record Group 112. Surgeon general's office to Dr Hess, July 20, 1906. Letter. No. 106047.

61. Donnally W. To the editor. *Dental Register.* 1906;60:594.

62. [Bethel LP]. Dental surgeons for Army and Navy—New Legislation. *Dental Summary.* 1906;26:137.

63. *Congressional Record, 59th Cong, 2nd Sess.* Vol 41. Washington, DC: Government Printing Office; 1907: 40.

64. US Congress. House. *Letter from the secretary of war, submitting recommendations as to an additional dental surgeon at the United States Military Academy.* 59th Cong, 2nd sess, 1906. H Doc 78.

65. Hyson JM Jr. *The United States Military Academy Dental Service: A History 1825–1920.* West Point, NY: United States Military Academy; 1989: 46–48, 60–64.

66. National Archives and Records Administration. Record Group 395. Sweet to military secretary and Haan to commanding officer 28th Infantry, December 26, 1906. Telegram and reply. No. 389-B. Box 8. Entry 977.

67. National Archives and Records Administration. Record Group 395. Sweet to BD Taylor, January 10, 1907. Letter. No. 389-B. Box 8. Entry 977.

68. National Archives and Records Administration. Record Group 395. BD Taylor to Sweet, January 12, 1907. Letter. No. 389-B. Box 8. Entry 977.

69. National Archives and Records Administration. Record Group 112. Captain Edward F Geddings, Medical Corps, to surgeon general, USA, May 27, 1908. Letter. No. 116484. Box 797. Entry 26.

70. National Archives and Records Administration. Record Group 395. Captain TW Wise, Medical Corps, to adjutant general, Army of Cuban Pacification, May 18, 1908. Letter. No. 1171-E. Box 15. Entry 977.

71. National Archives and Records Administration. Record Group 395. Comment "THB" on special orders No. 31, Headquarters, Army of Cuban Pacification, Havana, Cuba, February 18, 1908. No 1171-E. Box 15. Entry 977.

72. National Archives and Records Administration. Record Group 165. Surgeon General O'Reilly to chief of staff, April 1, 1907. Memo. Report no. 984. Box 8. Entry 5.

73. National Archives and Records Administration. Record Group 112. Jean C Whinnery (through channels) to inspector general, June 7, 1907. Letter. No 78773. Box 519. Entry 26.

74. National Archives and Records Administration. Record Group 112. John L Chamberlain, third endorsement, June 7, 1907. Letter. No. 78773. Box 519. Entry 26.

75. National Archives and Records Administration. Record Group 112. Lieutenant Colonel RG Ebert, Medical Corps, to adjutant general, Department of the Columbia, December 24,1908. No. 78773. Box 519. Entry 26.

76. National Archives and Records Administration. Record Group 94. Major General Greely to adjutant general, November 18, 1907. Telegram. No. 524625.

77. National Archives and Records Administration. Record Group 94. Surgeon General O'Reilly to adjutant general, November 19, 1907. Endorsement.

78. National Archives and Records Administration. Record Group 94. Adjutant general to Major General Greely, November 21, 1907. Telegram. No. 524625.

79. National Archives and Records Administration. Record Group 165. Major General William P Duvall, assistant to the chief of staff, to assistant secretary of war, December 26, 1907. Memo. Report no. 1637. Box 13. Entry 5.

80. National Archives and Records Administration Record Group 112. Surgeon general's office to chief surgeons of departments, November 20, 1906. Letter. No. 77614.

81. National Archives and Records Administration Record Group 112. Colonel CL Heizmann, chief surgeon, Department of California, to surgeon general, December 7, 1906. Letter. No. 77614.

82. National Archives and Records Administration Record Group 112. Torney to surgeon general, December 23, 1907. Letter. No. 77614.

83. National Archives and Records Administration. Record Group 94. Millikin to the surgeon general, April 16, 1908. Letter. No. 1371229. Box 5342. Entry 25.

84. National Archives and Records Administration. Record Group 112. O'Reilly to the adjutant general, May 15, 1908. Letter. No. 47516. Box 276. Entry 26.

85. Fifth endorsement, O'Reilly to the adjutant general, May 15, 1908, to letter, Millkin to the surgeon general, April 16, 1908. No. 1371229.

86. National Archives and Records Administration. Record Group 165. Memorandum for the acting secretary of war, Major General William P Duvall, assistant to the chief of staff, general staff, May 21, 1908. Memo. Report no. 2516. Box 22. Entry 5.

87. United States War Department. *General Orders and Circulars, Adjutant General's Office.* Washington, DC: Government Printing Office; August 12, 1908: No. 128.

88. National Archives and Records Administration. Record Group 165. Memorandum for the assistant secretary of war, Brigadier General WW Wotherspoon, War Department general staff, March 1, 1909. Report no. 3716. Box 34. Entry 5.

89. National Archives and Records Administration. Record Group 165. Memorandum for the assistant secretary of war, Brigadier General WW Wotherspoon, War Department general staff, August 3, 1909. Report no. 4354. Box 40. Entry 5.

90. National Archives and Records Administration. Record Group 94. John D Millikin, division hospital, Manila, to adjutant general, Philippines Division, April 13, 1909. Letter and endorsements. No. 1546722. Box 5856. Entry 25.

91. National Archives and Records Administration. Record Group 94. Millikin to adjutant general, November 27, 1909. Letter and endorsements. No. 1379686. Box 5364. Entry 25.

92. XYZ. Letter to the editor. *Dental Cosmos.* 1908;50:1443.

93. Ottolengui R. The situation in relation to Army and Navy legislation. An appeal for united effort to pass the bill. *Items of Interest.* 1907;29:94.

94. National Archives and Records Administration. Record Group 112. Dr Ottolengui to Secretary of War Taft, January 11, 1907. Letter. No. 106047.

95. [Johnson CN]. Army dental legislation. *Dental Review*. 1908;22:262.

96. San Francisco Dental Association [proceedings]. *Pacific Dental Gazette*. 1909;17:138–139.

97. Senator Edmund W. Pettus (1821–1907). Biographical directory of the United States Congress, 1774–Present. Website. Available at: http://bioguide.congress.gov/scripts/biodisplay.pl?index=P000279.

98. [Kirk EC]. What had become of it? *Dental Cosmos*. 1907;49:1201–1202.

99. [Kirk EC]. Army and Navy dental legislation. *Dental Cosmos*. 1907;49:1303–1304.

100. [Kirk EC]. A question of diagnosis. *Dental Cosmos*. 1908;50:87–91.

101. Smith BH. What has become of it? *Dental Cosmos*. 1908;50:143.

102. Fisher WC. RE the N.D.A. Committee on Army and Navy Dental Legislation. *Dental Cosmos*. 1908;50:38–39.

103. National Archives and Records Administration. Record Group 94. Surgeon general's office to Lieutenant Colonel George H Torney, Army General Hospital, Presidio of San Francisco, October 1, 1907, endorsement, Lieutenant Colonel Torney, October 7, 1907. Letter with endorsement. No. 70760.

104. National Archives and Records Administration. Record Group 94. Marshall to Surgeon General O'Reilly, October 10, 1907. Letter. No. 70760

105. National Archives and Records Administration. Record Group 94. Surgeon general's office to Marshall, October 14, 1907. Letter. No. 70760

106. National Archives and Records Administration. Record Group 94. Surgeon General O'Reilly to Marshall, October 17, 1907. Letter. No 70760.

107. National Archives and Records Administration. Record Group 94. special orders no. 5, par 21, War Department, January 7, 1908. No. 391988. Box 2730. Entry 25.

108. Biographical File of Colonel William HP Logan. Biographical Files, Research Collections, Office of Medical History; MEDCOM/OTSG, US Army. Falls Church, Virginia.

109. The Chicago-Odontographic Society [proceedings]. *Dental Review*. 1908;22:329.

110. National Archives and Records Administration. Record Group 94. Surgeon General O'Reilly to adjutant general, February 1, 1908. No. 70760.

111. National Archives and Records Administration. Record Group 94. BG Funston to adjutant general, March 5, 1908. Telegram. No. 1349490. Box 5288. Entry 25.

112. National Archives and Records Administration. special orders no. 29, par 11, War Department, February 4, 1908. No. 391988.

113. National Archives and Records Administration. Record Group 94. Commanding general, Philippines Division, to adjutant general, July 16, 1910. Cablegram. No. 1674931. Box 6200. Entry 25.

114. National Archives and Records Administration. Record Group 94. Surgeon general's office to adjutant general, September 13, 1910. Letter. No. 70760.

115. National Archives and Records Administration. Record Group 112. Colonel JVR Hoff, chief surgeon, Philippines Division, to adjutant general, October 24, 1908. Letter. No. 125782. Box 867. Entry 26.

116. National Archives and Records Administration. Record Group 112. Dr Marshall; Report on the need of dental prophylaxis in the United States Army, October 24, 1908. No. 125782. Box 867. Entry 26.

117. National Archives and Records Administration. Surgeon general's office to Marshall, December 1, 1908. Letter. No. 125782.

118. *Congressional Record, 60th Cong, 1st Sess.* Vol 42. Washington, DC: Government Printing Office; 1908.

119. [Ottolengui R]. Status of Army legislation; an appeal for a united effort on the part of the profession. *Items of Interest.* 1908;30:230–231.

120. US Congress. Senate, Reorganization of Corps of Dental Surgeons. S Report 130, 60th Cong, 1st Sess. Washington, DC: Government Printing Office; 1908: 1.

121. Bennett CG. Senate bill for reorganizing the Army Dental Corps. *Dental Cosmos.* 1908;50:302.

122. National Archives and Records Administration. Record Group 112. US Congress. Senate. 60th Cong, 1st Sess. January 30, 1908. S 4432. No. 106047.

123. [Ottolengui R]. The present status of Army and Navy Dental legislation. *Items of Interest.* 1908;30:151.

124. [Clapp GW]. Dental surgeons, the Army Medical Corps and recent legislation relating thereto. *Dental Digest.* 1908;14:239.

125. National Archives and Records Administration. Record Group 112. Dr Casady to Surgeon General O'Reilly, February 6, 1908. Letter. No. 106047.

126. National Archives and Records Administration. Record Group 112. Surgeon general's office to Dr Casaday, February 17, 1908. Letter. No. 106047.

127. [Kirk EC]. The Army dental bill: S. 4432. *Dental Cosmos.* 1908;50:292.

128. [Litch WF?]. Congressional action on the reorganization of the Army Dental Corps. *Dental Brief*. 1908;13:161.

129. National Archives and Records Administration. Record Group 112. Dr George E Hunt, dean, Indiana Dental College, to Secretary Taft, April 13, 1908. Letter. No. 106047.

130. National Archives and Records Administration. Record Group 112. Dr RJ Hood, secretary, Illinois State Dental Society, to Secretary Taft, June 5, 1908. Letter. No. 106047.

131. Rhein ML. Army dental legislation and the American Medical Association. *Dental Cosmos*. 1908;50:142.

132. Grady R. Letter to the editor of Dental Cosmos. In: Army and Navy Dental legislation. *Dental Cosmos*. 1908;50:720–721.

133. Rhein ML. Letter to the editor of Dental Cosmos. In: Army and Navy Dental legislation. *Dental Cosmos*. 1908;50:720–721.

134. National Archives and Records Administration. Record Group 112. Surgeon General O'Reilly to secretary of war, April 1, 1908. Letter. No 106047.

135. National Archives and Records Administration. Record Group 165. Senate Bill 4432, to reorganize the corps of dental surgeons attached to the Medical Department of the Army, March 24, 1908 [endorsement, Major General Bell to acting secretary of war, April 3, 1908]. Report no. 2222. Box 20. Entry 5.

136. National Archives and Records Administration. Record Group 112. Dr Donnally to Secretary of War Taft, April 9, 1908. Letter. No. 106047. Box 712. Entry 26.

137. US Congress. Congressional Record. *Act of 23 April 1908* [Army Medical Reorganization Act]. Sec 1, Stat 66. Vol 35.

138. National Archives and Records Administration. Record Group 112, Dr ML Rhein to Surgeon General O'Reilly, May 25, 1908. Letter. No. 106047.

139. National Archives and Records Administration. Record Group 112. Surgeon General O'Reilly to Dr Rhein, May 27, 1908. Letter. No. 106047.

140. National Archives and Records Administration. Record Group 112. Unidentified medical officer, May 29, 1908. Statement. No. 106047.

141. National Archives and Records Administration. Record Group 112. Frederick R Green, assistant to general secretary, American Medical Association, to secretary of war, July 10, 1908. Letter. No. 106047.

142. National Archives and Records Administration. Record Group 112. Unidentified contract dental surgeon to secretary, executive council, National Dental Association, September 9,1908. Letter. No. 106047.

143. National Archives and Records Administration. Record Group 112. Unidentified contract dental surgeon, September 21, 1908. No. 106047.

144. National Archives and Records Administration. Record Group 112. Unidentified contract dental surgeons, September 8, 14, October 20, 1908. Letters. No. 106047.

145. National Archives and Records Administration. Record Group 112. Donnally to O'Reilly, November 26, 1908. Letter. No. 106047.

146. National Archives and Records Administration. Record Group 112. O'Reilly to Donnally, December 16, 1908. Letter. No. 106047.

147. Sorber OM. The hindrances to effective dental service in the U.S. Army. *The Frater*. 1908. Quoted in: National Archives and Records Administration. National Record Group 94. Dr John D Millikin, Division Hospital, Manila, Philippine Islands, January 22, 1910. Letter. No. 524625. Box 3645. Entry 25.

148. National Archives and Records Administration. Record Group 94. Major General Weston to Major General Ainsworth, November 11, 1908. Letter. No. 524625. Box 3645. Entry 25.

149. National Archives and Records Administration. Record Group 112. Surgeon General O'Reilly to chief of staff, December 16, 1908. Memorandum. No. 106047.

150. National Archives and Records Administration. Record Group 165. Memorandum for the surgeon general, Major General J Franklin Bell, chief of staff, 24 November 1908. General staff report. No. 2222. Box 20. Entry 5.

151. National Archives and Records Administration. Memorandum for the second section, Major General JF Bell, chief of staff, December 22, 1908. General staff report no. 2222.

Chapter X

AN ARMY DENTAL CORPS AT LAST, 1909–1911

Introduction

When Brigadier General Robert O'Reilly retired from the Army on January 14, 1909, the dental surgeons and American dental community were no nearer their cherished goal of a commissioned dental corps than they had been in 1901. The new Army surgeon general, Brigadier General George Torney (1850–1913), benefited significantly from his predecessor's success with the Medical Department reorganization of the previous April and was free to focus on other pressing matters. Torney was also familiar with John Marshall and dental issues from his years as commander of the Presidio General Hospital (1904–1908) where Marshall practiced from September 1901 until March 1908, when he was transferred to the Philippines. However, the question was whether Torney would bring any change to the positions of the War Department and surgeon general's office toward the issue of commissioned status for the Army's contract dental surgeons.

Surgeon General Torney and Dental Legislation

On January 29, 1909, Torney had barely taken his chair as the new Army surgeon general when Representative John AT Hull, chairman of the House Committee on Military Affairs, sent him a copy of Bulkeley's bill (S 4432) and requested his views "as to the advisability of the proposed legislation" and for any suggested amendments.[1] After speaking with the secretary of war and reviewing O'Reilly's files on the bill, Torney wrote back on the 30th. He said O'Reilly's response of April 1, 1908, was appropriate, except that O'Reilly had "underestimated the item of expense." Torney explained:

> On Monday morning one of the best dental surgeons in the Army was in my office, and in a conversation he informed me that if a dental corps is ever organized on a proper basis to provide dental treatment for the Army as medical treatment is now provided, it will take a corps of at least 150 officers. I believe this statement is in no way an exaggeration and, in my opinion, the present bill to organize a commissioned dental corps of 50 officers is merely a stepping stone to that end. As you know, the Army is scattered throughout a great many posts, and for this reason a dental surgeon in the Army cannot treat as large a population as a dentist in civil life. If this estimate is not an exaggeration, and I do not believe it is, the cost of a dental corps large enough to satisfy the needs of the Army will be very much greater than was indicated in General O'Reilly's endorsement, dated April 1, 1908.[2]

Noting that the Army's current annual cost for the dental surgeons was $57,960, Torney enclosed two memoranda laying out the estimated annual costs for 50 dental surgeons and all of their associated support ($367,960), and 150 dental surgeons ($1,940,440). He concluded that "it rests with the gentlemen in Congress, who must provide the means for maintaining this Army, to decide whether it is practicable at this time to provide a commissioned dental corps."[2]

On February 18 Torney's January 30 letter to Hull sparked a major response from Dr Emory Bryant, former member of the National Dental Association (NDA) committee and President Theodore Roosevelt's personal dentist who had been discussing the dental bill intermittently with Chief of Staff Major General J Franklin Bell. Bryant's letter, however, did not go to the surgeon general or War Department, but rather directly to the president, who was then in the final month of his second term. Bryant attacked Torney's letter as "an erroneous understanding of the situation." He questioned the calculations of annual costs arrived at by Lieutenant Colonel (later Brigadier General) Jefferson Randolph Kean (1860–1950), the architect of O'Reilly Medical Department reorganization bills from 1903 to 1906. Kean had recently returned from the Army of Cuban Pacification to join Torney's staff as the chief of the sanitation division. Bryant contended that the number of dentists necessary would be 45, as in House Report No. 3642, or one per 1,000 officers and enlisted soldiers, as in the Senate version.[3] He wrote:

> I submit also, that the Army dentist can handle more patients than can the private dentists, all requiring services being at all times within call, while the private dental patients are scattered over a whole city or county: Therefore the idea that a Corps of 150 men will be required to give adequate service to the Army is based upon an assumption which is not justified by the facts, or conditions.[3]

Bryant turned briefly to the legislative background of the current bill before continuing his attack:

> It has had the support of the Surgeon-Generals of the Army from Sternberg up to the present incumbent, except that O'Reilly rearranged his ideas to some extent in the last year of his service AFTER the Medical Reorganization Bill was safely lodged in the Statutes beyond opposition. It can be safely asserted that the main opposition to this Bill giving the dental profession a recognized and dignified standing in the Army service is from the same Medical Officers that for years fought the Line Officers for proper recognition (Rank) and by every means possible impressed Congress and the Department that their contentions would benefit the service and obtain better men for their Corps, and we now find them persuing [sic] the same tactics they were loud in condemning when practiced against them. . . . I call your attention to the fact that it required a special message of your own as additional support to pass their reorganization Bill even as near as the present Congress. Under the circumstances the profession of dentistry feels it is not an imposition to ask for similar recognition by yourself, and only come to you when in the last extremity and urgency the situation demands.[3]

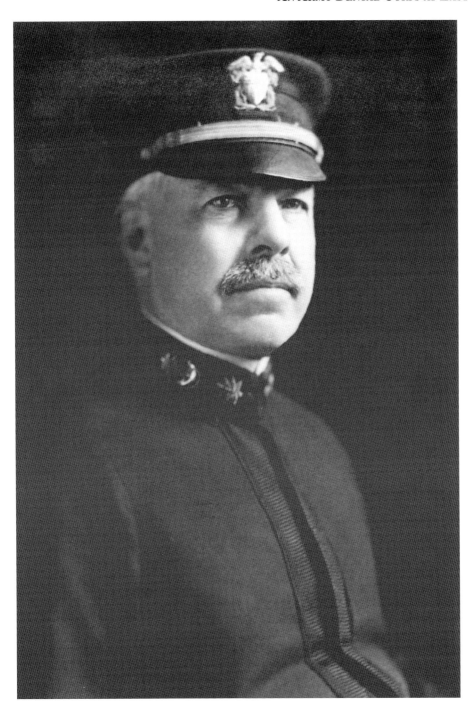

*Emory A Bryant, President Theodore Roosevelt's personal dentist,
during his World War I service in the US Navy Dental Corps.
Photograph: Courtesy of the American Dental Association.*

On February 21, 1909, Roosevelt endorsed the dental bill in a note to Representative Adin Capron of Rhode Island: "Can we not help along the army dental surgeon's bill? It seems to me to be an excellent measure and one that ought to be passed."[4,5] In the long run, little came from the president's support, but Kean now came to play a major role in the evolving struggle for a dental corps.

Lieutenant Colonel Jefferson Randolph Kean's Memorandum

Bryant's letter brought Lieutenant Colonel Jefferson Randolph Kean into play as Torney's lead staff officer working on the issue of commissioning dental surgeons. On March 23, 1909, Kean prepared a "Memorandum for the Surgeon General," subtitled "Being a study of the necessity for legislation conferring military rank on dental surgeons." Having served as the executive officer and a key assistant under O'Reilly from 1902 to 1906, Kean was familiar with the issues and how to get things done in the War Department, executive branch, and Congress. In putting together his memorandum, Kean drew heavily on John Marshall's numerous letters and memoranda to O'Reilly. The most important of these was Marshall's memorandum of December 16, 1904, which Kean believed contained "all the substantial arguments which have been advanced in the extensive correspondence on file in this office."[6,7]

Writing to the recently retired O'Reilly on March 25, 2 days after he gave Torney his memorandum, Kean noted:

> I have been amusing myself lately with the reading over of the entire literature on file in the office about dentists, and the preparation of an elaborate memorandum on the subject. I have gone into everything, even the study of the effect of the activities of the dental fraternity on the occurrences of the diseases of the digestive system by a comparison before and after their employment.[8]

Kean laid out Marshall's arguments (see Chapter 9, "Marshall's Draft Bill of December 1904") and analyzed them. He concluded: "That a commission is desirable cannot be disputed, but that it is essential to the dental surgeon for the proper performance of his work has not been demonstrated either by experience or by the great mass of argument on file in this office."[7] He then compared the "professional and administrative responsibilities of dental surgeons with those of medical officers," and the comparison did not favor the dentists.[7] In a single paragraph, Kean summarized the real reasons that the leadership of the Medical Department opposed granting commissions to dental surgeons, and they were dependant upon the deep-seated professional rivalry between dentists and physicians and the desire of the Medical Corps to retain complete control in the Medical Department:

> It seems evident, therefore, that the reasons why commissioned rank in its several grades is necessary for the administration of the great and complex organization of the medical service do not apply to dental surgeons, and that commissioned rank is not, therefore, *essential* to the performance of their duties. Still less reason is there for the possession of higher grades, since the dental service of the Army is without either complexity of organization or serious administrative responsibilities. An additional reason why any grade above that of First Lieutenant should not be given is that it

would place the dental surgeons above the officers of the Medical Reserve Corps, with the result that the latter would become discontented and the medical service at posts where they were stationed would be disturbed. It is feared also that the elevation in rank of dental surgeons above Reserve Medical Corps might not meet the approval of many distinguished physicians who have entered the Corps and to whose sympathetic interest and assistance the Surgeon General looks to secure well qualified men for the vacancies in the Medical Corps. The cheapening in any way of these commissions which have been accepted by many of the leaders of the medical profession in the United States would be a grave misfortune for the service. While these reasons militate against the conferring of dental surgeons of any higher grade than First Lieutenant, they do not prevent the giving of that grade, with the provision that dental surgeons shall rank next after all other officers of that grade [emphasis in original].[7(pp13–14)]

In his March 25 letter to O'Reilly, Kean explained the leadership's plan:

I have prepared a Bill which requires them to come in and serve the probationary period of at least three years under contract, and then authorizes a commission as first lieutenant after the [Medical] reserve corps. Nothing higher is to be given them, and I think it is pretty clear that we should fight to the last ditch on this proposition. The Navy has also conceded this much and we will work together to hold them down to it. It is much easier to kill legislation than it is to put it together, and I think we can choke them off from anything more if we keep our eyes open.[8]

To his memo, Kean attached the draft of an act, "To Improve the Status and Efficiency of the Dental Surgeons in the U.S. Army," that encapsulated these ideas and formed the basis for Torney's subsequent recommendations to the chief of staff in November.[7,9]

At the annual meeting of the NDA on April 1, 1909, in Birmingham, Alabama, the executive council's report thanked Doctors Donnally and Bryant for the help they gave the legislative committee during the past year. Furthermore, the council successfully proposed that it be the sole voice of the association and the profession when it came to issues of dental legislation for the Army.[10]

On April 9, 1909, Senator Bulkeley introduced a new bill (S 1530) to the 61st Congress, First Session, worded precisely as his earlier effort "to reorganize the corps of dental surgeons attached to the Medical Department of the Army," which was subsequently referred to the Committee on Military Affairs.[11,12] On July 5, 1909, Representative William Wiley (1842–1925) of New Jersey, a Civil War brevet major, introduced an identical bill (HR 11192) in the House.[11,13]

The Bulkeley and Wiley bills provided an opening for Torney to submit his own approach to organizing the Army's dental surgeons, which he had coordinated with the NDA.[5,9] On November 26, 1909, Torney submitted Kean's March draft bill to the Army adjutant general. The bill read:

Sec. 1. That, for the purpose of securing an efficient dental service in the army there shall be attached to the Medical Department a dental corps which shall be composed of dental surgeons and acting dental surgeons, the total number of which shall not exceed the proportion of one to each thousand of actual enlisted strength of the army: that the number of dental surgeons shall not exceed sixty, and the number of acting dental surgeons shall be such as may, from time to time, be authorized by law in accordance with the needs of the service.

Sec. 2. That all original appointments to the dental corps shall be as acting dental surgeons who shall have the same official status, pay and allowances as the contract dental surgeons now authorized by law.

Sec. 3. Acting dental surgeons who have served three years in a manner satisfactory to the Surgeon General of the Army shall be eligible for appointment as dental surgeons and after passing, in a satisfactory manner, an examination which may be prescribed by the Surgeon General, may be commissioned with the rank of first lieutenant in the dental corps to fill the vacancies existing therein. Officers of the dental corps shall have rank in such corps according to date of their commissions therein and shall rank next below officers of the medical reserve corps. Their right to command shall be limited to the dental corps and they shall be entitled to the respect and obedience of all enlisted men.

Sec. 4. That the pay and allowances of dental surgeons shall be those of first lieutenants not mounted, including the right to retirement on account of age of disability, as in the case of other officers: PROVIDED, That the time served by dental surgeons as acting dental or contract dental surgeons shall be reckoned in computing the increased service pay of such as are commissioned under this Act.

Sec. 5. That the appointees as acting dental surgeons must be citizens of the United States between twenty-two and thirty years of age, graduates of a standard dental college, of good moral character and good professional education, and they shall be required to pass the usual physical examination required for appointment in the medical corps and a professional examination which shall include tests of skill in practical dentistry and of proficiency in the usual subjects of a standard dental college course:

PROVIDED, That the dental surgeons attached to the medical department at the time of the passage of this Act may be eligible for appointment as first lieutenants, dental corps, without limitation as to age, and

PROVIDED FURTHER, That the professional examination for such appointment may be waived in the case of dental surgeons in the service at the time of the passage of this Act whose efficiency reports and entrance examinations are satisfactory to the Surgeon General.

Sec. 6. That the Surgeon General of the Army is authorized to appoint Boards of Examiners to conduct the examinations herein prescribed, one of whom shall be a surgeon in the army and two of whom shall be selected by the Surgeon General from the commissioned dental surgeons in the corps.[9]

In significant contrast to O'Reilly's last stated position, Torney accepted a commissioned dental corps, but only of first lieutenants. Moreover, a close reading of Torney's proposal reveals that, except for critical graded rank promotions, it gave the dental surgeons and the NDA most of what they had been seeking for years, including commissioned status, seniority for previous contract status, protection to those already in service, a military examining board, and a ratio of one to 1,000 enlisted troops, not to exceed 60.[9]

Several factors seem to have influenced Kean and Torney to reverse course so radically. In the four recent congresses, the House and Senate had repeatedly passed various dental bills but had never agreed on any one bill. Kean and Torney may have reasoned it was time to make the best possible deal rather than risk accepting provisions of rank that they did not want. Preventing dental surgeons from receiving rank higher than first lieutenant would limit problems among the new officers of the Medical Reserve Corps, who might have had personal and professional difficulty serving under a dentist. Above all, Kean and Torney were apparently trying to preserve the gains of the April 23, 1908, bill.

The day before Torney sent his memorandum to the chief of staff, Emory Bryant, representing the NDA, wrote to President Taft about the need for the War Department to support a dental corps bill. He endorsed Torney's current initiative, saying:

> The present Surgeon-General of the Army has drafted a Bill for a Commissioned Dental Corps, in which he grants every feature of the S.4432 heretofore referred to, with the exception of "graded rank promotion," making all commissioned as First Lieutenants unmounted, instead of grading from 1st Lieut. to Majors, as provided in S. 4432. . . . I have the honor to say that the terms of the draft of a Bill by the Surgeon General of the Army meets with the approval of the dental profession as a MINIMUM measure which it can consistently approve in justice to all concerned in consideration of the fact that all of the claims made by the profession of dentistry to recognition by our government has been approved by the Medical Department to which the Corps (Dental) will be attached.[5]

Bryant went on to ask President Taft for his personal involvement to push the bills through the War Department and Congress:

> The War Department is a large machine with complicated parts, and each part must fit perfectly to run smoothly. The dental corps is but one of the small "cogs" that go to make the complete machine, but it is out of place, as was the Contract Medical Corps. It required the aid of President Roosevelt to pass the Medical Bill, cannot the Dental Profession be equally fortunate in obtaining the aid of President Taft? We ask nothing more than the merits of the case demand and what has been acknowledged as our due, the only question involved is the manner and means of obtaining proper action. . . . Can you not give the matter your personal encouragement?[5]

On December 11, 1909, Torney recommended to the secretary of war that his proposed bill, if approved by the general staff, be endorsed by the War Department as a substitute for S 1530, which he believed "would be satisfactory to all parties concerned." The NDA concurred with this proposed change. On January 25, 1910, the general staff completed its study of S 1530 and recommended against its passage because the creation of a corps of dental surgeons was seen as "as a luxury rather than a necessity." Overall military policy was a more important issue at the time, and it had "become imperative to consider the needs of the Army as a whole before a further increase is authorized for any single arm, corps, or department." On January 31, 1910, the chief of staff, following the general staff's advice, recommended against passing S 1530.[14,15]

On January 31, 1910, Dr Emory Bryant appealed to Secretary of War Dickinson to pass the Dental Corps legislation. He was informed on February 23 that President Taft's demands for economy in the military meant the authorized strength of the Army for the next fiscal year was to be reduced by nearly 8,000. In this situation, the passage of any legislation that added a new corps of approximately 80 commissioned officers to the Army was not likely. Therefore, the War Department did not recommend passing S 1530 (and its identical bill, HR 11192).[16,17]

On February 10, 1910, Chief of Staff J Franklin Bell again reversed course, outlining the basic arguments for keeping contract dental surgeons rather than creating a corps of commissioned dental surgeons:

> The contract dental surgeons of the Army, employed under existing laws, are rendering satisfactory service to the Army, and the surgeons employed seem to be so well satisfied that so far no inconvenience has resulted to the service from their leaving the government employment; consequently there appears to be no urgent need at this time of creating a change in their status. Under existing law, the Army gets young, active dental surgeons, whose skill and knowledge are tested before their employment by a thorough examination. Should they demonstrate their unfitness, lack of skill, or become in any way undesirable, the War Department can discharge them and get others, for not only is the dental corps full, but many applications are on file for appointment to any vacancies which may occur.
>
> For these two reasons, i.e., that it is inopportune at this time to advocate an increase in the cost of the military establishment by the creation of a permanent commissioned Corps of Dental Surgeons, and that the operation of existing laws relating to dental surgeons in the Army is satisfactory to the War Department, it is thought that no bill having for its object the creation of a permanent Corps of Dental Surgeons in the Army should be recommended at this time for passage by Congress.
>
> There was a time when the attitude of the Surgeon-General toward the aspirations of dental surgeons, and when arguments by the Medical Department, were of such a character as to cause me to consider both attitude and arguments illiberal, and that the dental surgeons were in need of a friend at court and were deserving of sympathy and relief. I even thought they were entitled to more rank than they had expressed a willingness to accept and the Medical Department was ready to concede. I so informed Doctor Bryant.
>
> Since receiving orders from the Secretary of War, however, to submit this question to the General Staff for report, and since conference with the General Staff and listening to presentations of the other side of the question, I have concluded that my first impressions were incorrect, that the Medical Department was justified in most of its views, and that the General Staff is also justified in opposing this bill.[18]

On February 12, 1910, Surgeon General Torney sent a memorandum to the secretary of war advising him that HR 11192 was unacceptable to the War Department. Torney resubmitted his November 26, 1909, substitution as a counter proposal and recommended the secretary of war to advise the House Military Affairs Committee.[19,20]

Dental Treatment for Enlisted Soldiers and Dependents

The temporary nature of dental work and its limited applicability to conditions other than line-of-duty trauma remained a major issue within the Army. In March 1909, a request for special dental work for a member of the 6th Cavalry regimental band was refused. It was recommended that the soldier have the work done using the free materials the Medical Department furnished.[21]

On April 13, 1909, Dr John Millikin, contract dental surgeon, US Army, stationed in Manila, requested that he be allowed to work on dependents during regular hours (9 AM to 4 PM) using government materials. He also submitted a fee schedule for this work in order to "eliminate any possible complaint as to his right to charge." Millikin contended that after working from 9 AM to 4 PM, he did not feel that it was fair that he should be obliged to work on officers' families using his own dental materials and not be allowed to charge for this extra work. The fee schedule he submitted was considered reasonable and more affordable than the charges in civilian practice, and it accounted for the fact that the government provided the office and equipment.[22]

The chief surgeon of the Philippines Division, however, thought that changes were necessary in the regulations on dental care in his department. The surgeon general agreed but stated that the regulations did not forbid an officer or civilian employee from performing "outside work for which he receives compensation," as long as it did not interfere with his military duties. Therefore, no changes were necessary in the regulations.[22]

Regardless of where the dental surgeons served, the work loads remained enormous. A great source of continuing frustration was the lack of command emphasis on oral hygiene, assuring that many patients regressed after they were brought up to acceptable standards. Part of the problem lay in the time lost as a result of itinerancy. Criticized for his lack of productivity, Dr RM Hollingsworth pointed out that he had taken 2 days leave between 1907 and 1910 and had changed work locations 20 times in 30 months. He estimated he lost a week each time he had to relocate and set up his equipment, all of it time away from treating patients.[23]

In October 1910 Captain CF Morse, surgeon, 5th Cavalry at Schofield Barracks, Hawaii, submitted his criticism of the effect of itinerancy. He praised the work of George Graham, who had come on temporary duty from California, but pointed out that his schedule precluded sufficient treatment time. The deplorable condition of the men's mouths mandated more intensive treatment almost as a matter of accord. Forty or fifty soldiers with less than 18 months' service examined at random were found in need of serious emergency care with intensive follow up. Yet Graham was never at any site longer than a month as he made his rounds. Further compounding the delays was the fact that he was not authorized to bring a trained enlisted dental assistant from California, which meant that he had to train a new helper from the Hospital Corps at each work site. Captain Morse suggested more dentists be authorized and that permanent dental clinics be established wherever sufficient numbers of troops were concentrated. Both Morse and Graham urged greater command emphasis on dental hygiene.[24,25]

"Neither Fish, Flesh, nor Fowl": John Marshall and John Millikin
on the Status of Contract Dental Surgeons

In January 1910 Dr John Millikin, a contract dental surgeon since 1901 and stationed at the Division Hospital, Manila, expressed his views on the proposed reorganization of the Dental Corps. He reminded the adjutant general (through military channels) that 14 dental surgeons had left the service since 1904, nearly half the strength. Three (Bacon, Fisher, and Updyke) left during their original 3-year contract; seven (Decker, Foster, Rietz, Stone, Sorber, Rion, and Foster) left during their second contract (after six years' service); and four (Craig, Hussey, Waddell, and Ware) had left during 1909 alone. Lack of a pay increase, retirement for disability, and promotion had caused them to become discouraged over their futures. A return to civilian practice was the end result. Their replacements could be placed in three categories: recent graduates looking for experience, civilian dentists who were failures in private practice, and dentists lacking the finances to establish civilian practices. None of the above could replace the experienced dental surgeons who were lost.[26]

On January 31 John Marshall, now the chief of the dental service at the Division Hospital in Manila, endorsed Millikin's letter as follows:

> The present status of the dental surgeon is an anomalous one. He is an integral part of the Army, has to perform all the duties of a commissioned officer except sit on Courts Martial and make contracts for the Government, has to wear a prescribed uniform and conform in every respect to Army Regulations and yet by a decision of the U.S. Comptroller and of the Judge Advocate General he is not an officer but a civilian employee. In the words of President Taft applied to Contract Surgeons, "he is neither Fish, flesh, nor fowl" a sort of "Mex Officer."
>
> This status works to the great disadvantage of good discipline and often submits the dental surgeon to covert slights and sometimes to a thinly veiled insult. The dental surgeon if of real value to the Army should have a status equal to that of the other professions represented in the Army; viz, Divinity, Law, and Medicine. The dental surgeons of the U.S. Army all hold a well earned degree from recognized Universities. They are professional gentlemen and should be accorded a status commensurate with the dignity of a learned profession.
>
> The Army is entitled to the best dental service, but this cannot be longer secured under the present humiliating status. There is no inducement whatever for high class young men to enter the service. With a chance for advancement, increased pay, longevity pay, and retirement for disability and age, there would be no difficulty in securing the very best young men for the service. Military title could be waived and in its place establish three grades of status. Assistant dental surgeon, past assistant dental surgeon, and dental Surgeon with the pay and allowances of first lieutenant, Captain, and Major of the Medical Corps with promotion by seniority after examination. Many of the very best men of the Corps have asked for annulment of contract because they could not afford to give the best years of their lives to a service that made no provision for the future in case of disability or advanced age.[27]

On February 3 Lieutenant Colonel Charles Richard, the Manila Hospital commander, endorsed the correspondence, noting that: "The status of the contract dental surgeon is not satisfactory, and legislation necessary to remedy it would seem desirable." The division surgeon and Major General William Duvall, the commanding officer of the Philippines Division, added their favorable comments and sent the package to the adjutant general, who forwarded it to the surgeon general for comment. Torney replied on March 28 that his November 26, 1909, memorandum and draft bill "if enacted into law, would meet many of the points set forth in the enclosed communication."[28–31] Finally on May 5, 1910, the adjutant general notified Millikin that the War Department was currently considering the question of "a military policy" for the United States. The organization of the whole Army was to be worked out, and dental surgeons would "be considered" in these discussions. For this reason, no recommendation for dental legislation could be made at this time.[32]

Despite all the setbacks, a small palliative had been granted earlier on January 31, 1910, when the War Department issued Circular No. 3, which officially designated, "for the sake of brevity," Army dentists as "dental surgeons and not as contract dental surgeons."[33,34] Little real progress seemed to have been made in creating a proper dental corps and improving the status of the Army's dental surgeons.

The New Wiley Dental Bill: HR 23097

On March 16, 1910, Representative William Wiley renewed his efforts to change the military status of Army dentists by introducing another bill (HR 23097), which was actually Torney's draft bill of November 26, 1909, that had apparently reached Wiley via the NDA.[35,36] The bill was much more specific than the one he had previously submitted in conjunction with Senator Bulkeley. In his new bill, he proposed the appointment of dental surgeons and acting dental surgeons. Dentists would be authorized on the basis of one per 1,000 soldiers, but no more than 60 dental surgeons would be allowed. There could be as many acting dental surgeons as Army strength mandated. New entrants would be appointed acting dental surgeons at first with the same pay and status of the current contract dental surgeons. After 3 years' satisfactory performance, they could be commissioned first lieutenants eligible for retirement and disability pensions if vacancies existed. The dentists currently under contract would be eligible for immediate commissions, regardless of age, and their contracted time would be credited for longevity and pay. All new appointees would have to be between ages 22 and 30. They would have to pass physical and professional examinations conducted by a board appointed by the surgeon general and composed of one Army surgeon and two of the newly commissioned dentists. By adopting a compromise that the surgeon general and NDA had already worked out, Wiley's bill attempted to address the objections that had killed earlier legislative attempts.[35,37,38]

Indeed, a general staff paper of May 5, 1910, provided a glimpse of the actions over the recent past that led to the Wiley bill:

> The creation of a corps of Dental Surgeons is a matter which has been before the War Department for a number of years. The Dental Surgeons in the Army have been actively interested in this matter as is also the National Dental Association. There has been a considerable amount of correspondence between the War Department and Dr. Emory A. Bryant of the legislative committee of the latter association. . . . Bills have been

introduced in the 58th, 59th, 60th and 61st Congresses. There bills have differed in character and scope, but all contained some provision for giving Dental Surgeons commissioned rank. The Surgeon General, the Chief of Staff, and other officers of the War Department have from time to time made recommendations in favor of these bills, but no Secretary of War has recommended any of them. The last action taken by the War Department in this matter was in the latter part of February, 1910, when the Secretary of War, Mr. Dickinson, returned to the Chairman of the committees on Military Affairs of the House and Senate, respectively, bills introduced in the House by Mr. Wiley and in the Senate by Mr. Bulkley [sic], recommending "that this bill do not receive favorable consideration at the present session." The two bills referred to were in fact the same bill. The bill did not originate in the War Department and contained many features that were objected to by the Surgeon General and by the General Staff. A substitute bill was submitted to the Secretary of War by the Surgeon General [the November 26, 1909, draft bill], and it is understood a copy of this bill was furnished by the Surgeon General to the National Dental Association. It was introduced in the House on March 16th by Representative Wiley and has been referred to the War Department for recommendation.[36]

The General Staff's Position

On April 23, 1910, the general staff summed up the War Department's position on the proposed reorganization of the dental surgeons with commissioned rank. It referred to its memoranda of January 25 and February 10, 1910, which stated that the present time was not appropriate for legislation regarding rank for dental surgeons because of a continuing study it was making on the organization of the Army as a whole. Changing the status of a particular Army element should be deferred until completion of the study.[39]

On May 2, 1910, Brigadier General (later General and Chief of Staff, 1917–1918) Tasker Bliss (1853–1930), the acting chief of staff, informed the surgeon general that the secretary of war desired his opinion "as to whether you do or do not consider the maintenance of the present contract system for the employment of dental surgeons in the Army to be the best for the general interests of the service."[40] The same day, Surgeon General Torney replied:

> It is my belief that the contract system for Dental Surgeons, while it works fairly well, does not secure as good a class of dentists as might be secured if the candidates were given the prospect of a commission with the rank of 1st Lieutenant and the increase of pay for length of service provided by the Bill proposed by this office in November last which was submitted after very careful consideration of all the questions and interests involved. I, therefore, do not consider the maintenance of the present contract dental system to be the best for the general interest of the service.[41]

On May 4, 1910, the secretary of war (1909–1911), Jacob Dickinson, disregarded Torney's comments and informed Representative Wiley that he had returned his bill to the Military Affairs Committee with the recommendation that it not be approved. However, he left the door open for future legislation by saying, "My action at this time is without prejudice to the consideration of a suitable measure which may be proposed for a subsequent session."[42]

On May 5, 1910, Bliss sent Secretary Dickinson a memorandum that laid out the general staff's thoughts about what was best for the Army and also evaluated the Wiley bill. The general staff's position on commissioning dental surgeons was consistently negative over the years since 1903, and Bliss's memorandum strongly retained that position. Bliss noted that the NDA "claims that its purpose in advocating the commissioning of Dental Surgeons is to give prestige to the dental profession by recognizing Dental Surgeons as commissioned officers."[36] He disregarded this view, saying:

> It is possible that in giving commissioned rank to the representatives in the Army of other professions than the purely military one Congress may have given prestige to those professions. It is possible that this may have been done solely (as now desired by the Dental Association) for the purpose of giving added prestige and not with a single view to economy and efficiency of administration. If this be true, Congress must be the final judge as to its propriety. The only questions for present consideration are whether the bill will accomplish the avowed purpose and whether, if it does, the results will be for the best interests of all concerned.

> Assuming, however, that these titles give the desired prestige, it is obvious that the proposed law will accomplish nothing towards this end. It is proposed to give them, after three years' service, the grade of first lieutenant, and then forever to keep them below every other first lieutenant in the Army. Men who would accept such a proposition, or be willing to retain such a status very long, will need a great deal of arbitrarily conferred prestige, but manifestly they must seek it elsewhere than in this line. . . . It must appear so obvious to Congress that it is not intended to retain such a bob-tailed organization very long that it would seem almost trifling in the part of the War Department to recommend it. If the dental profession is to be assimilated to the medical profession, and if the hierarchy of military grades and rank and title is necessary for prestige of both of them, they should have the same organization, with a proportional number of the various grades.[36(p3)]

As to whether the proposed law was in the best interests of the Army, Bliss concluded that "it is plainly to the advantage of the government to follow the contract system as far as practicable."

> The only excuse for a permanent corps of medical officers is the fact that they sustain the closest relations with the troops in garrison and in the field and require many qualifications for military service which cannot be attained by practice in civil life. Even then, the contract system has been followed successfully for the lower grade officers in that department. . . . On the other hand, dentists require no qualification that they do not bring with them from civil life. The fresher from civil life and the dental college the better they are for our service.[36(p4)]

Bliss laid out a scenario in which the Army used contract dental surgeons who then returned to civil practice once they put aside sufficient funds. He reasoned:

> If the Army and Navy provided two or three hundred such places, to be occupied for a contract term of four years and thereafter at the same interval to be filled by new classes, it would be a boon to the profession. . . . The foregoing leads to the final and most important conclusion that the contract system for dental surgeons is the best for the military service. Under this system we got, or can get, the brightest young men

fresh from the best dental colleges, where they have learned the latest mechanical applications in a mechanical art. In the Army they have abundant practice of somewhat limited scope. But the Government does not, nor can it, probably, permit work of the more expensive and delicate kind that is common in civil life. There comes a time, therefore, when the professional qualifications of an army dentist are bound to deteriorate, to the disadvantage of his work, even of the more ordinary kind. The proposed bill, encouraging permanency in this position, deliberately contemplates bringing about this result.[36(p5)]

Bliss advised the secretary that the maintenance of the existing contract system was, "in the long run, the best for the dental surgeons, the best for the dental profession at large, and the best for the military service."[36] With the general staff unequivocal in its negativity toward a commissioned dental corps, it is not difficult to understand why Secretary Dickinson adopted a like posture on the Wiley bill.

The Dental Press's Position

In the May 1910 edition of *Items of Interest*, Dr Rodrigues Ottolengui reprinted Wiley's bill, along with Torney's November 26, 1909, memorandum to the chief of staff, in its entirety. His extensive, 6-page editorial, titled "The New Army Dental Corps Bill and the Surgeon-General's Opinion Thereon," pointed out that the Wiley bill, unlike its predecessors, had been drawn up with the guidance of the Army Medical Department and not solely by a committee of the NDA. He also referred to the fact that at the national meeting in Boston, the executive council of the NDA had scoffed at the idea that the Medical Department would ever present a bill for commissioning the dental surgeons or agree to the commissioning of the overage contract dental surgeons.[43–45]

At the same Boston meeting, it was argued that a provision of this kind would not be opposed by the department, and it was pointed out that an exactly similar clause appeared in the Medical Reorganization Bill passed by the last Congress. In spite of this argument, the contention was met with sneers and ridicule, and it was intimated to the executive council, in the presence of a large audience, that such notions resulted from utter ignorance of matters legislative and military.[43] Ottolengui concluded:

> Now that a bill, indorsed [sic] by the Medical Department of the Army, provides for the appointment of members of the preset dental corps, without limitations as to age, the dental profession may draw its own conclusions as to whether the opposite, and constantly iterated contentions of former National Dental Association Committees, have been based on ignorance, incompetency or some other cause.[43]

Dr Wilbur Litch, the editor of *Dental Brief*, recommended in his May 1910 issue that the dental profession urge their congressmen to vote for the bill, but noted that the bill did not provide for promotion beyond the grade of first lieutenant. This rank put the dental officer at a disadvantage compared with the medical officer. However, the bill would secure commissioned status, a "great gain for dentistry as a profession."[46]

In December 1910 Dr Ottolengui pointed out that the bill provided dentistry with a rank five grades lower than that of the physicians, lawyers, bankers, businessmen, teachers, and clergymen. The 170 first lieutenants in the Medical Reserve Corps even outranked the dentists.[47]

In 1911 Senator Henry Cabot Lodge of Massachusetts wrote Dr Emory Bryant of Washington, DC, saying that the main reason for the dental bill's failure in previous congressional sessions was not because of congressional "hostility to the measure," but because the individuals pressing its passage insisted that the dental examining board be controlled by civilians. Even to "friends" of the bill like himself, this was unacceptable. The service must control Dental Corps candidate selection. Also, Congress would reject any insistence on rank as high as captain and major.[48]

The 1911 Bulkeley Dental Bill: S 1530

On February 7, 1911, at the 61st Congress, Third Session, Senator Bulkeley of Connecticut, seeing a favorable opportunity, introduced his former bill (S 1530) as an amendment to the Army appropriation bill (HR 31237), which had already passed the House and was under consideration in the Senate. The bill "to reorganize the corps of dental surgeons attached to the Medical Department of the Army," gave commissioned status and graded ranks to the dental surgeons. In doing this, he was adding to the Army bill (HR 31237) a verbatim version of his earlier bill from the session before. It differed from Wiley's bill notably in providing for the promotion of some dentists to rank as high as major. It also failed to provide for any temporary strength increases via acting dental surgeons, as did Wiley's. The amendment was agreed to and referred to the Senate Committee on Military Affairs.[49]

The same dental bill had passed the Senate twice before and had been favorably reported in the House. It had the endorsement of the Army dental surgeons and the dental profession but not of the War Department, without which it had little chance of passing. The Army appropriation bill (HR 31237) was referred to the Conference Committee of the House and Senate.[49,50]

On February 8, 1911, Lieutenant Colonel JR Kean personally handed a memorandum from Surgeon General Torney to Major General Leonard Wood, now the chief of staff. In it, Torney endorsed the Wiley bill because contained these features:

(1) At least sixty dental surgeons: "this number is necessary to give each soldier one treatment a year."

(2) Officer status for dental surgeons: "since this is necessary to the self-respect and proper standing of professional men."

(3) Dental surgeons to rank below the officers of the Medical Reserve Corps: "because to give higher rank would cause discontent to the many distinguished physicians in civil life now commissioned in the Reserve Corps. Higher rank is not necessary since Dentists have no administrative responsibility, and command of men is not necessary."

could have been desired.[55,56]

The Act of March 3, 1911, not only created a commissioned dental corps but had a major impact on the status of dentistry as a profession. Before the enactment of the new act, the words "dentistry," "dental profession," and "dental surgeon" had no significance or recognition under the law. Now the United States government was committed to the "official recognition" of dentistry as a profession.[57]

The bill created a dental corps with a strength based on the ratio of one dentist for every 1,000 enlisted military personnel, a goal sought in the original dental bills of 1898 to 1900. In 1911, that came to about 95 dentists. After 3 years of service or appropriate waivers and exemptions, up to 60 of these dentists could be commissioned as first lieutenants, while the remainder would be acting dental surgeons. Those commissioned were entitled to all the pay and allowances of other officers in the same grade, although dentists ranked below all other officers in similar grade.[58] They still ranked below officers of the Medical Reserve Corps, who ranked below all first lieutenants in the Army. This meant that, among other things, a dental surgeon with many years' service could be "ranked out" of his quarters by a newly promoted first lieutenant or a newly appointed Medical Reserve Corps officer, even one on temporary duty for a few days or weeks. Also, with no promotion beyond first lieutenant, the maximum pay for a dental surgeon after 20 years would be $2,800, while a physician appointed as a first lieutenant was promoted to captain after 3 years' service, and then through the grades of major, lieutenant colonel, and finally colonel. His promotions were based on seniority.[59]

The status of the acting dental surgeon was difficult to define. Like contract status, it was of a "quasi-military" nature. Acting dental surgeons were civilians that wore the Army uniform without the shoulder straps. Enlisted soldiers were expected to give them the same courtesies and respect they gave to all officers, and they had all the allowances except disability retirement. After 3 years, if their services were satisfactory, they were eligible to take the examination for dental surgeon. If successful, they could be commissioned as first lieutenants in the Dental Corps if there was a vacancy.[60]

On May 10, 1911, Surgeon General Torney forwarded the list of 30 contract dental surgeons to be appointed first lieutenants in accordance with the Act of March 3 to the adjutant general. He certified that all had been examined except John Marshall, who would be retiring, and recommended that their relative rank in the Dental Corps be fixed according to the order of the date of their original contracts. This request spurred another round of exchanges between the adjutant general and judge advocate general on whether the new officers were to be commissioned as "First Lieutenant, Dental Corps" or "Dental Surgeons with the rank of First Lieutenant." On May 13, the judge advocate general opted for "Dental Surgeons with rank of First Lieutenant," and Major General Wood approved.[61–63] On June 6, 1911, the Senate confirmed the list of executive nominations for first lieutenants in the Army Dental Corps.[64,65] The first 30 contract dental surgeons had their contracts annulled so that they could accept commissions as "Dental Surgeon with the rank of First Lieutenant" from June 16 through August 1, 1911, with their relative rank based upon the date of their original contracts. Of the 30, 16 were original contract dental surgeons from 1901 and 1902, and 6 ultimately served as chiefs of the Dental Corps in the years from 1919 to 1946 (Table 10-1).[61,66,67]

TABLE 10-1

THE FIRST DENTAL CORPS OFFICERS

Name	Date of Rank	Date of Original Contract	Contract Annulled
John S Marshall[*][†]	13 April 1911	11 February 1901	16 June 1911
Robert T Oliver[*][†]	14 April 1911	11 February 1901	16 June 1911
Seibert D Boak	15 April 1911	15 April 1901	20 June 1911
Clarence F Lauderdale	16 April 1911	15 April 1901	19 June 1911
Franklin F Wing	17 April 1911	20 April 1901	19 June 1911
George L Mason	18 April 1911	15 May 1901	18 June 1911
Frank H Wolven	19 April 1911	1 June 1901	1 August 1911
John H Hess	20 April 1911	20 June 1901	20 June 1911
Hugh G Voorhies	21 April 1911	11 July 1901	10 June 1911
William H Chambers	22 April 1911	11 July 1901	16 June 1911
Alden Carpenter	23 April 1911	24 July 1901	16 June 1911
Charles J Long	24 April 1911	26 July 1901	6 July 1911
Edwin P Tignor	25 April 1911	17 August 1901	16 June 1911
John A McAlister, Jr.	26 April 1911	23 January 1902	19 June 1911
George H Casaday	27 April 1911	3 February 1902	16 June 1911
Julien R Bernheim[†]	28 April 1911	9 April 1902	20 June 1911
Rex H Rhoades[†]	29 April 1911	10 Nov 1902	20 June 1911
George E Stallman	30 April 1911	21 Jul 1904	11 July 1911
George I Gunckel	1 May 1911	16 Aug 1904	29 June 1911
Frank P Stone[*][†]	2 May 1911	28 May 1901	20 March 1907
		6 January 1911[‡]	27 June 1911
Raymond E Ingalls	3 May 1911	25 Mar 1907	21 June 1911
Harold O Scott	4 May 1911	4 September 1907	20 June 1911
John R Ames	5 May 1911	6 February 1908	18 June 1911
Edward PR Ryan	6 May 1911	11 January 1909	19 June 1911
Robert H Mills[†]	7 May 1911	17 May 1909	19 June 1911
Frank LK Laflamme[†]	8 May 1911	19 May 1909	18 June 1911
Minot E Scott	9 May 1911	19 September 1909	18 June 1911
George D Graham	10 May 1911	27 November 1909	6 July 1911
Robert F Patterson	11 May 1911	23 June 1910	19 June 1911
Samuel H Leslie	12 May 1911	12 August 1910	19 June 1911

[*]Original 1901 contract dental surgeon.
[†]Senior dental officers or chiefs, Dental Corps.
[‡]New contract.
Data sources: (1) National Archives and Records Administration. Surgeon General Torney to Adjutant General, 20 September 1911. Memo. No. 1829439. Box 6670. Entry 25. (2) National Archives and Records Administration. Henry P McCain, adjutant general, to Marshall, Oliver, et al, 15 June 1911. Letters. No. 1781254. (3) National Archives and Records Administration. Torney to adjutant general, 10 May 1911. Letter. No. 1781254.

Dr John S Marshall's Retirement: A Legacy Established

On June 13, 1911, while still stationed at Columbus Barracks, Ohio, the surgeon general informed John Marshall that his commission was at the White House ready for the president's signature. On June 17 Marshall accepted a commission as a first lieutenant with the date of rank from April 13, 1911, making him the first dentist to be commissioned in the US Army Dental Corps.[68,69]

On June 23, Chief of Staff Leonard Wood, acting on the War Department's instructions, directed the adjutant general to issue an order announcing Dr Marshall's retirement from active service under the requirements of a congressional act approved June 30, 1882. The retirement would take effect on the day Marshall accepted his commission as a first lieutenant in the Dental Corps. He was also to be nominated for an advanced grade under the provisions of the Act of April 23, 1904. Marshall's telegram of acceptance of his commission, dated June 17, 1911, was considered by the judge advocate general as his formal acceptance of the commission and hence his retirement date. Because Marshall was now 64 years old, he was retired by a requirement of law, not by presidential direction, so President Taft merely announced the departure. As the next step, the president nominated him to the Senate for advancement to the grade of captain on the retired list.[69,70]

On June 24, 1911, Dr John Marshall was officially notified of his retirement from active duty and ordered to proceed to his home in Berkeley, California. On July 6, 1911, the Senate approved his advancement in rank to the grade of captain (date of rank June 17, 1911) on the retired list under the provisions of the Act of April 23, 1904. On August 7, Marshall formally accepted his captaincy. In May 1913 Marshall volunteered as a recruiting officer for the Oakland, California, area, but his offer was declined. Again in March 1916, as the European war clouds began to drift toward the United States, he offered his services to the government. The surgeon general's reply was "should occasion arise where your services can be utilized you will be promptly informed." In February 1917 Marshall requested that he be placed on active duty and assigned to any position the War Department thought he was fit to fill. The War Department thanked him for his "patriotic offer." Marshall died of nephritis on November 20, 1922, in Berkley and was buried at the San Francisco National Cemetery.[71–79]

John Marshall, appropriately and affectionately known as the father of the US Army Dental Corps, had finally completed the original mission that Surgeon General George Sternberg had given him back in 1901—to establish a dental corps for the US Army (the world's first)—and had established a legacy along the way.

References

1. National Archives and Records Administration. Record Group 112. Representative Hull to Surgeon General Torney, January 29, 1909. Letter. No. 106047. Box 712. Entry 26.

2. National Archives and Records Administration. Record Group 112. Torney to Hull, January 30, 1909. Letter with memoranda. No. 106047. Box 712. Entry 26.

3. National Archives and Records Administration. Record Group 112. Emory A Bryant to [President Theodore Roosevelt], February 18, 1909. Letter. No. 106047. Box 712. Entry 26.

4. Bryant EA. A few facts about Army Dental Corps legislation. *Dental Brief.* 1911;16:440–441.

5. National Archives and Records Administration. Record Group 94. Bryant to President Taft, November 25, 1909. Letter. No. 1592137 (filed with No. 524625). Box 3645. Entry 25.

6. Biographical file on Jefferson Randolph Kean. Research Collections, Office of Medical History, OTSG/MEDCOM, Falls Church, Va.

7. National Archives and Records Administration. Record Group 112. Memorandum for the surgeon general, JR Kean, March 23, 1909. Letter with enclosure; An act to improve the status and efficiency of dental surgeons in the U.S. Army. No. 106047. Box 712. Entry 26.

8. JR Kean to O'Reilly, March 25, 1909. Letter. Brigadier General JR Kean Papers, University of Virginia Library, Charlottesville, Va.

9. National Archives and Records Administration. Record Group 94. Surgeon General Torney to adjutant general, November 26, 1909. Letter with enclosure; Memorandum for the chief of staff, and draft act. No. 1592137 (filed with No. 524625). Box 3645. Entry 25.

10. National Dental Association. *Transactions of the National Dental Association* [1909]. Philadelphia, Pa: The SS White Dental Mfg Co; 1910.

11. *Congressional Record, 61st Cong, 1st Sess.* Vol 44. Washington, DC: Government Printing Office; 1909.

12. National Archives and Records Administration. Record Group 112. US Congress. Senate. S 1530, 61st Cong, 1st sess, April 9, 1909. No. 106047. Box 712. Entry 26.

13. National Archives and Records Administration. Record Group 112. US Congress. House. HR 11192, 61st Cong, 1st sess, July 5, 1909. No. 106047. Box 712. Entry 26.

14. National Archives and Records Administration. Surgeon General Torney to secretary of war, December 11, 1909. Memo. No. 1592137 (filed with No. 524625). Record Group 94. Box 3645. Entry 25.

15. National Archives and Records Administration. Record Group 94. Memorandum for secretary, general staff corps, Lieutenant Colonel DA Frederick, chief, second secretary, general staff, January 25, 1910, with endorsement, Brigadier General Tasker H Bliss, assistant to chief of staff, to secretary of war, January 31, 1910. No. 1592137 (filed with No. 524625). Box 3645. Entry 25.

16. National Archives and Records Administration. Record Group 94. Dr Bryant to Secretary of War Dickinson, January 31, 1910. Letter. No. 1592137 (filed with No. 524625). Box 3645. Entry 25.

17. National Archives and Records Administration. Record Group 94. Secretary of War Dickinson to Dr Bryant, February 23, 1910. Letter. No. 1592137 (filed with No. 524625). Box 3645. Entry 25.

18. National Archives and Records Administration. Record Group 94. Major General Bell to secretary of war, February 10, 1910. Memo. No. 1592137 (filed with No. 524625). Box 3645. Entry 25.

19. National Archives and Records Administration. Record Group 112. US Congress. *Act to improve the status and efficiency of dental surgeons in the U.S. Army*. February 12, 1910. No. 106047. Box 712. Entry 26.

20. National Archives and Records Administration. Record Group 165. Memo. Senate bill 4432, to reorganize the corps of dental surgeons attached to the medical department of the Army. Surgeon General Torney to secretary of war, February 12, 1910. Report no. 2222. Box 20. Entry 5.

21. National Archives and Records Administration. Record Group 165. Brigadier General William W Wotherspoon, general staff, March 1, 1909. Memo. Report no. 3716. Box 34. Entry 5.

22. National Archives and Records Administration. Record Group 165. Brigadier General William W Wotherspoon, acting chief of staff, to assistant secretary of war, August 3, 1909. Memo. Report no. 4354. Box 40. Entry 5.

23. National Archives and Records Administration. Record Group 112. RM Hollingsworth to surgeon general's office, May 5 and May 20, 1910. Memo. No. 116290. Box 795. Entry 26.

24. National Archives and Records Administration. Record Group 112. Captain CF Morse, 5th Cavalry (through channels) to chief surgeon, Department of California, October 31, 1910. Letter. No. 125031. Box 862. Entry 26.

25. National Archives and Records Administration. Record Group 112. George D Graham to Surgeon Schofield Barracks, October 6, 1910. Letter. No. 125031. Box 862. Entry 26.

26. National Archives and Records Administration. Record Group 94. John Millikin to adjutant general, January 22, 1910. No. 524625.

27. National Archives and Records Administration. Record Group 94. First endorsement, Marshall, office of the examining and supervising dental surgeon, Division Hospital, Manila, January 31, 1910. No. 524625.

28. National Archives and Records Administration. Record Group 94. Second endorsement, Lieutenant Colonel Charles Richard, Manila Hospital Commander, February 3, 1910. No. 524625.

29. National Archives and Records Administration. Record Group 94. Third endorsement, chief surgeon, Philippines Division, February 8, 1910. No. 524625.

30. National Archives and Records Administration. Record Group 94. Fourth endorsement, Major General WP Duvall, commanding officer, Philippines Division, February 15, 1910. No. 524625.

31. National Archives and Records Administration. Record Group 94. Sixth endorsement, Torney, surgeon general, to adjutant general, March 28, 1910. No. 524625.

32. National Archives and Records Administration. Record Group 94. Adjutant general to Dr Millikin, May 5, 1910. Letter. No. 524625.

33. National Archives and Records Administration. Record Group 94. US War Department. Circular No. 3. January 31, 1910. No. 524625.

34. National Archives and Records Administration. Record Group 112. Endorsement, adjutant general to surgeon general's office request, January 28, 1910. No. 80285. Box 540. Entry 26.

35. National Archives and Records Administration. Record Group 112. US Congress. House. 61st Cong, 2nd sess, March 16, 1910. H Rep 23097. No. 106047. Box 712. Entry 26.

36. National Archives and Records Administration. Record Group 165.Memorandum for the secretary of war, Brigadier General Tasker H Bliss, acting chief of staff, May 5, 1910. Report no. 2222. Box 20. Entry 5.

37. *Congressional Record, 61st Cong, 2nd sess*. Vol 45. Washington, DC: Government Printing Office; 1910: 3264.

38. New Army Dental Corps bill. 61st Congress, 2nd Sess. H.R. 23097. *Items of Interest*. 1910;32:390–391.

39. National Archives and Records Administration. Record Group 165. Senate Bill 4432, to reorganize the corps of dental surgeons attached to the medical department of the Army. Lieutenant Colonel, DA Frederick, general staff, second section, to assistant secretary of war, April 23, 1910. Memo. Report no. 2222. Box 20. Entry 5.

40. National Archives and Records Administration. Record Group 165. Brigadier General Tasker H Bliss, acting chief of staff, to surgeon general, May 2, 1910. Memo. Report no. 2222. Box 20. Entry 5.

41. National Archives and Records Administration. Record Group 165. Surgeon General Torney to chief of staff, May 2, 1910. Letter. Report no. 2222. Box 20. Entry 5.

42. National Archives and Records Administration. Record Group 165. Secretary of War Dickinson to Representative Wiley, May 4, 1910. Letter. Report no. 2222. Box 20. Entry 5.

43. [Ottolengui R]. The new Army Dental Corps bill, and the surgeon-general's opinion thereon. *Items of Interest*. 1910;32:380–386.

44. Wiley's bill. *Items of Interest*. 1910;32:390–391.

45. Torney's memorandum. *Items of Interest*. 1910;32:391–399.

46. [Litch WF]. 'A bill to improve the status and efficiency of dental surgeons in the United States Army.' *Dental Brief*. 1910;15:365–366.

47. [Ottolengui R]. Army Dental Corps. *Items of Interest*. 1910;32:875–876.

48. Bryant EA. Further facts relating to the establishment of the Army Dental Corps. *Dental Brief*. 1911;16:832–833.

49. *Congressional Record, 61st Cong, 3rd sess*. Vol 46. Washington, DC: Government Printing Office; 1911.

50. [Ottolengui R]. Bills affecting dentists enacted by the last Congress. *Items of Interest*. 1911;33:310–311.

51. National Archives and Records Administration. Record Group 112. Surgeon General Torney to chief of staff, February 8, 1911. Memo. No. 106047. Box 712. Entry 26.

52. National Archives and Records Administration. Record Group 94. Secretary of War Dickinson to Senate Committee on Military Affairs, February 8, 1911. Memo. No. 524625. Box 3645. Entry 25.

53. National Archives and Records Administration. Record Group 112. Endorsement, Surgeon General Torney to secretary of war, February 14, 1911. No 106047. Box 712. Entry 26.

54. US Congress. Senate. *Reorganization of Corps of Dental Surgeons*. Congressional Record, 61st Cong, 3rd sess, 1911. S Rep 1201.

55. [Kirk EC]. Commissioned status for Army dental surgeons. *Dental Cosmos*. 1911;53: 482, 484-85.

56. [Litch WF]. The new Army dental law. *Dental Brief*. 1911;16:267.

57. Crenshaw W, Rodgers CW, DeFord WH. Report on Army and Navy dental legislation. In: *Transactions of the National Dental Association* [1913]. Philadelphia, Pa: The SS White Dental Mfg Co; 1914: 34–35.

58. Leslie SH. Dental service in the Army. *J Allied Dent Soc*. 1916;11:238.

59. [Kirk EC]. The Army Dental Corps. *Dental Cosmos*. 1914;56:1372–1373.

60. Ingalls RE. The Army Dental Corps. *Dental Digest*. 1915;21:424.

61. National Archives and Records Administration. Record Group 94. Torney to adjutant general, May 10, 1911, approved by Major General Leonard Wood. Letter. No. 1781254. Entry 25. Box 6515.

62. National Archives and Records Administration. Record Group 94. First endorsement, Henry P McCain, adjutant general, to judge advocate general, May 12, 1911.

63. National Archives and Records Administration. Record Group 94. Second endorsement, EH Crowder, judge advocate general, to adjutant general, May 13, 1911, approved by Major General Leonard Wood. No. 1781254. Box 6515. Entry 25.

64. Bryant EA. Appointments in the Army. Executive nominations of May 18th, 1911. *Items of Interest*. 1911;33:551.

65. [Litch WF]. The executive nomination of dental surgeons in the Army confirmed by the Senate. *Dental Brief*. 1911;16:499.

66. National Archives and Records Administration. Surgeon General Torney to adjutant general, September 20, 1911. Memo. No. 1829439. Box 6670. Entry 25.

67. National Archives and Records Administration. Record Group 94. Henry P McCain, adjutant general, to Marshall, Oliver, et al, June 15, 1911. Letters. No. 1781254. Box 6515. Entry 25.

68. National Archives and Records Administration. Record Group 112. Surgeon general to Dr Marshall, June 13, 1911. Telegram. No. 70760. Box 449. Entry 26.

69. National Archives and Records Administration. Record Group 94. Dr Marshall to adjutant general (Army), oath of office, June 17, 1911. Telegram. No. 391988. Box 2730. Entry 25.

70. National Archives and Records Administration. Record Group 165. Major General Wood, chief of staff, to adjutant general, June 23, 1911, Brigadier General Enoch H Crowder, judge advocate general, June 23, 1911. Memos. No. 7040. Box 69. Entry 5.

71. National Archives and Records Administration. Record Group 94. Dr Marshall to adjutant general (Army), May 20, 1913, February 4, June 12, 1917. Letters. No. 391988. Box 2730. Entry 25.

72. National Archives and Records Administration. Record Group 94. Adjutant general to Dr Marshall, February 12, June 29, 1917. Letters. No. 391988. Box 2730. Entry 25.

73. National Archives and Records Administration. Record Group 112. Dr Marshall to

surgeon general's office, March 16, 1916. Letter. No. 138035. Box 204. Entry 25.

74. National Archives and Records Administration. Record Group 112. Surgeon general's office to Dr Marshall, March 23, 1916. Letter. No. 138035. Box 204. Entry 25.

75. Vail WD. John Sayre Marshall, pioneer Army dental surgeon (1846–1922). *Dental Bulletin Supplement to the Army Medical Bulletin*. 1940;11:122.

76. National Archives and Records Administration. Record Group 92. Cemetery records, April 3, 1923. Box 2987. Entry 1942.

77. National Archives and Records Administration. Record Group 94. Special orders, no. 147, par 43, War Department, June 24, 1911. No. 391988. Box 2730. Entry 25.

78. National Archives and Records Administration. Record Group 94. Special orders no. 159, par 30, War Department, July 10, 1911. No. 391988. Box 2730. Entry 25.

79. National Archives and Records Administration. Record Group 94. Dr Marshall to adjutant general (Army), August 7, 1911. Letter. No. 391988. Box 2730. Entry 25.

Chapter XI

FROM A NEW CORPS TO A WORLD WAR, 1911–1917

Introduction

The creation of the US Army Dental Corps on March 3, 1911, did not immediately resolve the key issues that had confronted the Army's contract dental surgeons since 1901. Neither did it completely fulfill the aspirations of the National Dental Association (NDA) or America's dental community. Instead, the 1911 act was a compromise that probably left too much to be worked out later. Although the status of Army dentists was markedly different after March 3, 1911, than it was before, enormous challenges still lay ahead.

Implementing the New Law

The March 3, 1911 act establishing the Dental Corps brought in its wake a degree of uncertainty about some of its provisions and how they would be implemented in the Army, as well as many changes in the policies and procedures governing dental care. Surgeon General George Torney moved swiftly to clarify these uncertainties and then to disseminate information on the new law throughout the Army and the American dental community. Because the language of the act left some aspects of the legislation ill-defined, Torney asked Adjutant General Colonel Henry McLain to clarify three specific things: whether the current contract dental surgeons were "officers of the Medical Department" and thus paid from general appropriations upon appointment; whether the surgeon general could hire acting dental surgeons upon the commissioning of the current contractors; and what grade of contract dental surgeon would be superseded when the present members were commissioned.[1] On April 6, LP Mitchell, assistant comptroller of the treasury, replied to the adjutant general's inquiry on behalf of the surgeon general, saying that yes, the commissioned dental surgeons become officers in the Medical Department and are paid out of general appropriations. He also replied that 31 acting dental surgeons were authorized for hire upon the commissioning of the current contractors and that the acting dental surgeons supersede and replace those authorized in the acts of February 2, 1901, and March 2, 1907. Chief of Staff Major General Leonard Wood, along with the secretary of war, approved these decisions on April 10.[2]

While that inquiry was in process, Torney turned to replacing the April 6, 1905, memorandum "Concerning the Employment of Dental Surgeons in the United

States Army" with a new "Circular of Information" for prospective applicants based on the changes resulting from the Act of March 3, 1911. A completed draft of the circular was forwarded to the secretary of war for review and approval on April 15, 1911, igniting a series of exchanges that lasted until June and far exceeded Torney's original intention.[3,4] At Wood's request, on April 22 McClain directed Torney to rewrite paragraph 17 of the draft circular to conform to Paragraph 1422 of the existing 1910 Army Regulations, noting that "as the present law provides that dental surgeons shall be commissioned officers, no limitation can be imposed on their 'hours of official duty.'" He also directed the submission of "a draft of such amendments to Army Regulations as are made necessary by that portion of the Act approved March 3, 1911, that established a dental corps."[5,6] Paragraph 17 was lifted virtually intact from the 1905 memorandum and paraphrased the existing Paragraph 1422 Army Regulations:

> [Paragraph 17] Members of the Dental Corps are required to serve only the officers and enlisted men of the Regular and Volunteer Army and contract surgeons. The families of officers and enlisted men and civilian employees and their families are not entitled to free dental service. The hours of official duty are from 9 a.m. to 4 p.m. daily, except in cases of emergency. During other hours the dentists are allowed to operate upon persons not entitled to free services, but Government material may be used only upon persons entitled to free treatment.[3]

> [Paragraph 1422, Army Regulations] Dental Surgeons will operate between the hours of 9 a.m. and 4.p.m. upon those officers and enlisted men who are entitled to their services. They may operate upon others, not entitled to free service, before and after these hours, when their services are not required by those entitled to them, but material issued to them by the Government will be used only in operations upon officers and enlisted men of the Army. Emergency work, whether for officers or enlisted men, shall at all times have precedence over the work for those not entitled to free service, without regard to the hours of duty.[7]

Torney resubmitted his package with the proposed amendments on April 25. However, determining the revisions and publishing them Army-wide was a more pressing requirement than issuing the "Circular of Information" because basic Army Regulations governed virtually every aspect of soldiers' lives. Most of the changes that Torney submitted were simple editorial substitutions, such as replacing "dental surgeon" with "members of the Dental Corps" and adding "and acting dental surgeons" as appropriate. However, he also proposed changes in Paragraphs 1421, 1422, and 1425 of the Army Regulations. While 1425 was mainly administrative and minor, 1421 and 1422 raised major problems.[7-9]

The process of simple revisions disappeared when the surgeon general's proposed changes to Paragraphs 1421 and 1422 were addressed:

> *1421.* In accordance with the Act of Congress authorizing their employment, members of the Dental Corps will "serve the officers and enlisted men of the Regular and Volunteer Army." The families of officers and enlisted men, and the civilian employees of the Army and their families, are not entitled to free dental service.

1422. Members of the Dental Corps will operate upon those officers and enlisted men who need their services. Materials issued by the Government will be expended only in operations upon officers and enlisted men of the Army. Emergency work, whether for officers or enlisted men, shall at all times have precedence over other work.[7]

Paragraph 1421 raised no concerns for Torney because military families had been exempt from free dental care consistently since February 2, 1901. In Paragraph 1422, however, Torney omitted the duty hours provision, as well as the part that read: "the present affirmative provisions authorizing the doing of private work." He argued "it is considered inadvisable to encourage it by affirmative provisions like those omitted in view of the fact that the work on Army patients will be quite enough as a rule to occupy most of the time of the dentists."[7] The change from contract dental surgeon to commissioned dental officer ended the previous practice of contracting private work for payment between the dental surgeons and Army personnel, dependents, and civilian employees during nonduty hours. Torney had campaigned against this particular issue since his letter to the surgeon general on December 23, 1905 (see "John Marshall's Work at the Presidio" in Chapter 9).[10]

After reviewing applicable legislation, though, the general staff saw that the situation was much more complicated than Torney had imagined. A July 5, 1884, act (23 Stat 112) stated that medical officers and contract surgeons "shall whenever practicable attend the families of officers and soldiers free of charge." On April 23, 1908, another act (35 Stat 66) included dental surgeons within the Medical Department, and the March 3, 1911 act (36 Stat 1054) attached the new Dental Corps, "composed of dental surgeons and acting dental surgeons," to the Medical Department, which Comptroller Mitchell's April 6 memo confirmed.[9,11,12] Hence, the general staff concluded: "Inasmuch as dental surgeons are now 'medical officers of the Army' it would seem to be incumbent upon them whenever practicable to give their services free of charge to the families of officers and soldiers.[8,9] Therefore, the general staff recommended adoption of the following amended Paragraphs 1421 and 1422, which eventually significantly altered Army dentistry's functions and patient population:

1421. Members of the dental corps will serve free of charge all those entitled to free medical treatment by medical officers.

1422. Members of the dental corps will operate upon those entitled to their services. Materials issued by the Government will be expended only in operations upon those entitled to free service. Emergency work for officers and enlisted men shall at all times have precedence of other work.[8,13]

On May 24, Brigadier General Enoch Crowder, the Army judge advocate general, completed his review of the draft general staff memo to the secretary of war and offered his legal opinion on the amended paragraphs:

As members of the dental corps are now either officers in the Med. Dept. of the Army . . . or acting dental surgeons employed under terms and conditions applicable to army contract surgeons, I am of the opinion that members of the dental corps may properly be required to serve free of charge those who are entitled to free medical treatment by medical officers; and it is therefore recommended that paragraphs 1421 and 1422 of the A.R. be amended as indicated.[8]

After receiving Crowder's opinion, the chief of staff forwarded the approved amendments to the Army Regulations to the adjutant general for promulgation.[13,14]

On July 21, 1911, Major General J Franklin Bell, commander of the Philippines Division, wrote to the adjutant general to complain about the inflexibility of Paragraph 1424 of the 1910 regulation, which was not changed in the 1911 revision then in progress. Bell contended that 1424 "at times almost amounts to cruelty under conditions like those in the Philippine Islands. . . ."[15] The offending paragraph dated back to Torney's proposal of December 1907 as follows:

> *1424.* For plate work or for the filling of teeth of enlisted men the materials supplied by the Government will be used and no other, and members of the Dental Corps are forbidden to enter into any financial agreement with enlisted men involving an obligation for payment for silver, platinum, or gold used for filling cavities in teeth, for the construction of bridge work, for the fitting of crowns, the making of artificial dentures, or other dental work.[16]

General Bell proposed an amended paragraph that added:

> Exceptions may be made to this paragraph in the Philippine Division, upon individual applications setting forth the necessity therefore, by the post commander. In such cases a deposit sufficient to cover the additional expense will be made with the post commander when application is made.[15]

On September 1, 1911, Surgeon General Torney agreed to the provision for the Philippines. Under previous provisions, contract dental surgeons were allowed to enter into contracts with officer and enlisted personnel and their families to do dental work outside of Army time. This situation led to incessant problems, and Bell's suggestion appeared to Torney as a possible solution:

> It is believed that with this arrangement the endless controversy between the Dentists and enlisted men as to the validity of charges for dental work on this character, will be avoided, and at the same time exceptional conditions demanding unusual service may be met. Under the customs which obtained before the establishment of the conditions brought about by paragraph 1424, Army Regulations, 1910, this office was constantly making effort to adjudicate claims between contracting parties, but it is believed that such difficulties will not ensue if the plan contemplated within is put into effect in the Philippines.[17]

General Wood accepted Torney's recommendation but advised the secretary of war that the amendment be more broadly written to include similar cases at "any point outside the territorial limits of the United States," including Cuba, Puerto Rico, Alaska, Panama, and Hawaii, where the services of qualified civilian dentists may not be available. The prohibition on contracts between dental officers and enlisted soldiers remained in force in the continental United States, and probably saved many soldiers from purchasing expensive dental work they could ill afford on their monthly salaries.[18] On September 30 Wood directed Adjutant General McClain to amend the existing restrictions in Paragraph 1424 by adding the following caveat:

> Beyond the territorial limits of the United States, post commanders upon receipt of written application by enlisted men, may authorize such enlisted men to receive any class of dental treatment from members of the Dental Corps which the best interests of the service my require. In such cases a deposit sufficient to cover the proper expenses involved will be made with the post commander by the enlisted men concerned when the application is made.[18]

This change was published in War Department General Order No. 135 on October 6, 1911.[19]

Implementing the Act of March 3, 1911, resulted in a significant obligation to the dental care of military dependents. When this act was completed in the fall of 1911, the basic policies and procedures under which new Army dentists worked were significantly different, especially in regard to private work (which was now forbidden except outside the United States and under extenuating circumstances), and the provision of free dental care to the dependents of military personnel; all of which might have doubled the dentists' workloads.

Seeking Those of "the Highest Professional Ability"

On April 10, 1911, even before Surgeon General Torney had received the secretary of war's approval for the new "Circular of Information," he acted to win over the dental community and recruit new Army dentists. He sent an information letter to various dental journals summarizing the new dental legislation so that the details would reach the broadest audience possible. He emphasized that the new law gave the dental surgeons increased status, pay, and allowances and should make the service more attractive to "young practitioners of the highest professional ability . . . as may think they would enjoy a military life."[20] He wrote:

> It has long been recognized by the Surgeon-general of the army and the War department that the dental corps is a valuable addition to the medical department of the army, and that the status of dental surgeons as authorized by the provisions of previous law were inadequate and insufficient to properly reward them for their services or to further tempt young practitioners of the highest ability to enter the service.[20(p560)]

He also pointed out the challenges of Army dentistry as an inducement to the more adventurous, self-confident young professionals:

> The army dental surgeon, if he is to fill his position with credit to himself and his profession, and with proper efficiency to the service, must be well educated, above the ordinary in technical ability, and well qualified in all departments of dentistry. The need of these requirements will be more readily appreciated when the statement is made that the dental surgeons of the army are very rarely associated at a post with

> a member of their own profession. Consequently they are thrown entirely upon their own professional resources and must exercise their own judgment in the treatment of their more difficult and serious cases, as consultations are practically out of the question.
>
> Furthermore, the surgeon of the post frequently refers cases involving diseases of the mouth and jaws with which he is more or less unfamiliar, to the dental surgeon, and expects to find, as he has a right to do, that the dental surgeon is not only capable of rendering a correct diagnosis, but competent to take charge of the case if required to do so; as in the treatment of fractures of the jaws, deep seated abscesses of the jaws associated with impacted teeth, facial neuralgia, empyema of the maxillary sinus, etc.[20(p561)]

Torney ended with an offer of a secure and comfortable retirement or disability separation, something contract dental surgeons had wanted for years:

> The position of a dental surgeon in the United States army is an honorable one, and should prove attractive to young men, as the pay and allowances now offered are good, and in the unfortunate event of broken health incident to the service, or upon reaching the age limit of sixty-four years, he retires from the service with three-fourths pay, which after twenty years or more of service would give him a year's income of $2160.[20]

Torney's letter attracted much attention in the dental press. In an editorial preface to the letter in the May 1911 issue of *Dental Brief*, editor Wilbur Litch wrote the letter was "most opportune in that it places before a large body of young men about to graduate from dental schools, and before recent graduates, a clear statement of the duties of the army dental surgeon and the compensation allowed him under the law. . . . Even for the best equipped of our young graduates or practitioners, this is a financial proposition worthy of consideration." While civilian private practice and military pay were relatively equal, Litch noted that "Army pay, however, has the very great advantage that there are no deductions for office expenses, cost of material, or bad debts to be taken into account."[21(p351)] Litch believed that the new members of the Dental Corps would emulate the record of the "pioneers" of the past decade who had shown the importance of military dentistry. His preface honored those:

> . . . whose professional fitness and faithfulness to duty have been such vital factors in breaking down the walls of prejudice and demonstrating the indispensable importance of skilled dental service for the military forces of the nation. All honor these pioneers who have blazed the way! May those who, under new and better conditions, join their ranks emulate their record and be equally a credit to the army service and to the dental profession.[21(p352)]

Two months later, Litch returned to the subject because he questioned whether the current dental school curriculum would adequately prepare a young graduate dentist for the Army's oral surgical standards. Torney's letter clearly intimated "that the examiners will not be satisfied with a merely theoretical examination in oral surgery, but will demand, in addition to a knowledge of surgical pathology, practical demonstration of surgical skill, and a knowledge of the most advanced surgical technique as applied to minor oral surgical operations."[22(p435)] Litch recommended that the dental course might have to be changed significantly and lengthened to provide sufficient training in the new skills. He predicted that in the event of a war, a dental corps possessing the additional skills he recommended would prove itself "an indispensable adjunct" to the military in the treatment of gunshot and other wounds of the jaws.[22(p436)]

The War Department Gets the Blame for the "One-Grade Corps"

Despite the significant step forward that the legislation provided, disappointment was still widespread among the dental profession over the absence of promotion possibilities. At the meeting of the NDA's southern branch in Atlanta in early April 1911, the group's legislative committee discussed its efforts on Capitol Hill. Appealing to his audience's professionalism, Dr William Crenshaw, chairman of the committee, explained how the "three-grade corps" was lost and called on every member to act when called upon to prevent such disappointments in the future:

> This amendment [Bulkeley's] I am positive would have succeeded in getting through Congress, and we would have had a commissioned dental corps in the army with three grades of lieutenant, captain, and major, had it not been for the interference of the War department in the conference committee. The two higher grades were struck out, so that we have a law which gives rank, but no higher grade than lieutenant, and perhaps lieutenant unmounted. But the bill puts the army dentists on a commissioned basis; we have secured that much. We are, however, not satisfied with the bill, and if we are to get what we want, the profession must give more material help to the Legislative Committee. Hereafter, when the Legislative Committee writes or telegraphs you, we ask you at once to get to work on congressmen and senators in the way the committee suggests. The committee cannot do more than any other small number of men, and unless you are all active and act as one man, we are not going to have the recognition that the profession asks and is entitled to.[23(pp1057–1058)]

He concluded with a call for professional equality with the Army's Medical Corps, saying: "The government is slowly finding out that it will never get the efficiency it needs in the dental corps until it gives adequate recognition to our profession, and until it puts a premium on our services such as is placed on the medical service."[23(p1058)]

After thanking Senator Overman for his achievements and for what he would have achieved "if circumstances had not interfered over which he had no control at the time, and of which he was not informed," the long-time NDA lobbyist, Williams Donnally, then took up the cudgel with stark bluntness:

> The effect of the opposition to which I refer was that two of the three grades of rank for which the dental profession has contended for nine years were omitted, and thus our measure, enacted several times by the Senate and approved by the House Military Committee, was reduced to a one-grade army dental corps. This was done in the secrecy of the conference committee through the extraordinary efforts of the

> War department, not only officially through the secretary, the chief of staff, and the surgeon-general, but by such means as a lobby of commissioned officers in citizens' clothes buttonholing members of Congress at the Capitol, and asking them not to give dentists any rank at all. Medical men tried to defeat this legislation, and a remark of a former medical officer, now the chief of staff of the army, is substantially, that the more dentists we have, the fewer surgeons we will have in the army, and therefore he would not do for army dentists as he had previously indicated he would.[23(p1058)]

By singling out Chief of Staff Wood, Donnally placed blame for the defeat at the highest level of the War Department. Crenshaw and Donnally had called attention to a fact that would continue into the post-World War I period—the War Department general staff remained opposed to granting rank and grade to the officers of the Dental Corps.[24–27]

In an article in the June issue of *Dental Cosmos*, Dr William Fisher, a former Army contract dental surgeon from 1901 to 1904 now practicing in New York City, also expressed disappointment that there was no provision for promotion under the new law. He believed that "nothing less" than a three-grade promotion should have been accepted. The "one-grade corps" would not attract and hold good dentists because it lacked a system of promotion; they would retire as first lieutenants while their associates in the other corps advanced in rank to captain and on to full colonel. Even the lowest ranking Medical Reserve Corps officers would outrank a dental surgeon of many years' service. The only advantage the new law gave was retirement from age or disability. Fisher also pointed out that there would be no improvement in the social status of dental surgeons because the contract dentists had always been eligible for membership in the officers' clubs at the various Army posts; commissioned status was not necessary for "social recognition." Fisher concluded that as long as the new Dental Corps remained "a tolerated appendage" of the Medical Department rather than "a dignified adjunct," a corps could not develop "that will honor our profession."[28]

On June 11, 1911, Dr Emory Bryant wrote a letter to the editor of *Dental Cosmos* that was published in July, responding to Fisher, whose views "are merely opinions based upon imagination rather than facts or conditions, or knowledge of dental corps legislation." Others in the profession shared Fisher's stance, so Bryant, who was involved in the entire legislative process that produced the bill, believed the letter should not go "unanswered." At a time when "many of the leaders in the dental profession itself had lost interest in the matter," Bryant said the successful passage of the dental bill was due to "the very compromise" that some now criticized, and that failure was "narrowly missed" by the insistence on the "three-grade" rank. Dr Bryant had letters from a number of key congressmen who insisted that any rank above first lieutenant would have resulted in the bill's defeat; all agreed that any effort for increased rank would have "jeopardized" the bill's passage and considered it fortunate that the Dental Corps got as much as it did.[29,30]

The 1911 annual meeting of the NDA, which was held from July 25 to 28 in Cleveland, Ohio, should have been a time to celebrate the March 3 act and the achievement of commissioned status for Army dentists. The Committee on Army and Navy Dental Legislation reported that although the act was not all that they had hoped for, commissioned military rank was an improvement for dental surgeons.[31]

While the result of our efforts is not as creditable a recognition of the dental profession, not as generous to its representatives in the military service, nor as beneficial to the army personnel, as we sincerely desired and labored to attain, yet it is a decidedly notable and important legislative uplift of the profession's representatives in the United States army service, from the nondescript and odious "contract" position to that of a grade of regular military rank common to all staff corps.[31]

Army Dental Care after 1911

Although the small number of dentists in the Army was one reason care was limited to prophylaxis and emergency work, the limited budget of the surgeon general's office primarily determined the policy. This was especially the case when officers and enlisted soldiers at sites without a dental surgeon sought civilian care. Even with the 1911 creation of a dental corps and its expansion to a full complement of 90 authorized dentists, the number of dentists was insufficient to meet all the Army's needs, especially with care extended to dependents. The new corps grew slowly, even as demand for its services rose at a great rate. But because the Medical Department did not have sufficient funds to provide comprehensive free care, the surgeon general's office decided to limit major dental procedures to gunshot wounds and trauma in the line of duty until Congress made its intentions clearer by law or increased appropriation. Until then, individuals still carried the main financial responsibility for their full dental care. This policy applied to the militia and continued until World War II; Army dentistry was not intended for "chronic" problems.[32]

In December 1911, the newly retired John Marshall reviewed his past 7 years at the Presidio of San Francisco and concluded that Army personnel had willingly accepted dental care. He had been in the position of seeing the "dirty mouths" and "decayed teeth" transformed into "healthy condition." He recalled telling his patients with unclean mouths: "If you have not a tooth-brush, I will excuse you until tomorrow. Get a tooth-brush and brush your teeth carefully and return to me, and I will take care of you." Also, he had some cards printed and displayed in the waiting room with mottoes such as "Clean Teeth Do Not Decay" and "Please do not ask the dental surgeon to treat your teeth until after you have brushed them."[33(p1438)]

Because of their limited numbers, Army dentists were still largely nomadic. Their relatively small number and the large population eligible for their services posed a major problem, especially when combined with the extensive distances they were often expected to travel. In 1911 Lieutenant Charles J Long was one of two dentists assigned to what was then the Department of the East, Governor's Island, New York. He and his colleague were responsible for the department's two circuits, one covering the Army installations in the northern half of the command and the other the southern half. At a time when many harbor and coastal defenses were very active in the department, Long's schedule for July 1 to December 31, 1911, kept him and his assistant, Private Vernon Beyer, constantly on the road, shipping their dental outfit out as soon as possible so it could be set up upon their arrival. During this time, they treated troops at Fort Ethan Allen, Vermont; Plattsburgh Barracks, Madison Barracks, Forts Ontario, Niagara, Porter, Jay, HG

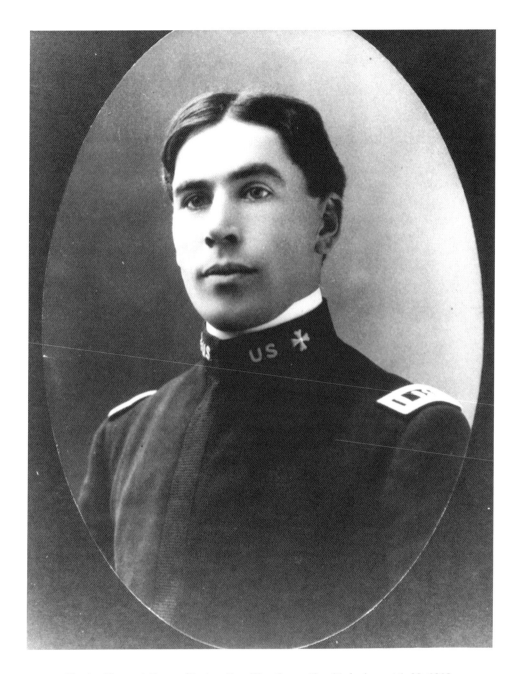

Charles J Long at Camp of Instruction, Pine Camp, New York, August 1–30, 1910.
Photograph: Courtesy of Colonel Charles J Long, III.

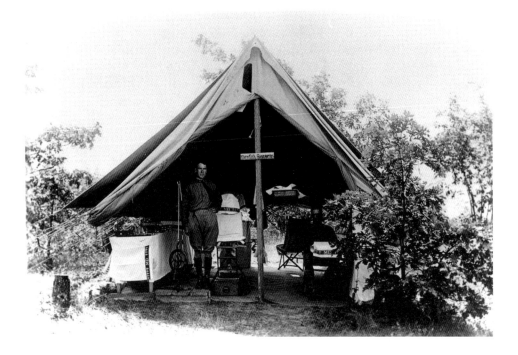

Charles J Long and his dental "office" at Camp of Instruction,
Pine Camp, New York, August 1–30, 1910.
Photograph: Courtesy of Colonel Charles J Long, III.

Wright, Terry, and Michie, New York; Forts Adams and Greble, Rhode Island; and Forts Rodman, Andrews, Banks, Warren, and Strong, Massachusetts.[34]

By 1912 the situation had only grown worse with reorganization. Colonel Louis Maus (who had established the first Army dental clinic for the V Corps in Jacksonville, Florida in 1898), now chief surgeon of the Eastern Division, faced a command spread from New England to the Gulf of Mexico. In May 1912 he informed the surgeon general that the four dentists assigned to his division had to serve a population of about 21,000 military and their 6,500 dependents at posts scattered from the Canadian border to Panama. As a result, he broke the work into four "districts" to place "the dental surgeons to the best advantage for the service of the command."[35]

In December 1912 he provided a detailed explanation to Major General Thomas Barry, the division commander. Even if the work could be divided evenly, Maus noted, each dentist would have about 7,000 patients "with the result that not more than 10% or 15% of the necessary work can be performed." The ratio was made worse because distance and local demand prevented the dentist in the Canal Zone from helping with stateside requirements, so Maus really only had three dentists available for most of his command. The presence of recruit depots in the division compounded the problem. Examination and care of the new recruits consumed so much time that care "of the old and valuable soldiers" in the command often could not be accomplished during the dentists' itineraries. Whenever emergencies detained a dentist on his circuit, his schedule often became so curtailed that units scheduled elsewhere were not visited. Maus added that the inordinate amount of time dentists had to spend traveling imposed personal expenses and made "personal conditions" for them "intolerable," especially if they had families.[36]

Maus pointed out that the 1911 law authorized the appointment of one dentist for every 1,000 enlisted soldiers, but the new Army Regulations specified that officers and dependents were also entitled to dental care. If these additional mouths were factored into the ratio, he estimated his division alone should have about 30 dentists (11 under the 1911 ratio), and the Army should have about 120 instead of the 45 allowed by the law. Unless the ratio was revised, he predicted severe problems in retaining quality dental officers, who would be driven out by the staggering workload. In the meantime he wanted the authority and funds to use local civilians whenever necessary. To get the most efficient use of the dentists he had, in the interim, he divided the division into four dental districts, each with roughly the same number of troops and travel dimensions.[36]

General Barry succinctly endorsed Maus's memo, saying, "this report shows a great deficiency in the number of dental surgeons required for this division, and it is recommended that if practicable some relief be obtained."[37]

The results were almost immediate. By June 1913 Maus had six dental surgeons serving just the United States portion and had six routes laid out that more equitably distributed the burden of dental care.[38] By December 1914 Maus, still the chief surgeon for what was now the eastern department, had assigned 14 dental surgeons and had reduced the routes so that no dentist served more than four posts .[39]

Militia Dental Surgeons: 1911–1914

On November 1, 1911, the chief of the Division of Militia Affairs, Brigadier General Robert Evans, issued a bulletin defining the effect of the new law on the status of militia dental surgeons:

> Section 3 of the Militia Law requires the Organized Militia to conform to the organization, armament, and discipline of the Regular Army. The Act of March 3, 1911, authorizes a Dental Corps to be attached to the Medical Department, prescribing certain limitations as to numbers of this corps. The Dental Corps is a part of the Regular Establishment, and in the opinion of this office, the Organized Militia would be authorized to attach to its Medical Department a Dental Corps in conformity with the proportion prescribed by the Act of March 3, 1911, and the officers of such corps, when on duty, would be entitled to pay out of the Federal funds allotted to the State.[40(p935)]

The militia affairs office was of the opinion that under the March 3, 1911, act, the members of the various state militia dental corps should be at once commissioned as first lieutenants, and that the contract feature of the act did not apply to the militia organizations.[40]

In 1913, however, the Division of Militia Affairs chief, in the office of the US Army chief of staff, reversed this opinion. In his 1913 report, he stated:

Dental surgeons are authorized at the rate of not to exceed one for each thousand of actual enlisted strength. All original appointments to the dental corps shall be as acting dental surgeons, and after three years' service in a manner satisfactory to the governor, or commanding general, District of Columbia Militia, such appointees may be appointed dental surgeons and be commissioned as first lieutenants in the dental corps.[41,42]

Like other volunteer officers, commissioned volunteer dental surgeons were not entitled to retirement under the federal law, but could acquire a pension if disabled "in the line of duty." The state regulated the pay of both acting and commissioned dental surgeons serving with the state militia, but while serving in federal camps of instruction or as United States volunteers, it was the same as the corresponding grades in the Regular Army.[42]

Out of the 48 state adjutant generals, by 1914 only 9 reported having any dental surgeons, and those 9 only had 14 among them. This prompted Edward Kirk, editor of *Dental Cosmos*, to urge the state dental societies to action in his editorial in the December 1914 issue:

In this connection it should be remembered that it is a function or should be a function of the several state societies to see to it that good representative men are appointed upon the dental surgeon corps by the adjutants-general of the several states militia, and in those states in which dental surgeons have not been appointed, the attention of the adjutants-general of such states should be called to the law of March 3, 1911, which gives authority to form such a corps in the proportion of one dentist (acting dental surgeon) to each one thousand men. It is somewhat surprising that the most progressive states in military affairs and with the largest state militias—for example, New York, Pennsylvania, Ohio, Indiana, and Illinois—have not appointed dental surgeons.[41]

The Dental Corps Falls Behind, 1912–1914

On June 30, 1911, the surgeon general reported a strength of 29 dental surgeons and 1 acting dental surgeon—the same number of contract dental surgeons authorized in 1901.[43] In early 1912 he announced that on Monday, April 1, examinations for the appointment of acting dental surgeons would be held at Fort Slocum, New York (later replaced by West Point); Columbus Barracks, Ohio; Jefferson Barracks, Missouri; Fort Logan, Colorado; and Fort McDowell, California. On that day, 59 candidates reported for the examinations to vie for the 29 positions to be filled. Nine candidates successfully passed the examinations for appointment as acting dental surgeons, and the papers of two or three more remained under evaluation. A large number of candidates failed the physical examination. The next examination was scheduled for October 7, 1912.[44,45] The Dental Corps ended its first full fiscal year with 28 dental surgeons and 10 acting dental surgeons, just 8 more than a year earlier.[46]

On September 11, 1912, at the annual NDA meeting in Washington, DC, First Lieutenant Edwin Tignor, representing the surgeon general, said that only 10 or 12 new dentists had been secured for the expanded 90-person Dental Corps. There had been no lack of applications, but few had passed the examinations, which

---

EXHIBIT 11-1

1914 DENTAL SURGEON APPOINTMENTS

By 1914 the adjutants general of the 48 states reported that dental surgeons had been appointed in their respective militias under existing federal militia legislation as follows:

- Michigan: one first lieutenant;
- Iowa: three first lieutenants and acting dental surgeons;
- Alabama: two first lieutenants;
- Texas: two acting dental surgeons;
- North Carolina: three first lieutenants;
- South Dakota: one first lieutenant;
- Oklahoma: one assistant dental surgeon;
- Nebraska: one first lieutenant acting dental surgeon;
- California and Maryland: one to be appointed in the near future;
- Idaho: less than 1,000 troops and none appointed for that reason;
- Utah: none appointed under present organization;
- Colorado: the military board in the near future would recommend the necessary changes be made in the code to include dental surgeons;
- Ohio: under the state laws no appointments of dental surgeons had been made;
- Delaware: the militia law of the state did not provide for a dental surgeon in the organized militia;
- North Dakota: code did not provide for the appointment of dental surgeons; and
- New York, Pennsylvania, Indiana, and Illinois: none appointed.

Data sources: (1) [Kirk EC]. The Army Dental Corps. *Dental Cosmos*. 1914;56:1375. (2) Boak SD. Militia dental surgeons. *Dental Cosmos*. 1914;56:1351–1352.

---

were not unduly difficult. This indicated that "a great many of the best men do not know that such openings exist and what this career means for the young man" and hence were not applying. Tignor offered to talk to anyone interested in a service career.[47]

At the annual meeting the next year, July 10, 1913, in Kansas City, First Lieutenant Alden Carpenter, the official representative of the corps, noted that there were currently 28 dental surgeons out of 60 authorized, and 23 acting dental surgeons of 40 available in the Army, representing a growth of 13 over the fiscal year.[48] This small group had to cover all the military posts in the United States, Alaska, Hawaii, the Philippines, Puerto Rico, China, and Panama. "So you may see, gentlemen," Carpenter said, "that the young man of active mind who longs for a change of scenery and climate may realize his ambition." It is difficult to determine the success of Carpenter's endorsement, but the next examinations for the appointment of acting dental surgeons were held on April 13, 1914, with 28 vacancies yet to be filled.[49,50] By the end of June 1914, the number of dental surgeons was still 28, but acting dental surgeons had grown to 39—an overall increase of 16 from 1913, 29 from June 1912, and 37 from 1911.[51] In a little more than 3 years, the Dental Corps had more than doubled in size (from 30 to 67), but it was still a long way from its authorized strength.

The European War: The American Ambulance, Neuilly, Paris, France, 1914–1916

The outbreak of the war in Europe in August 1914 between the Allied Powers (Great Britain and the British Empire, France, and Russia) and the Central Powers (Germany and Austro-Hungary) did not create any new urgency to resolve the status of the Army's military dentists, but it did spur voluntary American medical and dental involvement in assisting both the British and French. After a brief period of mobility, the fighting in France and Belgium settled into a stalemate in which opposing forces fought from trenches dominated by each other's artillery. Many Americans then in France, either as visitors or residents, wanted to show their sympathy for the suffering of the French people and their gratitude for France's contribution to America's war of independence. At the time, there was a small but

---

EXHIBIT 11-2

APRIL 1, 1912, EXAMINATIONS FOR THE APPOINTMENT OF ACTING DENTAL SURGEON

On April 1, 1912, examinations for the appointment of acting dental surgeon were held at Fort Slocum, New York; Columbus Barracks, Ohio; Jefferson Barracks, Missouri; Fort Logan, Colorado; and Fort McDowell, California. Of 59 candidates, only 9 passed the examination and were appointed. The successful candidates were:

- Dr Mortimer Sanderson of Philadelphia, Pennsylvania;
- Dr Albert Raymond White of Delaware, Ohio;
- Dr Charles Blanchard Seely of Montgomery, Pennsylvania;
- Dr Arthur Theodore Knoder of Columbus, Ohio;
- Dr John William Scovel of San Diego, California;
- Dr Arnett Percy Matthews of Pueblo, Colorado;
- Dr William Archer Squires of Grand Junction, Colorado;
- Dr Frank Coleman Cady of Fredonia, Kansas; and
- Dr John Howard Snapp of Columbus, Ohio.

Data source: (1) Examination of dentists for the Army. *Dental Cosmos*. 1912;54:260. (2) New appointments of acting dental surgeons. *Army & Navy Journal*. Quoted in: *Dental Cosmos*. 1912;54:851–852.

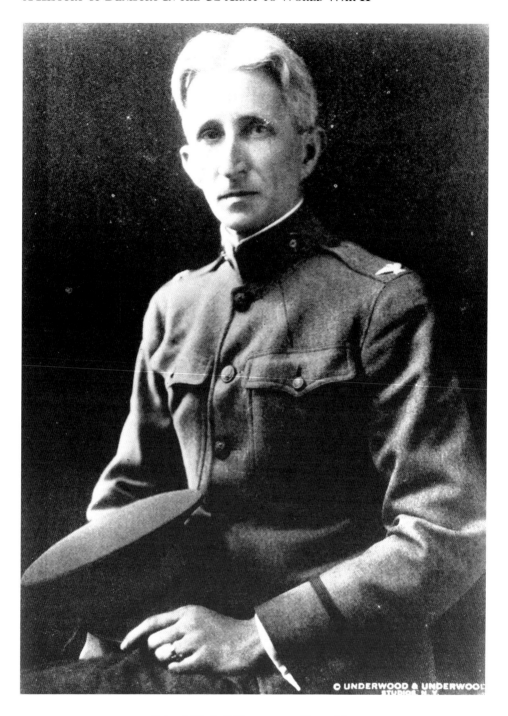

Colonel Edwin P Tignor as president of the
Association of Military Dental Surgeons of the US, 1917–1918.
Photograph: Courtesy of the National Library of Medicine.

complete American hospital at Neuilly, a suburb of Paris. This hospital formed the basis for the organization of an American hospital, called the American Ambulance (in French, "ambulance" means a military hospital).[52]

When the Americans, with the help of the US ambassador, Myron Herrick, proposed plans to organize a military hospital for the Allied wounded, the French minister of war placed at their disposal a large, four-story, nearly completed school building, the Lycee Pasteur, in Neuilly. Under the direction of an American architect and using the advice of American surgeons, the building was transformed into a modern, 400-bed hospital in less than 2 weeks. It was fitted out with operating rooms, a dental department, linen and bandage rooms, diet kitchens, and the latest in X-ray machines and ultra-violet ray filtering devices. On August 4, 1914, Dr George Hayes, an American dentist practicing in Paris, volunteered to organize the dental service for the hospital. On August 7 his offer was accepted and he was appointed to the medical board. This appointment was the first official recognition of the role of the dentist in a military hospital in the war. The hospital received its first wounded on September 7. The staff was made up largely of American and Canadian surgeons, physicians, dentists, nurses, and auxiliaries (the latter recruited from American women living in Paris). The hospital received no subsidy from the French government, the entire expense being borne by the United States.[52–55]

The American Ambulance dental service was under the charge of Hayes and his associate, Dr William Davenport. Hayes worked full time while Davenport worked 7 half days a week. Both men used their own instruments, chairs, engines, and supplies, while operating in a single room in the hospital. They immediately began prophylactic work. All laboratory work had to be sent to Paris because the hospital had neither room nor equipment for it. Shortly after they first starting seeing patients, the hospital's dental department became a center not only for operative and prosthetic dentistry, but also for wounds of the face and jaws. The stalemated, trench warfare that had descended over the western front meant that soldiers sustained head and jaw wounds at an alarming rate. It was estimated that by May 5, 1915, French and Belgian troops had suffered 55,770 facial wounds. Therefore, a high volume of these maxillofacial injury cases came to the hospital from other hospitals, severely taxing the endurance of Hayes and Davenport. Fortunately, other volunteers soon offered their services. In the end, Hayes had recruited a staff of 32, including 8 dentists, 8 dental technicians, 3 apprentices, 10 nurses or aids and 1 secretary.[53–57]

One volunteer dentist, Dr CM LeCron of Saint Louis, Missouri (and later London), reported working with a colleague, Dr WC Roberts, from 8 AM to 6 PM, 7 days a week. He said that it was

> difficult to get men who can conceive ideas for, and construct, appliances for fractured and horribly shattered jaws. . . . The general surgeons appreciate our work and give us due credit. This dental section is making much new history for dentistry and will certainly make the M.D.'s step down and admit that dentistry is an honorable and great profession.

Another volunteer, Dr William Potter (who later served with American forces in France) from the Harvard Dental School said that the oral hygiene program initiated at the hospital was "the most systematic work of the kind inaugurated in any military hospital." He described the facial wounds as follows:

The face is shot through from side to side, from above, below, in reverse and in all sorts of oblique directions. When so shot, either by a rifle ball, a shrapnel ball or a piece of shell casing, the bones of the upper and lower jaw are likely to be fractured. The teeth are often driven as projectiles into the face and there is usually a large loss of bony substance of the jaws.[58,59]

In June 1915 the Philadelphia Dental College sent a volunteer unit to the hospital, composed of Dr Simeon Guilford, dean of the college, and Doctors Dudley Guilford and D Morev Wass. They sailed for Europe on June 13 and arrived in Paris on June 29. Another member of the unit, Dr Carlton Russell, was delayed and left in late July.[60]

By December 1915 the hospital was accommodating about 600 patients, and by August 31, 1916, the dental department consisted of three operating rooms and a well-equipped laboratory. Some of the dental chairs and engines were donated by dentists and others where loaned by dental supply houses. In all, there were 10 dental surgeons, 8 laboratory technicians, and many nurses and assistants. All patients were examined, photographed, radiographed, had study models taken, and, in some cases, had face masks made for a permanent record of the results of treatment. A thorough prophylaxis was also performed and roots and badly decayed teeth were removed under local anesthesia, usually Novocain. Gold was unavailable, so amalgam was used to restore the posterior teeth. Vulcanite dentures were constructed for missing teeth or deformities. Patients with maxillofacial injuries came from other hospitals for treatment. Soldiers wounded at the front arrived for treatment within 48 hours of receiving their injuries. During the year ending August 31, 1916, 371 fractured maxillae cases were admitted to the hospital.[53–56]

American Institute of Dental Teachers: The 1915 "Relief and Aid" Fund

While the American Ambulance was being organized and outfitted, the dental profession in the United States gave increased attention to the events in Europe. On January 26, 1915, at the meeting of the American Institute of Dental Teachers held in Ann Arbor, Michigan, the organization voted to raise a "relief and aid" fund for the European soldiers who had suffered dental and oral wounds. A national committee of prominent dentists was appointed under the chairman, Dr Charles Koch, a Civil War veteran now at Northwestern University, to develop lithographed coupons certifying a contribution to the fund. Their plan was to distribute the contribution certificate booklets at $5 each to dental schools, dental societies, and the profession at large. The certificates were to be printed in lilac ink (the color of the dental profession) and have a red Geneva cross on their faces. It was hoped that a national distribution of the coupons would result in enough donations to help establish several special hospitals or wards for maxillofacial injuries. The Red Cross Society would distribute the funds.[61,62]

Concurrently, another appeal was launched in the United States for a fund to help the American Ambulance Hospital in Paris. The American Red Cross said it would supply disinfectants, gauze and cotton bandages, other hospital supplies, and some financial assistance. Dental supplies were contributed by such companies as the SS White Company, the Ritter Dental Manufacturing Company, and

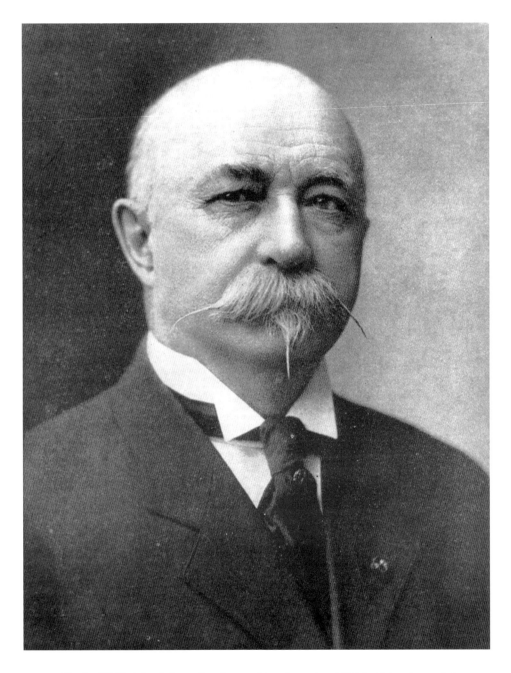

Charles RE Koch headed a national committee of prominent US dentists who created lithographed coupons certifying a contribution to the "relief and aid" fund for European soldiers who had suffered dental and oral wounds.
Photograph: Courtesy of the American Dental Association.

the Buffalo Dental Manufacturing Company. Dr Herbert Wheeler of New York was named the chairman of the national committee in America. In May 1916 Dr Wheeler reported that over $30,000 had been raised for the hospital and was on deposit in a New York City bank. The DuPont family in Wilmington, Delaware, was credited with raising a large portion of the money.[56,63,64]

Opportunities and Missed Opportunities

In a March 1915 editorial titled "Opportunity," Dr Edward Kirk, editor of *Dental Cosmos* and a long-time leader in the civilian dental community, called attention to the war in Europe and the need for "preparedness–readiness to take advantage of the opportunity when circumstances create the opportunity."[65] He repeated that call in another editorial titled "Again, Opportunity" in the November issue. As he saw it, the war in Europe was an ideal opportunity to prove the importance of the dental profession to the military once and for all:

> Suddenly the greater part of the civilized world is engaged in mortal combat; the most devastating war in the history of the human race is now in progress; gunshot wounds of the head and jaws in countless numbers require the skill and specially trained services of the oral surgeon and dental expert. The health and not infrequently the lives of soldiers are jeoparded (*sic*) by the lack of oral hygiene. Bodily infections in wounded soldiers arising from uncleanly mouths are unnecessarily increasing the death-rate in military hospitals, and the demand arises everywhere in connection with military hospitals for the special services that only dentistry and oral surgery can render. The opportunity needed to convince all concerned of the justness and practicality of the demand by the dental profession for the past half-century for a recognition of the importance and efficiency of the service which they are able to render under the circumstances existing is now signally in front of us. . . . Again, the question of successfully solving this problem involves the factor of preparedness upon the part of the dental profession to take advantage of the present opportunity.[65]

Kirk urged the profession to support efforts to establish dental hospital services in Europe on a humanitarian basis. He also urged the dental profession to seize the "opportunity" that the war presented to prove the "justness and practicality" of the profession's demand for the recognition of the importance of military dental surgeons.[65,66]

Dr William Fisher, a former Army contract dental surgeon, reminded American dentists that the US Army had had a dental corps, of sorts, for nearly 14 years, and that it behooved all dentists to support it and to impress their congressmen with the necessity of higher rank for dental surgeons. The "few good men" of the "old original corps," who hung on from year to year hoping for eventual promotion, needed the profession's backing. Each year their resignations created vacancies that became more and more difficult to fill with the "best type" of young dentists.[67]

Actually, the opportunity for military dental surgeons to understand Kirk's argument was already in preparation when his first editorial appeared in March 1915. In April 1915 the US Navy's Bureau of Medicine and Surgery dispatched

Surgeon AM Fauntleroy of the US Navy to France to gather information on the medical and surgical aspects of the war in Europe. Fauntleroy spent 4 months in France collecting valuable information on all medical and surgical areas and served on the operating staff of the American Ambulance for 2 months. Upon his return, the Bureau of Medicine and Surgery published his extensive observations as the "Report on the Medico-Military Aspects of the European War from Observations taken behind the Allied Armies in France" late in 1915.[68]

In the area of dental surgery, Fauntleroy described the work of Doctors Hayes and Davenport and the results they had achieved, noting "one of the most striking features of the value of a dentist in the organization of a military hospital is shown in the results obtained by surgical cooperation with dentists at the American Ambulance in connection with the mutilating wounds of the face."[68] On the growing importance of the dental surgeon in such surgery, he reported:

> One of the surgical advances of the present war has been the recognition of the dentist as a necessary unit in the organization of a military hospital. This has been brought about by the present-day trench warfare. The latter leads to the production of a large number of face and jaw wounds, involving usually a great loss of substance, in the form of bone, teeth, and soft parts. So valuable has this work become that every large military hospital now has its surgical dental department, which works in conjunction with the other surgical services and supplements certain procedures which are indispensable as regards bringing about a favorable result.[68(p100)]

Perhaps with Fauntleroy's recent visit in mind, as well as the visits from numerous other American medical and dental surgeons during the year, Dr Hayes offered to attach a dental surgeon from the Army and Navy to the American Ambulance for 4 months of first-hand experience. On December 19, 1915, Dr Hayes wrote to the US Ambassador in Paris, William Sharp, and asked him to assist with this offer. Hayes believed that the opportunity to gain valuable experience was great because "the work of the Department has developed to such an extent that at the present moment we have one hundred and nineteen cases of fractured jaws under treatment, and during periods of great activity over one fifth of the patients in the Hospital have been cases requiring the services of the dental surgeons for fractures and wounds of the face."[69] Hayes then outlined the extraordinary opportunity offered to study maxillofacial oral surgery:

> It seems to me of great and urgent importance that the proper authorities should become cognizant of the broad extension of this new field of service and of the advantages offered by experience acquired in this Department.

> To the Army and Navy dental Surgeons, who, far more than the ordinary practitioner, are liable to meet with similar fractures and mutilations caused by war projectiles, the American Ambulance through its Dental Department, offers an exceptional opportunity not only for active practical experience, but for study of over three hundred and forty cases treated up to the present, of which complete records are being kept including photographs, plaster models and masks, radiographs, histories and treatments, all of which are going to form a most valuable collection.[69]

Ambassador Sharp forwarded Dr Hayes's offer to the secretary of state, who forwarded it to the secretary of war on February 21, 1916. On March 2 Major General Hugh Scott, acting secretary of war following Garrison's resignation in February, replied to the secretary of state that he doubted the advantages to be gained by sending dental surgeons because of "the liability to violations of neutrality, also on account of the demand of all of our dental surgeons with troops, not to mention the considerable cost which would be involved." He said that all of these developments were already being recorded and taught in American dental schools and were appearing in medical journals. Despite the fact that numerous American military observers, including some from the Medical Corps, had already been in Europe for many months and that Fauntleroy had spent 4 months in France and produced a most valuable report, he believed it "inadvisable" to accept Hayes's offer.[70–72]

Other offers from Dr Hayes were received during 1916. Although no Dental Corps officer was ever sent to the American Ambulance to study its maxillofacial work or to Europe to observe military dental work, an Army medical observer in France after February 1916, Major James Church, Medical Corps (MC), filed several reports on dental topics. On November 17, 1916, he sent back a lengthy, illustrated report on the French Army's horse-drawn and truck-mounted mobile dental wagons that visited rest camps behind the front to care for oral and dental issues, allowing soldiers to return to their units as quickly as their problems allowed.[73] He noted:

> The French are now extending this policy of conservancy by employing specially fitted wagons or automobiles for the care of the men's teeth. Anyone who is familiar with the condition of the teeth of the average enlisted man in our service can appreciate the need of systematic care in any army.[73]

Church also visited the American Ambulance and saw Hayes's maxillofacial work up close. On December 6, 1916, he filed a report on dental surgery that covered the work in the American Ambulance and included photographs of patients and copies of Hayes's annual reports.[74,75] He wrote of Hayes's accomplishments:

> The extended use of Artillery in the present war has occasioned an increase in the wounds attended with extensive mutilation. Serious as these are whatever their anatomical location is, they are more deplorable perhaps when they involve the face, presenting, as they usually do, serious and oftentimes terrible disfigurement. It is not uncommon to see men with a considerable portion of the face shot away and, aside from the loss of function entailed, there is the added distress of being unsightly and hideous objects. . . . The process of repair of these lesions calls for the joint skill of the surgeon and the dentist, and the technical labor of the two professions meets on a common ground in the restoration of function and the repair from a cosmetic standpoint. It is my impression that this work was started by the American Ambulance and since scientific dentistry is a peculiarly American development, it is probable that this is so.[74]

While visiting the hospital, Hayes once again offered to receive an Army dentist attached to observe and work. After seeing the work that was being done, Church immediately realized what a valuable opportunity this was:

Dr. Hayes told me that he would be very glad to extend every facility to an Army Dentist sent here to observe the work: that he could have the opportunity of perfecting himself in this line which is really a new phase of Dental Surgery developed by the war. It is my opinion that the experience so gained would be of very real value to our Dental Corps. The experiences which even one man could acquire would be of value to the entire service. It is true that these methods will, at the proper time, be published, presumably in the form of a text-book, but the steady trend of modern technical teaching is toward a majority of clinical and a minority of didactic instruction. . . . Six months' practical experience at first hand in a clinic such as is offered here would be worth, I am sure, infinitely more than any knowledge gained from a text-book, no matter how good.[74]

Another extensive report on oral and dental surgery was filed by Majors Clyde Ford, MC, and William Lyster, MC, who were medical department observers with the British army. They visited the special maxillofacial surgical hospitals set up to handle those cases in France and England and observed the surgeons' work. They learned that at the beginning of the war, the British and French military and civilian surgeons were totally unprepared for the number and severity of mutilating facial gunshot wounds:

The first of these dreadful cases, falling into the hands of even skilful [sic] general surgeons, suffered a real neglect, not only because of the professional ignorance of surgical principles and operative technique, but on account of a lack of assistance of the dental surgeon. His art—involving the requirements of mechanical skill—is demanded in the treatment of almost all wounds of the face, complicated with fracture and invasions of the cavities of the mouth and nose.[76]

Ford and Lyster were particularly interested in the work at British General Hospital No. 22 in Etaples, France, as well as Stationary Hospital No. 13. Both were operated by volunteers from Harvard University ("The Harvard Unit"), the former under the direction of oral surgeon Varaztad H. (George) Kazanjian, and the latter under Major Valadier, an American dentist serving in the Royal Army Medical Corps (Territorial).[76] Of Kazanjian, they wrote::

The department of oral surgery at General Hospital No. 22, is conducted on a different principle from that of the American Ambulance at Paris, because the services lies wholly within the charge of a dentist, Dr. Kazanjian, who came out to France with the first Harvard Unit, and has remained for some time in charge of the service that he has developed. Dr. Kazanjian in civil practice in Boston confined his professional labors exclusively to dental surgery. It was only when the opportunity was presented by the great number of face injuries of this war that he attempted the plastic work that is associated with the restorative operations on wounds of the face in connection with injuries to the jaw and facial cavities. He has developed an operative technique, in connection with the application of his mechanical devices for support, that is unique in the practice of surgery. Many of the methods employed in the way of restoring the tissues to their normal sites are of such mechanical complication that only a dentist trained in mechanical methods could apply them. The surgeon's resources are certainly limited in comparison with those of a dentist, who has acquired a surgical technique which permits him to do the plastic operations of the face. So much is this the case that it seems apparent, in viewing a large number of badly mutilating wounds of the face which require mechanical methods of restoration, that a good dentist with some surgical technique possesses a better equipment for treatment of these cases than a good surgeon with no mechanical technique. Dr. Kazanjian's cases, which exhibit the results of his treatment, seem to justify this opinion.[76]

During their visits, those in charge of these hospitals offered "to admit Dental Surgeons of the U.S. Army to these clinics, and the promise to give them every assistance in acquiring the technique for this new treatment of these wounds."[76] However, none were ever sent.

On October 26, 1916, when asked to respond to one of the offers that came via the NDA, Colonel Henry Birmingham, acting surgeon general, acknowledged that the idea of sending a dental surgeon to Paris was "very desirable" and recommended First Lieutenant Minot Scott, Dental Corps, then at Fort Sam Houston, Texas, should such a detail be approved. Four days later, the adjutant general turned down the NDA's offer with virtually the same letter that General Scott had sent to the secretary of state on March 2.[77–82] Unfortunately, President Wilson's strict neutrality policy and the War Department's apparent disinterest prevented any active duty Dental Corps officers from going overseas to learn from the experience at Neuilly.[83,84] Although the reports by Church, Ford, and Lyster were probably useful, firsthand experience gained in these hospitals might have paid enormous dividends for the wounded when the American Expeditionary Forces (AEF) arrived in France the next summer and had to build a maxillofacial surgical service from the ground up in 1917 and 1918.

The Dental Corps, 1915–1916

The war in Europe stimulated some interest in the Army Dental Corps among the nation's young dentists. In December 1914 Dr Philip Scheiman of New York wrote to Edward Kirk at *Dental Cosmos* requesting information on the corps. He wanted to know what attracted dentists to the corps, the nature of the services they performed, what experience was necessary, and how many vacancies there were. In May 1915 First Lieutenant Seibert Boak replied to Scheiman's letter, telling him that the Army dental surgeons did all the work that any general practitioner in civilian life would perform, provided they were stationed at a post with a complete operatory. In the field or on an itinerant assignment, they had to limit their work to oral prophylaxis, fillings, and other minor procedures. Of the 92 candidates for the previous three examinations, only 29 had passed, and their average length of time in civilian practice was 2 years and 8 months. Although 10 candidates successfully passed the last examination, only 7 were given contracts because the law made provision for only 40 acting dental surgeons.[85,86]

In March 1915 the surgeon general announced that the next examination for the appointment of acting dental surgeons would be held on April 12, 1915. There were now only nine vacancies to be filled. In July the surgeon general announced that the examinations for appointment as acting dental surgeon would be held on October 18, 1915, with 12 vacancies to be filled.[87] By the end of June 1915 the Dental Corps numbered 34 dental surgeons and 35 acting dental surgeons.[88]

Army dentists spent a great deal of time traveling among the widely scattered posts in the United States and overseas. Itinerant dental surgeons suggested that it would save valuable time if the post surgeons did preliminary oral examinations of the command prior to their arrival at the post to determine which cases demanded immediate treatment. On December 14, 1915, the general staff recommended that the Medical Department adopt this policy. Three days later, the surgeon general's office concurred and issued the memorandum to the various department surgeons. It is not known how medical officers received the news of this extra responsibility, but more pressing to dentists was the small number of dental surgeons available to care for far-flung soldiers.[89]

In addition to this problem, the Army began to slowly expand in 1915 as the conflict in Europe continued. In September 1915 Edwin Tignor wrote that the majority of men then entering the service came from the rural and urban working classes, with a few small-town Americans sprinkled in. Most of these recruits arrived with "pathological mouths." They had never practiced any kind of oral hygiene, nor had they ever used a toothbrush. Each received an oral and physical examination and was given thorough training in all aspects of personal sanitation during the 2 months they were held at the recruit depot. Included in this period was intensive dental care, getting their mouths up to acceptable conditions, and toothbrush issue. Tignor said by the end of their training, most recruits had become conditioned to receiving routine, proper care, forming a lifetime habit that could not but redound to the overall benefit of quality professional dentistry once they reentered civilian life.[90,91]

In 1916 the dental requirements for recruits for the US Army were as follows:

> An applicant must have at least six serviceable double (bicuspid or molar) teeth, two above and two below on one side, and one above and one below on the other side, and so opposed as to serve the purpose of mastication; otherwise he is rejected. Deformities interfering with mastication or speech, chronic ulceration, fissure or perforation of the hard palate, are all causes for rejection.[92(p1071)]

By June 1916, as operations along the Mexican border began, there were 40 first lieutenants and 35 acting dental surgeons in an Army Dental Corps that was authorized 100 total, based on the one-dentist-per-thousand-troops formula.[88] The actual proportion of dentists to soldiers was approximately 1 to 1,300, not including the dependents and civilians entitled to treatment. By contrast, the British army in the field in France in 1916 had only 43 dental surgeons (excluding those with the Canadians).[90,93]

The National Dental Association's Renewed Campaign, 1915–1916

Perhaps spurred on by the war in Europe, in January 1915 the NDA and dental profession renewed their lobbying of Congress and the War Department to reorganize the Dental Corps and give higher ranks to Army dental surgeons. Both the Association of Military Dental Surgeons and the NDA petitioned and met with Surgeon General Brigadier General William Gorgas toward this end. Dr Homer Brown, chairman of the NDA's legislative committee, left a draft of a bill to reorganize the Dental Corps with the surgeon general for consideration. The proposed bill authorized one colonel as the chief of the corps, a number of majors equal to 25% of the corps' authorized strength, and captains and first lieutenants to an extent of 1 to each 1,000 of the Army's authorized strength, including the Hospital and Quartermaster Corps. This proposal would result in 1 colonel, 26 majors, and 81 captains and first lieutenants. Most of the 27 first lieutenants then in service would become field-grade officers, and the remainder of the first lieutenants and 11 acting dental surgeons would become captains. Afterward, a dental surgeon would become captain after 3 years' service, as in the Medical Corps. A recent dental graduate could be commissioned a first lieutenant at 22, captain at 25, and major at 32. The bill also provided for a dental reserve corps similar to the Medical Reserve Corps that had existed since 1908.[94–97]

The surgeon general forwarded the proposed bill to the chief of staff for review. On February 1, 1915, the chief of the War College Division, Brigadier General Montgomery Macomb, recommended to the chief of staff that the War Department reject the proposed bill. He claimed the bill's "effect will be to promote a class of professional men out of the grade and status in which it will be deemed appropriate and proper to extract and fill the teeth of enlisted men." While he admitted that dentists were valuable and necessary for the troops' health, what Macomb really wanted was "presence with troops of dentists who have not such military rank and grade that they will be tempted to prefer supervision to performance." A close reading of Macomb's response to the chief of staff indicates that the general staff preferred the pre-1911 situation to granting commissioned status, and that "continuance of the status of employment which existed prior to 1911, as recommended by the chief of staff in 1910, would have been a safe policy, and the action of the general staff in refusing to approve the bill is vindicated." The general staff articulated a policy position that it continued to use in the years to come. On February 4, the secretary of war, acting on Macomb's recommendation, advised the adjutant general that he did not approve of any legislation for organizing a dental reserve corps or the promotion of dental surgeons to higher grades.[97,98]

Having received no official reply from the surgeon general on the proposed dental bill of January, Homer Brown wrote to him on July 29, 1915:

> We made no effort to have the proposed legislation introduced in the last Congress, because we appreciated your generous reception of our representatives and our specific suggestions, as well as your attitude in general. Therefore, we would much prefer to cooperate with your Department, and the Honorable Secretary of War, to the end that the service be placed upon the highest possible basis, and, at the same time extend to the members of the Army Dental Corps adequate rank and promotion which will be in keeping with the importance of the service and the dignity of our profession, which is endeavoring to cooperate in every possible way with the medical profession's vigorous campaign against disease, of which you have been, and are, an illustrious exponent.[99]

On August 7 Brown wrote to Surgeon General Gorgas again informing him that he had not received any notice as to the general staff's action on the NDA bill, although he had "heard reports regarding their action." He continued, saying, "but will be very glad to be officially advised as to their position in the matter." With the NDA's 1915 meeting scheduled for San Francisco early in September, Brown wanted to be able to provide the members with information. "I think this will be advantageous to all concerned," he said, "as I am particularly anxious to cooperate with your Department and to have the united support of our organization of nearly twenty thousand members." Brown finally received an answer from Major (later Major General) Robert Noble, MC, of Gorgas's staff on August 10: "The provisions contained in the bill submitted were disapproved and no change in the organization of the Dental Corps was recommended by the General Staff."[100,101]

After 17 years of similar responses, the NDA's legislative committee knew enough to push on, regardless of the opposition. On November 3, 1915, the committee met "at some length" with Secretary of War Lindley Garrison and Major General Tasker Bliss to discuss the status of Army dental surgeons. According to Bliss in a memo to the chief of staff, Major General Hugh Scott, Garrison gave "them his views which were generally to the effect that he did not see the necessity of saddling the Government with additional expense in order to secure reasonably good dental service in the Army" on December 6.[102]

Bliss then laid out the details of Garrison's arguments:

> The arguments against the proposed legislation were clearly presented by the Secretary of War to the legislative committee of the National Dental Association when the members of it conferred with him in his office. He then told them that it was not believed to be necessary to create an expensive Corps, with high grades, actual rank and privilege of retirement in order to secure the character of dental service required in the Army; that high grade men, fresh from dental colleges and without an established practice in civil life, even now enter the Army and save money out of their pay during three or four years' service with which they are enabled to set themselves up in civil practice; that it is very likely that men of the highest grade (the class who when they become established in practice are able to charge a fee of perhaps twenty dollars an hour) will leave the service; that if such class of men could be tempted to remain in the service by merely calling them captains and majors or giving them slight increase of pay, they would probably deteriorate rather than advance; that their leaving the service is not an essential loss to the service, because what we need in the Army is simply the professional skill of the ordinary country practitioner; and that if our entrance examinations do not, as they should not, require more than that degree of professional skill, there will be no difficulty in securing all the dental service that is required in the Army.[102]

Bliss concluded that Garrison still disapproved of dental legislation and had not changed since his statement of February 4.[102] Undeterred by Garrison's response and in compliance with his request for a written report, the same day the committee submitted its list of recommendations on how to "increase the efficiency" of the Dental Corps and secure "a more equitable recognition" for the dental profession. It wanted the formation of a dental reserve corps similar to the existing Medical Reserve Corps, which would replace the existing "acting dental surgeons." The committee envisioned that after 2 years of service, some of the dental reservists would be selected for Regular Army commissions as first lieutenants to fill any vacancies in the Dental Corps. Dentists would be promoted to captain after a total of 7 years service in any category (contract, reserve, regular), and the top 25% would become majors. They further urged that one of the senior dentists be commissioned colonel to serve a 4-year term as chief of the Dental Corps. Finally, they accepted the Dental Corps strength ratio of one dentist per thousand soldiers.[103,104]

The NDA draft legislation was forwarded to the surgeon general, War College Division, and the judge advocate for review and comment. Brigadier General Macomb reiterated his division's stand of February 1, concluding:

> Dental surgeons do not require military rank for proper discharge of their duties. As the profession develops, young graduates in touch with the latest methods are offered in the army the opportunity to acquire practice and accumulate savings until they decide upon a location in which to build up practice in civil life. . . . Life tenure, with ultimate place on the retired list, would not tend to stimulate professional zeal.[105]

Macomb cited his February 1 memo in favor of approving only such legislation as would "repeal of so much of the Act of March 3, 1911, as authorizes appointment of dental surgeons with military rank, in order that the number of dentists now holding military rank and grade be not increased."[105]

On November 9 Lieutenant Colonel Henry Fisher, responding for the surgeon general's office, agreed that the Dental Corps did not get the best dentists because of limited promotion potential. Rank was a problem and a dental reserve corps would be "a step in advance." He noted that the NDA committee already knew all of this from a recent visit with Surgeon General Gorgas. His concluding comment on the necessity for a dental colonel was as follows:

> The creating of the grade of Colonel and Chief of the Dental Corps is entirely unnecessary. The duties of such an officer would be limited to recommending the assignment of Dental Surgeons to stations. When such assignments are made the duties of the office would be nominal.[106]

The most balanced analysis came from Brigadier General Enoch Crowder, the judge advocate general of the Army, who recommended entirely redrafting the provisions to present them "in a more logical and coherent manner than is done in the present draft." He apparently accepted the personal and professional arguments being advanced:

> An enactment along the general lines of this draft would undoubtedly be of benefit to the service. It is said that under the present law the best dental college graduates are reluctant to enter the Army, and certainly nothing is more calculated to deaden zeal and reduce efficiency than the knowledge, which the army dental surgeon has now, that no promotion is open to him.[107]

Despite the exchanges going on among the secretary of war, chief of staff, surgeon general, War College Division, and judge advocate general, no one replied to Dr Brown, the chairman of the NDA's legislative committee. On January 14, 1916, Brown, referring to his previous meeting in November, again approached both Secretary of War Garrison and Surgeon General Gorgas regarding rumors in the press of the "reorganization" of the Army and the Dental Corps. Brown understood that "corrective legislation is being considered for the other various departments of the Army," and wanted Garrison and Gorgas to know that "our committee feels that the Army Dental Corps must necessarily receive some favorable consideration under any plan of reorganization of the Army." The dental profession hoped that Garrison and Gorgas would endorse the recommendations that it thought would improve "the service and give to our profession recognition in accordance with the importance of the service rendered."[108]

On January 21 Major General Hugh Scott replied to Brown, writing, "… relative to the changes in the Dental Corps of the Army, the whole matter of increasing the efficiency of the Army is now before Congress, where it must be worked out as a single problem, and it is not practicable at this time to predict just what will be done."[109]

On February 20 Brown sent a telegram to Gorgas opposing recent legislation that he had proposed before the House Committee on Military Affairs on January 26. Brown wrote that "we consider this discriminating as unnecessary and humiliating and must insist that our representatives in the Army be accorded dignified recognition and actual rank in keeping with importance of service rendered." On February 21 Surgeon General Gorgas replied that his "desire is to increase the efficiency of the Dental Corps and to provide for the proper flow of promotion." He posed no objection to the "same provision regarding rank" as was authorized for the Medical Corps.[110,111]

Also on February 20 Dr John Millikin, a former contract dental surgeon and now the president of the Association of Military Dental Surgeons of the United States, chided the surgeon general on the professional inequity in the new proposed Army bill introduced before Congress on January 26. The bill required a dental surgeon to serve 19 years before making major, whereas the medical surgeons would be promoted to major in less than 12 years. To make captain, the dentists would have to serve 9 years, but their counterparts only had to serve 3. And the dental captain would not be a "real captain; only a hybrid." Millikin reminded the surgeon general that the "line" had been trying for many years to deprive "staff" officers of actual military rank. He considered the new law an "entering wedge" for the line and consequently an eventual menace to the Medical Corps.[113]

At the request of the chairmen of the Senate and House military affairs committees, Doctors Brown and Gifford of the NDA's legislative committee appeared before the committees on February 2 and 3, 1916, to testify on the pending general defense legislation and to make sure that their recommendations would not be eliminated. First Lieutenant Edwin Tignor, Dental Corps, joined them for the House testimony. The main efforts of the NDA to date had been directed at securing the support of the secretary of war, chief of staff, surgeon general, and chairmen of the military affairs committees for the incorporation of the association's recommendations in their general defense program. These included the Dental Reserve Corps (DRC) to replace the "acting dental surgeons," appointments from the DRC with 2 years of service at ages 23 to 30, promotions to captain with 7 years total service, majors not to exceed 25% of the corps and promoted by seniority, a colonel as chief of the Dental Corps, strength to be one per 1,000 enlisted strength (as at present), and the right to command limited to Dental Corps and DRC and enlisted dental assistants. [113]

In March 1916 an editorial in *Journal of the National Dental Association* noted that officers of the adjutant general's department, judge advocate general's department, ordnance department, Corps of Engineers, Quartermaster Corps, Signal Corps, and the Medical Corps were all staff officers. They all "have rank the same as all other officers and have had rank for many years, and surely no one has ever contended that either their efficiency or the efficiency of the line of the Army has suffered thereby."[114]

On March 23, 1916, Dr William Crenshaw, the president of the National Association of Dental College Faculties, wrote Senator Lee Overman of North Carolina, requesting that he support the dental amendments of the pending Army reorganization bill to accord appropriate rank for the dental surgeons. On April 10 Crenshaw's letter was presented in the Senate by Senator Smith of Georgia and ordered to be printed in the *Congressional Record*.[104] The War Department's continued opposition to any meaningful new dental legislation meant that Congress would have to step forward to make the changes. As when the Philippine Insurrection opened the way for contract dental surgeons in 1901, it would once again be a present or impending national emergency that forced changes to be made.

Senator Atlee Pomerene's Amendment, 1916

Responding to the NDA's active interest, on April 14, 1916, Senator Atlee Pomerene of Ohio introduced an amendment to the dental provision of the National Defense Act then under discussion:

> The President is hereby authorized to appoint and commission, by and with the advice and consent of the Senate, dental surgeons at the rate of 1 for each 1,000 enlisted men of the line of the Army. Officers of the Dental Corps shall have the rank, pay, and allowances of first lieutenants until they have completed five years of service, when they shall be eligible for promotion to the grade of captain. Officers of the Dental Corps, after 15 years of service, shall be eligible for promotion to the grade of major: Provided, That the number of majors at no time shall exceed 22 percent of the strength of the Dental Corps: Provided further, That the officers of the Dental Corps shall have the rank, pay, and allowances, including the right to retirement on account of age, service, or disability, of officers of like grade in the Medical Corps of the Army, and that service heretofore rendered as contract dental surgeon shall be computed as commissioned service; And provided further, That examinations for promotion in the Dental Corps shall be governed by act of April 23, 1908, section 5, as prescribed for the Medical Corps, except that the examining and review boards shall consist of one medical and two dental officers.[104(p6125)]

Pomerene's amendment was essentially the same as the Senate Military Affairs Committee's provision for Dental Corps promotions to lieutenant, captain, and major, except for the length of time dental officers had to serve before they were entitled to promotion. Pomerene thought the dental profession was due the same rank and recognition that the medical profession enjoyed and that the higher rank would attract the "best of the young men" in the profession. Under the proposal, dental surgeons would have to serve 10 years as first lieutenants before they could be promoted to captain, and 25 years before promotion to major. Pomerene's amendment shortened these periods for promotion to 5 and 15 years respectively.

The amendment was debated quite vigorously; like Senator Pomerene, the majority of the senators taking part in the April 14 debate were supportive of the dental profession. Finally, the Senate agreed that the Pomerene amendment should replace the military committee's amendment.[104,115]

During the final phases of hammering out the new National Defense Act, Homer Brown wrote to Surgeon General Gorgas to congratulate him on how well the Medical Department had fared in the pending bill and to thank him for cooperating with the NDA in the legislative process:

> In the first place I wish to congratulate you upon the favorable consideration given your Department, or at least it would seem to me that you fared particularly well. While all our recommendations were not incorporated in the Dental Corps provisions, yet I think some very positive improvements have been secured. Further, I think this generally harmonizes with your views, as expressed from time to time, and feel confident that you have always had in view the raising of the efficiency of the Corps to its highest possible standard. Under this legislation you will be in a position to bring about results which we hope will be fairly satisfactory to all since we appreciate your fairmindedness. The real point of difference between you and myself has been that I have always contended, as long as other non-combatant Corps have rank, there should be no discrimination made of the Dental Corps and am very glad that this point has seemingly been established by this Congress.[116]

The National Defense Act June 3, 1916, and the Beakes Bill

More than a year into the first world war, an extended debate on American national and military preparedness took place, which ultimately led to a restructuring of the Regular Army and the National Guard. During the months of debate in 1915 and 1916, it became evident that the Army would undergo substantial growth, which would mandate expansions in every branch of the service. The approved bill ultimately provided for large strength increases, expansion and integration of the National Guard's structure with that of the regulars, and the creation of a federal Organized Reserve to back up both components.[117]

Although some of what that the Dental Corps and NDA gained by the National Defense Act was still a compromise, the act provided many things that had been debated in the years since March 3, 1911:

Sec. 10, 39 Stat. 173: Dental Surgeons

Rank, pay, allowances, qualifications, and number of—The President is hereby authorized to appoint and commission, by and with the advice and consent of the Senate, dental surgeons, who are citizens on the United States between the ages of twenty-one and twenty-seven years, at the rate of one for each one thousand enlisted men in the line of the Army. Dental surgeons shall have the rank, pay, and allowances of first lieutenants until they have completed eight years' service. Dental surgeons of more than eight but less than twenty-four years' service shall, subject to such examinations as the President may prescribe, have the rank, pay, and allowances of captains. Dental surgeons of more than twenty-four years' service shall, subject to such examinations as the President may prescribe, have the rank, pay, and allowances of major.[11(p717)]

A May 1916 editorial in the *Journal of the National Dental Association* said:

> While the legislation secured is not altogether satisfactory, it was the best that could be obtained at this time. The Legislative Committee and others worked indefatigably to secure the adoption of an equitable and at the same time conservative bill, but it was found necessary to concede some important features in order to procure the enactment of a dental provision that would grant at least some of the more important objects sought.[115(p212)]

The "centralized handling" by the "well organized" dental association that coordinated the efforts to pass the bill and the elimination of the "cross-purpose" efforts that had caused the defeat of previous congressional dental legislation were the basic reasons for this year's success.[115]

On June 9 Representative Samuel Beakes of Michigan introduced a bill (HR 16355) to amend the section relating to the appointment and promotion of dental officers. The same day, the bill was referred to the Committee on Military Affairs and ordered to be printed. The bill read as follows:

> The President is hereby authorized to appoint and commission, by and with the advice and consent of the Senate, dental surgeons, who are citizens of the United States between the ages of twenty-one and thirty years, at the rate of one for each one thousand enlisted men of the line of the Army. Dental surgeons shall have the rank, pay, and allowances of first lieutenants until they have completed eight years' service. Dental surgeons of more than eight but less than twenty-four years' service shall, subject to such examination as the President may prescribe, have the rank, pay, and allowances of captains. Dental surgeons of more than twenty-four years' service shall, subject to such examination as the President may prescribe, have the rank, pay, and allowances of major: Provided, That the total number of dental surgeons with rank, pay, and allowances of major shall not at any time exceed fifteen: And provided further, That all laws relating to the examination of officers of the Medical Corps for promotion shall be adapted and made analogously applicable to dental surgeons: And provided further, That in computing the length of service of dental surgeons for promotion and other purposes, all such dental surgeons as are otherwise eligible and had service under contract before their appointment as dental surgeons with the rank of first lieutenant under the provisions of the Act approved March third, nineteen hundred and eleven, shall be given credit under this Act for the length of such contract service in addition to credit for service as first lieutenant under the said Act approved March third, nineteen hundred and eleven: And provided further, That all acting dental surgeons who on June third, nineteen hundred and sixteen, were serving under contract the three years' probationary service required by the said Act approved March third, nineteen hundred and eleven, shall, at the expiration of their respective periods of probationary service, become eligible to appointment to the rank of first lieutenant, subject to the examination hereafter required for original appointments under this Act.[118]

On June 10 the bill was referred to the surgeon general's office for comment. Although this amendment did not include all the improvements recommended and supported by the NDA, it was decidedly better than the existing legislation. If and when the new legislation became fully operative, it was estimated that the Dental Corps' strength would increase from its current 75 members (36 first lieutenants and 39 acting dental surgeons) to approximately 200 (full quota) to support an army of 211,000.[119]

On June 30 the surgeon general's office responded that it favored a change in the last two provisions of the bill because of some problems they created in promoting acting dental surgeons.[120,121] On July 6 the secretary of war agreed and informed Representative James Hay, the chairman of the Committee on Military Affairs, that the War Department disapproved of some of the provisos in the bill. It felt that these clauses would work as a "grave injustice" to the acting dental surgeons already in the Army as of June 3, 1916, because the wording prevented their prior service from being counted toward promotion, while prior service would be counted for those already first lieutenants. This resulted in incumbent acting dental surgeons serving another 3 years before promotion, while a dentist just entering service could be commissioned immediately. As a result, the War Department did not recommend the passage of the Beakes bills.[122]

On July 14, 1916, Colonel Henry Birmingham, MC, the acting surgeon general, again recommended that to avoid an injustice to the current acting dental surgeons and also "to provide a probationary term [analogous to that provided in Section 23, Act June 3, 1916, for second lieutenants of the line], " the last two provisos of HR 16350 be changed to include all contract and acting dental surgeon time be credited:

> That hereafter all appointments to the grade of first lieutenant in the Dental Corps shall be provisional for a period of two years, at the close of which period such appointment shall be made permanent if the appointee shall have demonstrated, under such regulations as the President may prescribe, his suitability, and moral, professional and physical fitness for such permanent appointment, but should any appointee fail so to demonstrate his suitability and fitness his appointment shall terminate.[123]

This report was sent to Congress as the War Department's stand on HR 16355.[124]

In June 1916 the adjutant general ruled that the acting dental surgeons currently in the Army could be appointed as first lieutenants in the Dental Corps in the order of their contract, without further examination. This ruling would give them date of rank over the dental surgeons to be commissioned as first lieutenants under the examinations to be held on July 10, 1916, as a result of the new law.[125,126] The law invalidated its 1911 predecessor, which placed all dental first lieutenants below all officers of the Medical Reserve Corps. Judge Advocate General Enoch Crowder concluded that subordinating captains and majors below lieutenants was "untenable under the theory of military rank."[127]

Some other minor changes followed. On June 26, 1916, Senator Miles Poindexter of Washington submitted an amendment to change the maximum age limit for commissions in the Dental Corps from 27 to 30 years. On June 28 Senator Henry Myers of Montana submitted an amendment to allow the commissioning of dental surgeons who were between the ages of 21 and 30. On July 21 Senator Pomerene submitted an amendment allowing service as a contract or acting dental surgeon be credited in computing length of service for promotion and for other purposes under the June 3, 1916, act. These were added in some form to the Army appropriation bill (HR 16460).[104]

The National Defense Act also provided for an Officers' Reserve Corps: "Said corps shall consist of sections corresponding to the various arms, staff corps, and departments of the Regular Army." Under this provision, the surgeon general organized a dental section in the Officers' Reserve Corps. Members of the corps were to be appointed and commissioned by the president as first lieutenants and had to respond to any "call for service in time of war or during any pending National crisis." Officers were appointed for a 5-year period, at the end of which they could be recommissioned subject to any further examinations and qualifications that the president might prescribe. While on active duty, they were entitled to the pay and allowances of their rank, including pension for disability, service incurred; they were not entitled to retirement pay. Appointees had to be between the ages of 22 and 55, graduates of standard dental colleges, and at the time of appointment in active practice in the states in which they resided. They had to pass a prescribed physical and a professional examination conducted by a board of one medical and two dental officers designated by the War Department.[128,132] Although many dentists were eager to get into the Dental Reserve, the surgeon general's office wrestled with procedures well into the fall before implementing that part of the law.[132]

Another feature of the bill was the states' authority to appoint dental surgeons in the National Guard. A state governor could now appoint and commission dental surgeons on the same basis as specified in the Regular Army, namely one to 1,000 enlisted members of the line. Any qualified applicant between the ages of 21 and 35 years of age could be commissioned a first lieutenant.[128]

The effects of the Act of June 3, 1916, on dentists included the following:

- The grade of acting dental surgeon was superseded and all acting dental surgeons were to be commissioned as first lieutenants with date of rank from June 3, 1916, subject to passing the examination.

- Service as contract dental surgeon under the Act of February 2, 1901, and service in the Dental Corps as acting dental surgeon or first lieutenant, under the Act of March 3, 1911, were to be reckoned in computing increased pay, promotion, and retirement.

- Dental surgeons were to rank in the Army according to the date of their commissions in the three existing grades of first lieutenant, captain, and major.

- A dental section in the Officers' Reserve Corps was created.

- Dental surgeons were to receive mounted pay (including costs associated with maintaining a horse).[132]

Some dentists, including the former Army contract dental surgeon, Dr John Millikin, the president of the Association of Military Dental Surgeons, believed that the regulation allowing dentists to enter the Officers' Reserve Corps or the militia only as first lieutenants was unfair to the profession. In the other branches of the Army (with the exception of the chaplain and veterinary sections), commissions were given up to and including the grade of major.[132] However, *Dental Summary* heralded the "advanced recognition" the new law gave to the dental profession and saluted Senator Pomerene and Congressman Julius Kahn, its sponsor in the House, for their efforts. It also praised the NDA for its role.[133]

One dentist, Dr Arthur Hackett, the chairman of the Army and Navy Legislative Committee of the California State Dental Association, condemned the new bill, calling it a "complete failure." He based his argument on the following points:

- The bill had not eliminated the "abominable contract status" because the new members of the corps had to serve for 3 years before being eligible for commission as first lieutenants.

- There was a medical head of the corps, not a dental.

- Under the new law the dental examining boards would consist of not less than three medical officers. One or two dental officers could be on the board also, but the law would be in effect with three medical appointees only. Heretofore, the boards had been composed of one medical officer and two dental surgeons.[134]

Furthermore, Hackett compared the new legislation for the Medical and Veterinary Corps to the Dental Corps. The new provision for the Medical Corps had the effect of promoting every officer below major to that grade "within four years." For the newly established Veterinary Corps, all "former governmental service" was to be counted toward promotion. All were to be major after "twenty years' service." This meant that 35 medical officers not yet in the service would be majors by July 1, 1920, and some veterinarians would be majors in 5 years; whereas it would take 19 years for a dental surgeon to make major.[134]

Hackett commented on the congressional debate:

> Note what some of the Senators had to say. None of our friends knew exactly what we had nor what we wanted. Senator Pomerene, who introduced the bill did not know whether he was asking for more than the Chaplains had or not. Mr. Gallinger believed that our profession already had as much as the Medical Corps and thought we ought to be satisfied with that, when in reality we have not a quarter of what the Medical Corps has nor have we ever asked for half what they have. Mr. Meyers believed our men were enlisted as soldiers and ought to have better recognition. The whole debate shows that Congress does not know our present status nor know what we are asking for. We doubt very much if two per cent of the profession know anything definite about the status of the Dental Corps or made any attempt to aid in this legislative campaign. If we cannot get the constituent societies to work on legislators while the latter are at home, it will be impossible for the National Committee to get results in Washington. An educational campaign should be started right now for the next session of Congress.[134(p640)]

Despite the successes of 1916 the board of trustees of the NDA recommended to its house of delegates that additional changes in Army dental legislation were required to bring the Dental Corps into alignment with the Medical Corps within the Medical Department.[135]

381

The Preparedness League of American Dentists, 1916

As Congress debated the fate of the National Security Act of 1916 and the battle of Verdun raged relentlessly on the western front, several Buffalo, New York, dentists initiated a new "Preparedness League of American Dentists" in association with the NDA in March 1916. Led by Dr J Wright Beach, the league's purpose was to assist the War Department during an emergency by providing its members voluntary service to the Army Dental Corps. Its members agreed to prepare the mouth of at least one Navy or Army recruit to meet military standards of service. Qualified league members were encouraged to apply for entry into the Dental Reserve and to assist in the formation of hospital and Red Cross dental units intended for overseas service. The league also decided to educate the government, universities, and their colleagues on the value of dental surgeons and the need for comprehensive courses dealing with the subject.[136]

Dr Beach and his associates mailed 20,000 circulars to members of the NDA and got a favorable response. Within a year, over 1,500 soldiers and sailors had received free care before entering service, and several hundred league members had served with National Guard units on the Mexican border. Courses on the treatment of maxillofacial war injuries were developed and presented in regional classes, which Beach believed would ultimately be the league's major contribution to the war effort. All league services were on a humanitarian basis with no compensation to the volunteers. There were two types of members, active and associate, the former paying a $1 fee.[136,137]

The incidence of head trauma in the war spurred a renewed emphasis on oral surgery and orthodontic training and the need for all dentists to expand their knowledge in the field. In *Dental Cosmos*, Dr Edward Kirk called for "oral war surgery" to be given "the status and dignity of a distinct specialty." He endorsed the league's view that dental school curricula should include graduate training in this field in order to properly prepare the nation's dentists for military duty. Not only was the proportion of gunshot head wounds much greater in modern war than in previous wars, but the damage done was much greater, resulting in more serious injuries. In 1917 the league (now with a membership of 25,000) responded to Dr Kirk's appeal by arranging for "War Dental Surgery" lectures, such as the ones given weekly from April 10 to June 26, 1917, by the unit located in San Francisco, California. Guest lecturers included Captain Frank Wolven, Millikin, and retired Captain John Marshall.[138–141] By May 1918 the league members countrywide had performed 236,115 dental operations for service members. It was estimated that another 150,000 procedures had been done but not officially reported to the league.[142]

Dental Support on the Mexican Border, 1916–1917

Events along the US-Mexican border from 1915 to 1917 provided the opportunity for the Army to gain additional insights into the demands of modern warfare and formed a demanding field test for the fledgling Dental Corps. Tensions between the Wilson administration and the changing governments in Mexico led

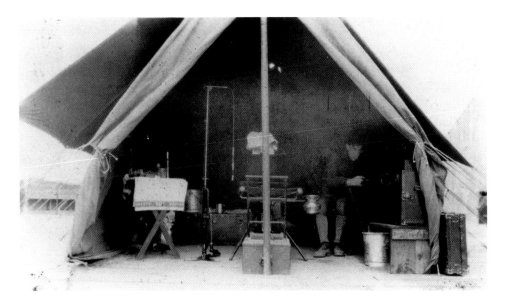

First Lieutenant Raymond W Pearson's dental office was in a tent
during the Punitive Expedition in Mexico.
Photograph: Courtesy of Colonel Raymond W Pearson.

to the assignment of growing numbers of Regular Army units to points along the border. After Pancho Villa's infamous raid on Columbus, New Mexico, on March 8, 1916, the National Guard trained and performed local security while Brigadier General John Pershing led regulars in the Punitive Expedition into Mexico. Although the Army had earlier experimented with the formation of large tactical units, this was the first time it had done so with the changes that the new National Defense Act initiated. The expanded Dental Corps was no exception.[143]

Medical personnel from other parts of the country were levied to support the enlarged forces whenever units deployed to the Mexican border or were formed for large tactical exercises. For example, when the experimental 2nd Division was formed in Texas City, Texas, in 1913, the surgeon general ordered that five dentists, along with their assistants and equipment, be reassigned temporarily from the central department. This team supplemented the five dentists already assigned to the southern department, which was headquartered at Fort Sam Houston, Texas. One of these assigned dentists was at Fort Sill, Oklahoma, and could support the border forces only indirectly by caring for the troops staging through. Of the two dentists based at Fort Sam Houston, one remained there while the other traveled along the lower Rio Grande. There was a dentist each at Fort Bliss, Texas, and at Fort Huachuca, Arizona, both of whom were pinned down by the work at their stations. Because it was unrealistic to expect these dentists to support additional troops, the department surgeon requested permanent assignment of at least three more dentists.[144,145]

To reduce the demands on southern department dentists, unit commanders

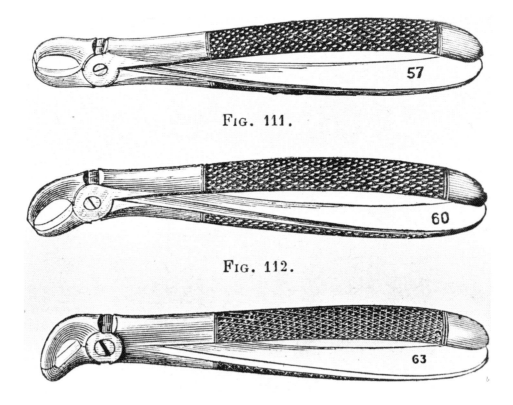

Instruments for tooth extraction, 1913.
Reproduced from: http://wwwihm.nlm.nih.gov/ihm/images/A/12/098.jpg.
Courtesy of: the National Library of Medicine.

were directed to assure that all of their soldiers underwent dental examinations every 6 months, as well as just prior to departure for duty along the border. They were authorized to leave behind, on a dentist's recommendation, all those requiring treatment or who had oral conditions that would take them out of the field before their unit's scheduled return. Four more dentists were assigned to the department and another three were expected, easing the workload. This was essential, as the Regular Army dentists had to provide support to Pershing's forces operating inside Mexico. By the end of 1915 two Regular Army dentists were at Fort Sam Houston, Texas and at Fort Bliss, Texas. Single dentists were assigned to Brownsville and Harlingen, Texas; and Forts Huachuca, Nogales, and Douglas, Arizona. Additional dentists were requested for Douglas, Harlingen, and Laredo.[146–149]

Passage of the National Defense Act almost concurrently with the National Guard mobilization inspired a flurry of interest in appointing dentists into the state formations. The Militia Bureau quickly issued guidelines saying dentists could be commissioned on the basis of one dentist per 1,000 troops and subject to examination by a board of three Medical Department officers from either regular or Guard components approved by the surgeon general's office. Applicants had to be between ages 21 and 35 and dental college graduates with at least 1 year of practice. States were enjoined to provide a roster of those who desired appointment and the Militia Bureau would undertake arranging the necessary boards. National Guard dentists commissioned under the 1914 law were automatically in the system without any further examination, as long as they agreed to take a new oath of office. Acting dental surgeons under the 1914 law had to take the examination, but once they passed, they would become credited with the time they served in the organized militia.[150]

Despite these efforts there was a shortage of dental officers at the border, especially within the federalized National Guard units. The Pennsylvania Guard, for example, was forced to employ a civilian dentist for its 13,000 troops while the appointment process was underway. Mrs George Childs Drexel, the president of the Pennsylvania Women's Division for National Preparedness, agreed to pay for the dental equipment and supplies for a dentist to work for 2 months. About 40 days after the Pennsylvanians had reached the border, Dr C Judson Hollister of Philadelphia arrived at their base, Camp Stewart, near El Paso, Texas. Hollister reported that he was kept quite busy because the 40 commissioned militia dental surgeons and their equipment that were supposedly "on the way" failed to appear. When he left after the 2 months were up, they were still not in camp. Hollister was critical of the poor dental health of the guardsmen he examined and treated.[151]

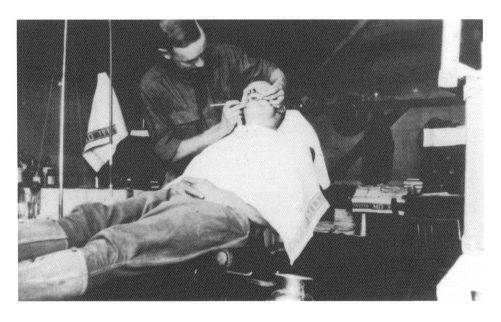

First Lieutenant Raymond W Pearson treats a patient during
the Punitive Expedition in Mexico.
Photograph: Courtesy of Colonel Raymond W Pearson.

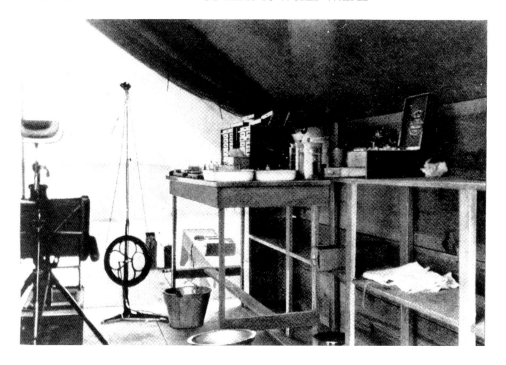

*Doctor C Julian Hollister, contract dentist with the 3rd Pennsylvania Infantry,
National Guard, on the Mexican border at Camp Stewart, El Paso, Texas, 1916.
His description: "A week later I was provided with a 14 x 14 wall tent and fly,
well floored and with shelves for instruments."*
Reproduced from: Dental Digest. *1917;23:3.*

One National Guard dental officer on the scene in 1916 was First Lieutenant Fred Malony, a Creighton University Dental College graduate. He was the dental surgeon for the 5th Regiment, Nebraska Infantry, and was on duty at Llano Grande, Texas. Malony said that there was only one dental outfit for the seven dentists stationed there. This equipment had been turned over to the militia dentists by a Regular Army dentist who took a furlough because of illness. Each dentist was allowed a little over an hour at the chair, and they saw 40 to 60 patients each day. Many soldiers had to go to outside to private civilian dentists to have their work done. The surgeon general's office had ordered 100 dental outfits in July 1916, but as of September, only five had reached the southern department. Malony was told that the heavy demand from Europe for dental material had caught the industry unprepared to cope with the surge of orders accompanying the border mobilization.[152,153]

Malony's dental outfit did not arrive until the end of November—over 7 weeks after he first arrived at the post. Even then, he was not impressed. Although of high quality, the "instruments were not practicable." It was obvious to him they had not been selected by anyone with dental training. Out of 11 pairs of forceps, only one was of any use. Likewise, most of the chisels and mirrors would never have been used in private practice. Because gold and porcelain work was not authorized, no instruments were included for that kind of work, assuring that soldiers desiring it would have to resort to civilian dentists.[153–156]

Malony was equally upset with the lack of command support. Although the soldiers were requested to have a toothbrush, its condition or use was a matter of indifference. Malony felt the command should issue quality toothbrushes just as it did tape for blisters and should stress proper brushing. Every week the soldiers underwent a medical inspection for bodily cleanliness, but only once in his 7 months on the border was there a "partial dental inspection." Ninety percent of the patients he examined had pyorrhea, but he could do little for them under existing conditions.[153]

He concluded his jeremiad by describing working conditions and their effect on patients:

> The dental office was in the farthest back room of an old hotel now being used as the Camp Hospital. I expect that room was 12 x 14 feet. Of course, when my outfit came there was not room in there for two chairs, so I was placed in the back part of the dispensary, and on windy days and cold days I had to stop work. Later on, in January, there was a little shack put up for a dental office which would accommodate two chairs. But by that time the men were so disgusted trying to get dental work done that we did not have many patients.[153(p346)]

First Lieutenant Ralph Irwin Parker of Burton, Ohio, who had been commissioned on August 28, 1916, and was assigned to the 5th Ohio Infantry as it left for El Paso, Texas, also found the dental condition of the border troops "deplorable." He too complained about not receiving his dental instruments. By the time he left in December 1916, he still had not received his own equipment, which he asked for when he joined his unit in September. Fortunately, he had brought a few of his own tools, enabling him to perform some procedures. He criticized the government instrument selection, saying it demonstrated "a lack of understanding as regards the needs of the dental surgeon . . . I told one medical officer that I could take the whole outfit and cut it down from five cases to three, and still have an outfit worthy of any first-class dentist." He felt the selection of instruments should be the responsibility of a Dental Corps officer, not a doctor in the surgeon general's office.[157–159] He also commented:

> When I first arrived the men were very antagonistic, and called us doctors "Butchers," and other names, quite in keeping with the above; but later, through tact and a little courtesy, I gained their good will, and they realized that I was doing the best that I possibly could for them. . . . Speaking frankly, I observed that too many dentists accepted their commissions as dental surgeons to the guard solely for the good time they anticipated, and considered the call an outing rather than one of serious consequence, the result being poorer dentists, and a never-ending friction between the troops and dental surgeons.[157(p343)]

On September 13, 1916, Lambert Oeder, a private then serving in Battery D, 2nd Field Artillery, New York National Guard and a graduate of the New York College of Dentistry, was commissioned a first lieutenant in the Dental Corps. He reported that an examination of the soldiers revealed that the average guardsman's teeth were in "dire need" of dental attention. Many had never seen a dentist, presuming they could let their teeth go and get "a false set some day."[160–166]

John Puffer, a graduate of the Indiana Dental College, was serving as a sergeant at Field Hospital No. 1 at Llano Grande, Texas when he was commissioned a first lieutenant, Dental Corps, Indiana National Guard, on October 6, 1916. He was appointed dental surgeon for the 2nd Regiment, Indiana Infantry. Puffer also complained of the dental inadequacies on the border. He stated that although the spirit of cooperation was high, the militia dental corps was not well organized when it reached the border, and there was a long wait for the dental equipment. Extraction was, for a time, the only treatment available. He said 94% of the 3,800 men he examined needed some kind of care, and most of the work should have been done before the militia was federalized. As it was, he estimated at least twice the number of dentists were required to meet the needs of all the soldiers.[167–169]

Private dental clinics, such as the Forsyth Institute and the Rochester Dental Dispensary, were also pressed into service under the auspices of the Preparedness League to treat the National Guard troops mobilized for the border but who were still in their armories. The Forsyth, by arrangement with the adjutant general of the Commonwealth of Massachusetts, treated over 409 recruits in a 2-day period. Sixty-five chairs were kept busy for 1962 fillings, 188 cleanings, 211 silver nitrate applications, and 271 extractions.[170]

The arrival of so many people new to military dentistry at a time of great stress underlined the need for some kind of training. Dentists had been dropped into the Army with little orientation since the first contractors, and those who had survived the experience thought that entry orientation was highly desirable. It was apparent that new dentists, regardless of component, required an introduction to the military, and with so many troops at the border, the time seemed right. Accordingly, Captain Robert Oliver, who was stationed at Fort Sam Houston, secured the authority of the surgeon of the El Paso District in September 1916 to establish a dental school.[171]

Oliver developed a modest curriculum and the first class began in late October. The school was established at Base Hospital No. 2 at Fort Bliss, and all dentists in the area were required to attend a weekly 2-hour session (physicians were also welcome). One hour was devoted to "Dento-Military" topics such as Army Regulations, paperwork, military justice, supply accountability, and field craft. The second hour focused on professional topics in which students shared experiences and treatment methods were discussed. The school served as a model for similar efforts in the mobilization camps after the April 6, 1917, declaration of war against Germany. By then the border crisis had passed. Pershing's force was back by January, and forces began to return to their home bases and armories.[172]

A World War Looms

The declaration of war resulted in the surgeon general's first request to identify dentists who could be spared from the border to go to induction and recruiting sites elsewhere. Five dentists were quickly identified and reassigned.[173] The lessons learned at Oliver's school and in the field were about to be applied under all the stresses of modern war. While some preparations for entry into the war had already been made, the Medical Department and its dental corps, like the rest of the US Army and the nation, were ill-prepared for the tremendous challenges of mobilization, training, supply, movement, and fighting the modern ground war that loomed ahead across the Atlantic Ocean in France.

References

1. National Archives and Records Administration. Record Group 112. Surgeon general to adjutant general, March 11, 1911. Memorandum. No. 136287. Box 956. Entry 26.

2. National Archives and Records Administration. Record Group 112. LP Mitchell, assistant comptroller of the treasury, to secretary of war, April 6, 1911. Letter. No. 136287.

3. National Archives and Records Administration. Record Group 112. George H Torney, surgeon general, to secretary of war, April 15, 1911. Letter with enclosure; Form 142, War Department, surgeon general's office, circular of information concerning the employment of dental surgeons in the United States Army. No. 136287.

4. National Archives and Records Administration. Record Group 112. Form 142, surgeon general's office. Memorandum concerning the employment of dental surgeons in the United States Army, April 6, 1905. No. 136287.

5. National Archives and Records Administration. Record Group 112. First endorsement, Henry P McClain, adjutant general, to Torney, April 22, to Torney to secretary of war, April 15, 1911. No. 136287.

6. National Archives and Records Administration. Record Group 94. Memorandum to the adjutant general, Major General Leonard Wood, chief of staff, April 21, 1911. No. 1773938 (filed in no. 524625). Box 965. Entry 26.

7. National Archives and Records Administration. Record Group 112. George H Torney to adjutant general. Memorandum of changes in Army Regulations made necessary by that portion of the act approved March 3, 1911, that establishes a Dental Corps, April 25, 1911. No. 136287.

8. National Archives and Records Administration. Record Group 112. Third endorsement, Brigadier General Enoch H Crowder, judge advocate general, to adjutant general, May 24, 1911. Letter with enclosure, "Draft memorandum for the secretary of war, chief of staff," May 1911 (no day). No. 1773938-A (filed in no. 136287).

9. National Archives and Records Administration. Record Group 165. Draft memorandum for the secretary of war, chief of staff, May, 1911. General staff report no. 6839. Box 67. Entry 5.

10. National Archives and Records Administration. Record Group 112. Lieutenant Colonel Torney, December 22, 1905, to Marshall to commanding officer, US Army Hospital, Presidio. Endorsement. No. 77614.

11. US Medical Department. Chap 19. *The Military Laws of the United States 1915. With Supplement Including the Laws of the Sixty-Fourth Congress, to March 5, 1917.* 5th ed. Washington, DC: Government Printing Office; 1917.

12. National Archives and Records Administration. Record Group 112. Mitchell to secretary of war, April 6, 1911. Letter. No. 136287.

13. National Archives and Records Administration. Record Group 165. Memorandum for the adjutant general, Major General Leonard Wood, chief of staff, May 26, 1911. General staff report no. 6839.

14. National Archives and Records Administration. Record Group 165. Memorandum for the adjutant general, Major General Leonard Wood, chief of staff, May 16, 1911. General staff report no. 6839.

15. National Archives and Records Administration. Record Group 25. Major General JF Bell, commanding, Philippines Division, to the adjutant general, July 21, 1911. Letter. No. 1379686. Box 5364. Entry 25.

16. National Archives and Records Administration. Record Group 165. Memorandum for the secretary of war, Major General Leonard Wood, chief of staff, September 11, 1911. General staff report no. 7671. Box 75. Entry 5.

17. National Archives and Records Administration. Record Group 94. Third endorsement, Surgeon General Torney to chief of staff, September 1, 1911, to letter, Bell to the adjutant general, July 21, 1911. No. 1379686.

18. National Archives and Records Administration. Record Group 165. Memorandum for the adjutant general, Major General William H Carter, acting chief of staff, September 30, 1911. General staff report no. 7671.

19. National Archives and Records Administration. Record Group 25. War Department general order no. 135, Major General William H Carter, acting chief of staff, October 6, 1911. No. 1379686.

20. Torney GH. Surgeon-General Torney on the new status of Army dental surgeons. *Dental Cosmos*. 1911;53:560–561.

21. Litch WF. Army dental service as a career. *Dental Brief*. 1911;16:351–352.

22. Litch WF. The dental school curriculum in its relation to Army dental service. *Dental Brief*. 1911;16:435–436.

23. National Dental Association Southern Branch [proceedings]. *Dental Cosmos*. 1911;53:1057–1058.

24. National Archives and Records Administration. Record Group 94. Memorandum for the chief of staff, Brigadier General Montgomery M Macomb, chief, War College Division, office of the chief of staff, February 1, 1915. No. 524625. Box 3645. Entry 25.

25. National Archives and Records Administration. Record Group 94. Memorandum for the chief of staff, Brigadier General Montgomery M Macomb, chief, War College Division, office of the chief of staff, November 19, 1915. No. 2349195 (filed in no. 524625). Box 3645, Entry 25.

26. National Archives and Records Administration. Record Group 165. Memorandum for the chief of staff, Brigadier General Joseph E Kuhn, chief, War College Division, April 9, 1917. General staff no. 8954-4 (filed in general staff no. 8954). Box 377. Entry 296.

27. National Archives and Records Administration. Record Group 165. Memorandum for the chief of staff, Colonel FE Lacey, Jr, acting director, War Plans Division, August 18, 1919. General staff no. 8954-25 (filed in general staff no. 8954).

28. Fisher WC. Another view of the new status of the Army dental surgeon. *Dental Cosmos*. 1911;53:690–691.

29. Bryant EA. Facts relating to the obtaining of commissioned rank for the Army dental surgeon. *Dental Cosmos*. 1911;53:830.

30. Bryant EA. Further facts about Army Dental Corps legislation. *Dental Brief*. 1911;16:499–502.

31. Crenshaw W, Deford WH, Rodgers CW. Report of the Committee on Army and Navy Dental Legislation. In: *Transactions of the National Dental Association*. Philadelphia, Pa: The SS White Dental Mfg Co; 1912: 28.

32. National Archives and Records Administration. Record Group 112. Brigadier General George H Torney, June 27, 1912. Memo. Box 54. Entry 242.

33. Public oral hygiene meeting. *Dental Cosmos*. 1911;53:1438.

34. National Archives and Records Administration. Record Group 393. Special order no. 125, George Andrews, adjutant general. Headquarters, Department of the East, June 5, 1911. No. 37233. Box 147. Entry 1486.

35. National Archives and Records Administration. Record Group 112. Colonel LM Maus, chief surgeon, Eastern Division, to the surgeon general, May 22, 1912. No. 142174. Box 1013. Entry 26.

36. National Archives and Records Administration. Record Group 112. Colonel LM Maus to commanding general, Eastern Division, December 1912. Letter. No. 142174. Box 1013. Entry 26.

37. National Archives and Records Administration. Record Group 112. Major General TH Barry, commanding, Eastern Division, to the adjutant general, January 2, 1913. No. 142174. Box 1013. Entry 26.

38. National Archives and Records Administration. Record Group 112. Colonel LM Maus, department of surgery, to surgeon general, June 23, 1913. Memo. No. 146076. Box 1044. Entry 26.

39. National Archives and Records Administration. Record Group 112. Special order no. 293, Colonel Edwin F Glenn, chief of staff, eastern department, December 18, 1914. No. 146076. Box 1044. Entry 26.

40. Bryant EA. The state militia dental corps. *Dental Brief*. 1911;16:935.

41. [Kirk EC]. The Army Dental Corps. *Dental Cosmos*. 1914;56:1375.

42. Boak SD. Militia dental surgeons. *Dental Cosmos*. 1914;56:1351–1352.

43. Office of The Surgeon General. *Annual Report of the Surgeon General, 1912*. Washington, DC: Government Printing Office; 1912.

44. Examination of dentists for the Army. *Dental Cosmos*. 1912;54:260.

45. New appointments of acting dental surgeons. *Army & Navy Journal*. Quoted in: *Dental Cosmos*. 1912;54:851–852.

46. Office of The Surgeon General. *Annual Report of the Surgeon General, 1913*. Washington, DC: Government Printing Office; 1913.

47. [Tignor EP]. National Dental Association, Wednesday: second session. In: *Transactions of the National Dental Association*. Philadelphia, Pa: The SS White Dental Mfg Co; 1913: 10.

48. Office of The Surgeon General. *Annual Report of the Surgeon General, 1914*. Washington, DC: Government Printing Office; 1914.

49. Carpenter A. Army Dental Corps. In: *Transactions of the National Dental Association*. Philadelphia, Pa: The SS White Dental Mfg Co; 1914: 13.

50. Examination of dentists for the U.S. Army. *Dental Cosmos*. 1914;56:408.

51. Office of The Surgeon General. *Annual Report of the Surgeon General, 1915*. Washington, DC: Government Printing Office; 1915.

52. Bacon R. The American ambulance: Neuilly-sur-Seine (Paris). *J Allied Dent Soc*. 1915;10:483–488.

53. Herrick MT. Dental service in the Army. *Dental Summary*. 1917;37:399–402.

54. Robinson F. A few remarks on the role of the American dentists in Paris during the Great War. *Dental Items of Interest*. 1923;45:213–214.

55. Guilford SH. American ambulance hospital and its work. *Oral Hygiene*. Quoted in: *Dental Record*. 1916;36:210–211.

56. Urgent appeal for the foundation of a special American dental hospital at Paris, for the relief of sufferers from wounds of the face and jaws sustained in the war. *Dental Cosmos*. 1915;57:1297–1298.

57. Ring ME. The life and work of Dr. George Byron Hayes, pioneer maxillofacial surgeon. *J Hist Dent*. 1999;47:105–109.

58. [LeCron CM]. Extracts from an interesting letter from France. *Am Dent*. 1915;1:9.

59. [Potter WH]. American dentists doing good work for wounded French soldiers. *Am Dent*. 1915;1:9.

60. Philadelphia Dental College sends new unit of dental surgeons to serve wounded French soldiers. *Am Dent*. 1915;1:9.

61. Red Cross fund for oral and dental injuries. *Dent Rev*. 1915;29:302.

62. Relief of soldiers dentally injured in European war. *Dent Reg*. 1915;69:149–150.

63. Special American hospital in Paris for wounds of the face and jaws. *Dental Summary*. 1916;36:81.

64. Wheeler HL. American hospital in Paris. *J Natl Dent Assoc*. 1916;3:198,215.

65. [Kirk EC]. Opportunity. *Dental Cosmos*. 1915;57:343–345.

66. [Kirk EC]. Again, opportunity. *Dental Cosmos*. 1915;57:1294–1295.

67. Fisher WC. The European war and the dental surgeon. *Dental Cosmos*. 1915;57:70–71.

68. Fauntleroy AM. *U.S. Navy, Report on the Medico-Military Aspects of the European War from Observations Taken Behind the Allied Armies in France*. Washington, DC: Government Printing Office; 1915.

69. National Archives and Records Administration. Record Group 94. George B Hayes, American Ambulance Hospital, to William G Sharp, American Ambulance, December 19, 1915. Letter. No. 2373021. Box 8111. Entry 25.

70. National Archives and Records Administration. Record Group 94. William G Sharp to secretary of state, January 15, 1916. Letter. No. 2373021.

71. National Archives and Records Administration. Record Group 94. Frank S Polly, State Department, to secretary of war, February 21, 1916. Letter. No. 2373021.

72. National Archives and Records Administration. Record Group 94. HL Scott, acting secretary of war, to secretary of state, March 2, 1916. Letter. No. 2373021.

73. National Archives and Records Administration. Record Group 165. Major James Robb Church; Vehicles for dental service in the French Army, November 17, 1916. Report. No. 9514-2, Army War College. Box 452. Entry 296.

74. National Archives and Records Administration. Record Group 165. Major Church; Dental surgery, December 6, 1916. Report. No. 9514-3, Army War College. Box 452. Entry 296.

75. Church JR. *The Doctor's Part: What Happens to the Wounded in War*. New York, NY: D Appleton and Co; 1918.

76. National Archives and Records Administration. Record Group 165. Majors Clyde S Ford and William J Lyster, Medical Corps; Oral and dental surgery and special hospitals, April 27, 1917. Report. No. 9514-4, Army War College. Box 452. Entry 296.

77. National Archives and Records Administration. Record Group 94. Dr Herbert L Wheeler to secretary of war, July 31, 1916. Letter. No. 2442571 (filed with no. 2194596). Box 7598. Entry 25.

78. National Archives and Records Administration. Record Group 94. PC March to Wheeler, August 16, 1916. Letter. No. 2442571 (filed with no. 2194596). Box 7598. Entry 25.

79. National Archives and Records Administration. Record Group 94. LaFayette L Barber, president, National Dental Association, to President Woodrow Wilson, October 9, 1916. Letter. No. 2373021.

80. National Archives and Records Administration. Record Group 94. LaFayette L Barber, president, National Dental Association, to President Woodrow Wilson, October 23, 1916. Letter. No. 2373021.

81. National Archives and Records Administration. Record Group 94. Colonel HP Birminghan, acting surgeon general, to adjutant general, October 26, 1916. Letter. No. 2373021.

82. National Archives and Records Administration. Record Group 94. Adjutant general to Barber, October 30, 1916. Letter. No. 2373021.

83. National Archives and Records Administration. Record group 112. First Lieutenant SD Boak to Major Robert Noble, surgeon general's office, March 23, 1915. Letter. No. 138037. Entry 26.

84. National Archives and Records Administration. Record group 112. Major Robert Noble, surgeon general's office, to First Lieutenant SD Boak. March 26, 1915. Letter. No. 138037. Entry 26.

85. Scheiman P. The Army dental surgeons corps. *Dental Cosmos*. 1915;57:72.

86. Boak SD. Information regarding the Army dental surgeons corps. *Dental Cosmos*. 1915;57:546.

87. Examination of dentists for the U.S. Army. *Dental Cosmos*. 1915;57:360,836.

88. Office of The Surgeon General. *Annual Report of the Surgeon General, 1916*. Washington, DC: Government Printing Office; 1916.

89. National Archives and Records Administration. Record group 165. Cooperation of medical officers at posts in making preliminary examinations, etc, December 14, 1915. Report no. 12232. Box 125. Entry 5.

90. Tignor EP. The educational value of oral hygiene in the Army. *Dental Items of Interest*. 1916;38:59–60.

91. Bernheim JR. Oral hygiene in the Army. *J Nat Dent Assoc*. 1917;4:501.

92. [Kirk EC]. Dental inefficiency. *Dental Cosmos*. 1916;58:1071.

93.   [Pedley FN]. The lack of dentists at the front. *NY Med J*. Cited in: *Tex Dent J*. 1917;35:32–33.

94.   National Archives and Records Administration. Record Group 112. Dr William C Fisher, president, Association of Military Dental Surgeons, to Surgeon General Gorgas, January 12, 1915. Letter. No. 106047. Box 712. Entry 26.

95.   National Archives and Records Administration. Record Group 112. Adjutant General McCain to Surgeon General Gorgas, February 5, 1915. Letter. No. 106047. Box 712. Entry 26.

96.   National Archives and Records Administration. Record Group 112. Dr Homer C Brown, chairman, legislative committee, National Dental Association to Surgeon General Gorgas, July 29, 1911. Letter. No. 106047. Box 712. Entry 26.

97.   National Archives and Records Administration. Record Group 94. Brigadier General Montgomery M Macomb, chief of War College Division, office of the chief of staff, to chief of staff, February 1, 1915. Memo. No. 524625. Box 3645. Entry 25.

98.   National Archives and Records Administration. Record Group 94. Chief of staff to adjutant general, February 4, 1915. Memo. No. 524625. Box 3645. Entry 25.

99.   National Archives and Records Administration. Record Group 112. Brown to Gorgas, July 29, 1915. Letter. No. 106047.

100. National Archives and Records Administration. Record Group 112. Brown to Gorgas, July 7, 1915. Letter. No. 106047.

101. National Archives and Records Administration. Record Group 112. Major Robert E Noble to Dr Brown, August 10, 1915. Memo. No. 106047.

102. National Archives and Records Administration. Record Group 94. Memo for the chief of staff, Major General Tasker H Bliss, chief, Mobile Army Division, December 6, 1915. No. 2349195 (filed with no. 524625). Box 3645, Entry 25.

103. National Archives and Records Administration. Record Group 94. Homer C Brown, et al, legislative committee, National Dental Association, to secretary of war, November 3, 1915. No. 2349195 (in no. 524625). Box 965. Entry 26.

104. *Congressional Record, 64th Cong, 1st Sess*. Vol 53. Washington, DC: Government Printing Office; 1916.

105. National Archives and Records Administration. Record Group 94. Memorandum for the chief of staff, Brigadier General MM Macomb, chief, War College Division, November 19, 1915. No. 2349195 (filed in no. 524625). Box 3645. Entry 25.

106. National Archives and Records Administration. Record Group 165. Lieutenant Colonel Henry C Fisher, acting surgeon general, to chief of staff, November 9, 1915. Memo. Report no. 11650. Box 122. Entry 5.

107. National Archives and Records Administration. Record Group 94. Memorandum for the chief of staff, Enoch Crowder, the judge advocate general, November 24, 1915. No. 2349195 (filed with no. 524625). Box 3645. Entry 25.

108. National Archives and Records Administration. Record Group 112. Brown to secretary of war and Surgeon General Gorgas, January 14, 1916. Letter. No. 106047. Box 712. Entry 26.

109. National Archives and Records Administration. Record Group 165. Major General HL Scott to Homer C Brown, legislative committee, National Dental Association, January 21, 1916. Report no. 11650. Box 122. Entry 5.

110. National Archives and Records Administration. Record Group 112. Brown to Surgeon General Gorgas, February 21, 1916. Telegram. No. 106047. Box 712. Entry 26.

111. National Archives and Records Administration. Record Group 112. Gorgas to Dr Brown, February 21, 1916. Telegram. No. 106047. Box 712. Entry 26.

112. National Archives and Records Administration. Record Group 112. Dr John D Millikin to Surgeon General Gorgas, February 20, 1916. Letter. No. 106047. Box 712. Entry 26.

113. Legislative Committee of the National Dental Association. Dentists in the Army and Navy. *Dent Reg*. 1916;70:184–187.

114. Why the dental profession is entitled to rank. *J Nat Dent Assoc*. 1916;3:108.

115. Recent Army dental legislation. *J Nat Dent Assoc*. 1916;3:212–214.

116. National Archives and Records Administration. Record Group 112. Homer C Brown, National Dental Association Legislative Committee, to Surgeon General William C Gorgas, May 25, 1916. Letter. No. 106047. Box 712. Entry 26.

117. Ganoe WA. *The History of the United States Army*. New York, New York: D Appleton and Co; 1924: 456.

118. National Archives and Records Administration. Record Group 112. HR 16355, 64th Cong, 1st sess, June 9, 1916. Bill. No. 106047. Box 712. Entry 26.

119. Brown HC. New legislation effecting the Army Dental Corps. *J Nat Dent Assoc*. 1916;3:200.

120. National Archives and Records Administration. Record Group 94. Adjutant General McCain to Samuel W Beakes, Medical Corps, June 10, 1916. Letter. No. 524625. Box 3645. Entry 25.

121. National Archives and Records Administration. Record Group 94. Endorsement, Colonel Henry P Birmingham, acting surgeon general, to Adjutant General McCain, June 30, 1916. Letter. No. 524625. Box 3645. Entry 25.

122. National Archives and Records Administration. Record Group 94. Secretary of War Baker to James Hay, July 6, 1916. Letter. No. 524625. Box 3645. Entry 25.

123. National Archives and Records Administration. Record Group 94. Colonel Birmingham to adjutant general, July 14, 1916. Memo. No. 524625. Box 3645. Entry 25.

124. National Archives and Records Administration. Record Group 94. Endorsement, Colonel Birmingham to adjutant general, July 29, 1916. No. 524625, Box 3645. Entry 25.

125. National Archives and Records Administration. Record Group 112. Surgeon General Gorgas to Adjutant General McCain, June 15, 1916. Letter. No. 106047. Box 712. Entry 26.

126. National Archives and Records Administration. Record Group 112. Endorsement, Adjutant General McCain to Surgeon General Gorgas, June 17, 1916. Letter. No. 106047. Box 712. Entry 26.

127. National Archives and Records Administration. Record Group 112. Judge advocate general, first endorsement to adjutant general's office, August 19, 1916. Letter. No. 162230. Box 1165. Entry 26.

128. Brown HC. Information relating to dental legislation and its application. *J Nat Dent Assoc*. 1916;3:317–318.

129. Information relating to appointments in the Dental Reserve Corps of the Army. *Dental Cosmos*. 1917;59:573.

130. National Archives and Records Administration. Record Group 112. First endorsement, to letter from EC Brachfield, DDS, September 27, 1916. Letter. No. 160906. Box 1159. Entry 26.

131. Army Dental Corps. *J Nat Dent Assoc*. 1917;4:185.

132. Millikin JD. Officers Reserve Corps. *J Nat Dent Assoc*. 1917;4:282.

133. New legislation affecting the Army Dental Corps. *Dental Summary*. 1916;36:519.

134. Hackett AE. Recent legislation affecting the Army Dental Corps. *Dent Items Interest*. 1916;38:639–640.

135. Our Army and Navy. *J Allied Dent Soc*. 1917;12:151.

136. Preparedness League of American Dentists. *Dental Summary*. 1916;36:519–520.

137. Beach JW. Preparedness League of American Dentists, our first birthday. *J Nat Dent Assoc*. 1917:363–364.

138. [Kirk EC]. Dental and oral war surgery. *Dental Cosmos*. 1916;58:1419–1421.

139. Patriotic duty of American dentists. *Tex Dent J*. 1917;35:40.

140. Conly TW. Dental preparedness. *Pacific Medical Journal*. 1917;60:348–349.

141. Value of the orthodontist in the military service. *International Journal of Orthodontia*. 1917;3:307–308.

142. Ash CE. Preparedness League of American Dentists. *American Dentist*. 1918;7:16.

143. Clendenan CC. *Blood on the Border: the U.S. Army and the Mexican Irregulars*. New York, NY: Macmillan Co; 1969.

144. National Archives and Records Administration. Record Group 112. Andrews to commanding general, central department, March 13, 1913. Telegram. No. 144904. Box 1036.

145. National Archives and Records Administration. Record Group 112. Department surgeon [Colonel WO Emby], to surgeon general's office, September 24, 1913. Letter. No. 146814. Box 1049. Entry 26.

146. National Archives and Records Administration. General order no. 30, October 27, 1914, headquarters, southern department. No. 154983. Box 1111.

147. National Archives and Records Administration. Record Group 112. Department surgeon first endorsement, December 23, 1915 to surgeon general's office letter, November 29, 1915. No. 146814. Box 1049. Entry 26.

148. National Archives and Records Administration. Record Group 395. Pershing to Farnsworth, September 28, 1916. Message. Entry 1187.

149. National Archives and Records Administration. Record Group 395. Farnsworth to Pershing, September 29, 1916. Message. Entry 1187.

150. National Archives and Records Administration. Record Group 112. Chief militia bureau to all adjutants general, June 23, 1916, dental surgeons, National Guard. No. 193261. Box 681. Entry 26.

151. Hollister CJ. With our militia at the border. *Dental Digest*. 1917;23:1–4.

152. National Archives and Records Administration. Record Group 112. Department surgeon to commanding general, southern department, September 22, 1916. Memo. No. 158779. Box 1142. Entry 26.

153. Malony FC. Dental conditions among state troops on the border. *Dental Summary*. 1917;37:344–346.

154. National Archives and Records Administration. Record Group 168. Nebraska dental surgeons. Brigadier General PL Hall, Jr, chief of staff, to adjutant general, Militia Bureau, September 27, 1916. Letter. No. 211., Box 177. Entry 12 A.

155. National Archives and Records Administration. Record Group 168. Nebraska dental surgeons. Colonel GW McIver, acting chief, Militia Bureau, to adjutant general of the Army, October 2, 1916. No. 211. Box 177. Entry 12 A.

156. National Archives and Records Administration. Record Group 168. Nebraska dental surgeons special orders no. 20, paragraph 13, adjutant general's department, State of Nebraska, September 27, 1916. No. 211. Box 177. Entry 12 A.

157. Parker RI. Dental conditions affecting state troops on the border. *Dental Summary*. 1917;37:342–343.

158. National Archives and Records Administration. Record Group 168. Ohio dental surgeons. MG Albert L Mills, chief of the Militia Bureau, to adjutant general of the Army, August 25, 1916. Letter. No. 211. Box 177. Entry 12 A.

159. National Archives and Records Administration. Record Group 168. Ohio dental surgeons. Adjutant General McCain to commanding general, central department, August 29, 1916. Telegram. No. 211. Box 177. Entry 12 A.

160. Oeder LR. Dental conditions on the border. *Dental Cosmos*. 1916;58:1165.

161. Militia dental surgeons. *J Nat Dent Assoc*. 1917;4:116.

162. National Archives and Records Administration. Record Group 168. New York dental surgeons. Adjutant General Louis W Stotesbury, State of New York, to chief of the Militia Bureau, August 29, 1916. Letter. No. 211. Box 177. Entry 12 A.

163. National Archives and Records Administration. Record Group 168. New York dental surgeons. Endorsement, September 13, 1916. Letter. No. 211. Box 177. Entry 12 A.

164. National Archives and Records Administration. Record Group 168. New York dental surgeons. Stotesbury to chief of the Militia Bureau, September 18, 1916. Telegram. No. 211. Box 177. Entry 12 A.

165. National Archives and Records Administration. Record Group 168. New York dental surgeons. Colonel GW McIver, acting chief of the Militia Bureau, to adjutant general of the Army, September 19, 1916. Letter. No. 211. Box 177. Entry 12 A.

166. National Archives and Records Administration. Record Group 168. New York dental Surgeons. Adjutant General McCain to commanding general, southern department, September 21, 1916. Telegram. No. 211. Box 177. Entry 12 A.

167. Puffer JW. A dentist with the militia. *Dental Summary*. 1917;37:219.

168. National Archives and Records Administration. Record Group 168. Indiana dental surgeons. Adjutant general, State of Indiana, to chief of the Militia Bureau, October 6, 1916. Letter. No. 211. Box 176. Entry 12 A.

169. National Archives and Records Administration. Record Group 168. Special orders no. 269, paragraph 1, adjutant general's office, State of Indiana, October 6, 1916. No. 211. Box 176. Entry 12 A.

170. Belcher WW. The dental dispensary in peace and war. *Oral Hygiene*. 1916;6:1001–1006.

171. Oliver RT. Address delivered at the graduating exercises of the Army medical and dental schools. *Milit Dent J.* 1923;6:61.

172. Dental school of instructions. *J Assoc Milit Dent Surg US.* 1918;2:24–26.

173. National Archives and Records Administration. Record Group 112. Surgeon general's office and reply commanding general, southern department, April 12, 1917. Telegram. No. 146814. Box 1049. Entry 26.

Chapter XII

PREPARING THE DENTAL CORPS FOR FRANCE, 1917–1918

Introduction

Relations with Germany deteriorated rapidly in early 1917. The United States declared war on April 6, joining Great Britain and the British Empire, France, Italy, and Russia in the war against Germany, Austria-Hungary, and the Ottoman Empire. Although the Army had learned some valuable lessons during the Punitive Expedition, the country and its army had a long way to go before they could make a meaningful contribution to the war effort. It became apparent very quickly that a large army would have to be raised and deployed to Europe if the United States was to play a significant role in the war. The War Department had envisioned a gradually expanding defensive force in its 1916 plans, but little thought had been given to dealing with the magnitude of demands that prevailed in 1917. The country now embarked on a mad scramble to raise and equip the massive force suddenly required.[1,2]

Organizing the Dental Corps for the War in Europe

Despite its experience on the Mexican Border, the US Army Dental Corps was no exception to the general unpreparedness of the Army and the United States. In April 1917, 86 officers composed the entire Regular Army Dental Corps. While a number of the Regular Army and National Guard dentists were fresh from field experience along the border, they had little formal military instruction and training. Prior to the war, the Dental Corps offered no military, technical, or professional training either upon entering the service or later, unlike the Medical Corps, which provided extensive military and professional training for officers in the Regular Army, Medical Reserve Corps, and National Guard. Aside from the National Guard units with assigned dental surgeons, unit training for dentists was nonexistent because there were no Army dental units and dental surgeons were not assigned to any units in the Regular Army at that time.[3–5]

The Army's basic directives on doctrine and organization for combat operations in a theater of war after mobilization were laid down in its 1914 *Field Service Regulations and Tables of Organization*.[5] These documents, and other applicable doctrine, formed the basis for the *Manual for the Medical Department, United States Army, 1916*,[6] which detailed the medical doctrine, organization, functions, policies, procedures, reports, and medical and dental equipment and supply tables.

This manual provided a carefully honed doctrine for the employment of the Medical Department's tactical elements with the field armies and divisions in times of peace and war. It paid special attention to the responsibilities of its hospitals on the supporting lines of communication and the zone of the interior. The manual called for only one Dental Corps officer and an enlisted assistant for each base hospital, just as the 1914 *Tables of Organization* had. However, it also listed one Dental Corps officer and enlisted assistant for the dental service in the four existing Army general hospitals, which were not covered in the tables. The only officially authorized position for Dental Corps officers within the field structure of the Army was in the base hospital. This deficiency and the failure to correct it during the war eventually had serious and lasting consequences. Even if there had been a structure to fill, though, the War Department was still working out how those interested could apply for commissions in the Dental Reserve Corps (DRC; later renamed the Dental Officers Reserve Corps [DORC] as part of the Officers Reserve Corps established by legislation in June 1917, but still commonly referred to as the DRC throughout the war years) that the National Defense Act authorized June 1916. Consequently, as of June 30, 1917, 88 dentists had accepted DRC commissions but only 20 were on active duty, all of them assigned to mobilized Red Cross Army base hospitals, 6 of which were already in England or France.[3,5,7–14]

With the Dental Corps largely missing from the Army's doctrinal and organization documents and the *Manual of the Medical Department*, Army dentists looked to French and British wartime experience to shape much of their organization, supply, and clinical procedures. The military structure that the War Department built to raise, train, deploy, support, and lead the US Army into combat against the Germans in France and Belgium determined the requirements for dental surgeons and assistants in mobilization and training camps, on the lines of communication, and in the combat divisions. Although the Army had experimented with infantry and cavalry divisions and brigades since 1911, and despite the fact that the National Defense Act of June 1916 had made them permanent organizations for operations, the Army of 1917 was still largely organized in small units scattered at posts around the country and overseas. The Army had prepared and published tables of organization and doctrine in 1914 in Field Service Regulations for Regular Army and National Guard divisions and a field army, but no permanent divisions had been organized when the United States declared war. To fight the war in Europe, the entire US Army had to be reorganized.[1,5,9]

While the Army's tables of organization laid out the Medical Department's overall allocations, grades, and positions for officers and enlisted soldiers in the field army, divisions, and lines of communication, they specifically identified only one Dental Corps first lieutenant in the base hospital on the lines of communication. In the absence of any official dental organization for the division, Captain Robert Oliver, the senior Dental Corps officer in the Army and then on duty along the Mexican Border, proposed one in an article in the April 1917 issue of the *Bulletin of the Association of Military Dental Surgeons of the United States*. Dropping the standard ratio from one to a thousand enlisted troops to one to fifteen hundred, he outlined a structure of 15 operating dental surgeons and one executive to administer the divisional dental service. The dentists would be distributed throughout the division to provide the full range of dental care in camp, but on campaign they would move from the tactical units to the division's headquarters, field hospitals, field ambulance companies, and a dental laboratory, where they could provide better support. A new, well-equipped field dental outfit, with all essential instruments for handling emergency treatment and gunshot wounds of the jaw, was needed to replace the existing portable outfit, which was too heavy for use with the division in the field. Oliver wrote:

> Thus equipped the dental surgeon, may if necessary, accompany his command anywhere the smallest unit of mobile sanitary material can go; as the entire outfit can be packed for transportation on any vehicle of the Sanitary or Combat train or carried by pack mule similar to the Regimental Aid Station. . . . making each division independent and competent to take care of itself from a dental and oral surgical standpoint, and able to conserve its effective strength by retaining services of men otherwise lost through being sent back for prosthetic treatment the length of the line of communications (to the base) occupying transportation that could oftentimes be more profitably utilized.[15(p4)]

In his introduction to Oliver's proposals, John Millikin, the editor of the *Bulletin*, lamented that "many of this nature have heretofore come from the Dental Corps of the Army only to be 'pigeon holed' by the Medical Department. We trust ere long to have an Army Dental Surgeon in the Surgeon General's office to make proper use of these valuable suggestions." The fate of Oliver's proposed divisional dental organization is not known, but his ideas surely accompanied him when he arrived in France in August 1917.

On May 3, 1917, within a month of American entry into the World War, the War Department published new tables of organization for the division. Because of sustained operations and the projected heavy casualties of trench warfare, this division was very large, including 28,256 officers and enlisted soldiers. It contained two brigades of two infantry regiments each, three artillery regiments, an engineer regiment, and supporting ammunition, supply, and sanitary trains. On May 24, 1917, the War College Division planners revised this to an expeditionary division of 18,919, but the final decisions on the size and structure of the American force that would serve in Europe came from Pershing and his staff at General Headquarters (GHQ), AEF, after they reached France in June 1917. On July 11, 1917, Pershing submitted his General Organization Project, which called for a 30-division force (1,372,399 soldiers), formed into five corps of six divisions (four combat, one training, and one replacement), to be trained and shipped to France in 1917 and 1918 to take the pressure off of the British and French combat forces.[1,9,10,16–19]

Pershing's GHQ also prepared all tables of organization for units destined for France because he and his staff had a more intimate understanding of the force and organizational requirements for ground combat and wanted the divisions tailored to their specifications. On August 8, 1917, the general staff issued a new division table of organization of 27,123 soldiers based on Pershing's input. With only minor adjustments, this became the basic division that saw action in World War I. Like preceding and succeeding tables, this August 8 version authorized a Medical Department component but did not specifically refer to or authorize the number of Dental Corps personnel or their placement within the division. As soon as tables of organization were issued for units destined for France, GHQ AEF specifically prohibited any changes without its approval.[1,9,16,20–22]

Based on the statutory ratio of one to a thousand troops, 27 Dental Corps officers and their enlisted assistants should have been allocated to these new divisions, but at first apparently only 20 of each were. This allocation may have resulted from the War College Division's expeditionary division of May 24, or because the AEF allocated 20 of the first dental officers to arrive in France to the First Division, which disembarked and assembled during the summer of 1917. When the AEF submitted its "Services of the Rear" plan to the War Department in Washington on September 18, 1917, it stated that the dental service would be on the line of communications and that the number of dentists and dental assistants would be one each per 1,000 soldiers. Having only arrived in Paris on August 22, Oliver's plans for the dental service were then still in gestation, but it was already clear to him that 20 dental officers were insufficient for a division of 28,000 soldiers. On November 14, 1917, the AEF mandated in its modification of Item M-415, Schedule of Priority of Shipments, that 25 dentists and 25 assistants would "accompany," not be assigned, to divisions going to France, in addition to the line of communication allocation. By specifying that dental personnel were attached or would accompany an organization and were not assigned to it, the War Department gave Pershing and GHQ AEF the maximum flexibility in using the service troops where they considered the need was greatest rather than tying them down in any fixed organizational structure once they reached France. Such a policy placed a heavy burden on Oliver and his small staff to allocate dental personnel among the competing requirements as they arrived in France.[10,11, 17,18, 23–26]

In the absence of documentary evidence, it remains unclear exactly how dental personnel were allocated to the division and used within its authorized medical structure. With no formal guidance on where the dentists were to be placed within the division either in the United States or France, they were apparently allocated to the larger infantry, artillery, and engineer regiments and the divisional trains at the statutory ratio and distributed in the same manner as the assigned Medical Corps officers. For the initial force of 30 divisions, this meant 25 dental surgeons and 25 dental assistants per division, or a total of 750 dental surgeons and 750 assistants, who had to be trained, equipped, and shipped with these combat divisions. Considering that the Regular Army Dental Corps of April 6, 1917, consisted of 86 dental surgeons, none above the rank of captain and no reservists, and lacked central leadership presence at the Office of The Surgeon General until August 1917, recruiting and training this dental force for France was an enormous challenge.

A major shift from the Dental Corps' previously authorized operating and treatment procedures took place as dental care was incorporated within the new divisions in the United States and largely replaced the former itinerancy practice. In accordance with prewar tables and doctrine, the division's major combat elements, the infantry, artillery, and engineer regiments, received an organic medical section staffed with Medical Corps officers and enlisted Medical Department personnel who handled sick call and routine health care when in camp, and care and evacuation of the wounded and sick on the battlefield. Twenty-five dental officers and their assistants were added to those numbers. Each infantry regiment eventually had a regimental dental surgeon who directed a regimental dental infirmary under supervision of the regimental surgeon. By 1918 a dental surgeon and assistant were assigned to each of the three battalions of the regiment, with the dental surgeon often acting as the assistant battalion surgeon and normally stationed at the battalion aid station when in combat. For the smaller divisional units without their own dentists, a few of the excess dental officers not allocated to the larger units provided care in the field on itinerant rounds while dental infirmaries and base dental units provided care in established mobilization camps and training areas. A divisional sanitary train of four field hospitals and four ambulance companies, one for each infantry regiment, was responsible for care and evacuation of sick and casualties. A dentist and assistant were added to each of the field hospitals, which had no authorization for dental personnel in the 1914 tables of organization or the 1916 *Manual of the Medical Department*.[5,8,10,11,16,17,27]

As a result of the Act of October 6, 1917, which created parity between the Medical and Dental Corps (see below, "Amending the Act of June 3, 1916—S 1786 and HR 4897"), significant changes took place in the ranks of Dental Corps officers, the dental command structure (especially in the AEF), and in the allocation of dental officers and assistants to the divisions. Effective October 6, Robert Oliver, then a captain and the AEF's senior dental surgeon, was promoted to colonel of the Dental Corps and became the chief dental surgeon. On October 12, upon receiving notification of the act, Oliver immediately directed an increase to 31 dental officers, including a division dental surgeon, per division in France from available and arriving assets. Many divisions never reached these allocation levels during the war. Oliver later said "though the organization which the Dental Corps finally developed was begun early in the history of the American Expeditionary Forces, its completion in a satisfactory manner was not practicable until after this bill reorganizing the corps became a law on October 6, 1917."

Discounting the division dental surgeon, this translated into a ratio of approximately one dental surgeon per 904 enlisted personnel for the divisions about to embark for France, and provided dental coverage for all of the division's numerous and often widely scattered subordinate units.[10,11,17,18,20,18,29] A single division now had as many dental surgeons as had been authorized to care for the entire US Army from 1901 to 1911.[21,24]

The AEF policy of attaching rather than assigning Dental Corps officers and assistants to the divisions determined War Department policies and left many organizational problems to be resolved for the remainder of the war. In December 1917 the division surgeon of the 78th Division recommended a new dental company composed of a chief dental surgeon and three units each of 10 dentists, 18 enlisted soldiers, and one 2-ton truck as part of the sanitary train. On February 7, 1918, the surgeon general proposed a change in the infantry division table of organization to provide 31 dental surgeons (one to be the division dental surgeon) and 32 assistants, as Oliver had authorized to be done in France. The War Plans Division reviewed both proposals and rejected them. The 78th Division proposal was counter to Pershing's policy of not adding small units to divisions and existing organizations. The surgeon general's recommendation was turned down because it was "in conflict with the general principles of organization enunciated by General Pershing," and insisted "that the proper place for the dental service is in the line of communications." Colonel William Logan, chief of the dental division of the surgeon general's office, informed the War plans division that ". . . he would have no serious objection to this disposition of dental personnel provided arrangements are made so as that when a division is ordered overseas there shall be attached thereto 31 dental surgeons and 32 enlisted assistants." The war planners agreed, pending Pershing's approval, which was soon received. On March 26, 1918, Brigadier General William Graves, assistant to the chief of staff, cancelled the November 1917 priority shipment schedule of 25 dentists and 25 dental assistants per division and authorized an increased allowance to 31 dental officers, one of whom served as the division dental surgeon, and 32 enlisted dental assistants.[21,24,25]

In April 1918 the War Plans Division rejected a proposal to add dental surgeons to numerous corps and Army troops then headed for France using the same reasoning it had used in February. Again, Colonel Logan stated that dental personnel were now shipped to France attached to each division and "as specifically requested from time to time by General Pershing." The war planners concluded:

> it appears that General Pershing has a constant flow of dental personnel to France and a positive means of getting more as needed to carry out his project of September 18, 1917 [Services of the Rear plan]. In view of these facts the war plans division is of the opinion that no dental personnel should be attached or assigned to corps or army troops, and that none should be ordered to accompany any of them when designated for overseas service.[30]

In an April 20, 1918, memo to Adjutant General Colonel DW Ketcham, the acting director of the War Plans Division, made it very clear that the AEF's previous plans and directives controlled these issues:

> The approved A.E.F. organization project places the dental service in the line of communications and the program for the shipment of personnel therefore does not contemplate any of it accompanying organizations of corps or army troops designated for overseas service. In conformity with this policy, no dental personnel will accompany organizations of the above troops when ordered abroad.[31]

Confusion about the status of the dental surgeons and assistants pervaded the Army. On April 16, 1918, Major (later Major General and Chief of the Dental Corps, 1954–1956) Oscar Snyder (1895–1983), then the dental surgeon of the 28th Division, wrote to the War Department asking about the status of the dentists and their assistants and how they would travel to France with their equipment if they were not on the division's tables of organization. In the clearest explanation yet prepared, Brigadier General Lytle Brown, director, War Plans Division, told the chief of staff:

> Dental surgeons and assistants are not part of the division and their omission from Tables of Organization is in accordance with the general principles of organization indicated by General Pershing . . . The dental personnel indicated should accompany the division when it sails for overseas service and their status until arrival in France will be that of attached only. After arrival they should receive definite orders as to their future movements, it being the policy to use them at base hospitals on the line

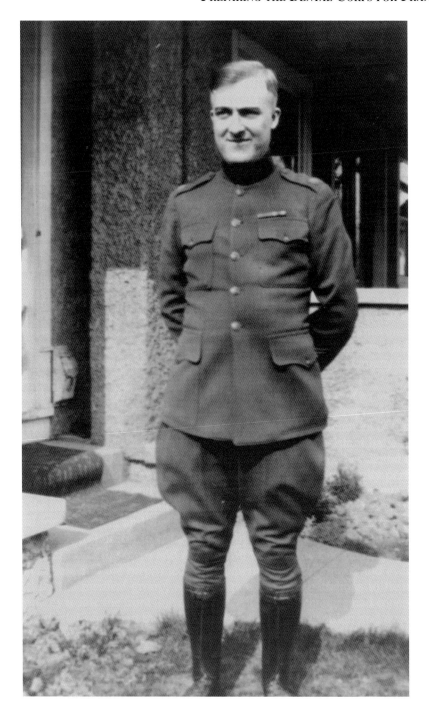

Major Oscar P Snyder, division dental surgeon, while stationed at
Camp Hancock, Georgia, with the 28th Division before it sailed for France in May 1918.
Photograph: Courtesy of Major General Oscar P Snyder.

of communication. . . . Until arrival in France they are administratively controlled by the division surgeon, through the division dental surgeon. As to whether they will remain attached to organizations enroute or go as a unit, should depend upon the division surgeon who will take into consideration the necessity for emergency dental service enroute. . . . The professional equipment should accompany them and be so stowed as to facilitate its separation from the division property proper, upon arrival. Their personal equipment should go with them in the same manner and should be that of any other unassigned noncombatant officer ordered for overseas service.[32,33]

Enlisted dental assistants were to be attached to the division in addition to the enlisted medical personnel provided by its tables of organization.[32,33]

It was not until June 19, 1918, when GHQ AEF issued General Order No. 99, that Dental Corps personnel and equipment within the division received formal structure and authorization (Table 12-1).[32,33] After the division dental surgeons reported having problems transporting their equipment, Oliver finally intervened and straightened out some of the confusion (see Chapter 13). The division now had 31 dental surgeons and 32 assistants, one of whom was assistant to the divi-

TABLE 12-1

AMERICAN EXPEDITIONARY FORCES ALLOCATION OF DENTAL PERSONNEL AND EQUIPMENT WITHIN THE DIVISION, 1918

Organization	No. of Units	Dental Officers	Enlisted Personnel	Portable Outfit (Complete)	Portable Outfit (Modified)
Headquarters	1	1	1	0	0
Infantry regiments (3 battalions)	4	12	12	4	8
Artillery regiments (3 battalions)	2	2	2	0	2
Artillery regiment (6 battalions)	1	2	2	1	1
Engineer regiment	1	2	2	1	1
Machine gun battalions	3	3	3	0	3
Field signal battalion	1	1	1	0	1
Train headquarters & military police	1	1	1	0	1
Ammunition train	2	2	2	0	2
Supply train	1	1	0	0	1
Sanitary train (field hospitals)	1	4	5	4	0
Total	**25**	**31**	**32**	**10**	**20**

Data source: General Orders No. 99, General Headquarters, AEF, 19 June 1918. In: *General Orders, GHQ, AEF, in United States Army in the World War 1917–1919*. Vol 16. Washington, DC: US Army Center of Military History; 1992: 351.

sion dental surgeon and was authorized 30 dental outfits and one dental laboratory in one of the field hospitals of the sanitary train. However, the GHQ AEF's policy on changes in tables of organization and unit organization, which allowed maximum flexibility of service forces, prevented any formal changes in tables of organization that would have codified this allocation guidance, so the basic structural problem remained unaltered. Based on the AEF's existing guidance, on July 26, 1918, the War Department general staff decreed that "there is no Table of Organization covering the organization of the Dental Corps, and it is not contemplated that one will be issued."[34]

By July 1918 the projected demands of the fighting in France forced Pershing to scrap his 30-division program for a plan of 80 divisions and 3,360,000 officers and enlisted in Europe by June 30, 1919. As estimates of the war's duration and intensity were revised, Pershing submitted a new plan for 100 divisions and 5,500,000 soldiers in Europe by June 30, 1920. In August War Department plans called for a total of 5,974 dental officers on active duty. Each of these programs carried new, larger requirements for dental officers and assistants and equipment not only for the combat divisions but also for the mobilization and training base in the United States and the line of communications in Europe. It was only the armistice of November 11, 1918, and Allied occupation of Germany that finally terminated planning for these enormous programs. Until that time, the efforts of the Army's Dental Corps in the United States during 1917 and 1918 were completely dedicated to selecting, training, and equipping dental surgeons and enlisted assistants to provide dental care for the force for the duration of its training in the United States and during combat operations in France.[1,9,20,35]

The Committee on Dentistry of the Council of National Defense in 1917

As part of the growing preparedness movement, Congress authorized the cabinet-level Council of National Defense in 1916. Aimed primarily at coordinating United States industrial production and personnel, the council spawned a large number of subordinate boards and committees, each focusing on a particular specialty. The general medical board dealt with military and civilian medicine, and under it fell the Committee on Dentistry, which was to mobilize all of the nation's dental forces for the war.[36]

With his committee at work since 1916, Dr Edward Kirk of Philadelphia, editor of *Dental Cosmos* and chairman of the Committee on Dentistry, issued the committee's first report on April 8, 1917. While it was too early to set any specific numbers, the committee recommended that enough dentists be appointed to fill the quotas for dental officers provided by law for the Army (one dentist per thousand enlisted) and Navy and for the DRC. The aid of the National Dental Association, state and local dental societies, the senior dental students, and the Preparedness League of American Dentists would greatly accelerate this process. The report urged establishing special courses of instruction in military dental surgery for prospective dental surgeons and placing dental school faculties and facilities at the disposal of the government for that purpose. The committee further suggested that all military hospitals be equipped with the necessary dental laboratory equipment to make prostheses for war injuries. It also wanted a survey of the dental instrument and supply industry to assure the flow of essential materials for both the government and civilian needs.[36]

A week later, the committee issued the findings of its subcommittees.[36] Their consensus was that dental faculty members should be deferred from the draft, as should dental students until they graduated. They further urged the War Department to provide instructors to the dental schools to cover military topics and to establish schools for newly appointed dental surgeons when they entered service. The committees suggested changes in Dental Corps application forms to improve standards for acceptance. They noted the need to revise the dental supply table and agreed with the need to coordinate with the dental manufacturing and supply industry. Finally, they emphasized that dental personnel levels should be premised on assuring that all members of the expanded force receive adequate dental care.[36]

At Dr Kirk's recommendation, a meeting was convened in Washington, DC, on May 12, 1917, of the deans of the dental colleges, the secretaries of the state boards of dental examiners, and the directors of dental infirmaries. At the meeting, which was held at the headquarters of the Council of National Defense, Kirk explained that the government needed trained specialists in all the various professions and wanted to avoid the mistakes that England, France, and other countries made when they placed their trained professionals "in the ranks," losing their special skills to service requiring less education and training, or worse, losing them altogether when they became casualties in the fighting. Estimating the number of annual hours available for a dental operator and the number of hours required to properly care for soldiers' dental needs, Kirk and the committee recommended an increase in the personnel in the Dental Corps to provide more efficient service. Rather than the present one per thousand troops, Kirk recommended one dentist for every 500 members of the line, which turned out to be an accurate prediction of the changes made in September 1918. After a discussion of all the existing wartime conditions affecting the dental profession and the military's needs, the group agreed to support the Committee on Dentistry and the general medical board. One of the key participants in this gathering was William HG Logan of Chicago (MD and DDS), the president-elect of the National Dental Association (NDA) for 1917–1918, a member of the Committee on Dentistry, and chairman of its committee on legislation and enrollment that was responsible for "devising ways and means for securing prompt enrollment of candidates in the Army and Navy Dental Corps." Logan returned to Washington in late May 1917 for the June 2 meeting of the general medical board and Council of National Defense, and in late June succeeded Dr Kirk as chairman of the Committee on Dentistry.[37–42]

Dr William HG Logan and Building the Wartime Dental Corps

In May 1917 the surgeon general announced that the examinations to fill 14 current vacancies in the Regular Army Dental Corps would be held on July 2, 1917, at Fort Slocum, New York; Columbus Barracks, Ohio; Jefferson Barracks, Missouri;

Fort Logan, Colorado; and Fort McDowell, California. He also said that on July 1, there would be 22 additional vacancies.[43] On June 12, 1917, Captain Robert T Oliver, the senior Dental Corps officer on active duty and stationed at Base Hospital No. 1, Fort Sam Houston, Texas, who had been on the Mexican border for the past year, reported that he had been very busy during the previous month conducting examinations for the Regular Army Dental Corps and the DRC. On average, he held two examination classes each week and predicted at least 50 successful candidates for the month, including six oral surgeons.[44] While Oliver's work was replicated by other Dental Corps officers throughout the Army, their efforts did not solve the real problem then facing the Army, the Medical Department, and the Dental Corps. Editorials in dental publications like *Dental Summary* revealed the true dimensions of the dilemma when it called for "ethical practitioners" to answer the government's request for one to two thousand dentists to apply for the DRC.[45]

The problem facing the Dental Corps and Medical Department was not how to fill positions in the Regular Army one or two at a time, but how to screen and select the thousands of trained dentists now so urgently required in the DRC to staff a rapidly expanding Army. Initially, the surgeon general's office employed an application and examination system not unlike its peacetime approach since 1901, which required a formal written application, a board examination, and a final decision. Often taking weeks to complete, this cumbersome system did not fill the pressing demands of the Dental Corps for trained dentists. When William HG Logan appeared in Washington in late May on Committee on Dentistry business, things immediately began to change. Logan was an 1896 graduate (DDS) of the Chicago College of Dental Surgery and a 1905 graduate (MD) of the Chicago College of Medicine and Surgery (in 1917 it became part of Loyola University's School of Medicine). Since 1902 Logan, a long-time acquaintance of John Marshall, had been a professor of oral pathology at the Chicago College of Dental Surgery. By the time of the war, he was one of the country's most distinguished oral and plastic surgeons and had a wide range of contacts within the American medical and dental communities, the administration, and Congress from his long career, role in the National Dental Association, and now membership on the general medical board.[42,46,47]

From his work on the Committee on Dentistry, Logan understood the problems of the current system of recruiting dental officers and knew it would never work. After looking at the existing procedures being used for commissioning, his committee realized it had to mobilize the American dental profession and had developed an organization and plans for recruiting dental surgeons for the Army and Navy. On June 1, 1917, Logan recommended to the surgeon general that well-qualified, experienced men of the dental profession throughout the country be designated to give "professional examinations to applicants desiring to be commissioned in the DRC." He later noted that "this request, although without precedent and most unusual, was granted the following day by Surgeon General Gorgas."[8,48–51] Logan went on:

> In the twenty-four hours that intervened between the presentation and the acceptance by Surgeon General Gorgas of the plan whereby preliminary dental examiners were to be officially appointed by the War Department, appropriate examiners were selected for each state so that no delay would be occasioned if final acceptance were

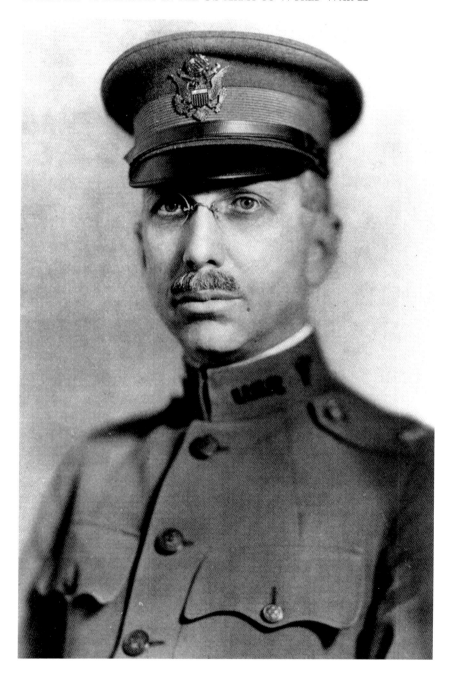

Major (later Colonel) William HG Logan, Medical Officers' Reserve Corps, became the first chief of the Dental Section, Personnel Division, Office of The Surgeon General, and thus the first de facto chief of the US Army Dental Corps, when he was appointed on August 9, 1917. He is pictured here as the incoming president of the National Dental Association.
Reproduced from: Journal of the National Dental Association. *1917;4(Dec):1280.*

secured. The men so selected and approved by the Surgeon General as preliminary dental examiners were the deans of well-recognized dental institutions throughout the United States, the secretary of each state dental examining board, and such additional dentists as the service demanded in certain localities.[48(p1952)]

All examinations completed by the preliminary dental examiners were forwarded to the surgeon general's office, where a Regular Army Dental Corps officer had the final approval authority.[48]

Logan's success developing the commissioning program for DRC officers during the summer clearly indicated the importance of having a strong, central direction of Dental Corps affairs within the surgeon general's office, as John Marshall had pointed out many years earlier. The surgeon general now made two critical decisions. On August 8, 1917, William HG Logan was commissioned a major in the Medical Reserve Corps, and the next day the surgeon general established a dental section within his Personnel Division, which had administered Dental Corps affairs prior to the war, and assigned Logan to head it. These actions made Logan the de facto head of the Dental Corps in the surgeon general's office (where no such representation had existed since dentists joined the Army in February 1901) and the first chief of the US Army Dental Corps. To enhance his influence and contacts with the American dental community in the new post, Logan wisely retained his positions as president-elect of the NDA and chairman of the Committee on Dentistry.[52]

Logan's system worked smoothly and efficiently. Only five DRC officers were commissioned during the first 2 months of the war. By June 30, 1917, only 20 were commissioned and on active duty, but by July 31, that number had quickly climbed to 598. On September 8, 1917, a little more than 3 months after Logan's recommendation was approved, the adjutant general discontinued all examinations for dental general practitioners as of September 18 at the surgeon general's request. On that date, the Regular Army Dental Corps numbered 178—19 captains and 159 first lieutenants—and the National Guard Dental Corps had 297 first lieutenants (not all on active duty). A sufficient number of commissioned officers were now in the DRC and enough completed applications were on hand to provide dental officers to care for an army of 5,000,000 troops "under the quota then authorized by law."[41,48,53,54] Logan concluded:

> It is of interest to record that the dental service of the United States Army was the only arm in the military organization that was built up through the aid of preliminary examiners, who gave liberally and gratuitously of their time to assist dentists desiring to enter military service. . . . The records show that through the hearty cooperation of the civilian members of the dental profession and the patriotic response of those desiring to enter military service, when war was declared there were eighty-six officers in the Regular Army, five had been commissioned in the Reserve Corps in the first two months of the war, and in the following three and one-half months the number had passed beyond 5,000. . . . These officers were secured without the holding of a single public meeting, without the presentation of a personal appeal by letter or by voice of any one in this nation, and, in this accomplishment, the dental profession established a record of which it may be justifiably proud.[48(pp1952–1953)]

Largely through Logan's recruiting innovations, by September 8, 1917, the Army had already procured enough dental officers for its immediate and future needs. Now, as a result of the Act of October 6, 1917, the DRC was also allowed the same grades and percentages within the grades as the law permitted for the Medical Reserve Corps. By the time that Logan spoke at the 21st Annual Meeting of the NDA in late October, he could report that the Army had received a total 6,251 applications for appointment in the DRC, had rejected 1,445 as unfit for physical or professional reasons, and had commissioned 4,695 new DRC first lieutenants. On November 18 Logan reported to the general medical board that 4,874 dental officers were now commissioned and subject to call up, more than enough for an army of 4,874,000 troops at the statutory ratio of one dentist per thousand soldiers. The DRC largely staffed Army dentistry during the war and provided dentists for the myriad new Army hospitals and the national Army divisions that were being organized and trained.[41, 55–58]

Meanwhile, those holding commissions but not yet called to active duty as dental officers were subject to being drafted by their local boards. If drafted, the dentist had to serve as a private until his orders for active duty as a dental officer were received. The drafted dentist who had not made application before September 18 likely lost any chance of securing a commission as a dental officer. However, on October 2, 1917, the law was changed to allow unassigned DRC officers to be deferred until called to duty as commissioned officers. The only recourse for those already in camps was to apply for a transfer to the Medical Department with duty as dental assistants until their active duty orders came in.[41]

When Dr Logan initially accepted his commission in the Medical Reserve Corps, some dentists accused him of "deserting dentistry" and severely criticized him. As it turned out, he had positioned himself where he could do dentistry the most good and then worked to achieve recognition for it on the same level as the medical profession. Dr CN Johnson, editor of *Dental Review*, quoted someone familiar with Logan and his work as saying "no dentist in the history of the profession has done more for dentistry than has Dr. W.H.G. Logan in 1917."[59,60]

These accolades did not spare Logan from criticism by some of his dental colleagues during and after the war, although little criticism ever appeared in the dental press. Some critics believed that using dental school deans and faculty to examine their own graduates for commissions placed them in a compromised position. In addition, older and more experienced dentists were needed throughout the Dental Corps for consultation and administrative positions. Unlike the Medical Officers Reserve Corps, which had ranks up to and including brigadier general to attract the most prominent civilian physicians and surgeons, the DRC was never able to obtain sufficiently high ranks for such eminent candidates and suffered from the fact that "older men of reputation, experience and patriotism were excluded from entrance, because sufficient rank was not offered to them and they were financially and professionally prevented from entering the service." Blame for much of this shortcoming was later placed on Logan, although even his critics admitted that "he had the contact with the Dental Profession, and with tact and energy he worked for success."[61]

Despite the criticisms, it was largely through Logan's efforts that the Dental

Corps expanded at the pace it did and the issues of supply, training, and personnel inequities were usually resolved in favor of the dentists. The bulk of the profession, in and out of uniform, came to appreciate his accomplishments on their behalf long before the war ended. Logan was promoted to lieutenant colonel on February 28, 1918, and to colonel on May 3, 1918. He was awarded the Distinguished Service Medal for his wartime efforts and was discharged from the Army on February 12, 1919. After the war, Logan returned to the Chicago College of Dental Surgery as professor of oral and plastic surgery and dean, affiliated it with Loyola University in 1923, and made it into a leading institution in maxillofacial surgery and dental research. He was a colonel in the Medical Officers' Reserve Corps from 1923 to 1933 and remained active in Dental Corps issues. He died on April 6, 1943. On October 16, 1970, the Logan Army Dental Clinic at Fort Belvoir, Virginia, was dedicated in Colonel William HG Logan's honor.[42,46,47,62]

Amending the Act of June 3, 1916: S 1786 and HR 4897

The swift slide toward war compelled Congress to modify the National Defense Act of 1916. In February 1917, even before war was declared, *Dental Summary* called for higher rank for dental officers, pointing out that the public throughout the United States would "accept and recognize" whatever Congress set as the "standard" for Dental Corps officers.[63] A proposed new law (S 1786) went to the War Department for comment on April 3, 1917. The section pertaining to the Dental Corps recommended the same rank structure as the Medical Corps with its size still based on one dentist for every thousand soldiers. As soon as the law was approved, the necessary promotions would occur on the basis of seniority in the present Dental Corps. The surgeon general also suggested adding to the bill a clause that restructured the Dental Corps and made Medical and Dental corps entry-level commissions as first lieutenant provisional for 2 years before becoming permanent. On June 1, the general staff recommended against the bill. It did not agree that Dental Corps grades should be distributed in the same ratio as those in the Medical Corps, did not envision the Dental Corps having any need for senior administrators, and wanted the 1916 structure to have more time to prove itself. Accordingly, on June 2, Major General Tasker H Bliss, acting chief of staff, informed the adjutant general that the secretary of war agreed with the general staff's position and requested that the bill be returned to Congress for further consideration.[64,65]

While this was going on, members of the dental profession and press offered various ideas for improving the Dental Corps. Dr Emmett J Craig, one of the original contract dental surgeons in 1901, recommended that the United States adopt the Canadian system, whereby the Dental Corps was awarded the same recognition as the Medical Corps and did not have to depend on the Medical Corps to select its members and supplies or to administer its affairs.[66]

In June 1917 Dr Rodrigues Ottolengui of *Dental Items of Interest* editorialized that a Dental Corps under a Medical Department head would have lower morale and efficiency than it would have under a dental head. Like Dr Craig, Ottolengui used the experience of the Canadian Dental Corps as support for his argument. He recommended that the NDA poll its members to see what the dental profession thought on the subject. Dr Homer C Brown, the chairman of the NDA's legislative committee, stressed the need for a chief of the Dental Corps, preferably with the rank of colonel. In *Dental Cosmos*, Kirk called the current war emergency a "golden opportunity" to demonstrate that dentistry was "a specialized department of the healing art, and not a sublimated form of artizanship [sic]."[67–69]

However, the general staff's June 2 action on S 1786 had not killed the initiative. On June 7, 1917, Representative Murray Hulbert of New York introduced a bill (HR 4897) in the House to amend the medical section of the National Defense Act of June 3, 1916. The bill provided "that during the existing emergency lieutenants in the Medical Corps of the regular Army and of the National Guard shall be eligible to promotion as captain upon such examination as may be prescribed by the Secretary of War." The purpose of the bill was to correct the inequity whereby initial appointments in the Medical Reserve Corps could be made as captain or major without any previous service, whereas, in the Medical Corps of the Regular Army and the National Guard, 5 years of previous service was required before promotion. The bill was referred to the Committee on Military Affairs, which recommended approval on June 21. The Senate began its work on the bill on June 26.[70,71]

On September 20, 1917, the committee reported back the Senate version of the bill (S Rept 131) with some substantial amendments. Finally, on October 5, the bill was introduced for consideration by the Senate. Senator Pomerene recommended the addition of an amendment affecting the Dental Corps, the former S 1786, which Senator Lodge of Massachusetts had previously suggested. The amendment read:

> *Provided*, that hereafter the Dental Corps of the Army shall consist of commissioned officers of the same grades and proportionally distributed among such grades as are now or may be hereafter provided by law for the Medical Corps, who shall have the rank, pay, promotion, and allowances of officers of corresponding grades in the Medical Corps, including the right to retirement as in the case of other officers, and there shall be one dental officer for every thousand of the total strength of the Regular Army authorized from time to time by law. *Provided further*, that dental examining and review boards shall consist of one officer of the Medical Corps and two officers of the Dental Corps. *And provided further*, That immediately following the approval of this act all dental surgeons then in active service shall be recommissioned in the Dental Corps in the grades herein authorized in the order of their seniority and without loss of pay or allowances or of relative rank in the Army.[70,72]

Pomerene said that in his view, the dental profession had been discriminated against in the Army. The types of injuries being reported from France highlighted the importance of the need for dental skills, which indicated to him that dentistry as a medical art was equal to any other and should be treated as such.[70]

Senator Francis E Warren of Wyoming, the father of Pershing's late wife, objected to the dental amendment, expressing the fear that the medical amendment for Medical Corps captains would fail to pass if the dental clause (Lodge amendment) was added to the bill. He felt that the medical clause was for "one distinct item," while the purpose of the dental clause was "to reorganize and change the whole dental service." Pomerene reminded his fellow congressmen that in the past, bills had come through for the "relief" of the medical profession with no "relief" for the

Dental Corps. Senator Overman of North Carolina recommended that the bill allow dental students to enlist in the Medical Department's Enlisted Reserve Corps, just as medical students could, and that it provide for Senate confirmation of the commission derived from the bill. The same day, October 5, all the amendments were agreed to and the bill was read three times and passed with the following title: "An Act to Provide for the Promotion of First Lieutenants in the Regular Army and National Guard to the Grade of Captain, and respecting the Dental Corps of the Army and Medical and Dental Students and for Other Purposes."[70]

The next day, October 6, the bill was sent to the House. Representative Stanley H Dent, Jr, of Alabama recommended that the House concur in the Senate amendments and pass the bill (HR 4897). The bill was vigorously debated, Congressman Dent defending it. Representative William H Stafford of Wisconsin raised the chief objections, protesting the speed of the process and questioning the appropriateness of a major restructuring evolving from amendments to what originally had been a simple bill to promote Medical Corps lieutenants to captains. He objected to giving dentists the same rank as medical officers because their responsibilities were less significant than those of their medical counterparts and because sufficient numbers of dentists were available without any promises of higher pay and rank.[70] Representative Horace M Towner of Iowa countered Stafford's comments by pointing out that Congress was not operating in normal times and that the changes had War Department approval. He believed that a widely organized "dental department" needed to be formed under the surgeon general.[70]

Indeed, the amendments did have War Department approval. Major William Logan, now head of the Dental Section, was deeply and personally involved as this dental legislation moved ahead. He recounted the story some years later:

> About 9 o'clock on the morning of Oct. 6, 1917, two representatives of the Senate and one of the House appeared at my desk in the Surgeon General's Office to ascertain whether it was my opinion that any ill effects would accrue to the Army or to the public needs if legislation were not provided whereby the dental students would be granted the same privilege of continuing in their studies as had been accorded to medical students. Otherwise, they would be called on to proceed to the camps when their numbers were reached by the various conscription boards, in quite the same manner as students in law, theology, engineering and the arts and sciences were conscripted. My reply was that, in my opinion, we could only safely consider the dental needs for an army of not less than 10,000,000 men in the ultimate, and furthermore, if the dental requirements of such an army were to be properly met, all important reparative work should be accomplished during the few months that the conscripted men were in training in our camps in the United States. For this purpose, we would need the assignment of two or three officers per thousand, and not to exceed one per thousand for the men in the field in France. To state this concisely, these representatives were informed that the best interests of the Army would be ultimately served if there was a minimum of two dental officers per thousand for the probable maximum strength of the Army. However, our department was of the opinion that not more than one officer per thousand could be assigned for a number of months to come, even though regulation authorizing two were granted, for the very practical reason that dental equipment was not available and it could not be made so for another six months.[48]

419

After their discussion with Logan, the congressional delegation decided to proceed with attaching the Senate amendment to the bill, even though it was the closing day of that session of Congress. They then completed their rounds of the War Department with visits to Surgeon General Gorgas, the secretary of war, and the judge advocate general. Logan was soon summoned:

> In a few minutes, I was called into conference by General Gorgas, in the presence of the committee, with regard to certain details of the question under discussion, at the end of which General Gorgas gave the full approval to the effort toward the passage of the dental bill and the attachment thereto of the amendment providing that dental students be treated with a consideration similar to that which had already been extended to medical students.[48(p1953)]

The delegation returned to Capitol Hill and that day, October 6, Congress voted on the measure. The amended HR 4897 passed the House and the president signed the act into law (Public No. 86).[48]

The dental profession was jubilant over this victory. *Dental Summary* called the act's passage "the greatest recognition the dental profession has ever received" because it gave dental officers the same standing as medical officers in the Army. Dr CN Johnson of *Dental Review* called the legislation a "red letter day for dentistry" and a "recognition to dentistry that it never before enjoyed." He credited Senators Lodge and Pomerene; the legislative committee of the NDA and its chairman, Dr Homer C Brown; the committee of deans of the dental colleges and their chairman, Dr Arthur D Black; and the thousands of dentists, dental students, and their friends who wrote letters to Washington supporting the bill's passage. But most of all, Johnson thought that the principal architect of all these efforts was really Major William HG Logan.[60]

Logan believed the amendment giving dental students the same rights as medical students was the deciding factor in the success of this legislation:

> Before dismissing the question of dental legislation of the year 1917, and its varied ramifications, I desire to express the opinion that had it not been for the attachment of the amendment to this bill that specified that "all regulations concerning the enlistment of medical students in the Enlisted Reserve Corps and their continuance on their college courses while subject to call to active service shall apply similarly to dental students," the bill that provided the "hereafter the Dental Corps of the Army shall consist of commissioned officers of the same grades proportionally distributed among such grades as are now, or may be hereafter, provided by law for the Medical Corps" would not have been passed on Oct. 6, 1917, which was the last day of that session of Congress. However, the conclusion should not be drawn that I did not feel that favorable action on this very same bill would probably have been reached in a subsequent Congress, because of the merit and justness of its demands, and the splendid efforts that had been put forth by all concerned to bring about a desirable end.[48(pp1957–1958)]

In a May 1919 speech to the Dental Society of the State of New York in Syracuse, Logan was very explicit about what this meant to the Dental Corps and the dental profession, as a whole:

Two important beneficial results followed this enactment. First, the allowing of advanced grades to members of the regular Dental Corps that they might perform their duties in the executive positions in which they were needed to assist as camp and division dental surgeons. The second benefit is found in the fact that many young practitioners of dentistry, who were well qualified, were attracted to the regular Dental Corps, because it assured them the same recognition for similar years of service as had been granted to members of the Medical Corps.[8(pp219–220)]

Speaking in 1921, Colonel Robert T Oliver, then the chief of the Dental Corps, eloquently summarized the importance of the act:

> . . . the Dental Corps of the Army has come into its own, has a voice in its control and has merged into and become a permanent fixture in the military establishment. We pioneers of the corps had strenuous service for a period of seventeen years, until finally upon enactment of a bill, October 6, 1917, the bursting dental chrysalis opened and a beautiful creation appeared to the world, resplendent with the radiance of realized hope and virile with knowledge of its autonomy. Its iridescent hues, however, soon merged into the familiar olive drab service color; and the Dental Corps, then composed of regular, national guard and reserve officers, soon found its equilibrium and began, with renewed energy and a contented heart, the great work that confronted it.[73(p13)]

Oliver's comments aside, the Act of October 6, 1917, was indeed a major milestone for the Dental Corps. Not only did it give the Dental Corps parity with the Medical Corps and professional recognition within the Medical Department, it almost immediately forced major changes in the allocation of dentists to the divisions as well as in the rank—and thus field—command structure for dentists, especially in the AEF. The act provided the crucial justification for increasing the allocation of Dental Corps officers for the divisions to 31. Effective October 6, the Dental Corps had 12 colonels (11 of them were the original contract dental surgeons of 1901 and 1902 and among the initial commissioned officers of 1911), all promoted from captain to colonel virtually overnight, including future Dental Corps chiefs Robert T Oliver (chief 1919–1924) and Julien R Bernheim (chief, 1928–1932). The corps also had 20 lieutenant colonels (including future chiefs Rex H Rhoades [chief 1924–1928, 1932–1934], Frank P Stone [chief 1934–1938], Robert H Mills [chief, 1942–1946], and Frank LK Laflamme [chief, 1919]), and 54 majors (including future chiefs Leigh C Fairbank [chief, 1938–1942], Oscar P Snyder [chief, 1954–1956], and Thomas L Smith [chief, 1946–1950]). This sudden explosion of rank meant that many Dental Corps officers soon occupied positions on Army, corps, and division staffs with sufficient rank and authority to direct and influence dental matters within those organizations. Moreover, these officers gained the command and administrative experience during the war that groomed them for the leadership of the Dental Corps for the next 40 years, through World War II and well into the postwar era.[11,74,75]

Many of the dentists who joined the DRC during the war saw great opportunities and remained in the Regular Army Dental Corps after the conflict to form its future leadership. One such officer was Walter D Love (1892–1991), who reported for duty at Camp Greenleaf, Georgia, in August 1918 and later served as assistant surgeon general (dental) and Dental Corps chief from April 1950 to April 1954.[8,76] Many other dentists returned to their civilian practices after the war but remained active in the Organized Reserves in the 1920s and 1930s and formed the expansion base for the enormous dental mobilization of World War II. Much that John Marshall had fought for had been achieved by his colleague from Chicago, William HG Logan.

The Threat of the Dental Student Draft

In 1917 many members of the dental profession presumed that the government intended to allow dental and medical students to continue in school until graduation. This was supposed to be a lesson learned from the British and French, who had decimated their future medical pool by sending partially trained students to the front as line combat personnel. However, once the draft started, the question of "class exemption" came up and the government announced that there would be no "special" regulations or exemptions except those provided by law. Immediately, the medical profession organized its case for exemption of medical students. Representative Henry Z Osborne of California introduced a bill (HR 5136) to defer medical students, even though an attempt to include an exemption provision for medical students in the National Army Act had previously failed. Finally, on August 29, 1917, Judge Advocate General Brigadier General Enoch H Crowder directed that second-, third-, and fourth-year medical students and hospital interns who were drafted could enlist in the Medical Department's Enlisted Reserve Corps and complete their courses. They were, however, subject to call up. At first it was assumed that dental students would be permitted the same option, but it turned out they were not included and continued to be subject to the draft. Dr Ottolengui, the editor of *Dental Items of Interest*, decried the policy, stating that the government must feel that a dentist was of greater value "with a gun or a spade" in his hands than his instruments.[77–79]

By fall 1917 a total of 1,341 dental students from the classes of 1918 and 1919 had already entered the Army through the first draft or as volunteers. It was estimated that the total loss due to this draft and subsequent second and third calls would be 1,121 students from the class of 1918 and 2,417 from that of 1919. Additionally, with the dental curriculum being lengthened from 3 to 4 years beginning in the fall of 1917, no graduation would take place in 1920. The freshman enrollment for fall 1917 for the class of 1921 was estimated to be only 1,330 students, or roughly one-third of the 4,184 freshmen matriculated in 1916. The class of 1917 had graduated 2,989 dentists. The average annual graduation rate from 1913 to 1917 was 2,497 dentists. The projection for the next 5 years was a total of 5,886 dentists—2,319 in 1918, 1,767 in 1919, practically none in 1920, 1,000 in 1921, and 800 in 1922. Thus, the average graduation would be only 1,177 per year. This total was unacceptable to the dental profession in view of the needs of the Army and the civilian population. Dental educators hoped that the class of 1918 would be allowed to complete its training and that the class of 1919 could be accelerated in order to graduate by January 1, 1919. On September 27, 1917, two letters from dental students requesting clarification of their status were read before the Senate.[70]

When HR 4897 finally passed on October 6, 1917, it allowed dental students (second, third, or fourth year only) to enlist in the Medical Department's Enlisted Reserve Corps and continue their college courses, the same as medical students. They were, however, subject to call up to active duty. At the end of each semester, the dean of their school had to submit a report to the surgeon general certifying that they had passed successfully to the next semester. Those who failed were called up to service. Those former students already in the National Army, National Guard, and Regular Army were eligible to be discharged to enlist in the Medical Reserve Corps to continue their studies.[49,59,80] Graduate dentists and physicians who had already been drafted into the Army as enlisted soldiers could apply for commissions in the Dental or Medical Reserve corps, but their applications would be kept on file until openings occurred. However, an important exception was made for those dentists who were "specially well qualified in the management of fractured jaws and oral surgery. . . ."[81(p522)]

In 1917 some civilian dentists applied for commissions in the DRC higher than lieutenant, even the rank of major. The *International Journal of Orthodontia* thought that these individuals made "the dental profession appear ridiculous." The journal pointed out that those who thought they would be performing a large amount of oral surgery were misled and that what the Army needed was the "general dentist" to get the recruits' mouths in proper order. However, the orthodontists would make excellent specialists for reducing and fixing jaw wounds due to their training and experience in applying bands and ligatures.[82,83]

War-Related Dental Training on Civilian Campuses

Soon after the war began, several dental colleges began giving courses in "war dental surgery." The College of Dental Surgery, University of Michigan, for example, gave such a course from May 28 to June 9, 1917. Three lectures were given daily and the afternoons were devoted to clinics and military drill. The course covered subjects such as head and face anatomy, oral sepsis, general and local anesthesia, oral prosthesis, military law and science, gunshot wounds, war dental surgery at the front, dental materials, diseases of Army life, plastic surgery, first aid, bandaging and splinting, tetanus treatment, bone grafting, and an introduction to the Army dental service. All the dental seniors and over 50 dental practitioners took the course.[84]

In September, Dr Herbert L Wheeler called for an increased emphasis on anatomy, histology, physiology, and mechanics of the maxillofacial bones in the dental curriculum and a "closer and more intimate relationship" between dentistry and the various medical specialties. The Army was in urgent need of dentists with a "knowledge of oral surgery and a genius for prosthetic restoration" to work with the surgeons in treating the large number of facial and jaw wounds encountered in trench warfare.[85] In October 1917 the surgeon general announced that he intended to establish a section of head surgery, including a division of plastic and oral surgery, in certain evacuation, base, and general hospitals. The division would treat all injuries and surgical diseases of the mouth and associated parts, including the facial bones and soft tissue, and the neck above the clavicle, except the diseases and injuries that fell under ophthalmology, otolaryngology, neurosurgery, and diseases of the thyroid. Oral surgeons with dual medical and dental degrees were to be placed in charge of these units. Because there would not be enough of these highly trained individuals, the remainder of the units would be under the command of a general surgeon with some experience in plastic and bone surgery and a dental oral surgeon as his associate.[86]

The government then defined the terms *plastic surgeon, oral surgeon, dental oral surgeon*, and *dentist* as follows: a plastic surgeon had an MD and did plastic work, bone grafting, and maxillofacial injury cases; an oral surgeon had both an MD and a DDS and a license to practice both medicine and dentistry; a dental oral surgeon had a DDS and was skilled in minor oral surgery; and a dentist had a DDS and acted as a dental oral surgical assistant.[41]

Accordingly, on October 15, 1917, facilities were set up for establishing a school for training in oral and plastic surgery with headquarters at the University of Pennsylvania Dental School. Branches were established at the Jefferson Medical College, its hospital, and the Baugh Institute of Anatomy; the Medico-Chirurgical Hospital; Philadelphia General Hospital; and Pennsylvania Hospital. Doctors

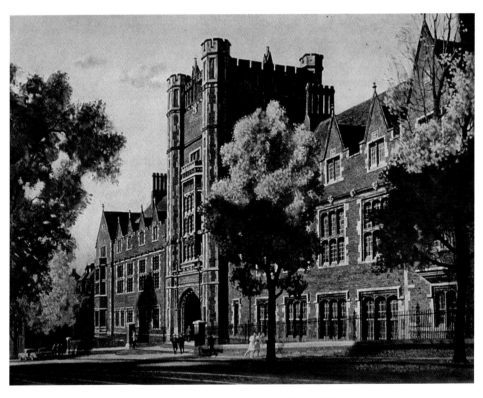

University of Pennsylvania School of Dental Medicine.
Reproduced from: http://wwwihm.nlm.nih.gov/ihm/images/A/26/814.jpg.
Courtesy of the National Library of Medicine.

Charles R Turner, dean, and Herman Prinz of the Evans Institute of Dental Surgery were placed in charge of organizing a teaching staff. Thirty-two medical and dental officers were detailed to Philadelphia to take the course. The medical officers were given special instruction in plastic surgery, bone transplantation, and blood transfusion. The dental officers received instruction in intraoral splint fixation, head and neck anatomy, and the systemic effects of focal infection. Similar schools were established at the Washington University Dental School in Saint Louis, Missouri; Northwestern University Dental School in Chicago, Illinois; and State University of Iowa, College of Dentistry in Iowa City, Iowa. In March 1918, after sufficient personnel had been trained, the courses were discontinued.[49,86,87]

Dr George Crile's Plan for Red Cross Army Base Hospitals

One of the major factors in the rapid transformation of the United States military medical system from peacetime to wartime was the new concept of the base hospital unit. After returning from a volunteer tour with the Lakeside Hospital/Western Reserve University Medical School of Cleveland, Ohio, at the American Ambulance in Paris (see Chapter 11) in October 1915, Dr George W Crile (1864–1943) conceived the idea and outlined the general scheme of the plan (Exhibit 12-1).[89] The concept was to organize military hospitals from existing civilian hospitals, medical schools, and medical centers, retaining their key personnel. In this manner, the best medical and surgical talent, already acquainted and accustomed to working together in civilian life, could be transported as a unit to the battlefield where they could still function as a unit. The American National Red Cross, through Colonel (later Brigadier General) Jefferson Randolph Kean, Medical Corps (who was then on detached duty to the American National Red Cross Headquarters from the surgeon general's office as director-general of the Department of Military Relief), immediately endorsed the base hospital plan and agreed to cooperate

---

EXHIBIT 12-1

DR GEORGE CRILE

Dr George Crile (1864–1943) served as an Army surgeon during the Spanish-American War and was founder of the American College of Surgeons. He was an authority on surgical shock and the means of preventing it through anesthesia and blood transfusions. He served as director of clinical research in the American Expeditionary Forces during World War I and successfully developed blood-banking techniques for military surgery 20 years before the practice became common in the civilian world. He also developed a pressure suit later used by fighter pilots in World War II. He remained a member of the Medical Officers' Reserve Corps and reached the rank of brigadier general.

Data source: Jones ET, ed. *Dictionary of American Biography, Supplement 3, 1941–1945*. New York, NY: Charles Scribner's Sons; 1973: 200–2003.

closely with the Medical Department on their organization, staffing, and equipping. By May 1916 seven hospitals were enrolled in what became known as the "affiliated medical units" program, and two others were prospects. The personnel were all enrolled in the Medical or Enlisted Medical Reserve Corps, and later in the Army Nurse Corps or DRC when they became functional. The minimum peacetime strength of the base hospital was 196 personnel. By the time the United States entered the war, 33 base hospital units were authorized and a number of them were equipped and trained for active duty with the US Army. An additional 14 were authorized in July 1917, and a total of 50 would eventually be formed during the war, with 49 serving in Great Britain or France. In *Dental Cosmos*, Dr Kirk called for the base hospital units being formed to make provision for competent dental surgeons on their staffs to treat jaw wounds. Because they had been trained and equipped since May 1916, the Red Cross base hospitals were the only Army hospitals ready for shipment to Europe when the Allies requested medical assistance. The first called and shipped to Europe were Base Hospital No. 2, the Presbyterian Hospital, New York; Base Hospital No. 4, the Lakeside Hospital, Cleveland, Ohio; Base Hospital No. 5, the Peter Bent Brigham Hospital, Harvard University; Base Hospital No. 10, the Pennsylvania Hospital, Philadelphia; Base Hospital No. 12, Northwestern University Medical School, Chicago; and Base Hospital No. 21, Washington University Medical School, Saint Louis. By June 1917 four base hospitals were already in England or France, two were en route to England, and four others were about to ship out.[91,92]

The medical staff of each standard, 500-bed base hospital unit consisted of one medical director, two administrative officers, one quartermaster, one adjutant, nine surgeons, seven physicians, two dental surgeons, and 50 nurses. Upon mobilization, the Army augmented the hospitals' regular staff with two Regular Army medical officers one to serve as the commanding officer and the other as the adjutant and 150 enlisted personnel. The total personnel, including nurses and civilian employees of each hospital, varied from 200 to 500 individuals depending upon the number of beds in the hospital.[92–94]

Staffing the Army Hospitals with Dentists

The Red Cross base hospitals were only one part of a complex of fixed and mobile hospitals that served the Army during the war. While Army dentists came to play important roles in most of them, prior to the war dentists were assigned to Army hospitals more by happenstance than by design. While dentists were often assigned to permanent hospitals, such as the General Hospital at the Presidio of San Francisco (renamed Letterman General Hospital in 1911), or the main hospital in Manila, their itinerant schedules took them to posts throughout their assigned areas in the geographic departments or divisions where civilian dentists were not readily available. Because there were so few dental surgeons, Army policy was to assign them to visit only "those stations where the services of a civilian dentist cannot be obtained."[95]

The Medical Department already had an established system of post, camp, and base hospitals in the departments or on the line of communications and in field and evacuation hospitals in the theater's forward zones of advance. The general hospitals in the United States and its territories supported these hospitals and came under the direct control of the surgeon general. The 1914 Army tables of organization and the 1916 *Manual for the Medical Department* allocated one dentist and one assistant to each 500-bed base hospital. In each of the four prewar general hospitals, the manual authorized a dental service of one dentist and one assistant.[5,8]

When the war came, the Medical Department had to staff and train all of these hospital units to support the mobilization and training bases in the United States and the AEF deployed in Europe. Base hospitals became the most important units because they would eventually supply almost all of the permanent hospitalization facilities for the AEF. The base hospital began the war as a 500-bed unit with one dentist (a first lieutenant), but instructions from the AEF soon changed it to a 1,000-bed hospital with a dental service of two Dental Corps captains and their assistants. A total of 165 numbered base hospital units were organized in the United States, of which 121 were eventually shipped with personnel and equipment to France and England (the AEF organized an additional 14 base hospitals from available resources), where they were operational during the war, temporarily supporting the camps at which they were training. In the United States camps and cantonments, the dental services of the 36 permanent camp base hospitals and 38 camp hospitals (virtually the same organizations) that were established to support the various mobilization and training camps provided dental care along with the dental infirmaries.[20,51,96]

Evacuation hospitals, which bridged the gap between base and camp hospitals and the frontline field hospitals, were established on the line of communications to care for the sick and wounded being evacuated to the rear areas. In 1916 no provision was made for dentists in these hospitals. In 1917 though, each evacuation hospital added one Dental Corps officer (a captain or first lieutenant) and an enlisted dental assistant. Like the base hospitals, evacuation hospitals were expanded to 1,000 beds and were then provided a Dental Service of two dentists and two enlisted assistants. Of the 60 evacuation hospitals organized in the United States, only 29 were shipped to France and saw action before the armistice (seven others reached France in November 1918).[8,20,51]

Dental officers experienced various difficulties mobilizing and shipping out. For example, in August 1917, Base Hospital No. 36 from the Detroit College of Medicine and Surgery, one of the Red Cross base hospitals, assembled at the state fair grounds, where the two dental officers, Captains Bion R East and Harry L Hosmer, provided care to unit members; otherwise, most of the group's time was focused on military basics and packing for shipment. When movement orders arrived, the dental officers were charged with supervising the loading and shipping of the hospital equipment and baggage in conjunction with a Regular Army Quartermaster Corps officer newly assigned to the hospital. At the port of Hoboken, New Jersey, in October, they monitored the transfer from railroad boxcars to their ocean transport. En route to England, they conducted daily sick call in the ship's pharmacy and attended various informal classes. East and Hosmer resumed their baggage responsibilities once in Liverpool and arranged for transfer of the goods across England to France and to their ultimate destination, the town of Vittel. The hospital's baggage included "complete equipment for two dentists bought in Detroit" and a dental laboratory, all of which arrived safely.[97]

General hospitals had no regularly assigned Dental Corps personnel until 1916. During the war, 34 additional general hospitals were opened around the country, so a total of 42 general hospitals were operational. The dental services handled routine dental examinations and treatment of patients who were in the hospital for medical or surgical care. Dental services were established on the ratio of one dentist to 1,000 beds, so there were several dentists in the larger hospitals. In September 1918, thanks to William HG Logan, the allocation for all hospitals was increased to three dentists per 1000 beds, but the war ended before it was fully implemented. Many of the larger general hospitals, which had a large patient load, also experienced significant expansion in the dental services. For example, Walter Reed General Hospital in Washington, DC, expanded from three to nine dentists during 1918, one of whom was on duty 24 hours a day to provide emergency dental treatment, and even opened a fully equipped dental department in a separate building. In addition, five female dental technicians worked in the hygienic sec-

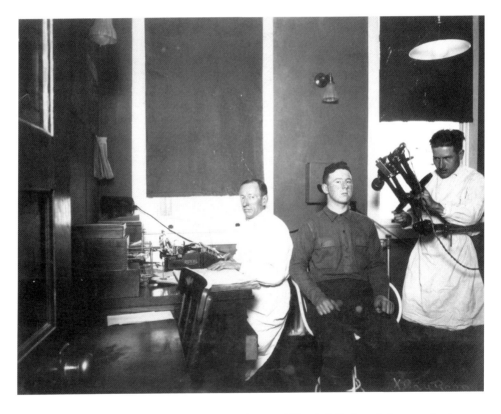

Oral surgery prosthetic room, Walter Reed General Hospital. Patients being examined.
Photograph: Courtesy of the National Museum of Health and Medicine,
Armed Forces Institute of Pathology. Reeve 34681.

tion of the department, thus freeing the dental officers to devote their full time to operating. A number of embarkation and debarkation hospitals were redesignated as general hospitals after November 1918 and additional general hospitals also opened after the armistice to handle the sick and wounded returning from France. A total of 43 numbered general hospitals and the original four hospitals were in operation at various times from April 1917 to March 1920.[6,8,20,39,40,96]

Women's Service

In 1917 the War Service committee of the Medical Women's National Association organized a group called the American Women's Hospitals, staffed by all-female personnel and officially a part of the Red Cross. This organization established the first American volunteer hospital unit for treating civilian casualties in France and Serbia. In December 1917, after American entry into the war, the Women's Hospital of New York equipped the first unit of female physicians that served as a base hospital at Ordway House, London, and at various places in France. The chairman of its dental service was Dr DeLan Kinney of New York.[98,99]

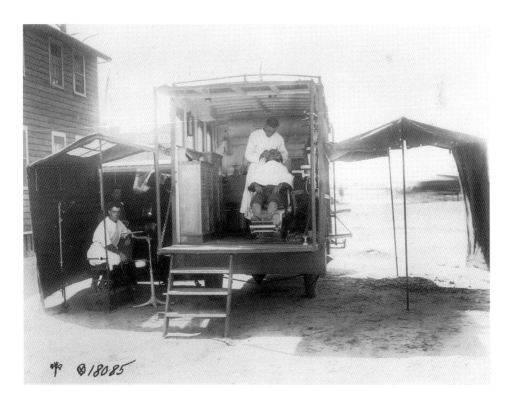

Dental motor car with patients, doctors working. Camp Upton, New York, 1918.
Photograph: Courtesy of the National Museum of Health and Medicine,
Armed Forces Institute of Pathology. Reeve 17664.

In April 1917 Dr Kinney had first applied to the surgeon general for appointment as a dental surgeon. A native of Nashville, Tennessee, she graduated from the University of Tennessee Dental School (1905) and the New York College of Dental and Oral Surgery (1916). She was an associate of Dr Rodrigues Ottolengui, editor of *Dental Items of Interest*, at the time of her application. In May the surgeon general's office replied that she was ineligible for the Regular Army Dental Corps because of her age (over 27), but could apply for the DRC. Her unusual first name originally hid the fact she was female, but when she reapplied, the surgeon general's office notified her that "women dentists" were not eligible for appointment.[100–106] Major Robert E Noble told her that "regardless of ability and eligibility," the law did not "provide for the commissioning of women, and nothing short of an Act of Congress would admit women," and recommended she join the American Women's Hospital Group.[99,107,108]

The Association of Military Dental Surgeons of the United States

The massive mobilization of American dentistry in support of the war effort and the large number of dentists now in uniform stimulated the growth of the Association of Military Dental Surgeons of the United States. Former Army contract dental surgeons of the initial 1901 group who were now in civilian practice originally established the association in 1913 as the dental equivalent to the Association of Military Surgeons of the United States (AMSUS) that Nicolas Senn had founded in 1891. In early 1915 the association's president was William C Fisher of New York City. John D Millikin of San Francisco was first vice president, William H Ware of San Francisco was second vice president, Charles J Long of Rock Island, Illinois, was secretary, and RW Waddell of New York City was treasurer. In the beginning, it was a rather small organization composed of members of the Regular Army Dental Corps and former contract dental surgeons.[109,110]

The association held its first annual meeting in 1915 in Washington, DC. It elected Dr John D Millikin president, replacing Dr William C Fisher. A former Army contract dental surgeon (1902–1912), Millikin was a vigorous advocate of Army dentistry. (Other officers elected were: Vice President Dr Charles J Long, Rock Island, Illinois; Secretary Dr Samuel W Hussey, Berkeley, California; Treasurer Dr Ralph W Waddell, New York City; and Member of Executive Council Dr Robert P Updyke, Pasadena, California, all of whom had served as original 1901 contract dental surgeons.) The association meeting in Louisville, Kentucky, in July 1916 coincided with that of the NDA.[111] During 1915 and 1916 Fisher and Millikin were both heavily involved in lobbying Congress, the War Department, and Surgeon General Gorgas on Army dental legislation (see Chapter 11). In October 1917 the association's annual meeting in New York City attracted more than 300 members of the armed forces. New officers elected in 1917 were: Captain Edwin P Tignor, president; Captain George Casaday, vice president; Dr Ralph W Waddell, secretary-treasurer; Dr John D Millikin, executive council member and editor of journal; Dr Edward PR Ryan, executive council member; and, Dr William C Fisher, associate journal editor and business manager. Honorary memberships were bestowed upon: Surgeon General Gorgas; Dr Homer C Brown of Ohio; Major William HG Logan of Chicago; Dr Lafayette L Barber of Ohio; Lieutenant Emory

Bryant, US Navy, of Washington, DC; and Dr Otto U King of Indiana.[112]

The association grew to include the dental officers of the National Guard, Navy, Public Health Service, and later the Veterans' Bureau, and was active as a lobbying force with the Department of the Navy, War Department, and Congress. In 1917 the association began publishing a journal, the *Bulletin of the Association of Military Dental Surgeons of the United States*, but changed the title the same year to *The Military Dental Journal*. Dr Millikin, who also served with William HG Logan on the Committee on Dentistry of the Council of National Defense's General Medical Board, was the editor of the journal, which carried articles and information specifically for military dentists. The organization, which was at its peak during World War I, had about 5,000 members and held regular annual meetings. The association and its journal were an important voice for Army and later military and government dentistry. After the war, however, membership fell off as the majority of uniformed dentists returned to civilian practice, and the association's influence waned. The journal ceased publication in 1924, following a congressional ruling forbidding Army officers to participate in this type of private professional enterprise. The association's decline continued throughout the 1920s and into the 1930s. With its membership down to 250 in 1938, the association amalgamated with the larger Association of Military Surgeons of the United States (AMSUS). A separate dental section was retained in the senior organization, which had already initiated its own dental section in 1936. Brigadier General Leigh C Fairbank (1889–1966), then the Dental Corps chief (1938–1942), was the driving force behind the merger.[109, 112]

Dental Equipment: Shortages, Improvisation, and Innovation

Because of the acute shortage of dental instruments in 1917, dental surgeons entering the service were asked to bring along certain instruments from their private outfits. The government agreed to purchase "dental outfits" in good condition from those on the short list at fair compensation. The new DRC officers were given instructions for equipping themselves in preparation for active duty.[113] The major reason for the equipment shortage was that the majority of dental instruments, including forceps, were made in Germany, with which the United States was now at war. Already heavily laden with orders from the Allies for the same reason, the American dental supply houses became swamped with large Army procurements and could not keep up with the increased demand. In addition to the portable dental outfits that were first developed in 1901 and had been the mainstay equipment for the prewar Dental Corps, the Army also began requisitioning stationary dental units for the National Army cantonments and National Guard mobilization camps. The medical supply depot in New York gave the contracts to the various dental manufactures, who tried their best to fill the orders. On May 25, 1917, the surgeon general directed the purchase of 500 portable outfits, followed by another order for 400 more on July 2 and a thousand late in August. During the war, the Army Medical Department bought a total of 4,030 portable outfits.[18,114–117]

Plans called for each dental surgeon in a division to be equipped with a portable dental outfit, an updated version of the outfit originally developed by John

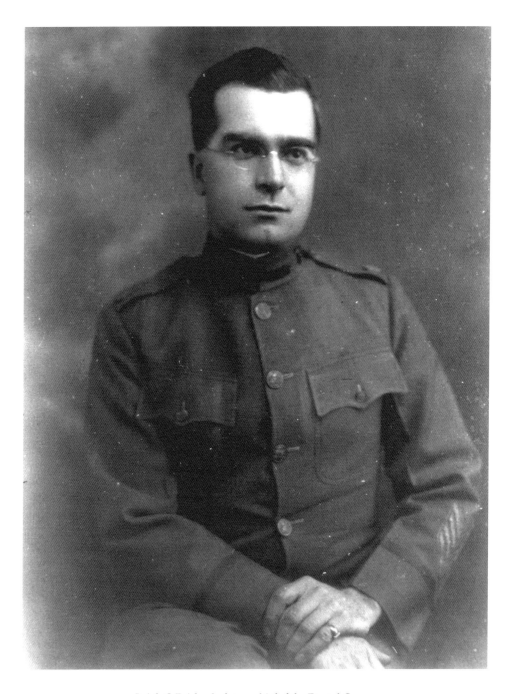

Leigh C Fairbank, future chief of the Dental Corps.
Photograph: Courtesy of Maryalice Minor, daughter of Leigh C Fairbank.

Marshall and Robert Oliver in 1901. When complete for overseas service, these portable outfits were not really so portable. Containing everything that the dentist actually required as well as supplies normally drawn from hospital stocks, the original outfit was made up of six packages: a dental engine in a chest, a collapsible dental chair in a chest, a field desk, two instrument chests, and a supply chest. Five additional packages were added for service in France: a portable stand and table, a single-burner coal-oil stove, a box of medicines, a box of miscellaneous supplies, and a box of alcohol. Altogether, the 11 packages occupied 39.3 cubic feet and weighed 775 pounds.[18]

After experiencing many problems with the shipping and frequent non-arrival of the portable outfits in 1917 and 1918, in June 1918 the surgeon general (on the advice of the AEF chief surgeon) directed all dental surgeons shipping out for France to take their outfits with them as personal baggage. This way, the surgeons were ready to work when they reached France and did not have to await his equipment. The ongoing problems with procuring and shipping dental equipment and supplies also left the AEF's medical supply depots without their full stock, often rendering them unable to fill requisitions for missing equipment.[10,18]

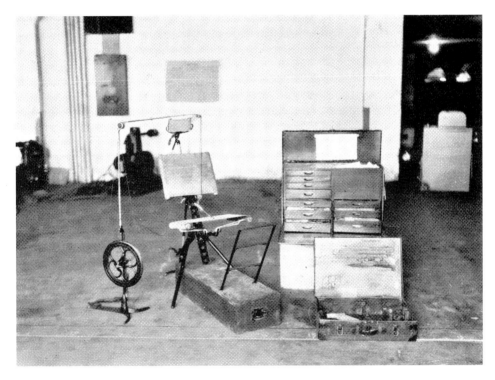

World War I portable dental outfit.
Reproduced from: Wolfe EP. Finance and Supply. In: The United States Army Medical Department in the World War. *Vol 3. Washington, DC: US Government Printing Office; 1928.*

a

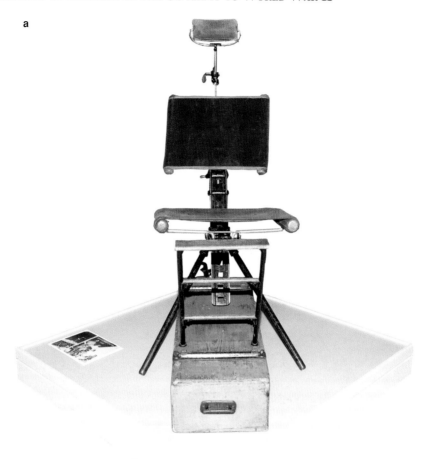

b

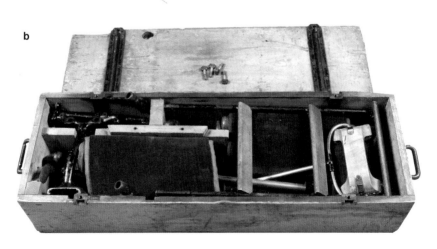

(**a**) *This portable dental chair was probably used through WWI.*
(**b**) *It breaks down to fit inside the wooden box to be transported.*
Photograph: Courtesy of US Army Medical Department Museum.

Stationed with the 28th Division at Camp Hancock, Georgia, First Lieutenant C Judson Hollister, Dental Corps, National Guard, who had recently served on the Mexican Border, stated that at the time of his arrival in the camp of almost 30,000 soldiers, there were 33 dental surgeons but only two dental outfits. In September 1917, another dental officer, First Lieutenant Harold Van Blarcom with the 116th Infantry Regiment, 29th Division, stationed at Camp McClellan, Alabama, complained that his unit had about 20 dentists but not one complete dental outfit between them. They spent "several weeks in shacks with nothing to do" but make friends, explore the camp, fill out forms, and try to learn the customs of the service. First Lieutenant HR Ludwig reported a similar situation upon his arrival at Camp Zachary Taylor, Louisville, Kentucky.[118–120] On the other hand, First Lieutenant J Crimen Zeidler, stationed at Camp Nicholls, Louisiana, reported that his dental infirmary had been established within 2 days of his arrival and his dental equipment was in place by the fourth day.[121]

Dental Ambulances

At least one valuable new piece of dental equipment entered the Army inventory during the war but saw little use in France. In 1915 Dr William C Speakman, a Wilmington, Delaware, dentist, performed several months of volunteer service with the American Hospital at Neuilly near Paris, France. In the course of his duties, he saw several British and French dental ambulances, basically van- or truck-mounted mobile dental clinics that had been donated by private groups on duty with tactical units. Impressed by the flexibility and mobility these vehicles provided for dental care at the front, Speakman was inspired to design his own dental ambulance while on the boat trip home. Through advertisements in local newspapers, he raised enough resources to have it fabricated on a Buick chassis and to take it back to France in early 1916. Fully equipped and attached to the American Hospital at Neuilly, Speakman's ambulance was heavily used. French authorities claimed that its services kept "soldiers to the number of a division and a half" at the front. Speakman later entered the DRC and served in France with Mobile Hospital No. 39 (Yale Unit). His ambulance design became the basis for later official action. After the US Army arrived in France, it took over the original ambulance itself as Dental Ambulance No. 1.[122,123]

In October 1917 the War Department adopted a standardized dental ambulance. The Cleveland Dental Motor Car Committee of the Cleveland Unit of the Preparedness League of American Dentists developed the basic design that the Committee on Dentistry of the General Medical Board accepted. The Brown Auto Carriage Company in Cleveland built the first three cars under the direction of Dr S Marshall Weaver, the chairman of the Preparedness League's Ambulance Committee. The chassis was the GMC Model 16, the only chassis used for ambulances overseas. The car was designed to provide for four dentists and a driver. In addition to a fully equipped operating room (chair, engine, bracket table, cuspidor, and the like) inside the truck, the outfit included two portable, waterproof tents, designed to be set up on each side of the chassis. Each tent had a wooden floor. The chair in the outfit was the model 1895 SS White portable dental chair. The vehicle had a 30-gallon water tank, compressed air tank,

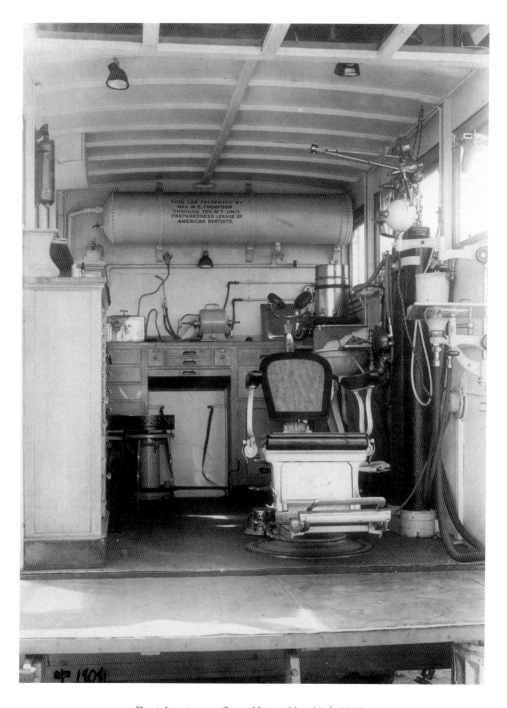

*Dental motor car, Camp Upton, New York, 1918.
Photograph: Courtesy of the National Museum of Health and Medicine,
Armed Forces Institute of Pathology. Reeve 017665.*

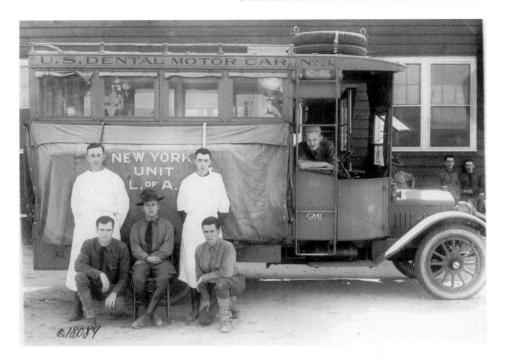

Dental motor car, Camp Upton, New York, 1918.
Photograph: Courtesy of the National Museum of Health and Medicine,
Armed Forces Institute of Pathology. Reeve 017666.

alcohol stove, and a sterilizer. The Cleveland unit donated the first car, and Dr Charles F Ash of New York donated the other two.[124]

In his final report, Colonel Robert T Oliver, chief dental surgeon of the AEF, wrote that:

> The need for dental ambulances, mobile dental offices, has been manifest through-out the entire dental service of the A.E.F. . . . The use of these dental ambulances with outlying commands or detachments within divisional training areas or in rear of combat sectors would have proven of great value inasmuch as the mobile units could proceed from place to place with little loss of time, either in actual transportation or in the unpacking and repacking of equipment ordinarily required of a dental officer on itinerary service.[10(p409)]

The Preparedness League of American Dentists had 25 completely equipped dental ambulances ready to be presented to the AEF, provided they could be shipped to France. However, neither Oliver nor the AEF chief surgeon's office could obtain the necessary tonnage priority allocation to get the dental ambulances on transports headed their way. Thus, the vehicles sat at ports of embarkation for months until they were finally removed and sent to the Army cantonments in the United States for use.[10,125]

437

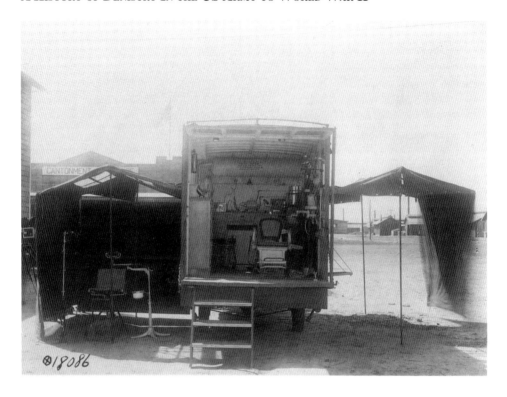

View from distance of dental motor car, door open, tent, chair,
spittoon beside. Camp Upton, New York.
Photograph: Courtesy of the National Museum of Health and Medicine,
Armed Forces Institute of Pathology. Reeve 17663.

Speakman's Dental Ambulance No. 1 operated extensively within the Zone of the Armies, but was one of only two such ambulances to actually serve in the AEF during the war. The American Red Cross donated the second ambulance, which functioned as Dental Ambulance No. 2 in support of aerosquadrons of the aviation service in the Advanced Section. Mobile dental offices were viewed as the "ideal type of dental equipment for Air Squadron Groups."[10(p409)]

Dental Standards for Conscripts and Recruits

In March 1917, with the imminent prospect of mass mobilization for the United States, *Dental Summary* mused about the implications to the dental profession of instructing millions of soldiers in the value of regular dental care. After the war, many believed that these men would continue to seek dental treatment and more dentists would be required to fill the new demand for service. Apparently, the new inductees' attitudes started to change when they arrived at the training depots and received among their equipment a "recruit kit," which included a toothbrush.[126,127]

a

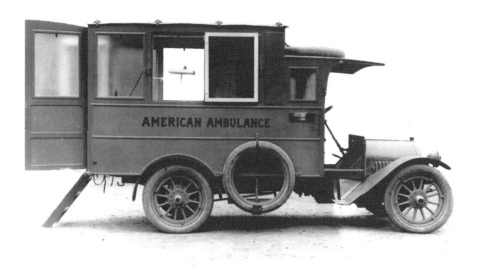

*American ambulance designed for William Speakman. (a) Exterior. (b) Interior.
Photograph: Courtesy of National Archives and Records Administration.*

b

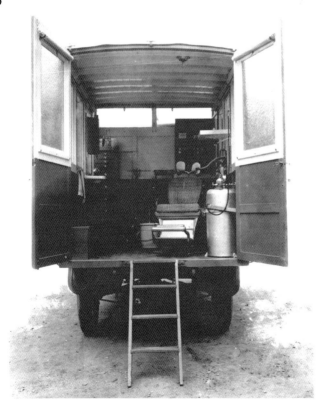

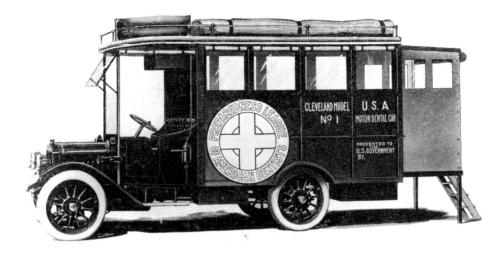

Cleveland Dental Ambulance. This design was the standardized War Department dental ambulance originally proposed by the Preparedness League of American Dentists in 1917. The original caption reads: "This is the car that has been designed and standardized by the Ambulance Committee of the Preparedness League of American Dentists, and accepted by the War Department. These cars are under construction and will be tried out in the various cantonments." Reproduced from: Dental Cosmos. *1918;24:10.*

With the introduction of selective service in 1917, some potential draftees opted to have their teeth extracted to avoid conscription, just as during the Civil War. The government deplored such actions and said that it would prosecute dentists who intentionally extracted teeth to disqualify a conscript. However, no reliable method was proposed to judge such actions.[128]

The huge growth of the forces compelled the Army to relax its dental requirements for recruits. The old requirement of four opposing molars was reduced in 1918 to three opposing molar teeth on the same side. Crowns, bridges, and partial dentures were counted as natural teeth, but full dentures were a cause for rejection. Still, about 50% of the rejected recruits were turned down because they did not have the required three molar teeth.[129] In addition to the six opposing molars, inductees had to have six opposing incisors. If any of the natural teeth were carious and could be repaired, they were considered adequate. The recruit could have the work done at home prior to induction or at the cantonment where he was ordered to duty. Even with the requisite teeth, those whose mouths showed conditions such as "deep pyorrhea pockets" or root infection (with or without a draining sinus) were referred to a medical advisory board for a decision. At the conclusion of an article on the subject extracted from the *Journal of the American Medical Association* and reprinted in *Dental Cosmos*, Edward Kirk wrote: "No registrants can be rejected on account of teeth defects."[130(pp274–275)]

These much looser wartime dental standards meant that many recruits who would have been rejected for peacetime service were now admitted. The new

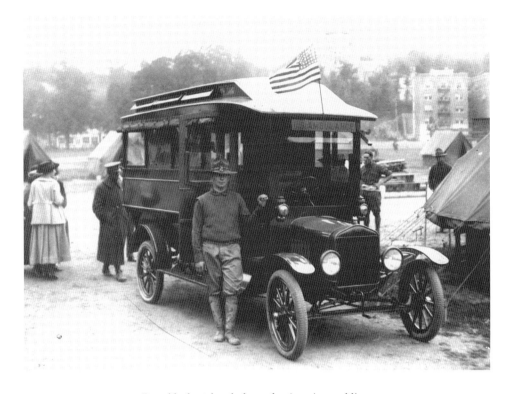

Portable dental ambulance for American soldiers,
circa February 1918, at Camp Meade, Maryland.
Photograph: Courtesy of National Archives and Records Administration.

troops' dental problems became the Army's dental problems, resulting in significant consequences for existing Army policies that only permitted emergency dental treatment and prohibited more refined dental work and materials. Dentures, bridges, restorations, and other serious dental deficiencies soon presented major problems at the mobilization and training camps and cantonments. In September 1918 Colonel Logan estimated that 90% of those who had entered the service required dental treatment.[18,131]

Establishing Dental Service at the Army's New Camps and Cantonments

As soon as war was declared, the Quartermaster General's Department embarked on a massive construction program to provide shelter to the millions of conscripts it anticipated being called up for training. Almost concurrently, National Guard units (26th through 42nd divisions) were recalled to federal service. These units were sent to 16 temporary mobilization camps, usually facilities in the south where the presumably milder climate allowed the greater use of tents. As guard units poured into the camps, 16 semipermanent cantonments with newly constructed wooden structures were hastily thrown together at sites throughout

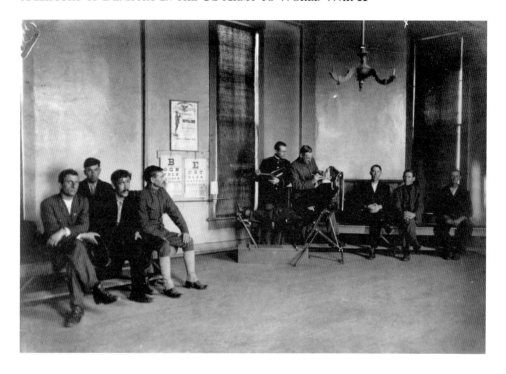

Dr Seibert D Boak, dental surgeon at Columbus Recruit Depot, Ohio,
from August 1915 to January 1918, completing a dental examination of a recruit.
Photograph: Courtesy of the family of Seibert D Boak.

the north in anticipation of hoards of draftees composing the so-called National Army (76th through 93rd divisions). Newly appointed dental officers were assigned to the cantonments both as part of the camp overhead and as members of tactical units in training. All too often these mobilization and training camps descended into chaos as soldiers, equipment, and supplies rarely arrived as planned or promised.[2,96,132,133] The dental story was certainly no exception to this rule.

The earliest concepts for dental treatment in the camps and cantonments included only emergency work like the kind the dental surgeons had done since 1901. Therefore dental equipment was limited to portable dental outfits for dentists in camp organizations and a base dental outfit for the base hospital, while the dental surgeons of the divisions in training brought their assigned individual portable outfits. By November 1917 it was clear that this approach was not working. The division and base hospital dental surgeons who trained in the camps either took their personal portable and unit dental outfits when they shipped out for France— leaving insufficient equipment for continuing camp requirements and requiring large-scale replacement—or went without their equipment if they left the outfits behind. Because of this totally unanticipated challenge, new dental infirmaries were authorized for each National Army cantonment and National Guard camp.[18,96]

The standard portable dental outfits were only intended for emergency care

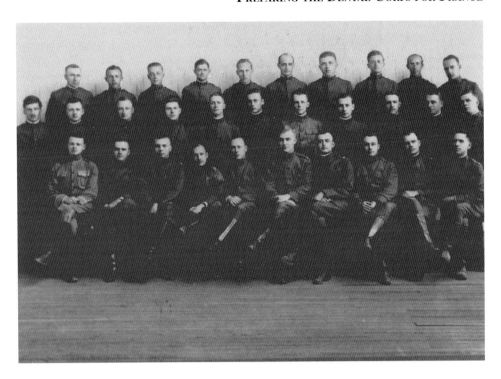

Oscar P Snyder (fifth from right) and dental surgeons of
28th Division at Augusta, Georgia, before shipping out to France, 1918.
Photograph: Courtesy of Major Oscar P Snyder.

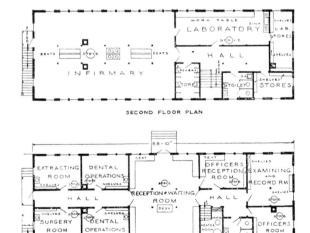

Construction drawing of a
standard camp dental
infirmary for a National Army
cantonment of 1917–1918.
Reproduced from: The
Medical Department of the
United States Army in the
World War. *Vol 5.*
Washington, DC: Government
Printing Office; 1923: 108.

FIG 63.

443

and were ill-suited to treat the more pronounced dental deficiencies that presented themselves. Thus, standard dental chairs, furniture, an electric dental engine
(where electrical power was available), an instrument cabinet, a laboratory outfit,
and some additional instruments together with the portable dental outfits were
used in general hospitals, at larger military posts, and in base hospitals to treat the
more complicated dental cases. Originally called the additional dental outfit, this
equipment package later became the base dental outfit used throughout the Army.
Unlike the portable outfits, heavy standard dental chairs and electric dental engines were readily available from civilian suppliers and the government procured
them for the infirmaries' base dental outfits. Each was designed for nine operating
dental surgeons and one orthodontist, and three units were sent to each camp and
cantonment in November 1917 for the newly authorized dental infirmaries. The
first 60 base dental outfits were authorized on August 14, 1917, and 400 chairs
and engines were required for all authorized dental infirmaries. From April 1917
to November 1918, the military purchased 1,550 chairs and 1,184 electric dental
engines. These acquisitions relieved the tension on the portable dental outfits and
the Army standards for dental treatment underwent a radical change.[18]

After the fall of 1917, when the camp's own base hospital included a dental
outfit, each training camp and cantonment had three or four dental infirmaries
"where the services of the dental surgeon could be fully utilized and practically
every kind of dental treatment needed could be furnished." Once these facilities
were equipped with the more complete base dental outfits, staffed, and operational, the dental surgeons could turn their portable dental outfits in to the camp
medical supply officer for refurbishing. The surgeon general's office then took
control of the outfits and could reissue them to deploying dental surgeons, thus
relieving the problem of availability of portable dental outfits. However, not all
dental infirmaries were operational until the late spring of 1918 and soldiers often
experienced inconvenience in obtaining treatment in some of the larger, more dis-
persed camps.[18]

The experiences of the dentists assigned to Camp Sherman, Chillicothe, Ohio,
were typical of the early problems of establishing dental services. Between August 13 and 22, 1917, seven dental reservists arrived at the camp, which was still
under construction. They spent a few days in temporary barracks until the post
hospital was completed. Three remained at the hospital while the others scattered to units located elsewhere on the post. They all shared the one dental outfit
of an Ohio National Guard unit. When First Lieutenant (later Major) Benjamin H
Sherrard reported as division dental surgeon on September 14, he sized up the
equipment situation and requested shipment of an unused set of field equipment
he had left behind at Jefferson Barracks, Missouri. His equipment arrived on September 17 and was set up in the officer's ward of the base hospital where most
dental services could be offered. More dentists arrived by the end of September.
They were quartered in the hospital until dental field outfits arrived, then joined
various organizations around the camp, eventually leaving five dentists to staff
the hospital. "Permanent quarters in the head surgery building were occupied
on or about October 10, 1917." Field equipment was used briefly, but by November 1, standard permanent equipment and furniture had been installed. There

were three operating rooms, a laboratory and an office, allowing full service dental and prosthetic operations. The unit received all oral surgery and prosthetic cases from the cantonment and provided all dental treatment to hospital patients and staff. Cordial mutual support quickly developed between it and the other medical departments.[134]

As the new recruits arrived at camp, the dental officers, who often lacked their equipment and had time on their hands, quickly introduced them to the latest advances in oral hygiene and preventive dentistry. Lieutenant Hollister of the 28th Division described a morning "tooth-brush" drill as "a great sight to see 150 men in line with cup, tooth-brush, and paste or powder in hands 'cleaning up' in a way that had been entirely unknown to most of them a few months ago." He estimated that at least 50% had never previously brushed on a regular basis.[118]

In March 1918 First Lieutenant Alvie R Livermore, a National Army dental surgeon stationed at Camp Zachary Taylor, Louisville, Kentucky, credited Army dentists with saving more teeth than their civilian counterparts because there was less chance for soldiers to have missing teeth replaced with bridges or dentures. Therefore, the forceps was not the "predominating instrument" of the military dentist, as was commonly believed outside the Army. Livermore praised his colleagues' ability to save teeth by restoration with amalgam and their success in treating periodontal conditions. First Lieutenant KF Smith, DRC, agreed, stating that the only difference between military dentistry and civilian dentistry was the type of restorative material available to the military dentist. It could be said that another reason for saving teeth in the Army was to dispel the reputation that came with the rumor, "if you got a toothache in the army, they pulled it out."[135,136] Later, the Camp Zachary Taylor dental clinic placed high in an "efficiency record competitive test" sponsored by the Association of Military Dental Surgeons of the United States in the first 3 months of 1918. Major William Mann, Dental Corps, who had entered the service in 1916, was in charge of the dental clinic. In January 1918 a record 9,554 total operations were performed.[117]

The dentists knew their job was to get their assigned units into the best possible oral health and ready for deployment. Once the soldiers were examined and their records made, the work began in earnest, with the most critical cases treated first. At Camp Dodge, Iowa, the oral problems of the forming 88th Division were identified and the troops ordered to treatment based on the dentist's recommendations, rather than their own or their unit's desires. Those failing to show up for treatment were checked on and disciplined if necessary. The unit dental officers accompanied their medical counterparts on fortnightly visits to the troops to follow up on treatments and to answer any questions their patients might have. Numbers of dentists were occasionally levied for reassignment to deploying units or as individual overseas replacements, and newly called up reservists had to replace them. Considerable turnover occurred between September 1917 and July 1918 when assignments finally stabilized, and, under the leadership of Lieutenant Colonel Frank P Stone, the dentists moved to France with the division.[137]

On July 3, 1917, most of the Pennsylvania National Guard was called into federal service and redesignated the 28th Division. During its training at Camp Hancock, Georgia, from August 1917 to April 1918, the division's medical department consisted of the 103rd Sanitary Train, ambulance companies numbers 109, 110, 111, 112, Headquarters, Field Hospital Section, field hospitals 109, 110, 111, 112, a mobile field laboratory, a veterinarian, Mobile Veterinary Section Number 109, and a medical supply unit. [138]

The 28th Division's medical department had a dental department consisting of 32 dental surgeons and 32 enlisted assistants. The assistants were selected for their adaptability for dental work. Shortly after mobilization, the dental surgeons were organized to work in three dental units, one in each brigade, to care for it and any auxiliary organizations in its locality. Parts of the previously built regimental infirmaries were used to house the dental units, the most central infirmary in each brigade being used, with a Dental Corps captain in charge of each unit. The captain's duties consisted of procuring the necessary supplies and equipment for the other dental surgeons and arranging for a system of appointments so that the dentists did not waste their time. The captain was also responsible for carrying out courses of instruction in subjects of importance to dental officers. Semimonthly inspections were held to evaluate the oral health of the soldiers. Each infirmary submitted a weekly report of the dental work performed to track the number of sittings, fillings, extractions, and the like. The local dental officers also gave talks to the enlisted troops on oral health. [139]

On August 30, 1917, First Lieutenant Oscar P Snyder joined the 28th Division at Camp Hancock as the dental supply officer. [140] On September 25, 1917, he reported to Major William HG Logan that there were only two portable dental outfits available for use in the camp for the 33 (counting himself) dental officers on duty, and only one base dental outfit had been shipped for use in a regimental infirmary. [141]

On October 20, 1917, Snyder reported that he had held triweekly meetings with the dental officers to discuss Army Regulations, Medical Department and courts martial manuals, and military writing and the various military forms to be filled out. In addition, he required each dental surgeon to write a paper on a dental subject to be read and discussed at the meetings. An oral examination of the enlisted soldiers revealed that 75% were in need of some form of dental attention. [142]

On November 24, 1917, Snyder reported that in compliance with the surgeon general's orders, division dental units numbers 1, 2, and 3 had completed organization and were composed of 8, 10, and 11 dental officers, respectively. The ratio of one dental surgeon to each thousand enlisted was as prescribed. In addition, there were two dental officers assigned to the Engineer Regiment, and Lieutenant Hollister with the "privately owned" dental ambulance. Snyder also reported that an additional 22 portable dental outfits had just arrived, therefore every dental surgeon in the division finally had his own equipment. [143] On January 4, 1918, Lieutenant Snyder reported to the division surgeon that there was a problem with the soldiers reporting for dental sick call. It seems they were not reporting early in the morning, but in some cases arrived as late as 8:45 or 9:00 AM. Snyder said the soldiers were "loafing around the place where sick call is being held until the last one when he might have been at the dental office, treated and out to duty by that time." He recommended that the surgeons holding sick call send all dental cases to the dental office before they proceeded with the actual sick call. In this manner the soldiers could be returned to duty quickly instead of wasting time at sick call.[144]

Broken appointments were also a problem for the dental surgeons because the training schedule made no provision to excuse those with dental appointments from drill, marches, kitchen police, or other duties. As a result, dental surgeons' hours were increased in order to do a greater amount of work.[143] In March 1918 sites for two new dental infirmaries for Camp Hancock, each 90-by-30 feet and two stories high, were selected and awaiting approval for construction by the construction quartermaster.[145,146]

In April 1918 the 28th Division's surgeon, Lieutenant Colonel William J Crookston, complained to the commanding general that there was "no such thing as enlisted dental personnel." It seems the dental assistants were working "on detached duty" and were carried by the organization to which they belonged. He felt that they should be permanently assigned to the Medical Department and detailed as dental assistants. By then, Camp Hancock had 28 dental assistants—17 from the line and 11 from the Medical department—and was still short four. Crookston recommended that these soldiers be authorized and recognized as dental assistants, assigned to the Medical Department, and detailed as dental assistants; that way they would accompany the regimental detachment and would be quartered and carried on the rolls of the different sanitary detachments.[147] Furthermore, he recommended that the "question of Dental Assistants be taken up with the Adjutant General, and that a definite decision as to their status be established."[148]

Snyder, by then a major (he was promoted on October 6, 1917), went to France in May 1918 as the division dental surgeon. The division's May 1918 personnel return stated that it deployed with its full quota of medical officers, but only 18 of the authorized 31 dental officers.[149]

One of the last big division cantonments to be completed was Camp Frémont, Palo Alto, California, the training site of the Regular Army's Eighth Division, giving it the advantage of learning from the preceding year's activities around the country. Major Charles M Taylor, Dental Corps, arrived in April 1918 and began organizing dental support for the camp as other dentists trickled in throughout May. Each was assigned to a fully equipped dental infirmary located in the dispensary of each thousand-person unit. A few of the infirmaries were in tents, but most were in buildings. Unit members received complete dental inspections and treatment began based on the degree of urgency. Among the first 14,339 soldiers inspected (about half the division), there were 21,402, carious teeth and 6,053 extractions were necessary. Nearly 4,000 troops had more serious oral problems. Permanent division dental infirmaries were completed in June, allowing full dental service of any complexity, while a laboratory allowed any category of dentures to be produced. The division dentists met twice weekly for classes on military and medical subjects and enjoyed close working relations with their medical colleagues.[150]

In 1918 First Lieutenant EH Scheifer described the dental department at Camp Grant, Illinois, which was located in a two-story building. The second floor had 18 chairs and cabinets, electric engines, sterilizers, atomizers, two air compressors, and a rest area for officers of the day. The first floor consisted of the reception room, extraction rooms, X-ray room, the commanding officer's office, and an examining room. All the dental units were finished in white enamel. In addition, there were eight or ten small clinics scattered throughout the camp, each with two or three dental outfits. About 70 dentists and an equal number of assistants were assigned to the camp. The majority of the assistants were dentists who were not commissioned. In October 1918 the clinics' 51 dental officers treated over 7,436 patients, inserted 9,084 permanent fillings, extracted 2,205 teeth, and performed 1,138 prophylaxes. Other work included root canal therapy, temporary fillings, and denture construction.[151]

In July 1918 the dental profession began a campaign to provide automobiles for to dental personnel at the various sprawling camps. Donated by private sources, these vehicles were eventually delivered to the dental services at Camps Upton, Greenleaf, Frémont, Sherman, and Merritt and allowed the dental officers to travel quickly to the various clinics on the bases. Previously, some dentists had to walk as far as 6 miles from one infirmary to another. The donations responded to a need first perceived during the Civil War by the Confederate Army, which found it expedient to provide official transportation for its hospital steward dentists to and from their assigned hospitals.[152]

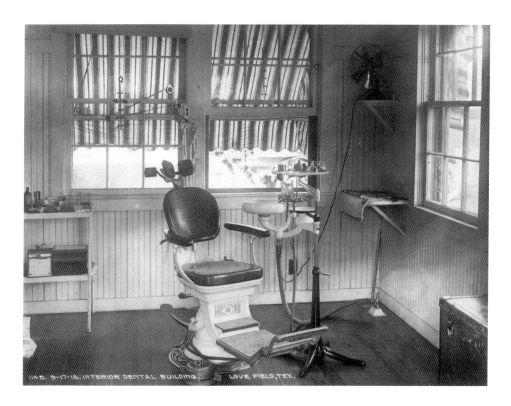

Interior of the dental buildingLove Field, Texas 1918.
Photograph: Courtesy of the National Museum of Health and Medicine,
Armed Forces Institute of Pathology. NCP 1338.

Dental Assistants

In 1918 the dental infirmary at Camp Sheridan in Montgomery, Alabama, was under the command of First Lieutenant William A Squires. By early 1918 dental facilities throughout the post were complete, and 21 dentists and 26 enlisted dental assistants were hard at work. A March 1918 news item in *American Dentist* described the dental work:

> Each dental operator has his own assistant who sterilizes each instrument immediately after use. The position of operator or assistant is no sinecure, as the infirmary handles from 250 to 300 patients daily. The regular schedule is from 7:30 a.m. to 5 p.m., but at all hours of the night men are kept on duty to attend emergency cases. Attendance at clinics and quiz classes, held two nights a week, is compulsory. Work in the dental infirmary is continuous instruction in the theoretical as well as the practical side of dentistry.[153]

The dental assistants at Camp Sheridan clearly played an important role in the installation's dental program, but the source of the dental assistants was as uncertain as it had been since the first contract dental surgeons entered Army service in 1901. At first they were soldiers of the Hospital Corps. After the Medical Department's Enlisted Force replaced the Hospital Corps as a result of the National Defense Act of 1916, the dental assistants had at least some dental training or interest in the field. They were usually accounted for on a separate muster roll along with the itinerant dentist, but they were still Medical Department personnel assigned at the will of the surgeon general's office. Close working relationships often evolved between the dentists and their assistants, and they were frequently reassigned together. However, such assignments were not policy and many dentists had to repeatedly train neophytes as they made their circuits. In 1915, for example, First Lieutenant Seibert D Boak asked that his assistant of 6 years be reassigned with him for the fourth time since 1909 because "I have trained him to my own methods of operating and disposition of instruments, which enables me to handle more patients per day." Major Robert E Noble in the surgeon general's office responded that the surgeon general no longer viewed it as "a good plan to make such transfers . . . for administrative reasons he does not think it desirable to make assignments permanent." The Mexican Border expedition and then the World War caused an unprecedented demand for dental care that gained recognition for skilled dental assistants and acknowledged them as a separate and required enlisted specialty. The National Defense Act of 1916 prompted a need to clarify the pay rates for Medical Department enlisted soldiers. On November 18, 1916, the secretary of war directed that privates first class on duty as dental assistants would be considered the same as surgical assistants for pay purposes. This decision made the duty more attractive and stabilized an enlisted career track.[154,155]

African Americans and Fort Des Moines, Iowa

On August 27, 1917, a special training camp was opened at Fort Des Moines, Iowa, for African American medical and dental officers. Before 1917 African American medical or dental officers did not exist, with the exception of a few isolated

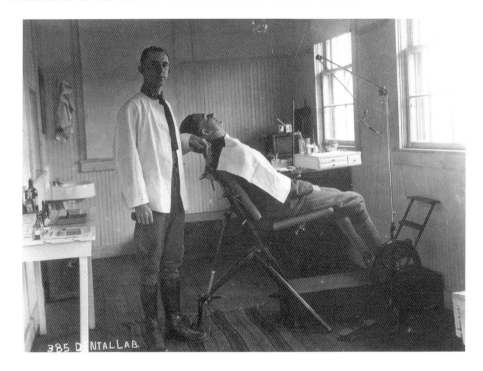

Interior of the dental building at Love Field, Texas, 1918.
Photograph: Courtesy of the National Museum of Health and Medicine,
Armed Forces Institute of Pathology. NCP 1609.

cases in African American National Guard units. Once African American combat divisions were approved for organization in the National Army, the need for medical and dental personnel became an urgent matter. There were already 1,200 African American enlistees in training at the reserve officers' training camp for service with the infantry. Thirty physicians from among this group were transferred at their request to the newly established medical training camp and commissioned in the medical section of the Officers' Reserve Corps. Soon there were 116 soldiers in training at the camp, including 12 dentists.[156]

Prior to the war, the surgeon general's office had not been receptive to the idea of African American commissioned medical personnel, claiming they could not itinerate in a segregated force and would be "social pariahs" because of their race and officer status.[157] During the war with Spain, Captain William T Jefferson, a black dentist from Chicago, had served as commander of D Company, Eighth Illinois Infantry, a segregated National Guard unit. In his spare time, he provided dental care to his and two other African American guard regiments, likely becoming the first African American to perform dentistry in the US Army.[158–162] He was among many black dentists who applied for an appointment in the new Dental Corps between 1901 and 1917 only to be rejected. Age or physical condition were often given as reasons for these rejections, while some applicants were turned down for lack of competence.[161,163–166] Once war was declared and the need for numbers of African

450

American medical officers could not be ignored, the surgeon general authorized their being commissioned in the inactive reserve to be called up as needed.[167]

It took most of July 1917 to develop a curriculum and prepare facilities before the first class began on August 27. The course lasted about 5 weeks and followed a mix of military and technical subjects. Dental officers took the same program as medical officers except for subjects wholly medical, for which dental topics were substituted. The *Journal of Allied Dental Societies* noted that the opening of the Des Moines camp marked "a new departure" in Army Medical Department policy toward "colored" medical personnel.[156,168–170] By June 1918 there were about 250 black medical and dental officers in the Officers' Reserve Corps providing care to the roughly 157,000 African American soldiers in the Army and in the 92nd and 93rd Divisions, both of which were then in France.[170,171]

Dental Officer Training

Training for all medical personnel gradually consolidated in the course of the war. By March 1918 there were 5,400 officers and enlisted soldiers, including dental personnel, in military medical training at the medical officers' training camp at Camp Greenleaf, Fort Oglethorpe, Georgia, and 3,800 at Fort Riley, Kansas. The

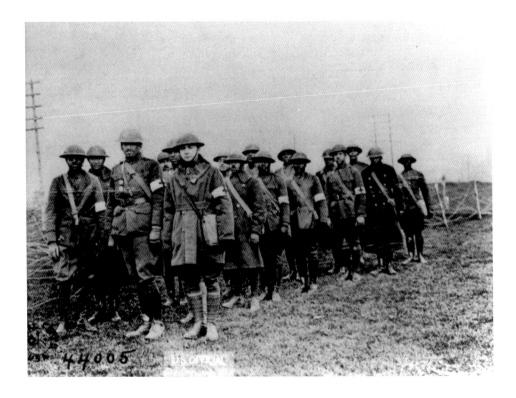

Dentists of the 92nd Division in the field at Millery,
Meurthe et Moselle, Lorraine, France. November 15, 1918.
Photograph: Courtesy of US Army Military History Institute. SC 44005.

Fort Riley camp had a capacity for 7,000 and Fort Oglethorpe for 5,500 medical personnel. Oglethorpe eventually grew to the same size as Fort Riley and became the single center for training and Fort Riley was phased out. Between June 1917 and March 1918, a total of about 9,000 officers and 20,000 enlisted soldiers graduated from the medical training camps or were still under instruction. The medical training camps at Fort Benjamin Harrison, Indiana, and at Fort Des Moines, Iowa, for African American soldiers were phased out first.[172]

Additional facilities were added at Camp Greenleaf, under the command of Brigadier General Henry P Birmingham, Medical Corps, National Army, to accommodate a 2-month course for dental personnel; one month was to be devoted to military training and one to professional training. Each class could include up to 165 officers and the same number of enlisted dental assistants, who were frequently selected from drafted dental college students. All recently appointed Regular Dental Corps officers and enough DRC officers to fill the class were ordered to take the course. On March 15, 1918, the first class of dental officers (50 Regular Army and 35 Reserve Corps) began their 2 months of instruction at Fort Oglethorpe. Lieutenant Colonel John H Snapp was the senior dental instructor, assisted by Majors Ben H Sherrard and E Henry Valentine, Dental Corps, and Major John D Eby, DRC. The staff already at the camp conducted the military instruction.[173–175]

During the first month of training, approximately 180 hours were devoted to general military subjects. The second month consisted of only 71 hours of military and 100 hours of dental subjects. The plan was to start a new class of about 85 dental officers each month. In March 1918 there were about 1,500 officers and 9,000 enlisted soldiers in camp from the various branches of the Medical Department: Dental Corps, Medical Corps, Sanitary Corps, and Veterinary Corps.[174]

Problems for Enlisted Dentists

Approximately 800 graduate dentists serving as enlisted soldiers passed though the medical officers' training camp at Camp Greenleaf during the war. The War Department called up more of them than could be accommodated or trained effectively. The enlistees were housed in converted mule stables and subjected to endless drill and fatigue duties as the school struggled to expand to train them properly. Dental Company No. 1, the dentists' training unit, fielded an undefeated football team as one of its few accomplishments. Most of the enlisted dentists were unable to use their skills, except for a fortunate few later selected for assignment as dental assistants in other camps.[173,174,176–178] In September 1918, when two dental officers were authorized per thousand troops, arrangements were made to examine those eligible for commissions in the DRC. But before the examinations could be held, the armistice was signed and the secretary of war ruled the commissions could not be issued. It was a bitter disappointment for the dentists involved who had understood that they would be commissioned even after the armistice was a reality.[179]

One of those victims of this "tragedy of Camp Greenleaf" was Dr Walter Dean Gearen of Racine, Wisconsin. He was a senior dental student at Marquette University who had enlisted in the Army so that he could continue his dental studies without interference from the draft. He graduated in 1918 with a DDS degree, took the Wisconsin dental boards and was licensed, and about 15 days later received his orders for active duty. He was assigned to Dental Company No. 1 at Fort Oglethorpe. In about 5 months, the company strength grew to some 450 enlisted soldiers, dental graduates from all over the country. "All Buck Privates," Gearen wrote, with a "scattering of one or two stripers, men who had some training in the this and that and knew a few of the tricks" of the military. Gearen described the training:

> Twice a day, five days a week, it was "fours right, left and Halt!" Saturdays was reserved for reviews . . . and inspections! Sundays was day off unless you had duties. The DDS's cooked, scrubbed, drilled, did guard duty . . . with latrine specialties, chased dogs off the streets, kitchen duties, office duty, shined the major's boots, this being considered a top assignment. If it was done in camp, it was done by dentists. But note that NOTHING was done about the SCHOOL of O[ral] & P[lastic] SURGERY . . . not one DAM thing! But By Gad we had the snappiest group in Parade daily that ever layed the dust of a drill field. FULL company in review daily at 5 PM.[180,181]

Some of the enlisted dentists got to serve as assistants for the commissioned dental officers in the dental clinic, a small "barracks-type building, located on the Dixie Highway, which ran right thru our area." It was equipped with three chairs (of an older make) and had no electricity, only foot engines. However, Gearen was never assigned to the clinic. He said, "I never touched a single dental instrument . . . or a tooth or layed my hands on a patient."[181,182]

In 1918 the Army had enough dentists for the AEF overseas. Therefore, it inducted all the 1918 dental graduates as privates and deferred commissioning them. If the war had continued and more troops were needed overseas, the Army planned to draw from this trained pool. Meanwhile, graduate dentists like Dr Gearen were kept in a holding pattern until the war was over.

Finally, in September 1918, Gearen was invited to take the examination for a commission in the DRC to fill vacancies created by the expansion of the Dental Corps and in military hospitals. He passed the examination and was notified in October 1918 that he would be receiving his commission as a first lieutenant. Yet, he did not get his commission until October 22, 1922. Though disappointed, Gearen went on to serve in World War II, spending over 2 years in New Guinea, and the Korean War, where he remained stateside. He eventually retired as a lieutenant colonel.[17,180]

Students' Army Training Corps, 1918

Congress created the Students' Army Training Corps on August 24, 1918, to provide personnel management and training of deferred students while they remained on campus.[183] In September 1918 all dental schools designated as "well recognized" by the surgeon general were allowed to apply for the establishment of a Students' Army Training Corps unit for their school. Students between 18 and 21 years old were eligible to enroll until the schools' prescribed quota was full. Each school was to be assigned a military director. The students' tuition would be paid by the government and they would be furnished uniforms and quarters as well as paid $30 a month. They would receive at least 6 hours of military drill a week and would be examined in military and professional subjects every 3 months. Those who failed would be sent to military camps for general duty. While in training, they would be subject to military law and discipline. The Army would furnish cots, blankets, and rifles for the program. The voluntary inductions into the Students' Army Training Corps were expected to start around October 1, and students had to pay their own expenses until then. By July 1, 1919, these students were providing some of the 9,200 dental officers needed for the planned Army of 4,500,000.[184–186]

After the armistice of November 11, 1918, the Students' Army Training Corps was demobilized without warning and began discharging its students the week of December 1, 1918. All discharges were completed by December 21. The abrupt ending to the Students' Army Training Corps program provoked an immediate response from the college administrators. The colleges had made up their 1919 budgets on the basis that the government had promised to pay fair compensation for the additional services they were to provide. Some thought that this reflected "bad faith" on the part of the military and that the colleges should be reimbursed for their efforts on the government's behalf. Others thought the program should be continued as part of universal military training.[187,188]

On December 6, 1918, the surgeon general announced that the dental graduates who were serving in the Army as privates could be commissioned as first lieutenants on the inactive list of the Reserve Corps prior to their discharge, provided their applications were started before November 11, 1918. They would be subject to recall for 5 years.[186,189]

A number of aspiring young dentists who were members of the Students' Army Training Corps eventually became Dental Corps officers after completing their postwar dental school educations. One such officer was James M Epperly (1900–1973), who served in the Students' Army Training Corps as a private from October 1 until the termination of the program on December 16, 1918. After the war, he continued his dental training at Saint Louis University School of Dentistry, joined the Reserve Officers' Training Corps program, and received his DDS. He was commissioned a first lieutenant on June 1, 1923, and entered active duty at Fitzsimons Army Hospital in Aurora, Colorado, on May 8, 1924. Capping his long career in the Dental Corps, Major General Epperly served as the assistant surgeon general (dental) and chief of the Dental Corps from December 1956 until July 1960.[190,191]

Dental Support to the Air Service

New technology generated an unusual departure from the Medical Department's normal policy of centralization. Medical personnel were attached to the aviation section of the Signal Corps because the War Department recognized the necessity of "giving efficient medical service to this rapidly developing new military arm." Aviation schools and installations were exempt from the local department commanders' oversight on the premise that the "administration of the

Aviation Section could best be accomplished by [its own] centralized control." The funds appropriated by Congress for the construction of flying schools included provisions for small hospitals of 40 or more beds at each installation. These hospitals were constructed "as part of the Aviation Section program and not as a part of the Medical Department program under the Surgeon General."[192]

Surgeon General William C Gorgas "appreciated that a rapidly developing aviation service could be more efficiently provided with medical service if a special medical service were assigned to this particular duty." Accordingly, he supported the designation of Lieutenant Colonel Theodore C Lyster (1875–1933), Medical Corps, as chief surgeon, aviation section, Signal Corps, US Army.[193] In October 1917 Gorgas further recommended that "in the interest of good administration" all Medical Department matters pertaining to the aviation section should be "under the immediate supervision" of Lyster who, in turn, was under the direct control of the commanding general, Air Division of the Aviation Section, Signal Corps.[192]

On May 20, 1918, President Wilson issued a proclamation establishing the Department of Military Aeronautics. Office Memorandum No. 1, Department of Military Aeronautics, dated May 21, 1918, established a medical division (or section) of the air service to "handle all matters pertaining to the administration of personnel, equipment, supplies, and all other matters affecting the Medical Department, which relate to the development, maintenance, organization, and operation of aeronautical personnel." Paragraph 2 of the memorandum established the medical branch as "a part of the Executive Section of the organization of the Department of Military Aeronautics," which included hospitals, medical research, medical personnel, care of pilots, and reports and returns.[192] Shortly thereafter, on May 27, 1918, dental officers First Lieutenant James F Dean (Mather Field, Sacramento, California); Captain Ralph Burkhart, (Eberts Field, Lonoke, Arkansas); First Lieutenant William Sankey, (Aviation Repair Depot, Dallas, Texas); and Captain George F Brand (Scott Field, Belleville, Illinois) were ordered for temporary duty to the places indicated.[194]

Captain Burkhart was sent to Eberts Field in response to the June 1918 complaints of its commander, Major Patrick Frissell, to the commanding general of the Southeast Department. He had to send his troops to the Base Hospital, Fort Logan H Roots, Arkansas, for dental X-ray work because his post had neither a dentist nor an X-ray machine. He had previously requested a dentist and sent in a requisition for an X-ray for his station without success. Because Fort Roots was about 30 miles away, his ambulance was gone an entire day and he had only two other ambulances, both of which had to remain at the flying field.[195]

When Captain Burkhart reported for duty, the post surgeon requested that everyone in the command go to the dental surgeon's office for "preliminary dental examination," at the rate of 100 patients per day, daily except Sunday, until the oral examinations were completed.[196] Such comprehensive screening showed that the dental situation at some of the aviation fields was so bad it inspired a search in October 1918 to locate any enlisted aviation section members who were graduate dentists and could help with the backlog of work.[197,198]

During crash landings, soldiers' faces were particularly prone to injury because of the flimsy construction of the wooden, fabric-covered aircraft. Because of frequent jaw injuries to flying personnel, it was decided in 1918 that study models be made of pilots' jaws to quickly fabricate intraoral splints in case of jaw fracture. Lieutenant William A Squires (1887–?), Dental Corps, said that eight out of every ten aviators that crashed and were not killed had their maxillae and perhaps their mandible fractured. He recommended taking good impressions and pouring them up in stone or metal with the aviator's name written on them. When the pilot made a change of station, he could take the models with him. Removable prosthetic appliances and fixed bridgework were regarded as "potential hazards" in the mouths of aviators because they could be "broken and/or loosened and forced into the soft tissue of the mouth, pharynx or trachea during rough flying or crash landings." It was recommended that extensive fixed bridgework should not be made for aviators and that removable appliances be "pocketed during flight."[199,200] Even in the 1930s, the Army took a dim view on unilateral partial dentures. Two deaths in the enlisted ranks by swallowing such a device were reported in the dental literature.[201]

From 1917 to February 1919, the medical section of the air service supervised 61 independent stations, with a total strength in 1919 in the United States of 41,000, and 45 hospitals with a bed capacity of 3,670. The air service of the surgeon general's office was discontinued effective March 14, 1919, and its functions, including the supervision of the commissioned and enlisted personnel of the Medical Department on duty with the air service, were transferred to the chief surgeon of the air service.[192]

The Dental Corps' Growing Strength

The Dental Corps expanded enormously during World War I to satisfy the demands of the vastly expanded US Army that grew to nearly 4,200,000 soldiers by November 1918. At first, however, that growth had been sluggish. At the end of July 1917, the Dental Corps numbered 933 dental officers on active duty—86 in the Regular Army, 249 in the National Guard, and 598 first lieutenants of the DRC. By June 30, 1918, the Dental Corps had ballooned to 5,837 officers—212 in the Regular Army, 253 in the National Guard, and 5,372 in the DRC (2,493 on active duty and 2,879 on inactive status), including 36 majors, 244 captains, and 5,092 first lieutenants. On November 30, 1918, the total number of commissioned officers in the Army Dental Corps reached 6,284, of which 4,620 (229 regular Army, 253 National Guard, and 4,138 DRC) officers were on active duty—the greatest number of dental officers actually on active duty at any one time during the wartime period. Of the 4,620 officers, 1,779 of were then in Europe (1,765 in the AEF). According to Oliver, the maximum number of dental officers who served in Europe during the war was 1,873 in November 1918, which included 1,861 Army Dental Corps and 12 US Navy Dental Corps officers assigned to support the US Marine Corps personnel in the Fifth and Sixth Marine Regiments of the Second Division. However, personnel reports from the AEF chief surgeon's office indicate that the highest number of Dental Corps officers in the AEF was 1,819, and that number was reached on January 11, 1919. The three tables below summarize the growth of the Dental Corps in commissioned officers in service by component and by rank as well as the growth of the DRC from April 1917 to November 30, 1918 (Table 12-2, Table 12-3, and Table 12-4).[10,17,35,202–204]

TABLE 12-2

COMMISSIONED DENTAL CORPS OFFICERS IN SERVICE BY COMPONENT, APRIL 1917 TO NOVEMBER 1918

	April 1917	July 1, 1918	November 30, 1918
Regular Army	86	211	229
National Guard	0	253	253
Dental Reserve Corps (DRC)	0	2,493	4,138
Total Temporary (National Guard and DRC)	0	2,746	4,391
Total in Service	**86**	**2,957**	**4,620**

Data sources: (1) Office of the Surgeon General. *Annual Report of the Surgeon General*. Vol. 2. Washington, DC: OTSG; 1919: 1111. (2) Office of the Surgeon General. *Annual Report of the Surgeon General*. Washington, DC: OTSG; 1918: 391.

On August 7, 1918, War Department General Order Number 73 consolidated the Regular Dental Corps, National Army and National Guard Dental Corps, and the DRC into the Dental Corps, US Army. The War Department order stated:

This country has but one army: The United States Army. It includes all the land forces in the service of the United States. Those forces however raised, lose their identity in that of The United States Army. Distinctive appellations, such as the Regular Army, Reserve Corps, National Guard, and national Army, heretofore employed in administration and command, will be discontinued, and the single term, The United States Army, will be exclusively used.[205]

TABLE 12-3

COMMISSIONED DENTAL CORPS OFFICERS IN SERVICE BY RANK, APRIL 1917 TO NOVEMBER 1918

	April 1917	July 1, 1918	November 30, 1918
Colonel	0	12	9
Lieutenant Colonel	0	19	17
Major	0	80	102
Captain	21	222	368
First Lieutenant	65	2,624	4,124
Total	**86**	**2,957**	**4,620**

Data source: Office of the Surgeon General. *Annual Report of the Surgeon General*. Vol. 2. Washington, DC: OTSG; 1919: 1115.

TABLE 12-4

GROWTH OF COMMISSIONED OFFICER STRENGTH IN
THE DENTAL RESERVE CORPS, APRIL 1917 TO JUNE 1918

Date	Commissioned Officers
April 1917	0
July 31, 1917	598
October 31, 1917	3,452
December 31, 1917	4,749
April 30, 1918	5,221
June 30, 1918	5,372

Data source: Office of the Surgeon General. *Annual Report of the Surgeon General.*
Washington, DC: OTSG; 1918: 391.

With the increase in the draft age to 45 in August 1918 (a result of projected personnel requirements for 1919 and 1920), some practicing dentists who had not already secured commissions in the now closed DRC faced the possibility of being drafted into the Army as privates, while many recent graduates held commissions. These dentists had not applied for commissions in the previous years, and now nearly 6,000 others were ahead of them in line. As of September 3, 1918, 5,981 dentists held active and inactive commissions, of which some 3,500 were already on duty, although all dentists serving in the Army were now known as members of the "Dental Corps, US Army" and no longer broken down by Regular Army, DRC, and National Guard. However, if the war continued, by July 1, 1919, the Army would need at least 3,000 more dentists for a total of more than 9,000 dental officers. First call for these openings would be given to the dentists already in the service serving as privates in the various camps and overseas units. After this group, commissions would be granted to civilian candidates successful in passing the examination for appointment as vacancies occurred (according to Army strength). If there was a surplus of dental officers, the enlisted dentists would be assigned as "dental mechanics [technicians]" to the camps and hospitals to help clear up the backlog of partial dentures.[39,140,184,206] Some members of the dental profession thought it was ridiculous to have experienced dentists serving as privates while "inexperienced, newly graduated" dentists were "wearing the officer's uniform." Others were of the opinion that the recent graduates could put the "older practitioners to shame" because of their special training in war surgery and fracture work.[207,208]

In his planning for the 80-division Army of 1919 and the 100 divisions of 1920, Colonel Logan developed new requirements for Dental Corps officers and assistants to be filled by July 1, 1919, which the surgeon general recommended to the general staff on August 22, 1918. Logan noted that to date, experience indicated that a minimum of one dental officer was required per 500 draftees in training in the United States because such a short time was available to prepare them for service overseas. The newly increased draft age of 45 would increase the number of

TABLE 12-5

INCREASE IN DENTAL CORPS OFFICER AUTHORIZATIONS FOR THE
EXISTING EMERGENCY (SEPTEMBER 28, 1918)

	Current Authorization	Increase	Total
98 divisions	1,395	1,643	3,038
Corps troops, American expeditionary forces	10	246	256
Army troops, American expeditionary forces	75	665	740
Lines of communication, services of supply	410	1,155	1,565
Required in US	1,308	2,299	3,607
Camps & cantonments	789	1,743	2,532
Military hospitals	98	451	549
Others	421	105	526
Total	**3,198**	**6,008**	**9,206**

Data source: National Archives and Records Administration. Decimal File 382, Dental Corps. Record Group 165. Memorandum for the chief of staff, Brigadier General Lytle Brown, director, War Plans Division, 8 September 1918, and memorandum for the adjutant general, General Peyton C March, chief of staff, 28 September 1918. No. 8954-20. Box 48. Entry 8.

those needing dental care, which was now running at 90%. Logan also added dentists and assistants for all Army and corps units, which the war plans division had specifically ruled out in April. The general staff reviewed the request and on September 8, recommended that for the duration of the existing emergency, the Dental Corps should be increased by 6,008 officers and 6,355 enlisted to a total authorized strength of 9,206 officers and 9,648 enlisted on active duty (Table 12-5).[209–211]

Once again, Logan was the catalyst for another vast expansion of the Army Dental Corps, which was achieved on September 28, 1918, when the chief of staff, General Peyton C March, approved the new authorizations. The ratio of one dentist per thousand enlisted strength was changed to one dentist per 500 enlisted soldiers, or two per thousand enlisted soldiers, as Kirk and then Logan had proposed in 1917. Camps and cantonments were increased by 1,743 dental officers from 789 to 2,532 because the majority of the dental work would be completed in their dental infirmaries. Each of 183 military hospitals in the United States was authorized three dental surgeons per thousand patients and increased from 98 to 549. While authorizing the adjutant general to make these changes, March also specifically restated the existing policy that "the recommendation therein is approved except that Dental personnel will not be assigned to any organization, but attached in order to leave the Commanding General, A.E.F. free to use such personnel where he considers for the best interest of the service."[212]

Speaking in Syracuse, New York, in May 1919, Logan explained how this change came about:

As most of you recall, efforts had been made since dentists sought entrance as officers in the United States Army, to have the quota of two per thousand authorized by law, but without avail, and here we find by authorization of the General Staff the granting of that which we had all sought so long. Why was it possible at that time to secure authorization for assigning two officers per thousand? It was because our civilian dentists banded themselves together to assist in making the selective service man dentally fit through the activity of that splendid patriotic organization the Prepared-ness League of American Dentists previous to his induction into military service; and because dentistry in posts, training camps and hospitals in this country, the base and evacuating hospitals, field service and far forward in the line had been tried and not found wanting, and the service of the dental officers had been proved worthy of ev-ery consideration. Therefore, the request for the authorization for doubling the quota was approved.[8(pp217–218)]

Because the number of commissioned dental officers was insufficient to cov-er the increased requirements, examinations were reopened on October 3, with the first opportunity for examination going to those graduate dentists already in the Army. The secretary of war stopped this process on November 9, when the impending armistice obviated the requirement for more dental officers. Only 10 new dentists were commissioned and ordered to duty out of the 800 to 900 applicants already acted on by the surgeon general. However, Colonel Logan intervened and convinced the War Department to give the successful applicants an opportunity to accept commissions in the DRC upon their separation from service.[48,182]

On To France

In less than 2 years, from April 6, 1917 to November 11, 1918, the US Army had expanded from a middling-sized total regular force of 133,000 to more than 4,200,000, equipped, trained, and flowing in large numbers (2,000,000) to France to fill the ranks of the American Expeditionary Forces under General John J Persh-ing. During the same period, the Medical Department expanded the Dental Corps from just 86 Regular Army dentists to a force of 4,620 dental officers on active duty in the United States and Europe and had received War Department approval for a dental corps numbering 9,206 officers and 9,648 enlisted soldiers for the even larger forces planned in 1919 and 1920. Orally and dentally, this Army was the fittest yet fielded by the United States because of the ceaseless efforts of the mem-bers of the Dental Corps—Regular Army, DRC, and National Guard. Drawing on French and British experience, oral surgeons had been carefully trained to handle the worst imaginable maxillofacial casualties in evacuation and base hospitals near the front. Dentists were in place and equipped throughout the divisions if not in the official tables of organization, and in their field hospitals and all along the chain of evacuation were ready to care for the American "doughboys" when and where needed. The preparations in the United States had readied the Medi-cal Department and Dental Corps for the struggle to save soldiers' lives from the frontlines to the hospitals in the rear.

References

1. Ferrell RH. *Woodrow Wilson and World War I, 1917–1921*. New York, NY: Harper and Row; 1985.

2. Kreidberg MA, Henry MG. *History of Military Mobilization in the United States Army, 1775–1945*. Washington, DC: Department of the Army; 1955.

3. Rhoades RH. The dental service of the Army of the United States. *J Am Dent Assoc.* 1928;15:264.

4. Office of the Surgeon General. *Annual Report of the Surgeon General, 1917*. Washington, DC: Government Printing Office; 1917: 293.

5. War Department. *Tables of Organization (Based on Field Service Regulations, 1914), United States Army, 1914*. Washington, DC: Government Printing Office; 1914.

6. War Department. *Manual for the Medical Department, United States Army, 1916*. Washington, DC: Government Printing Office; 1916.

7. Gillett MC. *The Army Medical Department, 1775–1818*. Vol 3. Washington, DC: Center of Military History, United States Army; 1981: 377–415.

8. Logan WHG. Dental service in the United States Army during the world war. *Dental Cosmos.* 1920;62:216–220.

9. Wilson JB. *Maneuver and Firepower: The Evolution of Divisions and Separate Brigades.* Washington, DC: US Army Center of Military History; 1998: 32–34.

10. Oliver RT. History of the dental service, AEF. In: Activities of the chief surgeon's office. In: *Reports of the Commander-in-Chief, Staff Sections and Services, in United States Army in the World War 1917–1919*. Vol 15. Washington, DC: US Army Center of Military History; 1991: 411.

11. Ford JH, ed. The dental section. In: *Administration American Expeditionary Forces, in the Medical Department of the United States Army in the World War*. Vol 2. Washington, DC: Government Printing Office; 1927: 116–117.

12. Brun BL. Oral surgery in the Army. *Dental Cosmos.* 1920;62:640.

13. Persons EE. Field service regulations, United States Army, 1914 and organization tables, United States Army, 1914. *Military Surgeon.* 1914;34:401–410.

14. Miller RB. The new manual for the medical department. *Military Surgeon.* 1916;38:300–319.

15. Oliver RT. Army Dental Corps. *Bulletin of the Association of Military Dental Surgeons of the United States.* 1917;1:3. Reprinted as: The Army Dental Corps of the U.S.A. *Br Dent J.* 1917:38:651–653.

16. Tables of organization for World War I infantry divisions of 1917–1918, Infantry division (combat). *American Expeditionary Forces: Divisions, in Order of Battle of the United States Land Forces in the World War*. Vol 3. Washington, DC: US Army Center of Military History; 1988: 446–447.

17. Office of the Surgeon General. *Annual Report of the Surgeon General, 1919*. Vol 2. Washington, DC: Government Printing Office; 1919.

18. Wolfe EP. Finance and Supply. In: *The United States Army Medical Department in the World War*. Vol 3. Washington, DC: US Government Printing Office; 1928.

19. Pershing JJ. *My Experiences in the World War*. Vol 1. New York, NY: Frederick A Stokes Company; 1931: 100-102.

20. *Zone of the Interior: Organization and Activities of the War Department, in Order of Battle of the United States Land Force in the World War, Part 1*. Vol 3. Washington, DC: US Army Center of Military History, 1988.

21. National Archives and Records Administration. Dental Corps, US Army (War Plans Division report no. 8954). Record Group 165. Memorandum for the chief of staff, Colonel DW Ketcham, assistant director, War Plans Division, general staff, 19 February 1918. No. 8954-8. Box 377. Entry 296.

22. National Archives and Records Administration. Dental Corps, US Army (War Plans Division report no. 8954). Record Group 165. Memorandum for the adjutant general, Brigadier General William S Graves, assistant to the chief of staff, 21 February 1918. No. 8954-8. Box 377. Entry 296.

23. National Archives and Records Administration. Dental Corps (decimal file 382). Record Group 165. Memorandum for the adjutant general, General Peyton C March, chief of staff, 28 September 1918. No. 8954-20. Box 48. Entry 8.

24. National Archives and Records Administration. Dental Corps, US Army (War Plans Division report no. 8954). Record Group 112. Memorandum for the chief of staff, Colonel D.W. Ketcham, assistant director, War Plans Division, general staff, 22 March 1918. No. 8954-10. Box 377. Entry 296.

25. National Archives and Records Administration. Dental Corps, US Army (War Plans Division report no. 8954). Record Group 112. Memorandum for the adjutant general, Graves, assistant to the chief of staff, 26 March 1918. Report No. 8954-10. Box 377. Entry 296.

26. National Archives and Records Administration. Record Group 112. Notes: AEF program for Medical Corps. Decimal File 320.2-1 (AEF). Box 5. Entry 31.

27. General Orders No. 99, General Headquarters, AEF, 19 June 1918. In: *General Orders, GHQ, AEF, in United States Army in the World War 1917–1919*. Vol 16. Washington, DC: US Army Center of Military History; 1992: 351.

28. Additional Dentists for Divisions. *Army and Navy Register*. Quoted in: *Dental Cosmos*. 1918;60: 460.

29. Biographical File on Colonel Robert T. Oliver. Available at: Research Collections, OTSG/MEDCOM, Falls Church, Virginia.

30. National Archives and Records Administration. Dental Corps, US Army (War Plans Division report no. 8954). Record Group 112. Memorandum for the chief of staff, Colonel D.W. Ketcham, acting director, War Plans Division, 18 April 1918. No. 8954-13.

31. National Archives and Records Administration. Dental Corps, US Army (War Plans Division report no. 8954). Record Group 112. Memorandum for the adjutant general, Colonel D.W. Ketcham, acting director, War Plans Division, 20 April 1918. No. 8954-13.

32. National Archives and Records Administration. Dental Corps (decimal file 382). Record Group 165. Memorandum for the chief of staff, Brigadier General Lytle Brown, director, War Plans Division, 10 May 1918. No. 8954-14.

33. National Archives and Records Administration. Dental Corps (decimal file 382). Record Group 165. Memorandum for Adjutant General Brown, 10 May 1918. No. 8954-14.

34. National Archives and Records Administration. Dental Corps (decimal file 382, War Plans Division report no. 8954-18). Record Group 165. Memorandum for the adjutant general, Brigadier General Lytle Brown, director, War Plans Division, 26 July 1918.

35. Clark CC. Great patriotic public sessions are big feature of twenty-second annual convention National Dental Association at Chicago. *American Dentist*. 1918;7:1.

36. [Kirk EC]. Committee on dentistry, general medical board of Council of National Defense. *J Natl Dent Assoc*. 1917;4:640–643.

37. Meeting of dental educators. *J Natl Dent Assoc*. 1917;4:642–656.

38. Allen CC. Meeting of deans and educators. *J Natl Dent Assoc*. 1917;4:657.

39. [Kirk EC]. Expansion of the Army Dental Corps. *Dental Cosmos*. 1918;60:935–936.

40. [King OU?]. Ten thousand dentists to be commissioned and assigned before July 1, 1919. *J Natl Dent Assoc*. 1918;5:1085.

41. Logan WHG. The dental profession's contribution in the present war emergency. *J Natl Dent Assoc*. 1918;5:239.

42. William Hoffman Gardiner Logan 1872–1943. *Dental Bulletin Supplement to the Army Medical Bulletin*. 1943;14:90–91.

43. Examination of dentists for the U.S. Army. *Dental Cosmos*. 1917;59:584.

44. Oliver RT. Letter from Captain Robert T. Oliver. *J Natl Dent Assoc*. 1917;4:786.

45. The Dental Reserve Corps. *Dental Summary*. 1917;37:385.

46. [Ottolengui R]. The man of the hour. *Dent Items Interest*. 1918;40:307–308.

47. US Army, Dental Activity (DENTAC), Fort Belvoir, Va. Dedication ceremonies Logan Army Dental Clinic to memorialize Col. William H.G. Logan. Fort Belvoir, Va: Dental Activity; 1970.

48. Logan WH. The development of the dental service of the United States Army in this country from April 8, 1917 to Feb. 12, 1919. *J Am Dent Assoc*. 1933;20:1952–1953.

49. Logan WH. Development of the dental service during the present war. *J Natl Dent Assoc*. 1918;5;996–999.

50. Kirk EC. Committee on dentistry, general medical board of the Council of National Defense, report no. 3, 13 May 1917. *J Natl Dent Assoc*. 1917;4:653–655.

51. Lynch C, Weed F, McAfee L. The surgeon general's office. In: *The Medical Department of the United States Army in the World War*. Vol 1. Washington, DC: Government Printing Office; 1923.

52. US War Department. Special orders no. 184, 9 August 1917. In: *Special Orders 1917*. Washington, DC: Adjutant General's Office; 1917: 5.

53. Logan WH. Report of committee on dentistry, general medical board, Council of National Defense, 9 September 1917. *J Natl Dent Assoc*. 1917;4:1135-37.

54. Office of the Surgeon General. *Annual Report of the Surgeon General, 1918*. Washington, DC: Government Printing Office; 1918: 391.

55. Logan WH. Report of committee on dentistry, general medical board, Council of National Defense, 18 November 1917. *J Natl Dent Assoc*. 1918;5:78–79.

56. National Archives and Records Administration. Record Group 165. Major General John Biddle, acting chief of staff, to the adjutant general, 3 November 1917. Report no. 12574. Box 131. Entry 5.

57. National Archives and Records Administration. Record Group 165. Memorandum for the chief of staff, Colonel PD Lochridge, acting chief, War College Division, 27 November 1917. Report no. 12574. Box 131. Entry 5.

58. Martin FH. *The Joy of Living: an Autobiography*. Vol 2. Garden City, NY: Doubleday, Doran & Company, Inc; 1933: 255.

59. [Bethel LP]. Congress gives dentistry the same recognition as medicine. *Dental Summary*. 1917;37:855–856.

60. [Johnson CN]. A red letter day for dentistry. *Dent Rev*. 1917;31:1008–1010.

61. Ryan EPR. President's address, Association of Military [dental] Surgeons of the United States. *J Assoc Milit Surg US*. 1919;3:164–165.

62. Biographical file on William HG Logan. Research Collections, OTSG/MEDCOM, Falls Church, Va.

63. [Bethel LP]. Anent Army and Navy dental surgeons. *Dental Summary*. 1917;37:162.

64. National Archives and Records Administration. Record Group 165. Memorandum for the chief of staff, Brigadier General Joseph E Kuhn, general staff, 1 June 1917. Report no. 13349. Box 140. Entry 5.

65. National Archives and Records Administration. Record Group 165. Memorandum for the adjutant general, Major General Tasker H Bliss, acting chief of staff, 2 June 1917. Report no. 13349. Box 140. Entry 5.

66. Craig EJ. The Army and the dentist. *West Dent J*. 1917;31:33.

67. [Ottolengui R]. Legislation in regard to the Army Dental Corps. *Dent Items Interest*. 1917;39:470.

68. Brown HC. New and proposed legislation affecting the Navy and Army Dental Corps. *J Natl Dent Assoc*. 1917;4:386.

69. [Kirk EC]. Our golden opportunity. *Dental Cosmos*. 1917;59:658.

70. *Congressional Record, 65th Cong, 1st Sess*. Vol 55. Washington, DC: Government Printing Office; 1917.

71. US Congress. House. *To Amend Section 10, National Defense Act*. 65th Cong, 1st sess, 1917, H Rept 84.

72. US Congress. Senate. *Promotion of First Lieutenants in the Medical Corps*. 65th Cong, 1st sess, 1917, S Rept 131.

73. Oliver RT. *Transactions of the Dental Society of the Sate of New York, 53rd Annual Meeting*. 1921:13.

74. Army promotions. *Dent Dig*. 1918;24:165–166.

75. Biographical Files on Oliver, Bernheim, Rhoades, Stone, Laflamme, Mills, Fairbank, Snyder, and Smith. Research Collections, OTSG/MEDCOM, Falls Church, Va.

76. Biographical File on Walter D Love. Research Collections, OTSG/MEDCOM, Falls Church, Va.

77. Black AD, Morgan HW, Friesell HE, Logan WHG, Castro FM. Why drafted dental students should be permitted to finish their courses. *Dental Summary*. 1917;37:773–776.

78. [Ottolengui R]. Unjust discrimination against dental students by the War Department. *Dent Items Interest*. 1917;39:780.

79. National Archives and Records Administration. Record Group 165. Representative Osborne to Secretary of War Baker, 4 August 1917, endorsement, judge advocate general to chief of staff, 10 August 1917, Secretary of War Baker to Representative Osborne, 14 August 1917. Letters. Report no. 13709. Box 145. Entry 5.

80. National Archives and Records Administration. Record Group 165. Colonel PD Lochridge, general staff, to chief of staff, 14 November 1917. Memo. Report no. 13709. Box 145. Entry 5.

81. Barrett L, comp. Our Army and Navy [Army Dental Corps]. *J Allied Dent Soc*. 1917;12:522.

82. Dentists in the Army. *International Journal of Orthodontia*. Quoted in: *Dent Dig*. 1917;23:609.

83. The value of the orthodontist in military service. *Dent Dig*. 1917;23:506.

84. The profession and war. *Dental Register*. 1917;71: 253–255.

85. Wheeler HL. The relation of the surgeon and the dentist in face and jaw injuries. *Dental Cosmos*. 1918;60:224.

86. [Blair JP]. Oral and dental surgeons for the Army. *Dent Reg*. 1917;71:494.

87. Barrett L, comp. Our Army and Navy [United States Dental School in Philadelphia]. *J Allied Dent Soc*. 1917;12:516.

88. Iowa dentists organize course in war oral surgery. *American Dentist*. 1917;5:12.

89. Jones ET, ed. *Dictionary of American Biography, Supplement 3, 1941–1945*. New York, NY: Charles Scribner's Sons; 1973: 200–2003.

90. The base hospital unit. *JAMA*. Quoted in: *Dent Dig*. 1917;23:534–535.

91. [Kirk EC]. Preparedness--mobilization—efficiency. *Dental Cosmos*. 1917;59:557.

92. Development of Red Cross Medical Department units. In: *The Surgeon General's Office, the Medical Department of the United States Army in the World War*. Vol 1. Washington, DC: Government Printing Office; 1923.

93. Ellis WH. Dental surgery in the Red Cross base hospitals. *Oral Hyg*. 1917;7:755.

94. US War Department. *Regulations Governing the Employment of the American Red Cross in Time of War*. Washington, DC: Government Printing Office; 1917: 7.

95. National Archives and Records Administration. Record Group 112. Colonel John L Phillips, commanding officer, Walter Reed General Hospital, to surgeon general, 13 July 1914, and first endorsement, Colonel Charles M Gandy, surgeon general's office, to commanding officer, Walter Reed General Hospital, 31 July 1914. Letter. No. 149731. Box 1070. Entry 26.

96. Weed FW. Military hospitals in the United States. In: *The Medical Department of the United States Army in the World War*. Vol 5. Washington, DC: Government Printing Office; 1923: 118–126.

97. *A History of the United States Army Base Hospital No. 36 (Detroit College of Medicine and Surgery Unit)*. NP; 1919 : 68–70.

98. Kinney D. American women's hospitals organized by war service committee of the Medical Women's National Association. *J Natl Dent Assoc*. Quoted in: *Pacific Dental Gazette*. 1917;25:774.

99. Barrett L, comp. Our Army and Navy [Unit of Women for France]. *J Allied Dent Soc*. 1917;12:516.

100. National Archives and Records Administration. Record Group 112. Kinney to surgeon general, 26 April 1917. Letter. No. 172478, Box 1223, Entry 26.

101. National Archives and Records Administration. Record Group 112. Ottolengui to surgeon general, 28 April 1917. Letter. No. 172478. Box 1223. Entry 26.

102. National Archives and Records Administration. Record Group 112. Kinney to Major General J Franklin Bell, 2 May 1917. Letter. No. 172478. Box 1223. Entry 26.

103. National Archives and Records Administration. Record Group 112. Surgeon general's office to Kinney, 4 May 1917. Letter. No. 172478. Box 1223. Entry 26.

104. National Archives and Records Administration. Record Group 112. Kinney to surgeon general, 28 May 1917. Letter. No. 172478. Box 1223. Entry 26.

105. National Archives and Records Administration. Record Group 112. Surgeon general's office to Kinney, 11 July 1917. Letter. No. 172478. Box 1223. Entry 26.

106. Dow TD, Jones M, comp. *History of the Tennessee State Dental Association*. Nashville, Tenn: Tennessee Dental Association; 1958.

107. Kinney D. What women dentists are doing in the present crisis. *J Natl Dent Assoc*. 1918;5:1048–1049.

108. National Archives and Records Administration. Record Group 112. Kean to surgeon general, 11 June 1917. Memo. No. 192485. Box 1357. Entry 26.

109. Hume EE. *The Golden Jubilee of the Association of Military Surgeons of the United States: a History of its First Half-Century, 1891–1941*. Washington, DC: The Association of Military Surgeons; 1941.

110. National Archives and Records Administration. Record Group 112. Fisher to Gorgas. Letter. No. 106047. Box 712. Entry 26.

111. Military officers elect officers. *American Dentist*. 1915;1:6.

112. Association of Military Dental Surgeons of the United States. *J Natl Dent Assoc*. 1918;5:64–66.

113. Necessary field equipment for Dental Reserve Corps Officers. *Dental Cosmos*. 1917;59:1067–1068.

114. [US War Department]. Memorandum regarding dental apparatus and supplies. *J Natl Dent Assoc*. 1917;4:812.

115. National Archives and Records Administration. Record Group 165. Purchase of dental outfits, 25 April 1917. Report no. 13278. Box 139. Entry 5.

116. Ryan EPR. The Dental Corps: Our responsibility. *J Natl Dent Assoc*. 1918;5:759.

117. Bayley MW. The dental clinic in the national Army cantonment. *Dental Cosmos*. 1918;60:705.

118. Hollister CJ. Dental service at Camp Hancock: headquarters twenty-eighth division. *Dent Dig*. 1917;23:770.

119. Van Blarcom H. Experiences in camp life. *NJ Dent J*. 1917;6:365–366.

120. Ludwig HR. With the Army. *Oral Hyg*. 1918;8:145.

121. Zeidler JC. Giving them the up and down. *Oral Hyg*. 1918;8:711.

122. Speakman [W]C. War dentistry. *Oral Hyg*. Quoted in: *Dent Rec*. 1918;37:140-43.

123. Speakman MAV. *Memories*. Wilmington, Del: Greenwood Bookshop; 1937.

124. [Weaver SM, Henahan JP]. The Cleveland Motor Dental Car for Army Use. *Amer Dent*. 1918;6:6–7.

125. National Archives and Records Administration. Record Group 120. Endorsement, Colonel Walter D McCaw, Medical Corps, chief surgeon's office, American Expeditionary Forces Headquarters, to Fourth Section, general staff, General Headquarters, AEF, 31 October 1918. No. 703. Folder 18. Box 5149. Entry 2065.

126. [Bethel LP]. Universal military training and its bearing on dental conditions of our young men. *Dental Summary*. 1917;37:236.

127. Bernheim JR. Oral hygiene in the Army. *J Natl Dent Assoc*. 1917;4:501.

128. Extraction of teeth to avoid military service. *Dominion Dental Journal*. 1917;29:293.

129. Healy TF. Examining the drafted men. *Amer Dent*. 1918;6:9.

130. Physical examination of registrants in the Army. *JAMA*. Quoted in: *Dental Cosmos*. 1918;60:274–275.

131. National Archives and Records Administration. Dental Corps (decimal file 382, War Plans Division report no. 8954-20). Record Group 165. Logan, cited in memorandum for the chief of staff, Brigadier General Lytle Brown, director, War Plans Division, 8 September 1918.

132. Ayres LP. *The War with Germany: a Statistical Summary*. Washington, DC: Government Printing Office; 1919: 26–28.

133. Coffman EM. *The War to End All Wars: the American Military Experience in World War I*. New York, NY: Oxford University Press; 1968: 54–85.

134. Wood CA. A history of the base hospital, Camp Sherman, Chillicothe, Ohio. *Mil Surg*. 1918;43:457–458.

135. Livermore AR. Army dentistry. *Oral Hyg*. 1918;8:267–268.

136. Smith KF. The practice of dentistry in the Army and in civil life (a comparison). *J Natl Dent Assoc*. 1918;5:408.

137. Huber CF. Letter with enclosure, dental history of the 88th division. Washington, DC: US Army Center of Military History.

138. National Archives and Records Administration. Record Group 120. Schedule 1165, 28th Division. Box 3626. Entry 2144.

139. National Archives and Records Administration. Record Group 120. Headquarters, Twenty-Eighth Division, Camp Hancock, Augusta, Ga. No. 703. Box 3630. Entry 2144.

140. National Archives and Records Administration. Record Group 120. Return of medical officers, etc., serving in the 28th Division, Camp Hancock, Augusta, Ga, during the month of August 1917. Box 3627. Entry 2144.

141. National Archives and Records Administration. Record Group 120. First Lieutenant Oscar P Snyder, Dental Corps, dental surgeon, Camp Hancock, Ga, to Major William HG Logan, surgeon general's office, Washington, DC, 25 September 1917. Report. No. 703. Box 3630. Entry 2144.

142. National Archives and Records Administration. Record Group 120. First Lieutenant Oscar P Snyder, dental surgeon, Camp Hancock, Augusta, Ga, to Major William HG Logan, surgeon general's office, Washington, DC, 20 October 1917. Report. No. 703. Box 3630. Entry 2144.

143. National Archives and Records Administration. Record Group 120. First Lieutenant Oscar P Snyder, dental surgeon, Camp Hancock, Augusta, Ga, to surgeon general, Washington, DC, 24 November 1917. Report. No. 703. Box 3630. Entry 2144.

144. National Archives and Records Administration. Record Group 120. First Lieutenant Oscar P Snyder, division dental surgeon, 28th Division, to division surgeon, Camp Hancock, Ga, 4 January 1918. Report. No. 703. Box 3630. Entry 2144.

145. National Archives and Records Administration. Record Group 120. Major Oscar P Snyder, division dental surgeon, 28th Division, to division surgeon, 18 March 1918. Memo. No. 703. Box 3630. Entry 2144.

146. US War Department. *Official Army Register 1918*. Washington, DC: Government Printing Office; 1918: 111.

147. National Archives and Records Administration. Record Group 120. Lieutenant Colonel William J Crookston, Medical Corps, division surgeon, 28th Division, Camp Hancock, Ga, to commanding general, 28th Division, 4 April 1918. Memo. No. 703. Entry 2144.

148. National Archives and Records Administration. Record Group 120. Lieutenant Colonel William J Crookston, Medical Corps, division surgeon, 28th Division, Camp Hancock, Ga, 8 April 1918. Memo. No. 703. Entry 2144.

149. National Archives and Records Division. Record Group 120. Return of medical officers, etc, serving in 28th Division on the last day of May 1918. Box 3627. Entry 2144.

150. Blanquie RH. Camp fremont Dental Corps notes. *Dental Cosmos*. 1918;60:1166–1167.

151. Scheifer EH. Life in the Dental Department at Camp Grant, Illinois. *Amer Dent*. 1919;8:7.

152. Ottolengui R. Report of Committee on Motor Cars for the Dental Service at Military Camps. *Dent Items Interest*. 1918;40:1002–1006.

153. Efficient dental work at Camp Sheridan, Montgomery, Alabama. *Amer Dent*. 1918;6:11.

154. National Archives and Records Administration. Record Group 112. First Lieutenant Seibert D Boak to Major Robert E Noble, 18 August 1915, and reply 20 August 1915. Letters. No. 138037. Box 975. Entry 26.

155. National Archives and Records Administration. Record Group 112. William M Criukshank, adjutant general, to commanding general, eastern department, 18 November 1916. Letter. No. 157271. Box 1131. Entry 26.

156. Barrett L, comp. Our Army and Navy (colored medical officers' training camp at Fort Des Moines). *J Allied Dent Soc*. 1917;12:515–516.

157. National Archives and Records Administration. Record Group 112. Surgeon general to president, 24 December 1904, profiles of 1898 black contract surgeons. Memo. No. 5. Box 468. Entry 242.

158. National Archives and Records Administration. Record Group 112. Jefferson to surgeon general, 24 February 1901. Application. No. 78832. Box 519. Entry 26.

159. National Archives and Records Administration. Record Group 112. Jefferson to surgeon general, 8 February 1901. Letter. No. 78832. Box 519. Entry 26.

160. National Archives and Records Administration. Record Group 112. Jefferson to Charles G Dawes, 1 March 1901. Letter. No. 78832. Box 519. Entry 26.

161. National Archives and Records Administration. Record Group 15. Pension record, William T Jefferson, declaration for pension, 4 January 1924, 31 October 1925. Cert. no. 969282.

162. McCard HS, Turnley H. *History of the Eighth Illinois United States Volunteers*. Chicago, Ill: E.F. Hartman; 1889: 45.

163. National Archives and Records Administration. Case files of persons examined for appointment as dental surgeons, 1900-17. Record Group 112. Charles C Fry. Box 344. Entry 101.

164. National Archives and Records Administration. Case files of persons examined for appointment as dental surgeons, 1900-17. Record Group 112. Andrew L Jackson. Box 348. Entry 101.

165. National Archives and Records Administration. Case files of persons examined for appointment as dental surgeons, 1900-17. Record Group 112. Robert G Johnson. Box 348. Entry 101.

166. National Archives and Records Administration. Case files of persons examined for appointment as dental surgeons, 1900-17. Record Group 112. Rufus P Beshears. Box 338. Entry 101.

167. National Archives and Records Administration. Record Group 112. Record card, Oliver to surgeon general, 20 June 1917, endorsement, surgeon general to department surgeon, southern department, Fort Sam Houston, 4 July 1917. No. 188808. Box 283. Entry 25.

168. National Archives and Records Administration. Record Group 112. Surgeon general to commandant, Medical Officers' Training Camp, Fort Des Moines, Iowa, 30 July 1917. Course of progressive instruction medical officers' training camp, Fort Des Moines. Telegram. No. 187170. Box 1322. Entry 26.

169. National Archives and Records Administration. Record Group 120. Surgeon general to department surgeon 14 May 1917. Memo. No. 320.2. Box 7. Entry 1241.

170. Hyson JM. *African-American Dental Surgeons and the U.S. Army Dental Corps: A Struggle for Acceptance, 1901–1919*. Located at: Research Collections, Office of Medical History, Washington, DC, or http://history.amedd.army.mil/ameddcorp/African-AmericanDentalSurgeons/frameindex.html. Chapter 4.

171. Barrett L, comp. Our Army and Navy (157,000 negroes in Army). *J Allied Dent Soc*. 1918;13:288.

172. Medical Corps instruction extended. *JAMA*. Quoted in: *Dental Cosmos*. 1918;60:275.

173. Training medical personnel. *Army and Navy Register*. Quoted in: *J Natl Dent Assoc*. 1918;5:326.

174. Medical Department training: dental officers. *Army and Navy Register*. Quoted in: *Dental Cosmos*. 1918;60:367.

175. Barrett L, comp. Our Army and Navy (enough Army dentists). *Army and Navy Register*. Quoted in: *J Allied Dent Soc*. 1918;13:292.

176. Medical department training. *Army and Navy Register*. Quoted in: *J Natl Dent Assoc*. 1918;5:415.

177. Waite SC. Dental Company No. 1. In: *Dental Alumni News, University of Buffalo (Winter 1988)*. Buffalo, New York: University of Buffalo; 1988 : 1-2.

178. Letter, Sheridan C Waite to Dr John M. Hyson, Jr, 27 January 1989.

179. Green JC. Dental Company No. 1. *Mil Dent J*. 1922;5:103.

180. Gearen WD. World War I Research Project: Army Service Experiences Questionnaire. Available at: Department of the Army, US Army Military History Research Collection, Carlisle Barracks, Pennsylvania.

181. Letter. Walter D Gearen to Dr John M. Hyson, Jr, 17 September 1979.

182. Letter. Walter D Gearen to Dr John M. Hyson, Jr, 30 January 1980.

183. US War Department. General orders no. 79, par. 2, 24 August 1918. In: *General Orders and Bulletins*. Washington, DC: Government Printing Office; 1919: 1.

184. [Ottolengui R]. The present status of dental service in the United States Army, and the effect of war conditions upon dental education. *Dent Items Interest*. 1918;40:825–826.

185. US Army, General Staff, Committee on Education and Special Training. Students' Army Training Corps. *J Natl Dent Assoc*. 1918;5:1093.

186. King OU. Dental Reserve Corps commissions to be granted enlisted dentists. *Tex Dent J*. 1919;37:3–6.

187. [King OU?]. Demobilization of the Student Army Training Corps between December 1 and 21, 1918. *J Natl Dent Assoc*. 1918;5:1288.

188. The S.A.T.C. and the Army Authorities. *Army and Navy Register*. Quoted in: *Dental Cosmos*. 1919;61: 93.

189. Enlisted dentists will get commissions. *Evening Mail*. Quoted in: *J Allied Dent Soc*. 1918: 523.

190. Biographical file on Major General James M Epperly. Available at: Research Collections, OTSG/MEDCOM, Falls Church, Va.

191. US War Department, Adjutant General's Office. *Official Army Register, January 1, 1938.* Washington, DC: Government Printing Office; 1938: 225.

192. National Archives and Records Administration. Record Group 341. Review of the development and the organization of the medical service of the Army Air Forces, 26 August 1944. Box 356. Entry 48.

193. US War Department. Special Orders No. 207, September 6, 1917.

194. National Archives and Records Administration. Office of the Director of Air Service. Record Group 18. Personnel orders no. 68, 28 May 1919. No. 703. Box 1237. Entry 166.

195. National Archives and Records Administration. Record Group 18. Major Patrick Frissell, commanding officer, Signal Corps Aviation School, Eberts Field, Lonoke, AK, to commanding general, southeast department, Charleston, SC, 27 June 1918. Letter. No. 703. Box 1360. Entry 393.

196. National Archives and Records Administration. Record Group 18. Samuel M Strong, Medical Reserve Corps, post surgeon, Eberts Field, to commanding officer, Eberts Field, Lonoke, Arkansas, 10 July 1918. Memo. No. 703. Box 1360. Entry 393.

197. National Archives and Records Administration. Record Group 18. Major Albert L Sneed, Signal Corps, to commanding general, southern department, Fort Sam Houston, Texas, 18 October 1918. Letter. No. 211.19. Box 1888. Entry 465.

198. National Archives and Records Administration. Record Group 18. Second Lieutenant Virgil C Thomas, adjutant, Squadron "C," to commanding officer, Love Field, Dallas, Texas, 14 October 1918. Letter. No. 211.19. Box 1888. Entry 465.

199. Squires WA. The advisability of recording the models of the jaws of aviators. *J AS-MUS*. 1918;2:169–170.

200. Mitchell DF. A history of aviation dentistry: with emphasis on development in the AAF during World War II. *Ann Dent*. 1946:1–2.

201. [Dental Subdivision, Office of the Surgeon General]. Dangers from the use of removable unilateral prosthetic dental appliances. *Dental Bulletin Supplement to the Army Medical Bulletin*. 1933;4:173–175.

202. V[ail] WD. The Dental Reserve Corps. *Dental Bulletin Supplement to the Army Medical Bulletin*. 1936;7: 19–20.

203. National Archives and Records Administration. American Expeditionary Forces Weekly Reports (decimal file 200). Record Group 120. Personnel, medical department, 30 November 1918. Boxes 4908, 4909. Entry 2065.

204. National Archives and Records Administration. Personnel, medical department (decimal file 320.2-1). American Expeditionary Forces. Record Group 112. Medical department personnel on duty in AEF, May 1919. Box 5. Entry 31.

205. US War Department. General orders no. 73, par. 1, 7 August 1918. In: *General Orders 1918*. Washington, DC: Government Printing Office; 1919.

206. [King OU?]. Sources of new dental officers. *Dental Cosmos*. 1918;60:1168.

207. Clark RA. Professional capability and dental commissions. *Dental Cosmos*. 1918;60:918.

208. Daniels B. Professional capability and dental commissions. *Dental Cosmos*. 1918;60:1129.

209. National Archives and Records Administration. Decimal file 382, Dental Corps. Record Group 165. Memorandum for the chief of staff, Brigadier General Lytle Brown, director, War Plans Division, 8 September 1918, and memorandum for the adjutant general, General Peyton C March, chief of staff, 28 September 1918. No. 8954-20. Box 48. Entry 8.

210. National Archives and Records Administration. Dental Corps, US Army (War Plans Division report no. 8954). Record Group 165. Memorandum for the chief of staff, Ketcham, acting director, War Plans Division, 18 April 1918. No. 8954-13.

211. National Archives and Records Administration. Dental Corps, US Army (War Plans Division report no. 8954). Record Group 165. Memorandum for the adjutant general, Ketcham, acting director, War Plans Division, 20 April 1918. No. 8954-13.

212. National Archives and Records Administration. Decimal file 382, Dental Corps. Record Group 165. Memorandum for the adjutant general, March, 28 September 1918. No. 8954-20.

Chapter XIII

THE DENTAL SERVICE IN THE AMERICAN EXPEDITIONARY FORCES IN FRANCE, 1917–1919: ORGANIZATION, ADMINISTRATION, PERSONNEL, TRAINING, AND SUPPLY

Introduction

The Allies had been fighting the war against Germany, Austro-Hungary, and the Ottoman Empire since August 1914, and Europeans on both sides were skeptical of the ability of the United States to make a meaningful contribution to the outcome. American planners themselves first anticipated a token ground effort, with greater naval activity and substantial logistical and financial support. When the Anglo-French Balfour Mission arrived in Washington in April 1917 and frankly described their horrendous losses and immediate needs, US leaders were quickly disabused of this naïve vision. Russia was on the verge of collapse, Britain's personnel resources were drying up at an alarming rate, and the French army was in a state of near mutiny. American planners realized concrete gestures needed to be taken quickly and that it would be necessary to raise and deploy a huge land force to Europe to shore up the Allies.[1]

Pershing and the Initial Echelon of the American Expeditionary Forces

President Woodrow Wilson appointed Major General John J Pershing commander-in-chief of the American Expeditionary Forces (AEF) and gave him broad guidance to form a staff, go to France, and determine the size and composition of the American contribution to the ground war. Pershing's small AEF headquarters group sailed for Liverpool, England, on May 28, 1917, on the *SS Baltic*. Hastily constructed plans called for the equally quickly formed 1st Division to follow a few weeks later as a token force to raise Allied morale. Accompanying the party was Colonel (later Major General and Surgeon General, 1918–1931) Merritte W Ireland (1867–1952), Medical Corps (MC), post surgeon at Fort Sam Houston, Texas, where Pershing's southern department was headquartered. A long-time acquaintance of Pershing's dating back to the Spanish-American War and the Santiago campaign, Ireland led the initial contingent of medical officers and physicians from Johns Hopkins Base Hospital No. 18. Among the physicians was Dr Hugh Hampton Young, a leading American urologist and an expert on venereal diseases.

During the trip across the Atlantic, Young described the problems of venereal disease in a series of lectures to Pershing and his staff and spelled out the poten-

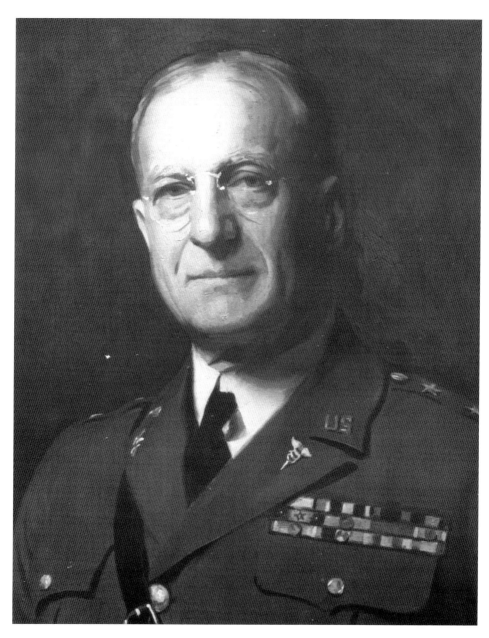

Merritte W Ireland, surgeon general 1918–1931.
Photograph: Courtesy of the National Museum of Health and Medicine,
Armed Forces Institute of Pathology. NCP 3569.

tially debilitating consequences for the AEF if such diseases were not controlled from the very beginning. Pershing agreed and even before he arrived in France had decided on a strong program of venereal disease control to be headed by Young, who later became the chief consultant in urology to the AEF chief surgeon. In addition to the medical lectures, briefings on various topics took place between discussions on grand strategy and efforts to revive long-forgotten memories of high school and college French.[2–4]

The surgeons from Johns Hopkins Hospital were members of Red Cross Base Hospital No. 18, one of a number of Army hospitals requested in April 1917 by the Allied delegation for immediate deployment to the western front to augment British medical facilities. Six such base hospitals were overseas and in operation by the end of June. Each had at least two dental officers on staff, for a total of 13 dentists in place with the general hospitals serving the British.[5]

Dental Unit Number 1

While the Army hospitals were on their way, on June 12, 1917, Pershing's headquarters in Paris requested the assignment of Captain Robert T Oliver, the senior officer of the Dental Corps, to the AEF chief surgeon's staff as well as the assignment of sufficient dental officers to support the troops arriving in France. As with Ireland, the request for Oliver was no mere coincidence. At the time, Oliver was assigned dental surgeon at Fort Sam Houston's Base Hospital No. 1 and had known and treated Pershing in the Philippines and on the border. Ireland and Oliver had probably first become acquainted in 1901–1902, while Ireland was in charge of the medical supply depot in Manila and medical purveyor for the Philippine Division, and Oliver was the supervising contract dental surgeon. The War Department issued confidential orders to Oliver on June 25. Oliver then requested that the surgeon general approve formation of a six-dentist unit, including himself, to deploy with him for duty with the AEF. Designated Dental Unit No. 1, the small group assembled in New York between July 10 and July 15. It consisted of five dentists from the Regular Army—Captains Oliver, Rex H Rhoades, and Raymond E Ingalls, and First Lieutenants George D Graham and William S Rice—and one Dental Reserve Corps (DRC) officer, First Lieutenant John B Wagoner, as well as two sergeants and three privates from the Medical Department.[6]

The unit joined the personnel from Base Hospital No. 18 and troops from the 5th and 7th US Artillery Regiments on board the US Army transport *Saratoga* for the trip overseas. As the ship steamed out of New York harbor on July 30, an inbound ship, the US Army transport *Panama*, accidentally rammed it and the *Saratoga* had to be abandoned. Tugs towed the sinking vessel to a shallow area where it settled into the water off Bay Ridge, Brooklyn. Although the dentists saved much of their personal property, all of the unit dental equipment was a total loss. The marooned soldiers spent several frantic days procuring new supplies and equipment, some of which was donated by the SS White Dental Supply Company of Philadelphia. Finally, on August 7, they loaded the *SS Finland* and sailed once again for the war zone. The trip across the Atlantic proved largely uneventful, and Oliver filled the time with daily classes on Army procedures and customs of the service for his unit and five DRC officers from other units who were on board. The *Finland* docked at Saint Nazaire, France, on August 21, where the unit was temporarily attached for support to AEF Base Hospital No. 1 (Exhibit 13-1).[7]

Oliver's orders were to report to General Pershing himself, so the unit remained in Saint Nazaire only long enough to transfer its equipment from the docks onto a train and for the soldiers to exchange their dollars for francs. They left Saint Nazaire the next day, and Oliver reported to AEF General Headquarters (GHQ) the morning of August 23. Oliver had known Pershing since their time together in the Philippines in 1902, and they had last seen each other when Oliver treated Pershing at Colonia Dublán, Mexico, in September 1916.[8] Pershing expressed pleasure at the unit's arrival and directed Oliver to report to the AEF chief surgeon, Colonel Alfred E Bradley, MC, to plan the assignments of unit members and to identify the requirements for theater dental support. On August 29 orders named Oliver as the AEF's senior dental surgeon and assigned him to the personnel division of the chief surgeon's office. Lieutenant Wagoner remained with him as "prosthetic assistant," along with Sergeants Wade and Henry. Captain Rhoades and Private First Class John E Carr went to the artillery training center at La Valdahon. Captain Ingalls and First Lieutenant Rice, along with Privates First Class Russell and Oldring, went to the 1st Division at Gondrecourt. First Lieutenant Graham assumed the duties of theater dental supply officer at Cosne.[7,9]

The responsibility for building the AEF's dental service from scratch fell to Oliver, whose years of supervisory experience since 1901 would now be tested. He immediately began planning for a comprehensive dental service for the combat and support forces that were anticipated, to include all personnel and equipment requirements. In this capacity, he functioned as a part of the AEF chief surgeon's personnel division. At the same time, he oversaw the establishment of a dental clinic and laboratory with the AEF headquarters in Chaumont and made technical visits to those dentists already at work with units throughout France. Not only did direct dental service to the troops have to be considered, but the support overhead

---

EXHIBIT 13-1

DENTAL UNIT NO. 1

Dental Unit No. 1 included: Captains Robert T Oliver, DC, Rex H Rhoades, DC, and Raymond E Ingalls, DC; First Lieutenants George D Graham, DC, William S Rice, DC, and John B Wagoner, DRC; Sergeants Lee Wade and MF Henry; Privates First Class John E Carr, William J Oldring, and Erskine Russel. The other dental officers, all first lieutenants, DRC, were Albert M Applegate and William M Irving, Base Hospital No. 8; JB Watson and HL Bull, Base Hospital No. 9; and RK Thompson, 1st Engineers.

Data source: Ingalls R. Diary of a dental officer. *Dental Bulletin Supplement to the Army Medical Bulletin.* 1939;10:1–18.

also had to be determined. Oliver had to identify the administrative and logistical positions in the supporting line of communications (LOC, later redesignated the services of supply [SOS] in February 1918) which required dentists at depots, headquarters, and hospitals. Further, in conjunction with medical personnel, Oliver began to detail and select "oro-dental specialists" to augment hospital surgical staffs. Oliver relied on his Mexican border experiences to develop and distribute an informal correspondence course on Army administration to all incoming dentists. This sufficed until a more formal school opened in the 1st Division on September 15, 1917.[6]

The Structure of American Expeditionary Forces Dental Support

Oliver and his miniscule staff struggled to build dental support and the proper distribution of dentists as the AEF's structure gradually emerged. The two major parts of the AEF quickly came into view—the Zone of the Armies containing the combat units and direct supporting elements and the LOCs that received, transported, stored, and distributed all supplies to the Army. The LOC was ultimately divided into 10 geographic areas—eight base sections in France (one being Paris and its environs) and the United Kingdom, an intermediate section of depots and storage, and an advance section with the Zone of the Armies that provided the direct logistical support to the fighting troops. The bulk of the medical support and hospitalization was sited within the LOC, with all of the camp and base hospitals, hospital centers, and main medical supply depots. The divisions, corps, and armies and supporting units of the AEF and their medical units, including evacuation and divisional field hospitals, were in the combat zones. They handled routine and battlefield care as well as evacuation of the sick and wounded.[6,10]

The initial combat divisions, such as the 2nd, 26th, 41st and 42nd, that followed the 1st Division in 1917, reached France with 20 or fewer dentists attached. The October 6, 1917, dental reorganization bill allowed Oliver to increase the number to 31, but many of the divisions arriving in 1918 often had far fewer than that. For example, the 2nd Division already in France in October 1917 had only five dental surgeons assigned. One of them was Lieutenant (junior grade) Alexander G Lyle, Dental Corps, US Navy, assigned to support the 5th and 6th Regiments, US Marine Corps, that composed one of the division's two infantry brigades, and who would later receive the Navy Medal of Honor in 1918 for heroism, serve as chief of the Navy Dental Corps during World War II (1943–1946), and become the only service dental officer ever to reach three star rank when he was promoted to vice admiral in 1948.[11] The senior dental officer was also designated division dental surgeon, who was responsible to the division surgeon for the supply, technical supervision, assignment, and evaluation of the division's dentists. The AEF's dental service grew proportionally with the force, with dental administrators assigned at each level of command, starting with Colonel Oliver at AEF GHQ. In the forward Zone of the Armies conducting combat operations against the Germans under GHQ, the First and Second Armies, and later the Third Army in November 1918 for occupation duties, had a chief dental surgeon who supervised the corps dental surgeons. The corps dental surgeons watched over divisions' dental surgeons and activities.[6,12–14]

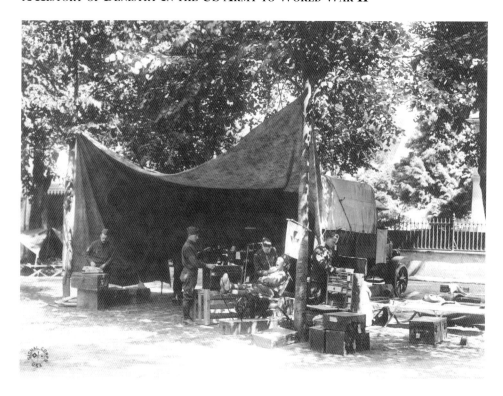

First Lieutenant CB Ray, Dental Officers' Reserve Corps, Ammunition Train,
26th Division, working on a patient in the dentist's chair of this motorized dental unit.
La Ferte, France, July 9, 1918.
Photograph: Courtesy of US Army Military History Institute. SC 18277

In the LOC area, supervising dental surgeons were eventually assigned to each of the eight base sections as well as the intermediate and advance sections. Their job was to coordinate dental service in their geographical areas through inspection and technical supervision and to render reports on their actions and findings to Oliver's office, which maintained overall technical control but not command. They further organized central dental laboratories and clinics in their areas and developed necessary technical training. Finally, they operated a centralized dental supply system for their areas, processing requisitions and issuing materials. A hierarchy of inspections was instituted throughout the system to assure standards and respond to requirements.[5,6]

Many of the dentists arrived in the AEF accompanying divisions or medical hospital units, but larger numbers also arrived monthly as bulk shipments of casuals and replacements earmarked for the LOC according to the AEF's M-415 shipping priorities. Although Oliver worked hard to achieve structure and coherence, his efforts in the beginning were largely transient, in part because of the novelty of the situation and the apparent inability of senior officers to envision the dental support that was required. Oliver first recommended a hierarchy of care, stretching from forward units back through the base hospitals to the general hospitals in the United States. The nature of the work anticipated and the dispersion of the units also prompted him to recommend increasing the old ratio of one dentist per thousand troops. On September 6, 1917, he wrote to the chief surgeon, then Colonel (later Brigadier General) Alfred E Bradley, MC:

> The number of Dental Surgeons for the Army under existing laws, is based upon a ratio of one to one thousand; which would give from twenty-five to twenty-eight for a Divisional organization under the provisions of the last table of organization. In as much as there is bound to be a vast number of all classes of Dental and Minor Oral surgical cases occurring among this number of troops it becomes readily apparent that this ratio of Dental Surgeons must be exceeded in order to provide adequate Dental attention for the Officers and men, and that the scope and character of treatment rendered must be such as to insure a degree of Dental fitness which will last thru the period of the War and thus assist in maintaining the greatest number of effectives for active duty.[15]

Bradley deferred Oliver's suggestions in favor of consideration for "one large dental plant" at Neufchâteau Hospital far forward in what became the advance section, instead of individual "divisional plants." Experience and practicality soon favored Oliver's approach, as did the October 1917 bill reorganizing the Dental Corps.[6,16]

The October 6, 1917, law gave dental students the same exemptions from the draft as medical students and, more importantly, gave the Dental Corps officers the same grades and percentages within grades as the Medical Corps. As a result, the War Department officially authorized an increase to 31 dentists in each division in March 1918. However, these changes did not produce any immediate growth in the number of dental surgeons in the AEF, which a little more than doubled from 130 on November 17 to 282 on April 6, 1918. The influx of 29 US divisions and supporting forces from April through August 1918 resulted in a steady build up of the Dental Corps in the AEF (Table 13-1). From April 6, the strength grew to 739 by July 6, 1,081 by August 3, 1,345 by September 7, and 1,606 by October 5. Officers of the DRC accounted for the bulk of dental surgeons in the AEF. After the armistice in November 1918, there were 1,779 Army dental officers in Europe supported by more than 2,000 enlisted soldiers serving as dental assistants, mechanics, or laboratory technicians.[6,17]

Personnel for the American Expeditionary Forces' Dental Corps

The AEF's Dental Corps grew from many sources simultaneously. Shortly after Oliver established himself in the chief surgeon's office, he was approached by several US dentists practicing in Europe who offered their services. Oliver recommended that dental boards be established and examination dates set to consider these dentists and any others who might apply for the Reserve or Regular Dental Corps or for dental officers who were eligible for promotion. Five highly qualified dentists were soon obtained from this source. Some foreign nationals trained at American dental colleges also applied but had to be turned away because they were not US citizens.[18]

The pressure to provide dental care to the soldiers in the units pouring into

TABLE 13-1

DENTAL CORPS OFFICER STRENGTH IN THE AMERICAN
EXPEDITIONARY FORCES, NOVEMBER 1917–SEPTEMBER 1919

Date	Officers	AEF	BEF	USAAS/F	USAAS/I	Total
November 17, 1917	DCRA	8				8
	DCNG	27				27
	DRC	95				95
	Total	**130**	**0**	**0**	**0**	**130**
February 2, 1918	DCRA	17				17
	DCNG	58				58
	DRC	149				149
	Total	**214**	**0**	**0**	**0**	**214**
April 6, 1918	DCRA	20				20
	DCNG	68				68
	DRC	194				194
	Total	**282**	**0**	**0**	**0**	**282**
June 1, 1918	DCRA	29				29
	DCNG	89				89
	DRC	345	10	1	0	356
	Total	**463**	**10**	**1**	**0**	**464**
July 6, 1918	DCRA	51				51
	DCNG	128				128
	DRC	547	12	1	0	560
	Total	**722**	**12**	**1**	**0**	**739**
August 3, 1918	DCRA	57				57
	DCNG	144				144
	DRC	868	12	2	1	883
	Total	**1,069**	**12**	**2**	**1**	**1,081**
August 7, 1918	All DC					
September 7, 1918	DC	1,330	12	2	1	1,345
October 5, 1918	DC	1,591	14	2	1	1,606
November 30, 1918	DC	1,765	11	2	1	1,779
January 4, 1919	DC	1,803	11	2	1	1,817
February 22, 1919	DC	1,712	12	2	1	1,727
April 12, 1919	DC	1,537	2	1	1	1,541
May 31, 1919	DC	1,113	0	1	0	1,114
June 28, 1919	DC	681	0	0	0	681
July 19, 1919	DC	312	0	0	0	312
August 16, 1919	DC	125	0	0	0	125
September 13, 1919	DC	67	0	0	0	67

(table 13-1 *continued)*

AEF: American Expeditionary Forces
BEF: British Expeditionary Forces
USAA/F: US Army Ambulance Service with the French
USAAS/I: US Army Ambulance Service with the Italians
DCRA: Dental Corps Regular Army
DCNG: Dental Corps National Guard
DRC: Dental Reserve Corps
Data sources: (1) National Archives and Records Administration. Record group 120. American Expeditionary Forces, decimal file 200, Personnel, Medical Department. Boxes 4908 and 4909. Entry 2065. (2) National Archives and Records Administration. Record group 112. Decimal file 320.2-1 (AEF), "Personnel, Medical Department, AEF." Box 5. Entry 31.

France was constant. For example, on August 15, 1917, the surgeon of the 29th Provisional Aero Squadron at Issoudun asked for immediate care for at least six of his soldiers and possibly others. The chief surgeon's office could only reply 6 days later that one of the few dentists available was going on his rounds at bases in the vicinity of Issoudun and would be on hand as soon as possible.[19]

Medical units in the field often dealt with the situation by detailing to their dental sections enlisted soldiers who were graduate dentists. This happened to

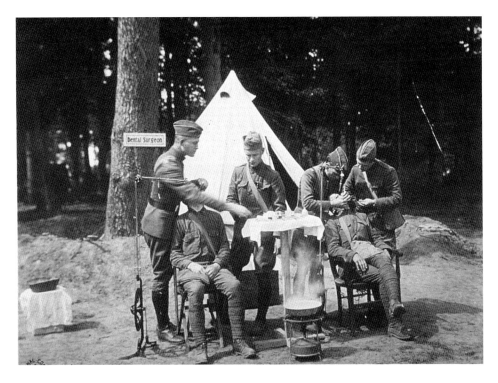

Field dental station, Saulty, France.
Reproduced from: http://wwwihm.nlm.nih.gov/ihm/images/A/22/436.jpg.
Courtesy of the National Library of Medicine.

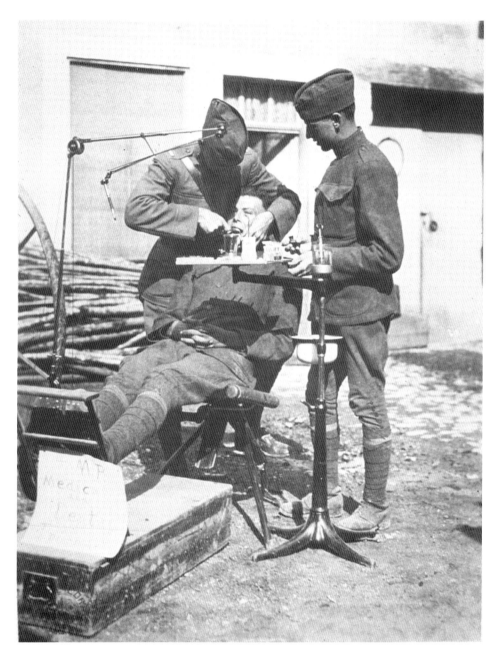

Teeth of a soldier being taken care of in the field hospital near Rimacourt, France.
Reproduced from: http://wwwihm.nlm.nih.gov/ihm/images/A/22/437.jpg.
Courtesy of the National Library of Medicine.

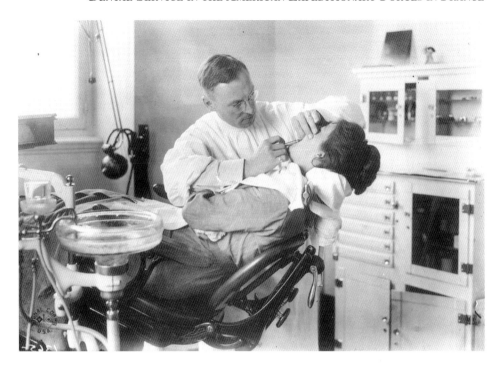

*Captain EG Barkley, dental surgeon, operates on a patient in the dental
department of Base Hospital No. 17 (Harper Hospital, Detroit, Michigan unit)
at Dijon, France. September 5, 1918.
Photograph: Courtesy of US Army Military History Institute. SC 28123*

Private Oscar Johnson at Base Hospital No. 36, who was originally sent to the hospital as a patient. The hospital's two dental officers were thrilled to learn that Johnson was a graduate of the University of Minnesota with a practice in Minneapolis. With Oliver's approval, Johnson remained at the hospital, took over a third chair in the clinic, and served as a dentist there for the duration of the war. Dr Johnson is presumed to be Oscar H Johnson, a 1916 graduate of the University of Minnesota College of Dentistry.[20,21] In other cases, the hospitals found they had brought some dental talent with them. For example, Sergeant Harold F Lafayette was a third-year student at Harvard who enlisted in his college's hospital unit, Base Hospital No. 5, and deployed before he formally graduated. He was assigned to the dental laboratory making splints and dentures at British Hospital No. 11 and No. 15. However, as soon as his formal notice of graduation caught up with him in November 1917, Lafayette's supervising dental officer, First Lieutenant William H Potter, successfully recommended him to Oliver for examination and commissioning in the DRC.[22]

During 1918, 92 graduate dentists were still serving in the line or as dental assistants in the AEF. All were encouraged to apply to be examined for commissions in the DRC.[23] These examinations were similar to those given by the regular dental examining board. In lieu of a candidate's original diploma and license, the board accepted a certificate stating the candidate's school and date of graduation and the source and date of license to practice dentistry (issued by the State Board of Dental Examiners). The board rated an applicant's performance on all subjects and rendered a general report on each candidate. The president of the board could terminate a candidate's examination at any time the board was convinced of "said candidate's disqualifications." A duplicate report was sent to the surgeon general's office via the chief surgeon's office, AEF.[24] On November 17, 1918, the examinations for temporary commissions in the Dental Corps were discontinued and the examination papers for such commissions were placed on file and suspended in the AEF for "an indefinite period."[25]

Despite the moratorium, applications continued to arrive at the chief surgeon's office. On November 20, 1918, Colonel Oliver notified the president of the dental board that he had 57 sets of application papers from enlisted dentists for appointment in the DRC.[26] On December 7, 1918, Captain Charles F Huber, the 88th Division dental surgeon, reported that he had 16 "authorized dental assistants" who were graduate dentists in his division.[27]

The majority of graduate dentists serving in the Army as enlisted troops were eventually used as dental assistants. Some of them had tremendous experience, such as Private First Class James Loraine Shipley (Northwestern University Dental School, 1915), who stated on his application for a dental commission that he had "six months at Base Hospital, Camp Grant, Ill. Two months in operating pavilion. In that time gave about two hundred general anesthetics. Four months as dental assistant in dental infirmary."[28]

This procurement program concluded on February 20, 1919, when the AEF chief surgeon, Colonel Walter D McCaw, recommended that 88 enlisted dentists (86 privates and 2 sergeants) be appointed and commissioned as first lieutenants in the dental section of the Officers' Reserve Corps. These dentists (all dental graduates) had been examined during November and December 1918 and passed the prescribed professional and physical examinations too late for active AEF service.[29]

Dental Reserve Candidates for the Regular Army

During 1918 some of the DRC officers opted to transfer to the Regular Army Dental Corps. On March 1, 1918, eight reservists filed their papers for preliminary examination for the corps and were invited to appear before the Army Dental Board on March 11, 1918. One candidate, First Lieutenant Schuyler E Waller, a graduate dentist, was serving as an officer in the 101st Engineer Train, AEF.[30]

Conversely, the dental board also examined candidates for appointment in the DRC. On March 13, 1918, a Canadian Army Dental Corps officer, three civilian dentists (practicing in such diverse places as London, England; Bombay, India; and Berne, Switzerland), and 10 US Army enlisted soldiers filed their application papers and were invited to appear before the board on March 18. Of this group of 14, 10 completed the examination, three failed to report for the examination, and one was rejected for physical reasons. In May 1918 five more enlisted soldiers sent in their application papers and two were found qualified. In June 1918 seven more enlisted dentists and a Red Cross dental officer applied for commissions in the DRC.[31–35]

Army Dental Schools

From the beginning it was obvious that dental officers coming from such a variety of sources needed orientation on Army procedures and military dentistry. The first groups to arrive in France attended the impromptu 1st Division School, whose example was emulated by later arriving units. Topics covered included various administrative procedures, visits to Allied medical units, and briefings on the growing AEF system of dental support.[6] Greater structure was imposed in November 1917 when orders established the Army Sanitary School at Langres.

The mission of the dental section of the Army Sanitary School was simply stated as follows:

> The purpose of this school is to give dental surgeons attached to Combat divisions or the S.O.S. instruction in preparation for field service in the A.E.F., which will supplement that given in the training camps in the United States and with troops in France.[36]

The first dental faculty member was First Lieutenant William S Rice, Dental Corps (DC), a veteran of the *Saratoga* disaster and an original member of Oliver's Dental Unit No. 1. On December 7 Rice transferred from the 1st Division to the dental section at the Army Sanitary School, Langres, France. The same month, he successfully requested a complete base dental laboratory outfit for the school.[37–39]

Classes began in January 1918 under the direction of now Major Rice (Rice was promoted directly to major on October 6, 1917).[40] On January 16, the first students arrived from the 2nd, 26th, and 42nd Divisions.[11] The new group of 13 dental officers included Lieutenant (junior grade) Alexander G Lyle, US Navy, of the 5th Marines, 2nd Division (Exhibit 13-2).[11] The session ran from January 16 to January 29, 1918, and included classes in medico-military subjects, oral surgery, oral surgical prosthesis, oral and general hygiene, courts martial and military law, maps and map reading, organization of the sanitary department, military discipline, oral manifestations of systemic disease, first aid, bandaging and splinting, general anesthesia, operating room technique, and gas instruction (Exhibit 13-3).[42,43]

On January 26, 1918, Colonel Seibert D Boak, the first contract dental surgeon hired in 1901, reported as the dental section's new director.[44] One of his first innovations was to require each student to write a thesis, the grade of which was incorporated in a report of the student's standing submitted to the commandant of the Army schools, the chief of training session, and to the appropriate division dental surgeon. Toward this end, Colonel Boak requested that the dental section be furnished with its own copies of all special and general orders, bulletins, circulars, and memoranda from AEF GHQ and the post.[45,46] A new session began on February 4, 1918, and included field trips to the Army Central Laboratory (to study bacteriology techniques), an American evacuation hospital, and an advanced medical supply depot. The classes were scheduled every 6 weeks thereafter with about the same curriculum.[47,48] Each class graduating until the armistice had 25 to 30 students.[49]

Among the textbooks used by the students were Truman W Brophy's *Oral Surgery: a Treatise on the Diseases and Malformations of the Mouth and Associated Parts*[50]; and George Van I Brown's *The Surgery of Oral Diseases and Malformations: Their*

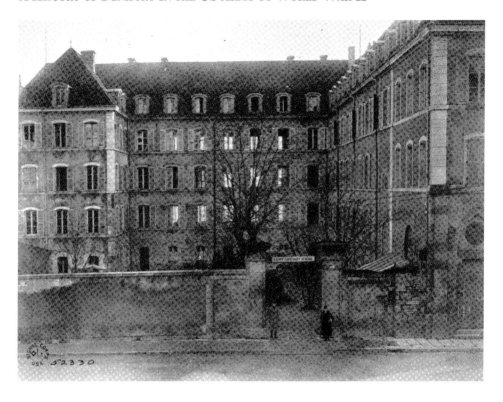

Army Sanitary School at Langres, France.
Reproduced from: Bispham WN. Training. Vol 7. In: Lynch C, Weed FW, McAfee L, eds.
The Medical Department of the United States Army in the World War.
Washington, DC: Government Printing Office; 1927: 601.

Diagnosis and Treatment.[51] The surgeons conceded that "the dentist is the logical man to look after all fractured jaw cases, for the wiring as applied by most surgeons is but a crude method that little or no attention is given the proper occlusion of the teeth."[52]

On March 25, 1918, Colonel Boak, Major Rice, and First Lieutenant William H Potter, DRC went to Paris to observe the trauma techniques used at the dental clinic of the former American Ambulance Hospital, now American Red Cross Military Hospital No. 1, at Neuilly, run by Doctors George B Hayes and William and Isaac Davenport (Exhibit 13-4).[53-55] The next day, they visited the dental department of the French Military Red Cross Hospital No. 65 (under the direction of Major Leon Frey of the French army). They then toured the stomatology service of the Val de Grace Hospital, one of the largest French military hospitals, and the Hospital Michelot under Dr Georges Villain. They returned to the dental clinic at Neuilly to study jaw fracture models for use in teaching at the Army Sanitary School.[56]

On May 5, 1918, led by the commandant, the class in session began a 2-week tour of observation and instruction at the French front while its successor started arriving at the school. From May 5 to May 18, 1918, this succeeding class, which in-

---

EXHIBIT 13-2

ALEXANDER GORDON LYLE

Alexander Gordon Lyle, Baltimore College of Dental Surgery, class of 1912, was commissioned a lieutenant (junior grade) in the US Navy Dental Corps in 1915. In 1917 he went to France with the 5th Regiment of Marines attached to the 2nd Division, American Expeditionary Forces. On April 23, 1918, under heavy shellfire on the French front at Verdun, Dr Lyle rushed to the assistance of Corporal Thomas Regan, who was seriously wounded, and "administered such effective surgical aid while bombardment was still continuing as to save the life of Corporal Regan." He was awarded the Navy Medal of Honor for "extraordinary heroism and devotion to duty." Dr Lyle participated in the Aisne Defense, the Aisne-Marne Offensive, Saint Mihiel Offensive, and the Meuse-Argonne Offensive. He received two Army Silver Star awards, the Italian "Merito de Guerra," and the Victory Medal with five bars. After the war, he was stationed with the 4th Marines in China. He then served on various ships and stations. From 1932 to 1936 he was chief of the dental service at the Newport Naval Hospital. In 1939 he was promoted to captain and served at Quonset, Rhode Island. In March 1943 he was commissioned a rear admiral and appointed the chief of the US Navy Dental Corps, the first dentist to hold flag rank in the US Navy. In 1946 he received a doctor of science degree from the University of Maryland. Admiral Lyle retired in 1947 after 32 years of service and in 1948 was advanced on the retired list to vice admiral.

Data source: Foley GPH, ed. *Proceedings of the 125th Anniversary of the Baltimore College of Dental Surgery March 4, 5 and 6, 1965 Baltimore, Maryland.* Baltimore, Md: Alumni Association and the Faculty of the Baltimore College of Dental Surgery, Dental School, University of Maryland; 1966: 188–189.

---

cluded six enlisted dentists, began a 2-week tour of the American front. Those of the previous class who had not been to the front were assigned to temporary duty with the 2nd, 26th, and 42nd Divisions, while those who had been went to temporary duty at Evacuation Hospitals No. 1 and No. 2. On May 18 the class reassembled at the sanitary school for the balance of the course. Transportation was furnished by the ambulance company attached to the Army schools.[57]

On July 2, 1918, Boak formally requested that Captain Fernand LeMaitre, surgical chief of French Maxillofacial Hospital No. 45, Vichy, be detailed to lecture to the dental section students on "The Importance of Cooperation between Surgeons and Dental Surgeons in the Treatment of Head Wounds." Boak wanted to show the students the prosthetic appliances, photographs, and masks that Dr LeMaitre had developed for facial wound emergency cases at Hospital No. 45.[58]

The next day, Boak's request was approved by Colonel Bailey K Ashford, MC, the commandant, who endorsed Captain Maitre's appearance as of the "highest importance" to the dental school.[59] The general staff passed the request on to the French Military Mission with the American Army, promising railway transportation on an American military train from Nevers to the school and arrangements for his "entertainment while at the Army Sanitary School."[60]

EXHIBIT 13-4

WILLIAM H POTTER

William H Potter, age 51, was professor of operative dentistry at Harvard Dental School and came to France with Base Hospital No. 5, landing in England on May 22, 1917, and in France on May 30, 1917. He served with this hospital in France at Camiers and at Boulogne until December 8, 1917, when he was assigned to the dental section of the Army Sanitary School as an instructor in oral surgery. His research and translations made both English and French maxillofacial procedures available to the student officers. First Lieutenant Potter was promoted to major, Dental Reserve Corps, on July 30, 1918 (with rank from February 9, 1918). On November 18, 1918, he was recommended for the Distinguished Service Medal. On December 5, 1918, after 18 months overseas service and with the closure of the sanitary school imminent, Major Potter requested he be allowed to return to his teaching position at Harvard.

Data sources: (1) National Archives and Records Administration. Record Group 120. Colonel SD Boak, director, dental section, Army Sanitary School, to commandant, Army schools, American Expeditionary Forces, 18 November 1918. Memo. Folder 2. Box 1780. Entry 395. (2) National Archives and Records Administration. Record Group 120. Major RA Dickson (for chief surgeon, American Expeditionary Forces, services of supply), to First Lieutenant William H Potter, 25 August 1918. Memo. Folder 2, Box 1780. Entry 395. (3) National Archives and Records Administration. Record Group 120. Major William H Potter, DC, to chief surgeon, American Expeditionary Forces, headquarters, services of supply (through military channels), 5 December 1918. Memo. Folder 2. Box 1780. Entry 395.

On July 7, 1918, Boak received permission for himself, Major Rice, First Lieutenant Potter, and an enlisted photographer, Sergeant John W Cooke, to visit the 82nd Division for 4 days to obtain material for instruction in the classroom (Exhibit 13-5).[61–71] Boak also visited the Ecole Dentaire at Paris to observe the war surgery work of Dr Georges Villain (Exhibit 13-6).[72] Colonel Boak was so impressed with Dr Villain's fracture work that on July 23, 1918, he requested that Villain, a dental graduate of the University of Pennsylvania, be invited to give the dental section a lecture called "Fractures of the Maxillae, and their Treatment." Boak emphasized that Villain had an "extra-ordinary ingenious grasp for the problem incident to facio-maxillary prosthesis" and that his lecture to the students was "highly desirable, if not a necessity."[73,74]

The same day, Boak requested that Dr Varaztad H Kazanjian (Exhibit 13-7), an American with General Hospital No. 20, British Expeditionary Forces, be invited to lecture on maxillofacial prosthesis and plastic surgery.[75] Dr Kazanjian had been serving with the British Army since the spring of 1915, and Boak believed that the students should "have the benefit of his experience."[73] Despite the approval of the school's commandant, Kazanjian's visit was disapproved by AEF GHQ because of the "travel and expense involved;" leaving the dental officers unable to experience the teaching of the dental surgeon called the "Miracle Man of the Western Front."[75,76] Meanwhile, apparently Captain LeMaitre's lecture on the French methods was so well received that on August 19, 1918, Boak

EXHIBIT 13-5

JOHN W COOKE

On February 8, 1918, Sergeant Cooke requested that he be transferred from the medical department to the dental section, Enlisted Reserve Corps, and returned to the United States to complete his dental education at Harvard. While a third-year dental student at Harvard (with an AB degree from Harvard, 1915), he had enlisted as a private, sanitary detachment, 101st Engineers, National Guard, at Boston on July 24, 1917, and was shipped overseas on September 24, 1917. He later transferred from the National Guard to the Regular Army and was assigned to duty at the dental section, Army Sanitary School, American Expeditionary Forces, on December 13, 1917. He was promoted to sergeant on January 19, 1918. Cooke cited General Bulletin No. 61, paragraph 5, War Department, dated October 23, 1917, as the basis for his request. This bulletin stated that "all regulations concerning the enlistment of medical students in the Enlisted Reserve Corps and their continuance in their college course while subject to call to active service, shall apply similarly to dental students." Although approved by his commanding officers, Colonels Boak and Ashford, Cooke's application was disapproved by the surgeon general, who decided on November 22, 1917, that the quoted legislation did not apply "under existing unusual circumstances to dental students abroad." On June 24, 1918, Sergeant Cooke requested permission to take the examination for commission in the US Army Dental Corps. Boak, for whom he had been working since Boak assumed command of the school on January 26, 1918, endorsed him as "capable and efficient" and having the "necessary educational and professional qualifications . . . as would make him a desirable candidate for the Regular Corps." Ashford also gave his approval. Finally, on July 1, 1918, Cooke was invited to take the examination given by the Army Dental Board on July 8 at Langres. Cooke completed a successful examination for appointment to the Dental Reserve Corps on July 12, 1918. In October 1918 First Lieutenant Cooke applied for a Regular Army commission and was directed to report to the examining board on November 1, 1918. He passed the examination. In November 1918 Cooke lectured the dental officers of the 82nd Division at Haute-Marne. On January 19, 1919, he was transferred from the sanitary school to Base Section No. 3, AEF.

Data sources: (1) National Archives and Records Administration. Record Group 120. Sergeant John W Cooke to commandant, Army Sanitary School, Army schools, American Expeditionary Forces, 8 February 1918. Letter. Folder 1. Box 1780. Entry 395. (2) War Department. Bulletin no. 61, par 5, 23 October 1917. In: *General Orders*. Washington, DC: Government Printing Office; 1917. (3) National Archives and Records Administration. Record Group 120. Colonel Robert T Oliver to Colonel Boak, 13 February 1918. Endorsement. Folder 1. Box 1780. Entry 395. (4) National Archives and Records Administration. Record Group 120. Sergeant John W Cooke to chief surgeon, American Expeditionary Forces, 24 June 1918. Letter, with endorsement. Folder 1. Box 1780. Entry 395. (5) National Archives and Records Administration. Record Group 120. Colonel Robert T Oliver (for chief surgeon, American Expeditionary Forces) to Sergeant Cooke, 1 July 1918. Letter. Folder 1. Box 1780. Entry 395. (6) National Archives and Records Administration. Record Group 120. Major WS Rice, recorder, Army Dental Examining Board, to surgeon general, US Army (through chief surgeon, American Expeditionary Forces), 12 July 1918. Folder 1. Box 1780. Entry 395. (7) National Archives and Records Administration. Record Group 120. Colonel Robert T Oliver, American Expeditionary Forces, to Lieutenant Cooke, 7 October 1918. Letter. Folder 1. Box 1780. Entry 395. (8) National Archives and Records Administration. Record Group 120. Alonzo G McCue, recorder, Army Dental Examining Board, to surgeon general, US Army (through chief surgeon, American Expeditionary Forces), 12 November 1918. Letter. Folder 1. Box 1780. Entry 395. (9) National Archives and Records Administration. Record Group 120. Colonel SD Boak, director, dental section, Army Sanitary School, to commandant, Army schools, American Expeditionary Forces, 28 November 1918. Memo. Folder 2. Box 1780. Entry 395. (10) National Archives and Records Administration. Record Group 120. First Lieutenant Cooke to chief surgeon, American Expeditionary Forces (through channels), 19 January 1919. Memo. Folder 1. Box 1780. Entry 395.

EXHIBIT 13-6

DR GEORGES VILLAIN

Dr Georges Villain was born in Paris in 1881 and graduated as Chirurgien Dentiste de la Faculte de Medicine de Paris in 1903. For 2 years he attended school in High Wycombe (England), where he acquired a complete command of the English language. Later, he entered the University of Pennsylvania, Department of Dentistry, and received his DDS degree in 1906. After returning to Paris, he became professor of prosthetics on the faculty of l'Ecole Dentaire. In 1914 he organized and directed the maxillofacial section at the school. He was one of the organizers of the Federation Dentaire Internationale in 1921. He died in an automobile accident on April 26, 1938.

Data source: Dr. Georges Villain, Paris, France (1881–1938). *Dental Cosmos*. 1938;25:1131.

---

successfully requested that he be invited back the week beginning September 8, 1918.[77,78] Boak thought so highly of Major LeMaitre that he recommended him for the Distinguished Service Medal on November 17, 1918, under the provisions of Confidential Memorandum, General Orders No. 26, GHQ, November 16, 1918. LeMaitre had not only assisted the sanitary school's dental section through lectures and onsite visits to French Maxillofacial Hospital No. 45, but had furnished photographs, radiographs, plaster models, and appliances used in the classroom.[79,80]

In September 1918 Boak, Rice, now Major Potter, and Sergeant Cooke visited Maxillofacial Center No. 6 at Lyons for 5 days to "obtain material for instruction purposes" at the school.[81,82] In October both Boak and Rice were assigned to tem-

---

EXHIBIT 13-7

DR VARAZTAD HOVHANESS KAZANJIAN

Dr Varaztad Hovhaness Kazanjian was a 1905 graduate of the Harvard Dental School. On June 26, 1915, he was commissioned a temporary honorary lieutenant, Royal Army Medical Corps, Harvard Surgical Unit, and assigned to General Hospital No. 22, British Expeditionary Forces, as the chief of the dental section. In July 1915 he organized a department of oral reconstructive surgery. In September 1915 he was transferred to General Hospital No. 20, British Expeditionary Forces. Dr Kazanjian was promoted to major in June 1916. His tour of duty was not completed until January 20, 1919. He was commissioned an honorary major, Royal Army Medical Corps, and awarded the Order of Saint Michael and Saint George.

Data source: Hapgood RL. *History of the Harvard Dental School*. Boston, Mass: Harvard University Dental School; 1930: 301.

---

porary duty at Mobile Hospital No. 6 for 3 days and Evacuation Hospitals No. 6 and No. 7 for 4 days each to get more current data.[83] The Army Sanitary School continued its dental section sessions through October 1918.[84]

In November 1918, after the armistice, Boak decided that it was important to record and fully document the activities of dental officers and the dental service in the combat divisions during the preceding 4 months of combat. He recommended that designated dental officers be ordered to report to the sanitary school sometime during the month of December 1918 to lecture the dental section on their experiences. Boak's request was approved by GHQ (Exhibit 13-8).[85,86]

The dental section of the Army Sanitary School, Langres, closed at the completion

---

EXHIBIT 13-8

DENTAL OFFICERS ORDERED TO REPORT TO THE SANITARY SCHOOL DURING DECEMBER 1918 AND THEIR ASSIGNED TOPICS

Dental Officer	Topic
Lieutenant Colonel Samuel H Leslie, chief dental surgeon, III Corps	The Corps Dental Surgeon
Major Gerald G Burns, division dental surgeon, 77th Division	The Division Dental Officer in Combat
Major Rea P McGee, Mobile Hospital No. 1	The Treatment of Maxillofacial Wounds
Captain John E Hughes, division dental surgeon, 29th Division	Transportation of Dental Equipment during Combat
Captain JA Corrizeau, division dental surgeon, 8th Division	Coordination of Dental Officers with Medical Department
Captain JT Ashton, division dental surgeon, 6th Division	Dental Administration in a Division
First Lieutenant Joseph H Jaffer, division dental surgeon, 3rd Division	The Duties of Dental Officers as Auxiliary Medical Officers during Combat
First Lieutenant MF Carney, division dental surgeon, 27th Division	Dental Service in the Rest Areas
First Lieutenant Leo Winter, Mobile Hospital No. 6	Duties of the Dental Officer with a Mobile Hospital

Data sources: (1) National Archives and Records Administration. Record Group 120. Colonel SD Boak, director, to G-5, general headquarters, American Expeditionary Forces (through channels), 19 November 1918. Letter. No. 3603-539. Box 1309. Entry 11. (2) National Archives and Records Administration. Record Group 120. Brigadier General Frank E Bamford, 20 November 1918. Endorsement. No. 3603-539. Box 1309. Entry 11.

of the course ending December 17, 1918.[87] Boak reported his departure on January 19, 1919, for reassignment to headquarters, Base Section No. 2, AEF, as supervising dental surgeon.[88]

Enlisted Support

The need for a large number of qualified enlisted assistants was met through the organization of schools at Saint Aignan and Neuilly. The former was established at one of the largest replacement depots, allowing numbers of enlistees to be screened. Many of these candidates had some medical or dental training prior to entering the Army. Most of them took a short course to become dental assistants prior to assignment throughout the theater, but others remained for more intensive courses at Saint Aignan to become "laboratory assistants-dental mechanics." Those who performed the most competently among these graduates were sent to a more advanced class at Neuilly, Army Reserve Corps Hospital No. 1. There they took 6 weeks of instruction in the manufacture of splints and dental prosthetics before being assigned to major hospitals where advanced maxillofacial surgery took place. One other school for enlisted soldiers was established after the armistice at Bordeaux, where training was given in oral hygiene and prophylaxis. Nearly 400 students graduated before the school closed in May 1919.[6]

Female Dentists Overseas

Some female dentists managed to see overseas service with the Red Cross base hospitals in England and France. On May 13, 1918, Dr Sophie Nevin of Brooklyn, New York, assigned to a refugee hospital under construction at Labouheyre, France, offered her services as a dentist to Brigadier General William S Scott, the commander of Base Section No. 2, Bordeaux, Gironde. It seems that while Nevin was waiting for her hospital to open, she began performing some dental treatment on the 4th Battalion, 20th Engineer Regiment, stationed at Mimizan, Les Bains, Landes. The engineer unit had no dental surgeon or any immediate prospect of having one assigned to it. Unfortunately, the available field dental equipment had also been removed. Dr Nevin felt that with the proper equipment, she could perform a valuable service while she waited for her duties to begin at the refugee hospital. The next day, May 14, General Scott sent a memorandum to the base surgeon outlining Nevin's proposal and recommending that it be accepted. On May 17, Colonel Henry A Shaw, the base surgeon, replied that the available Army dental surgeons in the area were "adequate" to furnish all necessary dental care for the 20th Engineers and he recommended that Dr Nevin's offer be declined. In notifying Dr Nevin of this decision on May 18, General Scott stated that he regretted that he could not make her "Commander-in-Chief and boss of all the dental work" for the district.[89–92]

In July 1918 Spanish-American War nurse, Dr Katherine Alice Doherty, who was practicing dentistry in Milwaukee, Wisconsin, went overseas to work at the American Women's Hospital No. 1 at Neufmoutiers, France. The hospital treated refugee children and young adults. Later, the hospital was moved to Luzancy. Dr Doherty was assigned to Boullay Thierry to treat a group of 86 refugee children

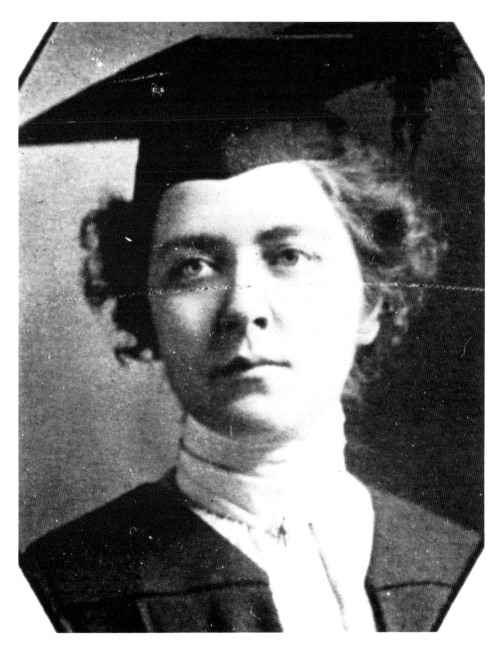

Katherine (Kate) Alice Doherty, graduate of Northwestern University Dental School (1901), went overseas to work at the American Women's Hospital No. 1 at Neufmoutiers, France. Photograph: Courtesy of Northwestern University Dental School Library, Chicago, Illinois.

and then to Viele Maisons to perform emergency work for the passing soldiers. She treated 472 patients alone. In February 1919 she was joined by Dr Kinney and Dr Edna Ward of Colorado. In 1 month at Luzancy, the three dentists treated 288 patients. Dr Doherty later received the Reconnaissance Francaise Citation from the French government for her 20 months of service.[93] Another dentist, Dr Marie J Hyman, also served with the women's hospital group.[94]

Female dentists in the United States also cooperated with the Preparedness League of American Dentists to treat the large number of draftees. In addition, dental hygienists also helped to clean up the recruits' mouths.[94]

Some female dental assistants applied to the Army in 1917. On May 2, 1917, Maude M Kerr of Ada, Ohio, asked the surgeon general if there was "a place for Dentists' assistants" in the Army. On May 19, 1917, Frances Weiland of Chicago, Illinois, wanted to know if there was such a position as "Female Dental assistant" in the war zone.[95] On June 16, 1917, Antonette Faytinger of David City, Nebraska, requested an application blank as a dental nurse or assistant in the Dental Corps. All three women were given the same reply: "women" were not eligible for appointment.[96]

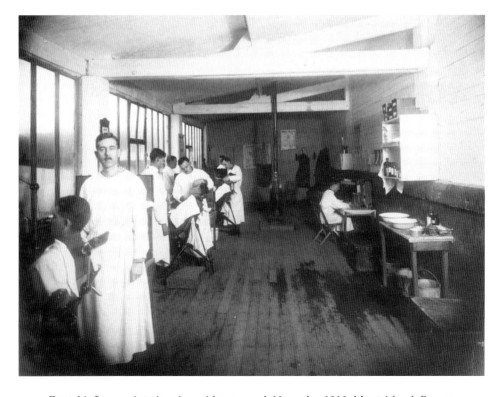

Dental infirmary, interior view with personnel, November 1918. Montrichard, France. Photograph: Courtesy of the National Museum of Health and Medicine, Armed Forces Institute of Pathology. Reeve 015397.

EXHIBIT 13-9

DR HELEN E MYERS

The first woman to be commissioned in the US Army Dental Corps under the Army Female Medical Department Act of 1949 (HR 4384) was Dr Helen E Myers of Philadelphia and Lancaster, Pennsylvania, who had received her DDS degree from Temple University in 1941. She was ordered to active duty on March 21, 1951, as a captain and assigned to Fort Lee, Virginia.

Data sources: (1) National Archives and Records Administration. Record Group 407. Precedent & History File 858. Press release, "First woman dentist in Army to report for duty March 21," 15 March 1951 [no. 354-51]. No. 44. (2) GI molars get feminine touch. *Ark Dent J*. 1953;24:50–52. (3) Cimring H. Something different in uniforms. *J Am Dent Assoc*. 1961;63:96–97. (4) Hyson JM, Jr. Female dentists in the U.S. Army: the origins. *Mil Med*. 1995;160:60–61.

On March 4, 1918, Major General Peyton C March, the acting chief of staff, said that "women physicians could not be commissioned" in the Medical Reserve Corps, and that it would take an "Act of Congress" for that to change. However, female physicians who wished to serve could apply to the Medical Department as laboratory technicians, anesthetists, and nursing instructors. Furthermore, he emphasized:

> Women physicians have not the physical qualifications which would be required for the performance of any duty which may be required of a medical officer. There are limitations both on the places in which their services may be utilized and the kind of services which they may perform. Therefore male physicians who are available for any and every duty that may fall to the part of a medical officer in any place whatsoever, are under the terms of the law commissioned as officers in the Medical Reserve Corps and female physicians being limited to special duties and to serving in special places are employed by contract.[97]

The same guidelines were invoked for female dentists applying to the Dental Corps, and the war ended without any appointments. No legislation for the commissioning of women was enacted until 1950, when the exigencies of the Korean War dictated a change in Army policy (Exhibit 13-9).[98–101]

Dental Supplies and Equipment

When the AEF first arrived in France, an obvious shortage of dental supplies and equipment existed in part because the US Army was competing with the Red Cross, which had established itself in Europe shortly after war began in 1914. In July 1917, for example, Dr Herbert L Wheeler of New York notified the Medical Department that 12 dental chairs, 12 fountain cuspidors, a supply of instruments for 4 or 5 chairs, and about $10,000 was to be made available in Paris for the AEF. However, all the property was diverted to the American Red Cross.[102]

The first dental surgeons sent to France had their portable dental outfits issued to them before they left the United States, and many were able to begin work as soon as they arrived at their stations. However, for reasons of limited shipping space, this policy was discontinued and the dental surgeons arriving later brought no dental equipment with them. For instance, the dental surgeons assigned to the 2nd and 26th Divisions were without equipment and none was available in the medical supply depot, where planners presumed it would be. Because most of the dental supplies in France were already depleted, the Army had to rely on the British for equipment. Unfortunately, the British had little stock and did not anticipate another delivery for 8 to 12 weeks. Consequently, the AEF chief surgeon's office at first decided to wait for supplies from the United States.[103–105]

Later, in March 1918, the medical purchasing officer, Major Daniel P Card, reported that a second large requisition for dental supplies and equipment submitted to the French Mission was again refused because of the scarcity of dental material in France. Likewise, the British War Office refused requisitions and recommended that the supplies be brought from the United States. In some instances, dental equipment was lost and accidentally found later, as Oliver noted on August 8, 1918: "50 odd boxes of freight, (chests and boxes), containing dental supplies, was found yesterday in the store-houses at Gievres where they have been for an indefinite period of time." Ten packages of dental supplies were found at Base Port No. 5 and several at Base No. 1 and No. 2. Oliver recommended that "steps be taken to unearth all dental supplies that may possibly be stored at the several depots of the medical supply department for the purpose of immediate shipment to Intermediate Medical Supply Depot No. 3."[108]

In August 1917 Lieutenant Colonel Clement C Whitcomb, MC, commanding the AEF Medical Supply Depot in France, reported in response to an August 16 requisition from the 5th Regiment, US Marines, that no dental supplies were in stock. A few days later he requested that a cable be sent to the surgeon general in Washington stating the urgent need for "twenty-five portable dental outfits" for stock at his depot. As a temporary measure, an emergency requisition was authorized for the eventual purchase of dental equipment, including instruments and supplies for 25 dental outfits in Paris. The AEF Medical Supply Division hoped to accumulate surplus stock from all possible sources prior to the arrival of large numbers of US units. On August 22, 1917, the medical depot in New York City shipped the first 20 portable outfits to the depot in France and continued to ship outfits throughout the war, shipping 391 complete outfits in the period June 1 to August 31, 1918, alone.[107–110]

Another significant problem the Dental Corps in France soon encountered was the fact that its supplies and equipment were being ordered by medical, not dental, officers. For example, Lieutenant Colonel Whitcomb questioned whether two base dental outfits for each of the 60 hospitals were necessary. In September 1917 he commented on a dental requisition: "If one base outfit, in addition to one portable outfit for each Dental Surgeon on duty there, is deemed sufficient for each hospital (and in my opinion that equipment is ample), it is requested that this requisition be returned."[111]

In other instances, the portable dental outfits assigned to travel with the dental surgeons to France were misplaced en route and when the dentists got to France, there were no tools available for them. In August 1917 First Lieutenant Reginald S Murdock, DRC, experienced this problem when he arrived at Camp Saint Martin, Boulonge, France.[21] Murdock, a 1915 graduate of Washington University, Dental School, was assigned to the infirmary, 12th Engineers (Railway) and assisted the only British dental officer servicing the sector of 75,000 troops. The regimental surgeon commented on the British dentist:

> His equipment is so scanty that amalgam fillings can be used only in the more favor-able cases, the greater part of his work consisting of extractions and cement fillings. Murdock is assisting him and doing what work he can for our troops, but is of com-paratively small value without equipment, and the British are not prepared to furnish it.[112,113]

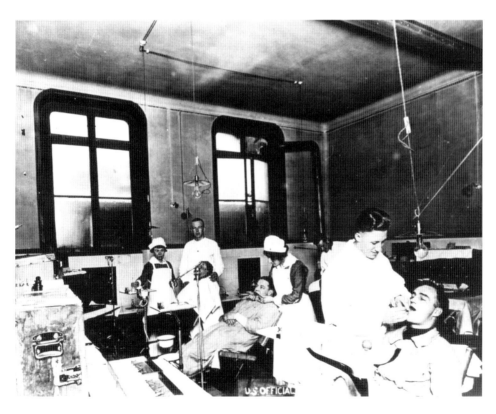

Dental infirmary at US Army Base Hospital No. 57, Paris, Seine, France, January 30, 1919. Left to right: First Lieutenant CH Nash; Ruth Dennis, assistant; Captain WW Cursler; Ruth Ivy, as-sistant; Private GW Charlton; and Private LW Stewart.
Photograph: Courtesy of US Army Military History Institute. SC 52129.

Another dental surgeon, First Lieutenant Agustin L Magruder, DRC a 1916 graduate of Tulane University of Louisiana, College of Medicine, School of Dentistry (New Orleans College of Dentistry), had the same problem upon his assignment to the 17th Engineers (Railway) at Camp No. 1, Section No. 1.[21] His equipment was aboard the ill-fated *Saratoga*, sunk in New York Harbor with its wartime cargo. Nothing could be done to resupply Magruder until "other material arrives from the United States." A requisition for his new equipment would be "filled as soon as practical."[114,115]

Even after the armistice, there was still a shortage of dental equipment at some AEF hospitals. On November 30, 1918, the surgeon at Camp Hospital No. 33 complained that many cases of "face wounds and fractured jaws" from the front arrived and the hospital still had only dental field equipment; therefore, it was "impossible to treat these men as they should be." In addition, they had no oral surgeon on duty with the "special training" required for that type of work. Certain dental equipment items were deemed essential to the maxillofacial service, like anatomical articulators, investment flasks, maxilar metal for cast splints, and maxilar flux powder.[116,117]

The shortage of divisional dental laboratory outfits was also a problem as late as June 1918. On June 27, 1918, Lieutenant Colonel James R Mount, MC, Medical Supply Depot No. 3, sent a memorandum to the chief surgeon, AEF, saying that the divisional dental equipment contained only "one laboratory outfit." He recommended that 50 complete outfits be requisitioned from the United States and that "provision be made to have this item made a part of the initial equipment of troops leaving the United States." In October 1918 First Lieutenant Stephen F French, DC, Base Hospital No. 43, reported that on October 12 he had used the last of his alloy and on October 15 the last of his oxyphosphate cement, and that he was "unable to obtain any more."[118,119]

In December 1918 Major Howard I Benedict, attending dental surgeon, advance section, complained to Colonel Oliver that he had reported for duty and found "no dental equipment of any nature" on hand. When he visited the newly arrived Evacuation Hospitals No. 3 and No. 12, and Field Hospital No. 301 and No. 303, he found they had no dental outfits. The 6th Infantry dental surgeons had "only a few instruments for emergency work." For his efforts, "one complete portable dental outfit" was shipped to him from the medical supply depot at Cosne. As late as January 1919 the 815th Pioneer Infantry at Glorieux, Meuse and the 816th Pioneer Infantry at Verdun, Meuse "badly needed" dental outfits.[120–122]

Throughout the war, dental surgeons continued complaining about the lack of dental outfits available. In February 1918 First Lieutenant William C Webb, Jr, at the II Corps school reported that he had "no personal equipment on hand" and had to share a colleague's for a week. On August 5, 1918, Major Raymond W Pearson, the 33rd Division dental surgeon, sent a memo to his division surgeon that three of the 129th Infantry Regiment's dental outfits were still stored at Le Havre and attempts to get them had been unsuccessful. Other dental outfits for the three infantry and two field artillery regiments of the division were still probably at Brest. The 33rd Division had no surplus outfits on hand to send to these units. In September 1918 Captain Walter L Wilson, DC, of the 5th Corps Replacement Battalion, reported that he had neither a portable dental outfit nor supplies.

One dental surgeon with the 2nd Corps Replacement Battalion at Pont De Metz, France, reported that he had been working without a contra angle handpiece from October 18 to the end of November 1918.[123–126]

Confronted by these shortfalls, Oliver's office did its best to find solutions. An automatic requisition system was put into effect in the summer of 1917 for every 25,000 troops reaching France, and dental supply officers were assigned to all depots handling medical material. Shortages still occurred because of accidents, congestion, and improper handling at the ports. Dental supply officers were assigned to places on the dates indicated: Cosne Depot, September 1, 1917; Advance Medical Supply Depot, Is-sur-Tille, March 1, 1918; Medical Supply Depot No. 1, February 1918; and Base Port, Base Section No. 1, Saint Nazaire.[5,6] Most of the maxillofacial material was misplaced on the Marseille docks and not recovered until 1919. Railroad personnel had to be educated to give dental equipment adequate shipping priorities.

Even with the best planning, the vagaries of war often intruded. When purchasing officers turned to European sources, they encountered the availability problems. When they finally shipped the dental laboratory equipment that had accumulated in England, the ship carrying it was torpedoed in the English Channel. Much more dental equipment was lost when a freighter from the United States was sunk off the Irish coast. A particular problem arose while attempting to procure the special equipment necessary "for maxillofacial surgery and for the prosthetic and reconstruction procedures required in the practice of that specialty." The dental section report told the story:

> Adequate consideration and study had been given this subject prior to the departure from the United States of specialists in this line, and provision had been made whereby special chests containing maxillofacial unit equipment would be shipped immediately on their departure. These plans failed and the much needed special equipment for this service was not received until after the signing of the armistice. It was found subsequently in the midst of a quantity of supplies at the port of Marseille.[6(p117)]

American medical supply specialists turned to French and British manufacturers to obtain much of the missing equipment, but not all of the requisitions could be met due to their own demands for these materials. Though this equipment was not available on many occasions when it was needed by the dental officers at evacuation hospitals, mobile hospitals, and a few base hospitals, the deficiency was well met by individual ingenuity and by improvisation.[6]

Problems with the Transportation of Dental Equipment and Supplies: The Origins of American Expeditionary Forces General Order No. 99

An enormous problem that developed at the division level was that the tables of organization did not include dentists or their assistants and equipment and were not modified during the war to include them. This meant that no trucks or road transportation were specifically dedicated to move the 6 tons of professional equipment that the division's dentists and their assistants needed to carry. In fact, they had to beg rides just for themselves. Thus, when urgent movements became more commonplace starting in the spring of 1918, huge amounts of dental equipment had to be abandoned or turned over for salvage. When the divisions reached their new locations, the dental surgeons flooded the medical supply depots with emergency requisitions for whole new dental sets.[5,6]

The postwar official history of the AEF's dental section, most likely written by Oliver, recounted this problem and its consequences:

> In combat divisions, the transportation of dental equipment and supplies was always a problem and when not carried individually, a source of irritation to division commanders, transportation officers, and division surgeons. This was largely due to the fact that no provision had ever been made in the Tables of Organization for dental personnel, commissioned and enlisted, or for dental equipment. Omission in these Tables of the Dental Corps and of provision for transport of its supplies resulted in the loss of much equipment and the consequent temporary lack of dental services in several divisions. The First Division on its movement into a combat area in May, 1918, found it expedient to abandon all its dental equipment on account of the lack of transportation, for the material had not been considered by its transportation officer in making his allowances for the rapid movement of equipment and supplies. This loss was immediately investigated and efforts were made for finding and salvaging the abandoned equipment. Though not found at the time it was subsequently redeemed through the salvage service. In the interim, through the efforts made at intermediate medical supply depot No. 3, the dental service of the division was reequipped with modified portable outfits.[6(pp116–117)]

While the issue was never fully resolved during the war, Oliver quickly realized what a serious problem it presented to effective dental care and took a number of steps to rectify the situation. The increased tempo of American operations in the late spring of 1918 brought the seriousness of the problem to a critical state in some front line divisions. On May 14, 1918, Colonel Walter D McCaw, acting in the absence of the chief surgeon, sent a memo (probably composed by Oliver) to the chief of staff, SOS, outlining the problem and laying out a recommended distribution of dental officers and equipment in a division. The basic problem remained the lack of dentists in the division table of organization:

> The Tables of Organization, Series "A", January 14, 1918, fail to mention the authorized personnel, commissioned and enlisted, of the Dental Corps. This omission has occasioned considerable difficulty in the adjustment of Medical Department personnel (both commissioned and enlisted) and recently in Divisions preparing to move into combat areas, has been the cause of much confusion with the problems of transportation and shipment of equipment. It seems the question of transportation has been estimated largely on citations made in the Table of Organization. There being no representation therein for dental officers, their enlisted assistants or their equipment, this excess of transportation facilities has been lacking.[127]

While Oliver did not achieve the inclusion of the Dental Corps in revised wartime tables of organization, he at least partially rectified this crippling oversight with AEF General Order No. 99 on June 19, 1918, which "for the first time" accounted for the dentists within the division (see Chapter 12, "Organizing the Dental Corps for the War in Europe").[6]

The problems of the division table of organization and transportation of dental equipment and supplies only further exacerbated the basic shortcomings of the portable dental outfit that the dental surgeons took to France. Originally created by John S Marshall and Robert Oliver in 1901 for use in the Philippines, this portable outfit was simply too heavy and bulky. Once American divisions entered the line and active ground combat operations in the late spring and summer of 1918, the existing portable dental outfits were quickly revealed as impractical "for active field service." Oliver's office determined that the complete portable outfits would be kept for use at camp hospitals and detached units of the SOS, which could more easily transport them. For the dentists in the combat divisions, a modified portable outfit was developed that could be packed into three chests or footlockers containing all of the essential equipment, including a dental engine, medicines, and supplies required for practicing dentistry under field conditions. On June 19, 1918, AEF GHQ published General Order No. 99, which allocated 10 complete and 20 modified portable dental outfits and directed their disposition within each division.[6]

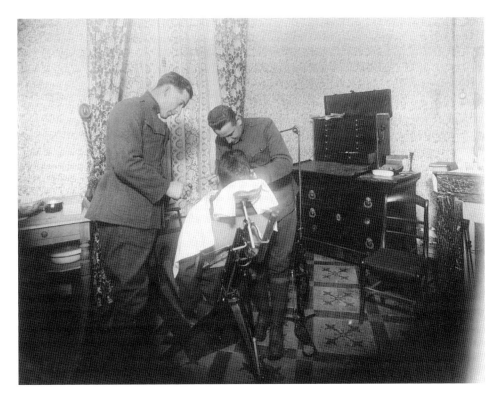

Dental infirmary, interior view with personnel, 1918. Meusnes, France.
Photograph: Courtesy of the National Museum of Health and Medicine,
Armed Forces Institute of Pathology. Reeve 015404.

Dental Emergency Kits

On May 11, 1918, in a memorandum to division dental surgeons from the office of the chief surgeon, AEF, Oliver developed other solutions to the problem of moving dentists and their equipment around front line tactical units and combat areas. Experience at the front had shown that even the newly slimmed-down dental outfits were not all that portable along the front lines, so they were consigned to the divisional rear areas and the field hospitals in the sanitary train. For divisions in front line battle areas, an even more stripped down outfit, called the "campaign equipment," was provided, which consisted of the dental engine chest and the dental emergency kit. Oliver designated the dental emergency kits as personal dental equipment and directed dental surgeons to carry two emergency kits with standardized contents with them at all times when accompanying their commands into combat areas. Two of the old style Hospital Corps pouches were adapted for carrying light canvas or khaki cloth instrument rolls. In the absence of this type of instrument roll, a tightly rolled hand towel secured with a rubber band was recommended. The dentists carried the 9 pound Pouch No. 1, which contained a small blank book with indelible pencil (for dental records) and three rolls. Roll number one had the extraction forceps and oral surgery instruments; number two carried the operating instruments; and number three contained the medicines and a small amount of supplies. The enlisted dental assistant carried Pouch No. 2, which weighed 8 pounds. This pouch contained roll number four, which included amalgam, cements, a glass slab, cotton rolls, ligature wire, towels, soap, and other miscellaneous supplies. Later, a 4 ½ pound folding aluminum trench chair was added and carried in a container slung over the dental assistant's shoulder.[128,129]

These kits were intended to be used strictly for emergency treatments for roughly a 2-week period. Oliver cautioned the dental surgeons: "It is not considered necessary to attempt more than emergency treatment for the relief of pain in the majority of cases however, should time and condition permit, plastic fillings (alloy or cement) may be accomplished in those cavities that permit of excavation by hand instruments." Individual preference could determine the exact content of the temporary kits, as would available stocks of supplies. Oliver instructed the dental surgeons to make arrangements with their regimental surgeons for evacuating dental cases that required more than emergency treatment. These cases were to be sent to the dental service at division field hospitals where modified portable dental outfits were installed. While the emergency kits helped solve the transportation problem, dentists and their assistants were left to shoulder the extra load.[128,129]

As a result of developing and pushing forward the dental emergency kits, the divisional dental service was significantly enhanced:

> Thus officers were enabled to render first-aid dentistry at all times for the relief of pain and for minor oral surgical and dental operations. This modification of dental equipment helped solve many of the transportation problems for the dental service in combat divisions, and while it increased the weight carried by dental officers, it proved advantageous by making it possible for anyone requiring dental service to obtain it at any time from the dental officer of his command.[6(p116)]

The whole issue of dental equipment and supply was referred to a dental equipment board in July 1918. Working within the larger medical equipment board, the dental board was expected to re-evaluate the equipment considered essential for dental officers in tactical units and hospitals in direct support of combat. It concluded substantial revisions were needed based on actual experiences and was in the process of modifying at the time of the armistice. In March 1919 Lieutenant Commander Cornelius H Mack, DC, US Navy, then the 2nd Division's dental surgeon, stated that the outfit "panned out so badly on account of transportation." He believed that a "more compact and less weighty" portable outfit would be an improvement over the current design. Oliver informed him that the dental equipment board was considering modifying the field outfit based on wartime experience. The board's findings carried over into postwar changes in field dental equipment and supplies.[5,130–132]

Captain Haymes's Wooden Chair Design

The persistent shortages in dental equipment and supplies inspired a great deal of inventiveness on the part of the hard-pressed dentists. Because of the shortage of dental chairs, in 1918 Captain John E Haymes, division dental surgeon, 36th Division, AEF, designed an improvised portable wooden dental chair for field use. The dental officers in the division used his chair "in the absence of the authorized chair." Oliver liked the idea because the chair could be constructed from materials readily found in the quartermaster department and in the locality of field operations. He promised to submit the description and diagram to the dental equipment board and give Captain Haymes "full credit for priority and invention of this chair in case it proves of practical value." From the diagram, it appears that Haymes's design served as the prototype for the all-metal World War II portable dental chair. The chair required about 12 feet of 1-by-10 or -12 lumber, a few yards of rope, and 5 hinges with screws. The hinges were placed so that when the chair was closed it would lie flat on the back board. A detachable headrest could be devised to be removed in transit.[133,135]

The "Amex War Denture"

In the early spring of 1917 a man with the standard removable vulcanite denture was barred from voluntary enlistment in the US Army on the basis that the dentures were a liability and subject to break. Consequently, the Army began experimenting with aluminum as a substitute denture base. Actually, aluminum had originally been introduced into the dental profession by Dr James Baxter Bean, the former Confederate dental surgeon who had organized the world's first military maxillofacial hospital ward in Atlanta during the American Civil War. In November 1866 Dr Bean exhibited his cast aluminum plate at the second meeting of the Maryland Association of Dentists in Baltimore. It was recorded in the minutes that this was the "first successful effort known to the association in casting aluminum as a base for teeth."[135–138]

In June 1917 First Lieutenant Edward H Raymond, Jr, DC, in conjunction with

First Lieutenant John B Wagoner, DRC, did the initial wartime work on casting aluminum dentures at the Base Hospital No. 2 (Presbyterian Hospital Unit), British Expeditionary Forces, in France. On August 8, 1918, Colonel Boak asked Lieutenant Wagoner to deliver a lecture and demonstration on the new all-aluminum plates to Army Sanitary School students. The Army called the new cast aluminum denture the "Amex Denture," and officially adopted it as the "war denture" for the AEF in France. Captain Raymond and Major Wagoner were given the credit for its development as a vulcanite substitute.[139,140]

In introducing the new denture, the Army cited the unusual wartime conditions as the reason for developing "a standard type denture sufficiently strong to withstand the hardships of masticating field rations, to resist fracture from all ordinary accidents and to prevent malicious distortion or mutilation." Because of the cramped space and poor lighting in tents, huts, and dugouts at the front, dentures that were removed for the night were broken far more often in military than in civilian life. Intentionally breaking one's dentures to get away from the front, like the self-inflicted wound, was probably rare, but the metal denture made it even less common.[135,141]

The Amex Denture was inexpensive, easily made of materials locally procurable, durable, light in weight, had good thermal conductivity, and was easy to clean; all of which commended its use. The denture consisted of a metal plate with metal teeth all cast together in one piece. The posterior teeth were always cast as part of the denture, but porcelain teeth could be used for the six anteriors, if time could be spared for vulcanizing. The objectionable appearance of full upper dentures with all-metal teeth had to be disregarded on the basis that war service efficiency outweighed aesthetic considerations. Clasps for partial dentures could be incorporated into the casting.[135]

The Amex casting flask was developed from a model made of a section of a "Soixante Quinze" (French 75-mm artillery) shell. The materials required for the denture were aluminum ingots, pink baseplate wax, casting wax for tooth forms, investment compound of pulverized silox and Plaster of Paris, and DuTrey's Anterior Diateric teeth. Old newspaper soaked to a pulp was used as a substitute for fiber asbestos in the lid of the casting flask. The average all-metal denture weighed 22 grams and cost about 6 or 7 cents for the metal. On November 7, 1918, all the AEF dental laboratories were ordered to begin fabricating the war denture. Apparently, the armistice of November 11, 1918, halted the mass production of these new "war dentures" so examples are very rare. In fact, the extensive denture collection of the National Museum of Dentistry in Baltimore, Maryland, does not include a single specimen. In the 1920s the aluminum base was highly touted by Dr Dayton Dunbar Campbell, special lecturer in dental prosthetics at the Kansas City Western Dental College and founder and president of the Campbell School of Prosthetic Technic.[135,142,143]

Invention of Carpule Syringe

Local anesthesia was introduced in 1905 with the synthesis of novocaine hydrochloride by Alfred Einhorn (1856–1917) of Germany. The drug was supplied in powder form, so dentists had to mix up a new solution each time they needed it.

This process was time consuming and awkward on the battlefield. Unfortunately, stock solutions deteriorated rapidly. Harvey S Cook, an Army surgeon from Valparaiso, Indiana, solved this problem by inventing the carpule. He was inspired by the cartridges used in Army rifles and made the first carpule syringe himself. He fabricated a brass syringe, which locked a double-pointed needle in place, cut the glass tubes, and used pencil erasers as rubber stoppers. He spent his evenings sterilizing the solutions and filling the carpules for the next day's work. His invention revolutionized the delivery system for all types of medication, particularly local anesthesia in dentistry.[144,145]

Prosthetic Treatment Policy

In general the provisions of Paragraph 1401, Army Regulations, provided for kind of treatment accorded the enlisted men in the AEF. Loss of teeth occurring "in line of duty" was to be replaced by "suitably constructed dentures (vulcanite)." Special treatment with "extra materials," which the dental officer provided, was authorized only in "exceptional cases" in the "best interests of the service." Crown and bridgework and gold for cast inlays was recommended for officers only. The dental surgeons were to keep this "special material" on hand and be reimbursed for the "cost of materials actually used," plus a small percentage to cover waste (Table 13-2).[146,147]

At least one medical officer, Colonel John W Hanner, commanding officer of Base Hospital No. 116, thought this process was unfair to the dental surgeons. In June 1918 he sent a memo to the chief surgeon, AEF, in which he stated,

> If the Government feels that it is for the best interests of the service that such work should be done, necessitating these extra materials, it seems just to me that the government should furnish the stock of materials that would be required for this work, and the dental surgeon should not be required to purchase them personally.[148]

Vulcanite or aluminum dentures were the only type of prosthetic service offered to the enlisted soldiers, gold was not authorized. If clasps were used, they had to be made of German silver or the French metal, Melchoir.[149] The prosthetic work was to be completed by the dental officer in charge of the division's portable dental laboratory. In combat areas, its usual location was at one of the field hospitals farthest removed from the front lines. In training areas, it was located at the headquarters dental office.[150]

French Centres de Prosthèse Dentaire

There was significant cooperation between the American and French Dental Corps throughout the war. In the absence of US Army dental surgeons, American soldiers billeted near French centres de prosthèse dentaire (centers of dental prosthetics) often received routine dental and prosthetic appliances from the French. The fee charged was 5 francs per tooth for appliances made of vulcanite with German silver clasps. Oliver believed this was fair and equitable, but recommended that American patients be transferred to American hospitals as soon as possible

TABLE 13-2

ALLOWABLE FEES FOR NONGOVERNMENT METALS

Metal	Price
Gold, simple	$2.00
Gold, compound	$2.50–$3.50
Gold inlays, simple	$3.00–$3.50
Gold inlays, compound	$4.00–$5.00
Gold shell crowns, bicuspids, swaged cusps	$5.00
Gold shell cast cusps	$6.00
Molars, swaged cusps	$6.00–$7.00
Cast cusps	$7.00–$8.00
Gold porcelain crowns (richmond, goslee, steele, or ash facings, and bridge dummies)	$5.00
Porcelain crowns, with cast gold base	$3.00
Bridges	charges based on components plus a charge for consolidation, not to exceed $1.00 for each interproximal space soldered

Data sources: (1) National Archives and Records Administration. Record Group 120. Special instructions governing the character of dental treatment accorded in the American Expeditionary Forces, chief surgeon, American Expeditionary Forces. Memo. No. 703. Folder 18. Box 5149. Entry 2065. (2) National Archives and Records Administration. Record Group 120. Circular no. 4, office of the chief surgeon, headquarters, American Expeditionary Forces, 22 December 1917. Box 5464. Entry 2072.

(without risk to the patient), and that only emergency dental treatment be given, except for unusual cases that could be retained for long periods. The American hospitals were treating the French soldiers in the same manner.[151–153]

On the Line of Communications: Base Section No. 1, American Expeditionary Forces

Dental operations at the base sections were different than in units and hospitals. The best example of its type is the office of the surgeon at Base Section No. 1, AEF, established at Saint Nazaire, France, on July 2, 1917, after the arrival of the first convoy of American troops. The office of supervising dental surgeon was established on April 18, 1918, when Colonel George H Casaday, one of the original contract dental surgeons, reported. His duties were to inspect all stations within the base section where troops were located to determine "whether defects exist in the treatment and management of dental work"; to determine the "sufficiency and quality of dental personnel and dental equipment"; to make reports to the base surgeon's office with suggestions as to "corrective measures necessary in case of personnel and equipment"; and to "tabulate reports of all work performed by Dental Officers in the Base Section and to make periodical consolidated reports of same to the Chief Surgeon, American E.F."[154]

In addition, Casaday was responsible at that time for the supervision of the dental activities for Base Section No. 2, No. 5, and No. 7, which required him to make occasional inspection trips. The scope of the dental work was limited because the organizations going through the ports remained only a short time and each had its own dental surgeons who accompanied it to its training area, where it prepared to enter the line. The number of dental surgeons remaining permanently in the base sections was limited because of the overall shortage of dental officers; consequently, the dental service for the section's assigned personnel was also limited.[154]

On December 17, 1918, Lieutenant Colonel Frank P Stone reported for duty as supervising dental surgeon. He immediately began enlarging the scope of the

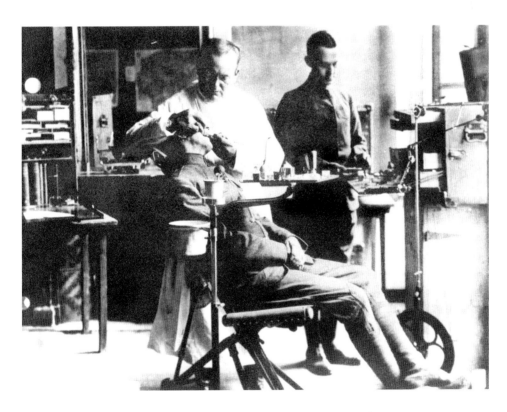

*Captain EE Courtwright, dental surgeon, IV Corps Headquarters,
in dental laboratory operating on patient. Toul, France, August 22, 1918.
Photograph: Courtesy of US Army Military History Institute. SC 22970.*

dental service and personnel to meet the increased demand caused by the influx of troops awaiting transportation back to the United States. Infirmaries were opened at Camps No. 4 and No. 5, at Camp Montoir, and an additional infirmary was built at Camp No. 1. The billeting areas around Nantes and Angers were supplied with additional dental surgeons and a local dental supervisor was placed in charge of each district. The character of the dental service began to change to meet the needs of the section. Dental officers were on duty at the reception camp and a dental inspection of each soldier preparing for embarkation was a part of the general physical examination. The soldiers were listed in order of the urgency of their dental needs and were sent to the dental clinic according to that list. The main embarkation camp at Camp No. 1 had the best-organized and most well-equipped dental infirmary in France.[154]

One unit of dental support overlooked until close to the war's end was the smaller logistical unit that was not authorized to have its own dentists. For example, in August 1918, the intermediate section of the SOS had about 85,000 troops, ex-

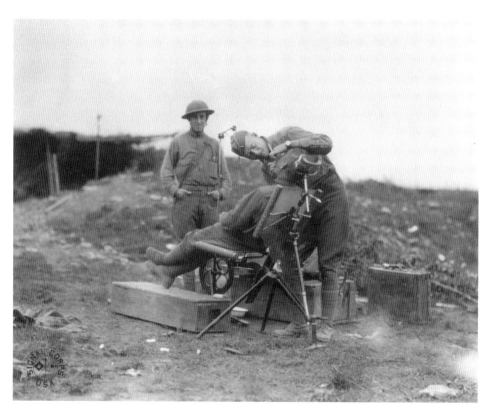

First Lieutenant RM McNulty, dental surgeon, 309th Field Artillery Regiment, 78th Division, with assistant Private JJ Cleveland, operates on a patient just back from the lines, Fey-en-Haye, Meurthe et Moselle, France. September 22, 1918. Photograph: Courtesy of US Army Military History Institute. SC 33390

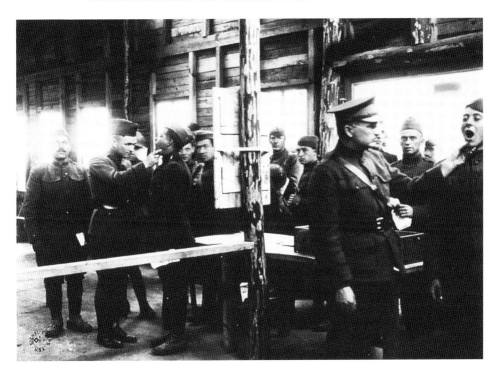

*Dental surgeons completing a dental examination of personnel of
the 83rd Division at Le Mans, France. October 6, 1918.
Photograph: Courtesy of US Army Military History Institute. SC 26030.*

cluding the depot division or replacement battalion troops, and only 40 dental surgeons were not employed with base hospital dental staffs. The units generated many requests for dental treatment and the dental situation had become "acute" in the opinion of the section surgeon. Furthermore, the few dental surgeons available were constantly being taken away and assigned to the Army Sanitary School for instruction and training.[155] On August 22, Oliver agreed to assign two dental surgeons and more "as they become available."[156] As a result of the continuing shortage of Dental Corps officers in the AEF, this was one of many times Oliver had to juggle his scant resources to provide dental care.

A Continuing Shortage of Dental Surgeons

Shortages of dental officers persisted at every echelon throughout the war, despite every effort to spread the talent or obtain more personnel. Because of the limitations imposed by AEF policies, the Dental Corps in the AEF never even reached its statutory ratio of one dentist per thousand enlisted personnel. By the time of the armistice in November 1918, there was a shortage of over 300 dental surgeons. The fundamental problem was that organizations under a thousand troops and

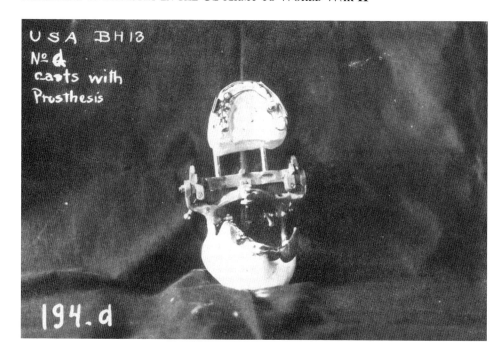

Base Hospital No. 13. Cast on articulator with dental/facial prosthesis.
Open view. Limoges, France.
Photograph: Courtesy of the National Museum of Health and Medicine,
Armed Forces Institute of Pathology. Reeve 012037A.

casuals arriving in France were not accounted for in the basic allocation of dental surgeons in accordance with the ratio. Soon a shortage occurred for the AEF as a whole, and this was especially true for units, such as engineer and service units, that expanded significantly after their arrival in France.[6]

On August 14, 1918, a frustrated Colonel James L Bevans, chief surgeon at III Corps headquarters, complained that his July 9 letter and July 25, 1918, telegram to the adjutant general, GHQ, for a dental surgeon had gone unanswered. He stated that an increasing number of both officers and enlisted personnel required dental treatment and that the assignment of a dental surgeon with his enlisted assistant and portable dental outfit was "urgently needed." Major General Robert L Bullard, his commander, recommended approval and Captain William Z Carroll, DRC, a 1911 graduate of the Northwestern University Dental School, was assigned as attending dental surgeon.[21,157–159]

In September 1918 Carroll reported that he was "continually instructing the men who come under my care in the importance of Oral Hygiene." He also complained, "Equipment with which I am working incomplete. Portable dental field equipment which arrived with me at Brest, France, August 7, 1918 has not been received to date." Finally, in October 1918 Carroll received his dental outfit that had been traveling from the New York medical dupply depot since about July 25, 1918.[160,161]

By then Carroll had sufficient experience with his unit to issue a memorandum on oral hygiene to the corps headquarters commandant:

1. Attention is called to the lack of care given their teeth by the men of this Command and of other organizations coming under my care.

2. It is of great importance under present conditions in the field that the teeth be thoroughly brushed, if possible, after each meal and, in so doing, prevent those diseases of the teeth and gums that are caused directly by food particles left undisturbed from day to day in the many crevices between the teeth and gums.

3. If tooth powder or paste is not available, the use of common salt instead will suffice, if the tooth brush is used two or three times daily.

4. The danger of contagion is greatly lessened in the individual if the mouth is kept clean.[162]

On August 17, 1918, Lieutenant Colonel EP Walser, the commanding officer of the I Corps Artillery Park, complained to the chief surgeon of the III Corps over the lack of dental care for his troops:

At full strength this organization has 1335 officers and men. At present we have over 1200 and we have no dentist either attached or permanently assigned to this organization. The condition of the teeth of many of the men is very bad as they have had no dental attention of any kind since leaving the United States and I urgently request that a dentist be at least temporarily assigned to this organization.[163]

The chief surgeon recommended that the request for a dental officer be approved. The corps commander concurred.[164]

Even the dental officers complained about the absence of dental care for the troops. On October 3, 1918, Captain Louis A Haffner, dental surgeon with the 4th Corps Replacement Battalion, sent a memo to his commanding officer. It read:

1. The need of dental treatment in an organization of this kind is greater than the average, for the personnel is ever transient, men arrive daily, after having been enroute several days, the hygienic condition of the mouth is demoralized on account of the lack of cleanliness. A lot of men are evacuated from hospitals and other organizations with temporary fillings in their teeth. Fully fifty per cent of my time is taken up with such work.

2. My records show that I treated forty patients during the first two days of October, which is without a doubt too many for one officer to handle and give the proper attention to each individual. There is ample need of another Dental Officer at this station for operating alone.[165]

The deficiencies in dental surgeons for the divisions of the Second Army from November 12 through December 3 indicate the problem for front line units (Table 13-3).[166]

TABLE 13-3

DENTAL SURGEON STAFFING IN SECOND ARMY DIVISIONS,
NOVEMBER 12–DECEMBER 3, 1918 (AUTHORIZED STRENGTH: 31)

Division	November 12, 1918	November 19, 1918	November 26, 1918	December 3, 1918
4th Division	18	18	Transferred	No report
7th Division	No report	18	18	18
28th Division	No report	21	21	22
33rd Division	No report	29	29	33
35th Division	No report	No report	22	26
85th Division	22	No report	17	16
88th Division	24	24	25	25
92nd Division	31	31	29	29

Data source: National Archives and Records Administration. Record Group 120. Colonel George H Casaday, chief dental surgeon, Second Army, 12, 19, and 26 November, and 3 December 1918, in File 319.1 "Dental Personnel." Reports. Box 3295. Entry 924.

Even as late as 1919, First Army headquarters was frequently reminded of the shortage of dental surgeons. On January 17, 1919, a plea came in from the captain of a military police battalion on detached service with the provost marshal, advance section, SOS:

> Request is made that a dental surgeon be assigned to this organization for a period of six weeks. This organization was on duty at the front, or on the move, from February 17, 1918 until September 20, 1918, and since the latter date has been on duty in the Army area. It has been possible to obtain dental treatment for only the serious cases, and as a result, the teeth of many of the men require attention.[167]

The request was approved by Major John G MacDonnell, provost marshal of the First Army, and a dental officer was ordered to report for temporary duty as soon as one was available.[168]

The continuing shortage of dental officers presented problems that were only resolved after the armistice, when Oliver adopted what was called "a general plan for equalization." He reduced the dental contingent of each division that was returning to the United States to a skeleton group capable of providing dental services on the voyage, retaining two thirds (approximately 20 or so for a fully staffed division) of the dental personnel in France. He then reassigned the retained personnel to provide dental care for those commands without any dental officers. Oliver's policy partly accounts for the slow drop in the overall numbers of Dental Corps officers in AEF from November 1918 (1,779) through April 1919 (1,537), when he discontinued this equalization plan because the number of American forces had so significantly declined that such levels of dental support were no longer necessary. By the end of May 1919, 1,113 dental surgeons remained in the AEF, but by mid-July that number was down to 312 and only 67 remained by mid September.[6,169,170]

The Medical College, Dental Section, American Expeditionary Forces University, Beaune

In November 1918, shortly after the armistice was signed, educational leaders in the United States and the AEF formulated plans whereby the soldiers could continue their educations if they had been interrupted by the war. In February 1919, after 2 months of planning, they made arrangements to establish the AEF University at Beaune, Cote D'Or, under the leadership of Colonel Ura L Reeves, with Dr John R Erskine of Columbia University as educational director.[171]

At first, all branches were taught except the medical sciences. Finally it was decided to establish a medical college with departments of medicine, dentistry, veterinary medicine, and pharmacy headed by Colonel Joseph H Ford, MC, and assisted by Colonel Louis Brechimin, Jr.[171] On February 28, 1919, the Medical Department issued a memorandum recommending that suitable officers of the Dental and Veterinary Corps be selected and assigned to duty as deans of the Schools of Dentistry and Veterinary Medicine, respectively. Lieutenant Colonel Otis H McDonald, DC, then attached to the V Corps as corps dental surgeon, was selected to command the dental section of the medical college.[171,172]

The chief difficulty with the school was putting together a competent faculty, scattered as qualified candidates were in France, England, Germany, Italy, and Luxembourg. However, McDonald, an "old-established practitioner," knew the ropes and came up with a competent faculty. It was composed of: Captain J Howard Gaskill (DDS, Pennsylvania College of Dental Surgery), instructor of dental pathology and fractures and splints; First Lieutenant Morris BS Fleischer (DDS, MS, University of Pennsylvania), instructor of bacteriology, pathology, and oral hygiene, adjutant; Captain Frampton W Farmer (DDS, Southern Dental College), instructor of operative dentistry; Captain Alva L Cowart (DDS, Atlanta Dental College), instructor in anesthesia and exodontia; First Lieutenant Raymond R Henry (DDS, University of Minnesota), instructor in operative technique; Captain Edward B Lodge (DDS, University of Michigan), and Captain H Morrow (DDS, University of Iowa), supervisors of dental education. The first lectures were given on March 13, 1919, to students gathered from all over the AEF.[171]

The dental section had an aggregation of 85 students, representing 54 different colleges and universities, and 12 had DDS degrees. Nine students had 3 years of dental school, and 18 had between 1 and 2 years of dental school.[170] The dental course was designed to prepare two types of students: those contemplating entering dental college, and dental undergraduates who were in need of review in order to qualify for admission to dental schools certified by the National Association of Dental Faculties. The course consisted of didactic lectures and laboratory instruction in anatomy, bacteriology, biology, chemistry, histology, metallurgy, microscopy, pathology, physiology, and clinical operative, oral surgery, and prosthetic dentistry. The dental course ran for 12 weeks and was taught by dental officers. The medical subjects were taught by the medical faculty in conjunction with the medical students. Captain Trueman J Slade, DC, was in charge of the clinical department.[173]

By March 6, 1919, a seven-chair dental clinic became operational. All AEF personnel, including civilians, were eligible for treatment according to Army Regulations. Treatment was rendered by commissioned dental officers only. Prior to closing in June 1919, the clinic accepted only emergency cases and those that could be completed in one sitting.[174]

The dental school closed on June 7, 1919, so that the dental officers could rejoin their units and render treatment to their personnel en route to the United States. They moved out with their enlisted assistants and portable dental outfits. However, the school had accomplished its mission by giving the students "an idea of the studies they elected, the difficulties that are most often encountered, and the interesting features of such studies." Each student received a certificate of attendance.[171,175] The closing of Beaune marked the termination of a remarkably effective wartime schooling system created in a very little time with few resources.

Postwar Dental Examination and Treatment

The pressure for dentists only abated when units began to return to the United States in the spring of 1919. Early in the embarkation from France, Oliver's office decided to classify the returning troops as follows:

(1) Class "A," mouth in hygienic condition.

(2) Class "E," dental work needed, but not immediately.

(3) Class "C," immediate dental work required. This included teeth to be extracted, large cavities to be filled, "pyorrhea" and Vincent's Angina.[176]

The dental surgeons on duty at the transient camps requested (in writing) that their commanding officer send 15 class "C" patients daily for treatment. When all the class "C" cases were completed, the class "E" should be substituted, so that all appointment time was utilized. Upon completion of the work, the commanding officer was expected to file a report to that effect to the office of the sanitary inspector.

Apparently, complaints were received in the surgeon general's office in Washington, DC, that some officers and enlisted soldiers returning from overseas were unable to get dental care while on board the transports. Lieutenant Colonel Frank LK LaFlamme at the surgeon general's office ordered that steps be taken to correct this problem by having dental officers "with the necessary portable equipment" on duty to take care of any emergencies that might arise on board.[177]

Oliver responded that a trimmed-down dental service consisting of eight dental surgeons was authorized to return with each division to render emergency treatment during the voyage home. In addition, each dental officer leaving France was to take with him one full and complete dental portable outfit to be carried as "extra baggage" on authority granted by SOS headquarters. This method was advocated as a means of both ensuring adequate professional service while traveling and transporting a large amount of portable equipment to the United States for retention in the service.[178]

To the Front

Robert Oliver's unremitting work to organize, equip, train, and supply the AEF's dental surgeons was aimed at one thing: providing the best possible oral and dental care for the American soldier, whether in the rear areas or the front line trenches. Of the 42 divisions that eventually reached France, 30 saw active combat operations or long stretches in the trenches. Accompanying the soldiers into combat as well as treating them in rear area hospitals, Dental Corps officers conclusively proved their value to the Army and Medical Department on the battlefields of France.

References

1. Coffman EM. *The War to End All Wars: the American Military Experience in World War I*. New York, NY: Oxford University Press; 1968: 10–11, 17.

2. Harbord JG. *The American Army in France, 1917–1919*. Boston, Mass: Little, Brown and Co.; 1936.

3. Young HH. *Hugh Young: a Surgeon's Autobiography*. New York, NY: Harcourt, Brace and Co; 1940.

4. Vandiver FE. *Black Jack: the Life and Times of John J. Pershing*. Vol 2. College Station, Tex: Texas A&M University Press; 1977.

5. US Department of the Army. *U.S. Army in the World War, 1917–1919, Reports of Commander-in-Chief, AEF, Staff Sections and Services*. Vol 15. Washington, DC: Historical Division; 1948.

6. Ford JH. *The Medical Department of the United States Army in the World War*. In: Administration American Expeditionary Forces. Vol 2. Washington, DC: Government Printing Office; 1927.

7. Ingalls R. Diary of a dental officer. *Dental Bulletin Supplement to the Army Medical Bulletin*. 1939;10:1–18.

8. National Archives and Records Administration. Record Group 395. Pershing to Farnsworth, 28 September 1916, and reply 29 September 1916. Telegrams. No. 1344. Box 22. Entry 1187.

9. National Archives and Records Administration. Record Group 120. Brigadier General Benjamin Alvord, memo for the chief of staff, 29 August 1917. Memo. No. 80. File 1-38. Entry 588.

10. Pershing JJ. *My Experiences in the World War*. Vol 1. New York, NY: Frederick A Stokes Co; 1931: 109–110, 321–322.

11. Foley GPH, ed. *Proceedings of the 125th Anniversary of the Baltimore College of Dental Surgery March 4, 5 and 6, 1965 Baltimore, Maryland*. Baltimore, Md: Alumni Association and the Faculty of the Baltimore College of Dental Surgery, Dental School, University of Maryland; 1966: 188–189.

12. National Archives and Records Administration. Record Group 120. Return of medical officers, etc, serving in the 2nd Division, during the month of October 1917. In: *Returns–Medical and Dental Officers, Medical Department, 2d Division*. Box 3412. Entry 2144.

13. Spaulding OL, Wright JW. *The Second Division American Expeditionary Force in France, 1917–1919*. New York, NY: The Hillman Press; 1937: 4–12.

14. US Navy. *The Medical Department of the United States Navy with the Army and Marine Corps in France in World War I: its Functions and Employment.* Washington, DC: Bureau of Medicine and Surgery, US Navy Department; 1947.

15. National Archives and Records Administration. Record Group 120. Captain Robert T Oliver to chief surgeon, "Divisional dental base units" 6 September 1917. Letter. File no. 449. Folder 16. Box 5122. Entry 2065.

16. National Archives and Records Administration. Record Group 120. Oliver to chief surgeon, 6 September 1917, handwritten comment, AEB [Alfred E Bradley, chief surgeon, American Expeditionary Forces]. Letter. File no. 449. Folder 16. Box 5122. Entry 2065.

17. Logan WHG. Our dental army at home and abroad. *Dental Summary.* 1920;40:716.

18. National Archives and Records Administration. Record Group 120. Captain Robert T Oliver, chief surgeon's office, American Expeditionary Forces, to chief surgeon, AEF, 1 October 1917, and notation, "Enrollment data-candidate EDW Dean," Captain Robert T Oliver. Memo. No. 211.2321-12. Folder 10. Box 4956. Entry 2065.

19. National Archives and Records Administration. Record Group 120. Surgeon, 29th Provisional Aero Squadron, to chief surgeon American Expeditionary Forces, 15 August 1917 and reply 21 August 1917. Memos. No. 166. Folder 28. Box 5466. Entry 2062.

20. *A History of the United States Army Base Hospital No. 36 (Detroit College of Medicine and Surgery Unit).* NP; 1919.

21. Polk RL. *Polk's Dental Register and Directory of the United States and Dominion of Canada.* 14th ed. Detroit, Mich: RL Polk & Co; 1928.

22. National Archives and Records Administration. Record Group 120. First Lieutenant William H Potter to Lieutenant Colonel Robert T Oliver, 28 December 1917. Letter. Folder 1. Box 1780. Entry 395.

23. National Archives and Records Administration. Record Group 120. Dental Corps (temporary) examination for (jacket A), 26 August–6 December 1918. No. 211.2321-12. Folder 9. Box 4955. Entry 2065.

24. National Archives and Records Administration. Record Group 120. Examination for appointment in the Dental Corps, USA (temporary), Colonel Robert T Oliver, DC, to president, dental board, Base Section No. 3, 18 October 1918. Memo. No. 211.2321-12. Folder 9. Box 4955. Entry 2065.

25. National Archives and Records Administration. Record Group 120. Dental Corps (temporary) examination for (jacket A), endorsement, Colonel Robert T Oliver, DC, to Private First Class George C Timmis, 2nd Cavalry, American Expeditionary Forces, 5 December 1918, and to Private Gale L Holmberg, Camp Hospital No. 52, 3 January 1919. No. 211.2321-12. Folder 9. Box 4955. Entry 2065.

26. National Archives and Records Administration. Record Group 120. Colonel Robert T Oliver to president, Army Dental Board No. 2, 1st Depot Division, American Expeditionary Forces, 20 November 1918. Memo. No. 211.2321-12. Folder 10. Box 4956. Entry 2065.

27. National Archives and Records Administration. Record Group 120. Captain Charles F Huber, division dental surgeon, 88th Division, American Expeditionary Forces, to chief surgeon, American Expeditionary Forces, Services of Supply, 7 December 1918, No. 211.2321-12. Memo. Folder 9. Box 4955. Entry 2065.

28. National Archives and Records Administration. Record Group 120. Application for appointment in the Dental Corps US Army, Private James Loraine Shipley, 24 December 1918. No. 211.2321-12, Folder 9. Box 4955. Entry 2065.

29. National Archives and Records Administration. Record Group 120. Colonel Walter D McCaw, chief surgeon, American Expeditionary Forces, to adjutant general, general headquarters, 20 February 1919. Memo. No. 211.2321-12. Folder 9. Box 4955. Entry 2065.

30. National Archives and Records Administration. Record Group 120. Colonel Robert T Oliver, office of the chief surgeon, headquarters, American Expeditionary Forces, to president, Army Dental Board, AEF, 1 March 1918. Memo. Folder 1. Box 1780. Entry 395.

31. National Archives and Records Administration. Record Group 120. Colonel Robert T Oliver, office of the chief surgeon, headquarters, American Expeditionary Forces, to president, Army Dental Board, AEF, 13 March 1918. Memo. Folder 1. Box 1780. Entry 395.

32. National Archives and Records Administration. Record Group 120. Major William S Rice, recorder, Army Dental Examining Board, American Expeditionary Forces, to surgeon general, US Army (through chief surgeon, AEF), 20 March 1918. Memo. Folder 1. Box 1780. Entry 395.

33. National Archives and Records Administration. Record Group 120. Colonel Robert T Oliver, office of the chief surgeon, headquarters, American Expeditionary Forces, to president, Army Dental Board, AEF, 8 May 1918. Memo. Folder 1. Box 1780. Entry 395.

34. National Archives and Records Administration. Record Group 120. Major WS Rice, recorder, 22 May 1918. Endorsement. Folder 1. Box 1780. Entry 395.

35. National Archives and Records Administration. Record Group 120. Chief surgeon, American Expeditionary Forces, to president, Army Dental Board, AEF, 26 June 1918. Memo. Folder 1. Box 1780. Entry 395.

36. National Archives and Records Administration. Record Group 120. Brigadier General Harold B Fiske, general staff, to commandant Army schools, American Expeditionary Forces, 20 July 1918. Memo. Folder 2. Box 1781. Entry 397.

37. National Archives and Records Administration. Record Group 120. Major WS Rice to commandant, Army schools, American Expeditionary Forces, 6 March 1918. Memo. Folder 2. Box 1780. Entry 395.

38. National Archives and Records Administration. Record Group 120. First Lieutenant William S Rice to surgeon general (through chief surgeon, American Expeditionary Forces), 7 December 1917. Letter. Folder 3. Box 1781. Entry 397.

39. National Archives and Records Administration. Record Group 120. Major James R Mount, Medical Corps, to First Lieutenant William S Rice, dental surgeon, Army school, 24 December 1917. Letter. Folder 1. Box 1780. Entry 395.

40. US War Department. *Official Army Register for 1920*. Washington, DC: Government Printing Office; 1920: 98.

41. National Archives and Records Administration. Record Group 120. Major William S Rice, director, dental section, Army Sanitary School, American Expeditionary Forces, to commandant, Army schools, AEF, through commandant, Army Sanitary School, AEF, 16 January 1918. Report. No. 3603-368, Box 1301. Entry 11.

42. National Archives and Records Administration. Record Group 120. Program, third session, dental section, Army Sanitary School, 16–29 January 1918. No. 3603-368. Box 1301. Entry 11.

43. National Archives and Records Administration. Record Group 120. Dental section, Army Sanitary School: program of instruction & record of course. Folder 1. Box 1781. Entry 397.

44. National Archives and Records Administration. Record Group 120. Major William S Rice, assistant director, dental section, Army Sanitary School, American Expeditionary Forces, to chief surgeon, AEF, 29 January 1918. Report. No. 3603-368. Box 1301. Entry 11.

45. National Archives and Records Administration. Record Group 120. Colonel SD Boak, director, to commandant, Army Schools, American Expeditionary Forces, 7 February 1918. Letter. No. 2028. Box 1676. Entry 352.

46. National Archives and Records Administration. Record Group 120. Army Sanitary School, dental section, third session, to chief surgeon, American Expeditionary Forces, 29 January 1918. Report. No. 3603-368. Box 1301. Entry 11.

47. National Archives and Records Administration. Record Group 120. Army Sanitary School, dental section, fourth session, to chief surgeon, American Expeditionary Forces, 4 February 1918. Report. No. 3603-368. Box 1301. Entry 11.

48. National Archives and Records Administration. Record Group 120. Colonel SD Boak, director, dental section, Army Sanitary School, to commandant, Army Schools, American Expeditionary Forces, 18 February 1918, 21 March 1918. Memos. Folder no. 2. Box 1780. Entry 395.

49. Boak SD. Letters from France. *J of the Nat Dent Assoc*. 1918;5:1089.

50. Brophy TW. *Oral Surgery: a Treatise on the Diseases and Malformations of the Mouth and Associated Parts*. Philadelphia, Pa: P Blakiston's Son & Co; 1915.

51. Brown GVI. *The Surgery of Oral Diseases and Malformations: their Diagnosis and Treatment*. Philadelphia, Pa: Lea & Febiger; 1912.

52. Brun BL. *Reference Book Written by Dr. B. Lucien Brun, World War I, 1917–1919, Sanitary School United States Army, France*. Located at: National Museum of Dentistry Archives, Baltimore, Md.

53. National Archives and Records Administration. Record Group 120. Colonel SD Boak, director, dental section, Army Sanitary School, to commandant, Army Schools, American Expeditionary Forces, 18 November 1918. Memo. Folder 2. Box 1780. Entry 395.

54. National Archives and Records Administration. Record Group 120. Major RA Dickson (for chief surgeon, American Expeditionary Forces, services of supply), to First Lieutenant William H Potter, 25 August 1918. Memo. Folder 2, Box 1780. Entry 395.

55. National Archives and Records Administration. Record Group 120. Major William H Potter, DC, to chief surgeon, American Expeditionary Forces, headquarters, services of supply (through military channels), 5 December 1918. Memo. Folder 2. Box 1780. Entry 395.

56. National Archives and Records Administration. Record Group 120. Report on a visit to Paris, March 25th to 30th, 1918, Colonel SD Boak, director, dental section, Army Sanitary School, to chief surgeon, American Expeditionary Forces (through medical channels), 16 April 1918. Report. Folder 2. Box 1780. Entry 395.

57. National Archives and Records Administration. Record Group 120. Colonel Bailey K Ashford, commandant, Army Sanitary School, American Expeditionary Forces, to Brigadier General James W McAndrew, commandant Army Schools, 27 April 1918. Letter. No. 3603-366. Box 1301. Entry 11.

58. National Archives and Records Administration. Record Group 120. Colonel Seibert D Boak, director, dental section, Army Sanitary School, to Colonel MAW Shockley, G-5, 2 July 1918. Letter. No. 3603-539. Box 1309. Entry 11.

59. National Archives and Records Administration. Record Group 120. Colonel Bailey K Ashford, commandant, Army Sanitary School, 3 July 1918. Endorsement. No. 3603-539. Box 1309. Entry 11.

60. National Archives and Records Administration. Record Group 120. Colonel Harold B Fiske, assistant chief of staff, G-5, to the French Mission, 7 July 1918. Letter. No. 3603-539. Box 1309. Entry 11.

61. National Archives and Records Administration. Record Group 120. Colonel SD Boak, director, dental section, Army Sanitary School, to Colonel MAW Shockley (through channels), 2 July 1918. Letter. Folder 1. Box 1780. Entry 395.

62. National Archives and Records Administration. Record Group 120. Sergeant John W Cooke to commandant, Army Sanitary School, Army schools, American Expeditionary Forces, 8 February 1918. Letter. Folder 1. Box 1780. Entry 395.

63. War Department. bulletin no. 61, par 5, 23 October 1917. In: *General Orders*. Washington, DC: Government Printing Office; 1917.

64. National Archives and Records Administration. Record Group 120. Colonel Robert T Oliver to Colonel Boak, 13 February 1918. Endorsement. Folder 1. Box 1780. Entry 395.

65. National Archives and Records Administration. Record Group 120. Sergeant John W Cooke to chief surgeon, American Expeditionary Forces, 24 June 1918. Letter, with endorsement. Folder 1. Box 1780. Entry 395.

66. National Archives and Records Administration. Record Group 120. Colonel Robert T Oliver (for chief surgeon, American Expeditionary Forces) to Sergeant Cooke, 1 July 1918. Letter. Folder 1. Box 1780. Entry 395.

67. National Archives and Records Administration. Record Group 120. Major WS Rice, recorder, Army Dental Examining Board, to surgeon general, US Army (through chief surgeon, American Expeditionary Forces), 12 July 1918. Folder 1. Box 1780. Entry 395.

68. National Archives and Records Administration. Record Group 120. Colonel Robert T Oliver, American Expeditionary Forces, to Lieutenant Cooke, 7 October 1918. Letter. Folder 1. Box 1780. Entry 395.

69. National Archives and Records Administration. Record Group 120. Alonzo G McCue, recorder, Army Dental Examining Board, to surgeon general, US Army (through chief surgeon, American Expeditionary Forces), 12 November 1918. Letter. Folder 1. Box 1780. Entry 395.

70. National Archives and Records Administration. Record Group 120. Colonel SD Boak, director, dental section, Army Sanitary School, to commandant, Army schools, American Expeditionary Forces, 28 November 1918. Memo. Folder 2. Box 1780. Entry 395.

71. National Archives and Records Administration. Record Group 120. First Lieutenant Cooke to chief surgeon, American Expeditionary Forces (through channels), 19 January 1919. Memo. Folder 1. Box 1780. Entry 395.

72. National Archives and Records Administration. Record Group 120. Colonel Seibert D Boak, director, dental section, Army Sanitary School, to Colonel Bailey K Ashford, medical representative, G-5, general staff, American Expeditionary Forces, 7 July 1918. No. 3603-366. Box 1301. Entry 11.

73. National Archives and Records Administration. Record Group 120. Colonel SD Boak, director, dental section, Army Sanitary School, to G-5, general headquarters, American Expeditionary Forces (through channels), 23 July 1918. Letter. No. 3603-539. Box 1309. Entry 11.

74. Dr. Georges Villain, Paris, France (1881–1938). *Dental Cosmos*. 1938;25:1131.

75. Hapgood RL. *History of the Harvard Dental School*. Boston, Mass: Harvard University Dental School; 1930: 301.

76. National Archives and Records Administration. Record Group 120. General head-quarters, American Expeditionary Forces, to commandant, Army schools, 29 August 1918. Endorsement. No. 3603-539. Box 1309. Entry 11.

77. National Archives and Records Administration. Record Group 120. Colonel SD Boak to G-5, general headquarters, American Expeditionary Forces (through channels), 19 August 1918. Letter. No. 3603-539. Box 1309. Entry 11.

78. National Archives and Records Administration. Record Group 120. Brigadier General HB Fiske, assistant chief of staff, G-5, to chief of French Mission, 29 August 1918. Letter. No. 3603-539. Box 1309. Entry 11.

79. National Archives and Records Administration. Record Group 120. Colonel SD Boak, director, dental section, to commandant (through director), Army Sanitary School, 17 November 1918. Letter. Folder 1. Box 1780. Entry 395.

80. National Archives and Records Administration. Record Group 120. Colonel Sanford H Wadhams, General Staff, to assistant chief of staff, G-5, 13 September 1918. Memo. No. 3603-539. Box 1309. Entry 11.

81. National Archives and Records Administration. Record Group 120. Colonel SD Boak, director, to G-5, general headquarters, American Expeditionary Forces (through channels), 29 August 1918. Letter. No. 3603-539. Box 1309. Entry 11.

82. National Archives and Records Administration. Record Group 120. Brigadier General Harry A Smith, commandant, 31 August 1918. Endorsement. No. 3603-539. Box 1309. Entry 11.

83. National Archives and Records Administration. Record Group 120. Special orders no. 274, par 80, general headquarters, American Expeditionary Forces, 1 October 1918. No. 3603-539. Box 1309. Entry 11.

84. National Archives and Records Administration. Record Group 120. First Lieutenant FP Hall, adjutant, Army Sanitary School, to G-5, general headquarters, American Expeditionary Forces, 23 September 1918. Memo. No. 3603-366. Box 1301. Entry 11.

85. National Archives and Records Administration. Record Group 120. Colonel SD Boak, director, to G-5, general headquarters, American Expeditionary Forces (through channels), 19 November 1918. Letter. No. 3603-539. Box 1309. Entry 11.

86. National Archives and Records Administration. Record Group 120. Brigadier General Frank E Bamford, 20 November 1918. Endorsement. No. 3603-539. Box 1309. Entry 11.

87. National Archives and Records Administration. Record Group 120. Colonel SD Boak to Major Lee S Fountain, headquarters, Base Section No. 1, 9 December 1918. Letter. Folder 1. Box 1780. Entry 395.

88. National Archives and Records Administration. Record Group 120. Colonel SD Boak to chief surgeon, American Expeditionary Forces (through channels), 19 January 1919. Memo. Folder 1. Box 1780. Entry 395.

89. National Archives and Records Administration. Record Group 120. Nevin to Scott, dental attendance & treatment Base Section No. 2, 13 May 1918. Letter. No. 703. Box 76. Entry 2361.

90. National Archives and Records Administration. Record Group 120. Scott to Shaw, 14 May 1918. Memo. No. 703. Box 76. Entry 2361.

91. National Archives and Records Administration. Record Group 120. Shaw to Scott, 17 May 1918. Endorsement. No. 703. Box 76. Entry 2361.

92. National Archives and Records Administration. Record Group 120. Scott to Nevin, 18 May 1918. Endorsement. No. 703. Box 76. Entry 2361.

93. The work of women dentists in France. *Dent Dig*. 1919;25:427.

94. National Archives and Records Administration. Record Group 165. Photograph caption, Dr Marie J Hyman. No. WW-245B-6.

95. National Archives and Records Administration. Record Group 112. Kerr to Surgeon General, 2 May 1917; Weiland to War Department, 19 May 1917; Surgeon general's office to Weiland, 3 July 1917. Letters. No. 158360. Box 1138.

96. National Archives and Records Administration. Record Group 112. Faytinger to surgeon general, 16 June 1917; surgeon general to Faytinger, 3 July 1917. Letters. No. 191004. Box 1349. Entry 26.

97. National Archives and Records Administration. Record Group 165. March to Senator John F Shafroth, 968 Medical Reserve Corps, 4 March 1918. Letter. No. 968-1. Box 107. Entry 8.

98. National Archives and Records Administration. Record Group 407. Precedent & History File 858. Press release, "First woman dentist in Army to report for duty March 21," 15 March 1951 [no. 354-51]. No. 44.

99. GI molars get feminine touch. *Ark Dent J*. 1953;24:50–52.

100. Cimring H. Something different in uniforms. *J Am Dent Assoc*. 1961;63:96–97.

101. Hyson JM, Jr. Female dentists in the U.S. Army: the origins. *Mil Med*. 1995;160:60–61.

102. National Archives and Records Administration. Record Group 120. Surgeon, base and line of communications, St Nazaire, to chief surgeon, American Expeditionary Forces, Paris, 24 July 1917. Memo. no. 449. Folder 16. Box 5122. Entry 2065.

103. National Archives and Records Administration. Record Group 120. Colonel Alfred E Bradley, chief surgeon, American Expeditionary Forces, to chief of staff, 6 October 1917. Memo. File No. 449. Folder 16. Box 5122. Entry 2065.

104. National Archives and Records Administration. Record Group 120. Chief surgeon, American Expeditionary Forces, to Lieutenant Colonel William J Lyster, liaison officer, Medical Corps, 2 December 1917. Memo. File no. 449. Folder 16. Box 5122. Entry 2065.

105. National Archives and Records Administration. Record Group 120. Colonel Lyster to chief surgeon, 11 December 1917, Francis A Winter, chief surgeon, line of communication, to chief surgeon, American Expeditionary Forces, 12 January 1918. Memo. File no. 449. Folder 16. Box 5122. Entry 2065.

106. National Archives and Records Administration. Record Group 120. Major Daniel P Card, purchasing officer, medical department, to chief surgeon, American Expeditionary Forces, 19 March 1918; and "in re dental supplies," Supply Division, chief supply officer, 8 August 1918. Memos. File no. 449. Folder 16. Box 5122. Entry 2065.

107. National Archives and Records Administration. Record Group 120. Lieutenant Colonel Clement C Whitcomb, MC, to chief surgeon, base group and line of communication, 22 August 1917. Memo. File no. 221. Folder 29. Box 5466. Entry 2062.

108. National Archives and Records Administration. Record Group 120. Lieutenant Colonel Clement C Whitcomb, MC, to chief surgeon, base group and line of communication, 3 September 1917. Memo. File no. 221. Folder 29. Box 5466. Entry 2062.

109. National Archives and Records Administration. Record Group 120. Major Thomas C Austin, MC, surgeon base group & line of communication, to officer in charge, Medical Supply Depot, 8 September 1917. Memo. File no. 221. Folder 29. Box 5466. Entry 2062.

110. Wolfe EP. Finance and Supply. In: *The United States Army Medical Department in the World War*. Vol 3. Washington, DC: US Government Printing Office; 1928.

111. National Archives and Records Administration. Record Group 120. Lieutenant Colonel Clement C Whitcomb, MC, Medical Supply Depot, France, to chief surgeon, base group & line of communication, 21 September 1917. Endorsement. No. 221. Folder 29. Box 5466. Entry 2062.

112. National Archives and Records Administration. Record Group 120. Major Albert S Bowen, MC, surgeon, Camp St Martin, Boulogne, France, to chief surgeon, American Expeditionary Forces, 19 August 1917. Memo. No. 271. Folder 30. Box 5466. Entry 2062.

113. National Archives and Records Administration. Record Group 120. Major Albert S Bowen, MC, surgeon, 12th Engineers (Railway), Camp St Martin, Boulogne, France, to chief surgeon, American Expeditionary Forces, 14 September 1917. Endorsement. No. 271. Folder 30. Box 5466. Entry 2062.

114. National Archives and Records Administration. Record Group 120. Surgeon, 17th Engineers (railway), to chief surgeon, base group & line of communication, Paris, 28 August 1917. Memo. No. 282. Folder 30. Box 5466. Entry 2062.

115. National Archives and Records Administration. Record Group 120. Colonel Francis A Winter, MC, surgeon, base group and line of communication, Paris, to surgeon, 17th Engineers (railway), 29 August 1917. Endorsement. No. 282, Folder 30. Box 5466. Entry 2062.

116. National Archives and Records Administration. Record Group 120. Surgeon, Camp Hospital No. 33, Base Section No. 5, to Colonel George H Casaday, supervising dental surgeon, Base Section No. 5, 30 November 1918. Letter. No. 282, Folder 30. Box 5466. Entry 2062.

117. National Archives and Records Administration. Record Group 120. Colonel Robert T Oliver, chief dental surgeon, American Expeditionary Forces, to Medical Equipment Board, 21 January 1919. Memo. File no. 449. Folder 15. Box 5122. Entry 2065.

118. National Archives and Records Administration. Record Group 120. Lieutenant Colonel James R Mount, MC, NA, to chief surgeon, American Expeditionary Forces, 27 June 1918. Memo. No. 449. Folder 15. Box 5122. Entry 2065.

119. National Archives and Records Administration. Record Group 120. Report of dental work at post hospital, casual officers' depot, APO 726, American Expeditionary Forces, October 10–31 1918, First Lieutenant Stephen F French, DC. Report. Box 3058. Entry 3026.

120. National Archives and Records Administration. Record Group 120. Major Howard I Benedict, attending dental surgeon, advance section, to Colonel Robert T Oliver, DC, 6 December 1918. Memo. File no. 449. Folder 15. Box 5122. Entry 2065.

121. National Archives and Records Administration. Record Group 120. Colonel Robert T Oliver, DC, to Major Howard I Benedict, attending dental surgeon, advance section, 16 December 1918. Telegram. File no. 449. Folder 15. Box 5122. Entry 2065.

122. National Archives and Records Administration. Record Group 120. Colonel James R Mount, MC, to chief surgeon, 29 January 1919. Telegram. File no. 449. Folder 15. Box 5122. Entry 2065.

123. National Archives and Records Administration. Record Group 120. Report of dental work, First Lieutenant William C Webb, Jr, February 1918. Report. Box 3383. Entry 1041.

124. National Archives and Records Administration. Record Group 120. Report of dental work, Captain Walter L Wilson, DC, 5th Corps Replacement Battalion, September 1918. Report. Box 3391. Entry 1147.

125. National Archives and Records Administration. Record Group 120. Dental report, First Lieutenant Roy B Slack, November 1918. Report. Box 3383. Entry 1040.

126. National Archives and Records Administration. Record Group 120. Major Raymond W Pearson, 33rd Division dental surgeon, to Lieutenant Colonel Levy M Hathaway, 33rd Division surgeon, 5 August 1918. Memo. Box 3383. Entry 1040.

127. National Archives and Records Administration. Record Group 120. Colonel WD Mc-Caw, to chief of staff, service of supply, 14 May 1918, in 82d Division dental surgeon. Memo. Box 3899. Entry 2144.

128. National Archives and Records Administration. Record Group 120. Colonel Robert T Oliver, "Dental emergency kits," 11 May 1918. Memo. Folder 1. Box 1780. Entry 395.

129. Oliver RT. History of the dental service, AEF. In: Activities of the chief surgeon's office. In: *Reports of the Commander-in-Chief, Staff Sections and Services, in United States Army in the World War 1917–1919*. Vol 15. Washington, DC: US Army Center of Military History; 1991: 411.

130. National Archives and Records Administration. Record Group 120. Lieutenant Colonel Cornelius H Mack, DC, USN, Division dental surgeon, 2nd Division, to chief dental surgeon, American Expeditionary Forces, 6 March 1919. Memo. File no. 449. Folder 15. Box 5122. Entry 2065.

131. National Archives and Records Administration. Record Group 120. Colonel Robert T Oliver, chief dental surgeon, American Expeditionary Forces, 24 March 1919. Endorsement. File no. 449. Folder 15. Box 5122. Entry 2065.

132. Revision of dental supply tables. *Army and Navy Journal*. 1918;55:1876.

133. National Archives and Records Administration. Record Group 120. Lieutenant Colonel George D Graham, DC, corps dental surgeon, I Army Corps, to chief dental surgeon, American Expeditionary Forces, 23 December 1918. Memo. File no. 449. Folder 15. Box 5122. Entry 2065.

134. National Archives and Records Administration. Record Group 120. Colonel Robert T Oliver, chief dental surgeon, American Expeditionary Forces, to Lieutenant Colonel George D Graham, DC, chief dental surgeon, 1st Army Corps, 19 January 1919. Memo. File no. 449. Folder 15. Box 5122. Entry 2065.

135. Raymond EH. A type of denture for Army use. *Dental Cosmos*. 1918;60:516.

136. Hyson JM Jr, and Foley GPH. James Baxter Bean: the first military maxillofacial hospital. *MSDA J*. 1997;40:77–81.

137. Maryland Association of Dentists. *Dental Cosmos*. 1867;7:376.

138. Bean JB. The aluminum base. *Dental Cosmos*. 1867;8:470–473.

139. National Archives and Records Administration. Record Group 120. Colonel Seibert D Boak, director, dental section, Army Sanitary School, American Expeditionary Forces, to G-5, general headquarters, AEF (through channels), 8 August 1918. Letter. Folder 1. Box 1780. Entry 395.

140. National Archives and Records Administration. Record Group 120. Colonel Robert T Oliver (for chief surgeon, American Expeditionary Forces), 7 November 1918. Memo. Folder 1. Box 1780. Entry 395.

141. National Archives and Records Administration. Record Group 120. The Amex Denture (cast aluminum), office of the chief surgeon, American Expeditionary Forces, 30 September 1918. Circular Letter no. 13-B. Folder 1. Box 1780. Entry 395.

142. National Archives and Records Administration. Record Group 120. Colonel Robert T Oliver (for chief surgeon, American Expeditionary Forces), 7 November 1918. Memo. Folder 1. Box 1780. Entry 395.

143. Campbell DD. The cast aluminum base. *Dental Summary*.1920;11:925.

144. Asbell MB. *Dentistry: A Historical Perspective*. Bryn Mawr, Pa: Dorrance & Co; 1988: 178.

145. Lufkin AW. *A History of Dentistry*. Philadelphia, Pa: Lea & Febiger; 1948: 346–347.

146. National Archives and Records Administration. Record Group 120. Special instructions governing the character of dental treatment accorded in the American Expeditionary Forces, chief surgeon, AEF. Memo. No. 703. Folder 18. Box 5149. Entry 2065.

147. National Archives and Records Administration. Record Group 120. Circular no. 4, office of the chief surgeon, headquarters, American Expeditionary Forces, 22 December 1917. Box 5464. Entry 2072.

148. National Archives and Records Administration. Record Group 120. Colonel John W Hanner, commanding officer, Base Hospital No. 116, to chief surgeon, American Expeditionary Forces, 24 June 1918. Memo. No. 703. Folder 18. Box 5149. Entry 2065.

149. National Archives and Records Administration. Record Group 120. Colonel Robert T Oliver, to dental surgeon, Base Hospital No. 24, 8 August 1918. Endorsement. No. 703. Folder 18. Box 5149. Entry 2065.

150. National Archives and Records Administration. Record Group 120. Colonel Robert T Oliver, chief dental surgeon, American Expeditionary Forces, to division dental surgeon, 5th Division, AEF, 5 June 1918. Memo. No. 703. Folder 18. Box 5149. Entry 2065.

151. National Archives and Records Administration. Record Group 120. Sous-secrétaire d'etat du service de santé militaire, to chief surgeon, American Expeditionary Forces (through general chief of the French Mission at headquarters, services of supply), 5 October 1918. Letter. File no. 703. Folder 18. Box 5149. Entry 2065.

152. National Archives and Records Administration. Record Group 120. Circular, sous-secrétaire d'etat du service de santé militaire, to MM directeurs du service de santé of all the regions, 5 October 1918. Letter. File no. 703. Folder 18. Box 5149. Entry 2065.

153. National Archives and Records Administration. Record Group 120. Colonel Robert T Oliver, DC, (for chief surgeon, American Expeditionary Forces), to sous-secrétaire d'etat du service de santé militaire, and to chief surgeon, AEF (through chief of the French Mission, headquarters, services of supply), 26 October 1918. Memo. File no. 703. Folder 18. Box 5149. Entry 2065.

154.   National Archives and Records Administration. Record Group 120. Colonel Charles L Foster, MC, General historical synopsis, services of supply, headquarters, Base Section No. 1, office of the surgeon, France. Report. File no. 117-43.1. Box 4. Entry 2255.

155.   National Archives and Records Administration. Record Group 120. Colonel Ernest L Ruffner, MC, surgeon, intermediate section, services of supply, to chief surgeon, American Expeditionary Forces, services of supply, 15 August 1918. Memo. File no. 211.19. Box 3030. Entry 2997.

156.   National Archives and Records Administration. Record Group 120. Colonel Robert T Oliver, DC, 22 August 1918, to surgeon, intermediate section, services of supply. Endorsement. File no. 211.19. Box 3030. Entry 2997.

157.   National Archives and Records Administration. Record Group 120. Colonel James L Bevans, chief surgeon, III Army Corps, to Major General Robert L Bullard, III Army Corps, American Expeditionary Forces, 14 August 1918. Memo. File no. 321.6. Box 76. Entry 1042.

158.   National Archives and Records Administration. Record Group 120. Major General Robert L Bullard, 14 August 1918. Endorsement. File no. 321.6. Box 76. Entry 1042.

159.   National Archives and Records Administration. Record Group 120. Brigadier General Merritte W Ireland, MC, National Army, 22 August 1918. Endorsement. File no. 321.6. Box 76. Entry 1042.

160.   National Archives and Records Administration. Record Group 120. Captain William Z Carroll, "Dental report," September 1918, headquarters, 3rd Army Corps, American Expeditionary Forces. Report. Box 3385. Entry 1071.

161.   National Archives and Records Administration. Record Group 120. Captain William Z Carroll, "Dental report," October 1918, headquarters, Third Army Corps, American Expeditionary Forces. Report. Box 3385. Entry 1071.

162.   National Archives and Records Administration. Record Group 120. Captain William Z Carroll, DC, office of attending dental surgeon, headquarters, 3rd Army Corps, American Expeditionary Forces, to camp commandant, headquarters, 3rd Army Corps, 1 October 1918. File no. 703. Box 1042. Entry 1042.

163.   National Archives and Records Administration. Record Group 120. Lieutenant Colonel EP Walser, 1st Corps Artillery Park, to chief surgeon, 3rd Army Corps, American Expeditionary Forces, 17 August 1918. Memo. File no. 211.19. Box 62. Entry 1042.

164.   National Archives and Records Administration. Record Group 120. Colonel James L Bevans, chief surgeon, 3rd Army Corps, 18 August 1918, Lieutenant Colonel George K Wilson (for corps commander), 20 August 1918. Endorsements. File no. 211.19. Box 62. Entry 1042.

165.   National Archives and Records Administration. Record Group 120. Captain Louis A Haffner, dental surgeon, 4th Corps Replacement Battalion, to commanding officer, 4th Corps Replacement Battalion, 3 October 1918. Memo. File no. 211.19. Box 60. Entry 1074.

166. National Archives and Records Administration. Record Group 120. Colonel George H Casaday, chief dental surgeon, Second Army, 12, 19, and 26 November, and 3 December 1918, in File 319.1 "Dental Personnel." Reports. Box 3295.Entry 924.

167. National Archives and Records Administration. Record Group 120. Captain Henry K Tice, Military Police Corps, First Army MP Battalion, to commanding general, First Army (through military channels), 17 January 1919. Letter. File no. 211.19. Box 155. Entry 763.

168. National Archives and Records Administration. Record Group 120. Major John G MacDonnell, provost marshal, First Army, 22 January 1919, Brigadier General William R Sample, 27 January 1919. Endorsements. File no. 211.19. Box 155. Entry 763.

169. National Archives and Records Administration. Record Group 120. Personnel, medical department, American Expeditionary Forces. Decimal file 200. Boxes 4908 and 4909. Entry 2065.

170. National Archives and Records Administration. Record Group 120. Personnel, medical department, American Expeditionary Forces. Decimal file 320.2-1 (AEF). Box 5. Entry 31.

171. Fleischer MBS. History of dental section, medical college, AEF University, Beaune, Cote d'Or, France. *Dental Cosmos*. 1921;63.

172. National Archives and Records Administration. Record Group 120. Colonel JH Ford, MC, to commanding officer, 28 February 1919. Memo. File no. 352.923. Box 1904. Entry 408.

173. National Archives and Records Administration. Record Group 120. Lieutenant Colonel OH McDonald, DC, director, dental section, American Expeditionary Forces University, 2 March 1919. Memo. File no. 352.923, Box 1909, Entry 408, RG 120, NARA.

174. National Archives and Records Administration. Record Group 120. Lieutenant Colonel OH McDonald, DC, director, dental section, medical college, to commanding officer, American Expeditionary Forces University (through medical channels), 6 March 1919 and 29 May 1919. Memos. File no. 703. Box 1909. Entry 408.

175. National Archives and Records Administration. Record Group 120. President, American Expeditionary Forces University, 5 June 1919. Telegram. File no. 703. Box 1909. Entry 408.

176. National Archives and Records Administration. Record Group 120. Major Lee S Fountain, DC, office of sanitary inspector & health officer, Nantes, to commanding officers of organizations billeted in area, 15 March 1919. Memo. File no. 703. Box 199. Entry 2130.

177. National Archives and Records Administration. Record Group 120. Lieutenant Colonel Frank LK Laflamme, the surgeon general's office, to chief dental surgeon, American Expeditionary Forces, 25 April 1919. Memo. File no. 703. Folder 18. Box 5149. Entry 2065.

178. National Archives and Records Administration. Record Group 120. Colonel Robert T Oliver, chief dental surgeon, American Expeditionary Forces, to surgeon general, US Army, 2 June 1919. Memo. File no. 703. Folder 18. Box 5149. Entry 2065.

Chapter XIV

The Dental Service in the American Expeditionary Forces in France, 1917–1919: Oral and Dental Care

Introduction

Within the limits of personnel, organization, and equipment that constrained their preparations, Colonel Robert Oliver and the dental surgeons in the American Expeditionary Forces (AEF) organized, equipped, and carried out their assigned missions as best they could. The real test for the Army dental officers and their assistants came in the AEF's hospitals, dental clinics, and especially in the front line combat divisions, where they faced the uncertainty and dangers of modern warfare. For many, that test came within weeks of their arrival on the French shores.

Dental Work in a Base Hospital

Medical units, including dental staff, flowed into France as Oliver worked to resolve the multitude of problems in administration and logistics confronting the dental service. These medical units were expected to meet their missions almost immediately, regardless of conditions. An example of the problems they faced can be drawn from the experience of Base Hospital No. 18 from Johns Hopkins University, which arrived at Saint Nazaire, France, on June 28, 1917. While the hospital was temporarily attached to Base Hospital No. 1 at Saint Nazaire, First Lieutenant Livius Lankford of the Dental Reserve Corps (DRC), the assistant dental surgeon, opened the first dental clinic in France for AEF soldiers. The history of Base Hospital No. 18 claimed that "the service rendered was of such character as to call forth praise from all those who received attention—and the appointment lists were always taxed to their capacity." On July 26, 1917, the unit finally reached its assigned location in the advance section to operate what was then called US Army Hospital No. 2 (it reverted to the designation Base Hospital No. 18 on September 21, 1917) at Bazoilles-sur-Meuse near Neufchâteau in the northwestern part of the Vosges Department in northeastern France. Once in place, the Hopkins unit was the most forward American hospital, and received its first patients on July 31.[1-8]

The dental department, however, did not open until August 26 because of a delay in the arrival and installation of equipment. First Lieutenant B Lucien Brun, DRC, and Lieutenant Lankford were both residents of Baltimore and members of the unit when it was called to active duty.[6-8] In August 1917 Brun reported the slow start up of the dental service:

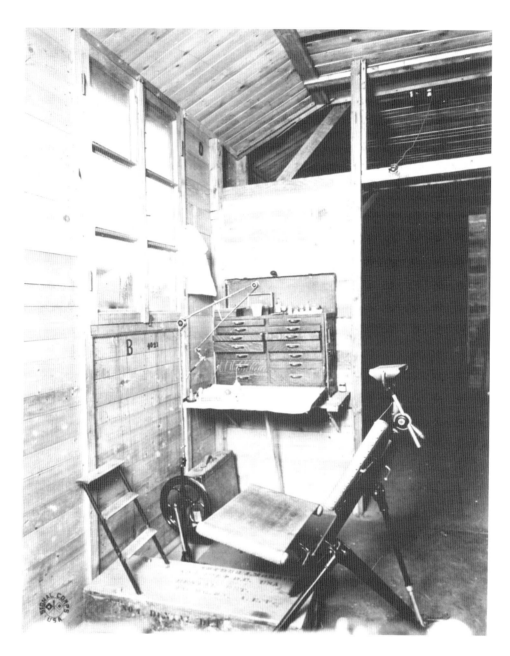

*Dental room at Camp Hospital No. 64, Chatillon, France,
January 1919, showing the portable dental outfit set up.
Photograph: Courtesy of the National Library of Medicine.*

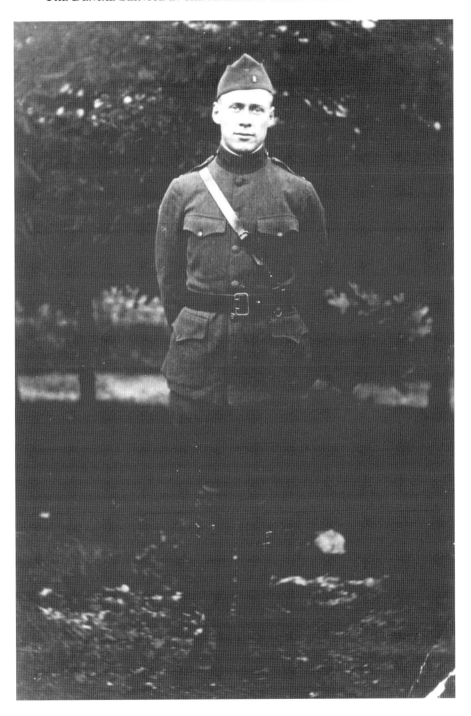

Doctor Livius Lankford at Base Hospital No. 18,
Bazoilles sur Meuse, France, November 1, 1918.
Photograph: Courtesy of Dr Lankford's daughter, Mrs Fred Henninghausen.

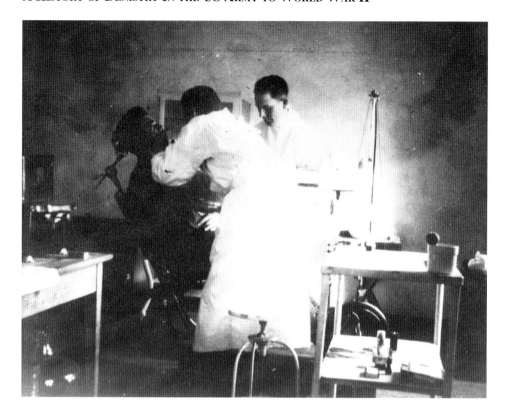

Doctor Livius Lankford with a patient in what he called
"my operating room at St. Nazaire," 1917.
Photograph: Courtesy of Dr Lankford's daughter, Mrs Fred Henninghausen.

Owing to fact that Government forms were not received by the Dental Department until August 29/17 no complete record was kept of work performed in Dental Department prior to that date, it not being known just what information was desired. Dental Department in operation but four days in present month, from Aug. 28 to Aug. 31, with incomplete outfit.[9]

Base Hospital No. 18 took over facilities that the French had built and used as a 1,000-bed war hospital since March 1916. Located on the grounds of an old chateau, the hospital consisted of 36 frame barracks grouped about the chateau, which served as an office and administration building. There were 25 buildings for the hospital proper; 20 were used as wards, then there was an operating room, receiving office and shower baths, clothing room, linen and supply room, and one barracks for the enlisted troops. Eleven general purpose buildings served as officers' barracks, six as more troop barracks, one each as kitchen and mess hall, carpenter shop, fumigation room and plumber's shop, storage building, and morgue.[2]

The Americans made some changes to the operating pavilion, namely, adding a dental department; eye, ear, nose, and throat department; laboratory; and

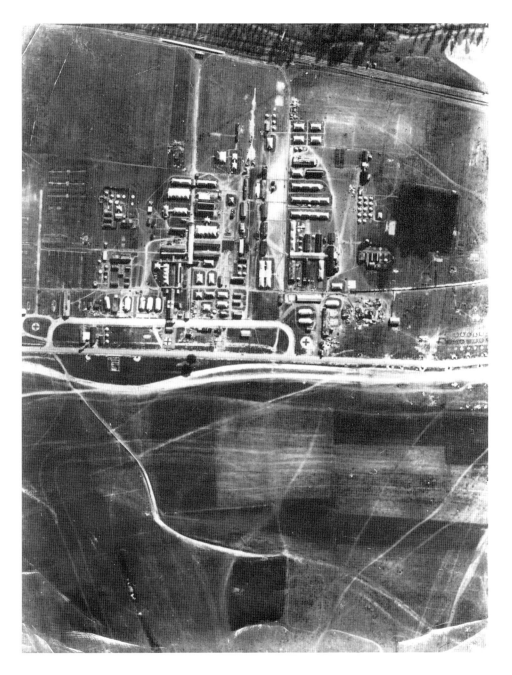

Base Hospital No. 18, aerial view.
Photograph: Courtesy of Dr John M. Hyson, Jr, Collection Office of Medical History.
Office of The Surgeon General, US Army, Falls Church, Virginia.

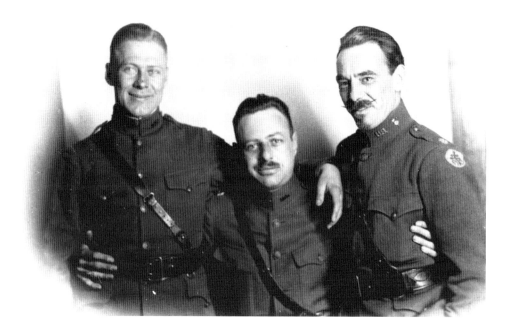

*Livius Lankford (left), unidentified officer, and
Major B Lucien Brun (right), at Base Hospital No. 18.
Photograph: Courtesy of Doctor Lankford's daughter, Mrs Fred Henninghausen.*

increased space for the X-ray department. Also, the large number of female nurses made it necessary to dedicate two of the French wards as their living quarters, and another as a combined kitchen, dining, and living room for them. There were two medical and two surgical wards, along with single wards for officers, patients with infectious diseases, neurological patients, and ambulant cases. The capacity of these wards was 375 beds.[2]

In the report of an inspection conducted on February 28, 1918, Colonel Henry C Fisher of the Medical Corps (MC), the AEF's general sanitary inspector, noted that Lieutenant Brun was in charge of the dental department where "excellent work being done," but that it was equipped only "for ordinary work, not for plastic work. No facilities for plate and bridge work."[10] In March 1918 Brun went to the Army Sanitary School for 2 weeks of special training, which included some maxillofacial surgery instruction under First Lieutenant (later Lieutenant Colonel) William H Potter (1856–1928). Potter was professor of operative dentistry at Harvard Dental School, formerly served on the staff of the American Ambulance at Neuilly, and had come to France in June 1917 with Harvard's Base Hospital No. 5, spending 6 months with the British Expeditionary Forces. Potter was thoroughly familiar with current British, French, and American practice for treating jaw fractures and wounds, which made him an ideal instructor for Brun.[11-14]

In May 1918 Brun began splinting and caring for fracture patients arriving at the hospital. From May 23 to June 16, Brun and Captain Harvey B Stone, MC, a surgeon, were sent to French military hospitals at Tours, Bordeaux, Lyons, and Paris and the American Red Cross Military Hospital No. 1 at Neuilly to observe the methods and equipment being used to treat face and jaw wounds. After his return and throughout the summer months, Brun handled an increasing number of maxillofacial cases in addition to his regular work in the dental clinic.[7,15]

In his next inspection report of June 20, Colonel Fisher noted that Brun was "especially interested in doing oral restoration work."[16] In June Major William C Speakman, DRC, a skilled dental surgeon who had arrived with Major Vilray P Blair's maxillofacial surgery team in April (see "Dr Vilray P Blair and Maxillofacial Surgery" below), temporarily joined the dental staff on an observational assignment until he was ordered to Lyons at the end of the month.[17,18] In July 1918 the monthly hospital return reported that "at this date, there is a very interesting clinic for this department, consisting of battle wound face and jaw cases, through and through gunshot wounds, and cases presenting much lost substance."[19]

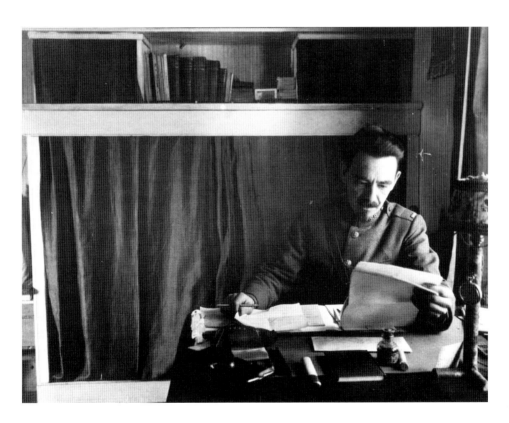

Lieutenant B Lucien Brun doing paperwork in his quarters at Base Hospital No. 18.
Caption from note with photo reads, "Here we have the 'Dent' Man Bruno of B.H. 18 —
Posing for that Celebrated Picture Cleaning up on his paper work."
Photograph: Courtesy of Brun's daughter, Lucille F Lane.

By mid 1918 the dental officers of Base Hospital No. 18, which became part of the Bazoilles Hospital Center in July, were experienced and well trained. The dental clinic was eventually replaced with a new clinic and laboratory that had "the most modern equipment" installed. Because of its location near the front, Bazoilles received many jaw and face wounds, and Lieutenant Brun and the new dental clinic took on the task of caring for the maxillofacial cases while the laboratory handled most of the splint work.

On September 10, 1918, now Captain Brun was appointed the supervisor of dental operations for the entire Bazoilles Hospital Center, in addition to his continuing dental duties at Base Hospital No. 18 and a growing workload of maxillofacial patients. In preparing for the upcoming Saintt Mihiel offensive, the hospital commander had decided "to utilize the service in the operating room of both Dental Surgeons at this post, one for day and the other for night duty."[20–22] Brun drew the night shift on Harvey Stone's team. In a personal diary, Brun jotted down his frenetic pace during the offensive's early days:

> Wednesday, Sept. 11. With Americans opening grand offensive all along line from Pont-a-Mousson to Verdun – advance had been made all along [Saint Mihiel] salient. Mont Sec has been taken. Weather conditions still very bad. Hard going for our boys. . . . Thursday, Sept. 12th. Drive continues with unabated fury & success. . . . Friday, Sept. 13th. First convoy of wounded received. Day & night teams start work. Much for me to do before starting in on night shift which runs from 8 P.M. to 8 A.M. — worked until 3:30 A.M. morning of Saturday, Sept.14 Weather cleared up. Very damp — arose at 6:30 had bath & breakfast and then over to 46-116 and 42 [Base Hospitals No. 42, 46, and 116] where I found seven jaw cases had come in. Got work started on them. Returned at 12:30, had lunch — then to office until 4 — to bed until 6:30 supper and to operating room all night — two more convoys arrive for us. Sunday, Sept 15th. . . . To all hospitals until 12 noon . . . Large convoy arrives at 8 P.M. Up all night — 50 odd operations today — to bed at 5:30. . . . Monday, Sept. 16. . . . To other hospitals between 9 & 1. Go "on" again tonight — almost all in. Day & night for nearly four days with but little sleep.[23]

Brun was treating maxillofacial cases in Base Hospital No. 46 and No. 116 as well as his own Base Hospital No. 18 and the designated specialty hospital of the Hospital Center, Bazoilles, Base Hospital No. 42, where Captain Hugh W Brent was assigned as the oral and plastic surgeon late in August. Cases were increasingly concentrated at Base Hospital No. 42 during the Saint Mihiel offensive in September, and laboratory equipment was moved there from Base Hospital No. 18. More and more, Brun's time was taken up with maxillofacial matters. On September 30 the hospital center commander formally directed Brun to assist Captain Brent with the maxillofacial cases received at Bazoilles. Brun worked heavily on these cases for the remainder of the year.[15]

While stationed at Bazoilles-sur-Meuse from August 1917 through December 1918, Brun and Lankford treated 3,500 officers and enlisted soldiers and 132 other patients in 6,577 individual sittings.[9,24] Base Hospital No. 18 rapidly curtailed its activities after the armistice, closed on January 17, 1919, leaving for the United States on January 31, 1919, and completed demobilization on February 25, 1919, at Camp Upton, Long Island, New York.[6]

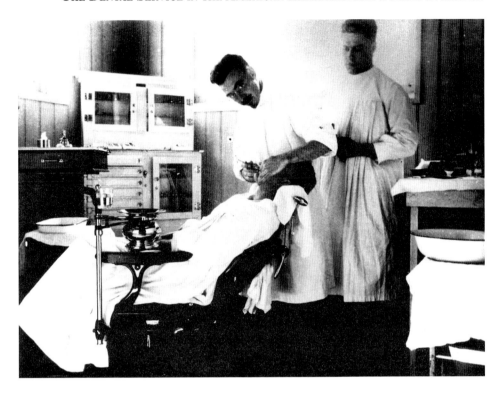

*Lieutenants B Lucien Brun and Livius Lankford in the
dental clinic at Base Hospital No. 18, France.
Photograph: Courtesy of Brun's daughter, Lucille F Lane.*

Base and Camp Hospitals

The experiences of the staff at Base Hospital No. 18 were duplicated across much of France where American hospital units were located. First Lieutenant George M Boehler, a 1908 graduate of Creighton University's College of Dentistry, assigned to Base Hospital No. 49 at Neufchâteau, wrote home that his unit was in comfortable surroundings.

My duties since arriving here have been many and varied. Besides my regular duties as Dental Surgeon, I am a Fire Marshall in one section of the Hospital Center, assist censoring mail, and last but not least, am Officer of the Day when my turn comes in my particular Unit. So you can readily understand that my time is well occupied in helping to do my bit.

The Dental Department when fully completed will be one of the important branches of the Hospital, as there is a great demand for dental service, for the "blessured" men who come here for treatment from the front, and the importance of dental attention is well understood and recognized by all the personnel of the Army.[25,26]

543

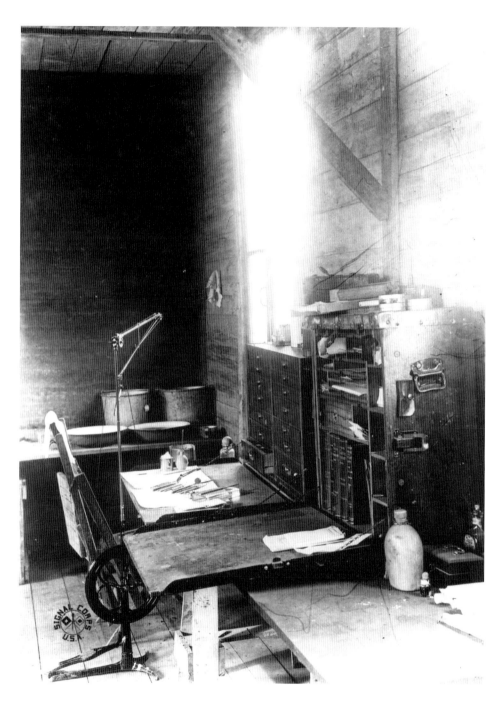

An interior view of the dental office at Camp Hospital No. 70,
Saint Florent-le-Viel, France, 1918.
Photograph: Courtesy of the National Library of Medicine.

First Lieutenant Theodore V Symanski, DRC, at Camp Hospital No. 26 at the First Replacement Depot at Saint Aignan noted that many casuals passing through the command, especially those from the front, needed dental care. He wrote home that his "Dental Department" shared a temporary barracks building with the central dental laboratory in the village of Noyen, about a mile from the rest of the hospital. Combined, the dental activity consisted of 82 officers and soldiers. All of the latter were either dentists without commissions or former dental students and technicians, while all but two of the dentists were members of the National Guard or Dental Reserve Corps. Symanski judged the available equipment as excellent. Twenty-seven chairs were devoted to operative work, four to prosthetic work, and two to oral surgery. A final two were in a separate "officers' operating room." The dental laboratory could turn out two dozen dentures a day, while the chairs handled 110 to 150 patients daily. Camp Hospital No. 26 closed on June 26, 1919, "and with it both the Dental Department and Central Laboratory."[27]

In addition to serving the large flow of replacements and casuals, Camp Hospital No. 26 itself served as a replacement pool. Requests for personnel sent to Oliver's office were filled mostly by drafts on the hospital staff. Dental personnel

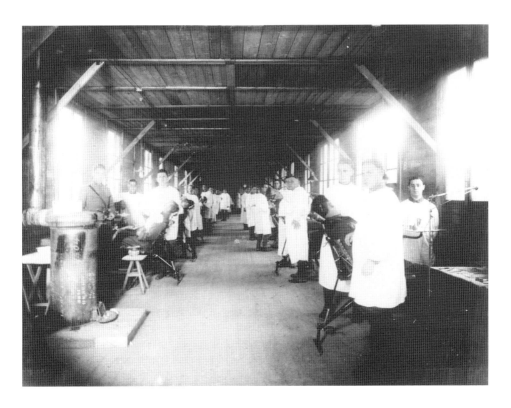

Dental Infirmary at Camp Hospital No. 26, 1st Depot Division, Saint Aignan, France.
Photograph: Courtesy of the National Library of Medicine.

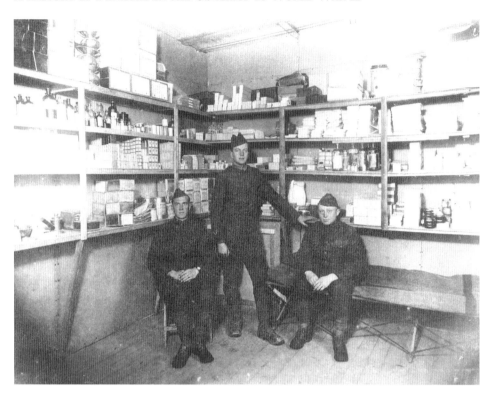

Dental supply room at Camp Hospital No. 26,
1st Depot Division, Saint Aignan, France.
Photograph: Courtesy of the National Library of Medicine.

from Camp No. 26 went to several infantry divisions as well as to other posts throughout the AEF. Newcomers from the United States took their places to become acclimated before serving as replacements for line units.[27]

Trench Mouth

Another specialized area that formal training could not address was Vincent's Angina, or "trench mouth." In February 1918 Lieutenant (junior grade) Douglas B Parker of the US Naval Reserve Dental Corps, a dental surgeon at the US Navy Base Hospital No. 1 in Brest, France, reported that he had noted "some ten cases of Vincent's Angina," which bacterial examination confirmed. While relatively rare during peacetime, this affliction of the throat, mouth, gums, and tonsils was widespread among British and French troops in the trenches, and came to be known as "trench mouth," "trench throat," or "trench gums." By the spring of 1918, the disease was quite prevalent in the AEF's camps and training areas and resulted in the hospitalization of a large number of soldiers; one hospital alone had more than 700 cases being treated at one time. While normally not life threatening, trench mouth was incapacitating and required several days to treat.[28–30]

First described by the French physician Henri Vincent (1862–1950) in 1898 and named after him, Vincent's Angina or Vincent's Disease was an ulcero-membranous disease characterized by swollen gums with a grey sloughing membrane that bled freely.[30,31] The symptoms were described as pain in the region of the gums and teeth accompanied by fetid breath and loose or painful teeth. Gums began sloughing away, became a shiny pus color, shredded easily and bled at the slightest touch, and finally sloughing occurred to the extent of showing the spaces between the teeth where the gums ought to be.[30,32] To prevent an epidemic, all infected soldiers had to be referred to their unit dentists, who instructed them in oral hygiene. Toothbrushes had to be cleaned, isolated, and covered after each use, and brushing itself could not abrade the gums. Alcoholic beverages were also discouraged. Finally, all eating and drinking utensils had to be cleaned thoroughly in very hot water and never shared.[31]

In May 1918 First Lieutenant John E Walker, MC, investigated the situation at Blois and Saint Aignan. Since April 26 at Blois, 25 cases had tested positive for the Vincent's organism among 3,000–4,000 troops. Several of these patients were also found to be carriers of the diphtheria bacillus. Four or five cases were considered serious enough for hospitalization. All cases had mouths that were in bad condition with calculus formation.[33]

The treatment for trench mouth consisted of a thorough prophylaxis, removal of retained roots, and cavity filling. After that, the gums were treated with silver

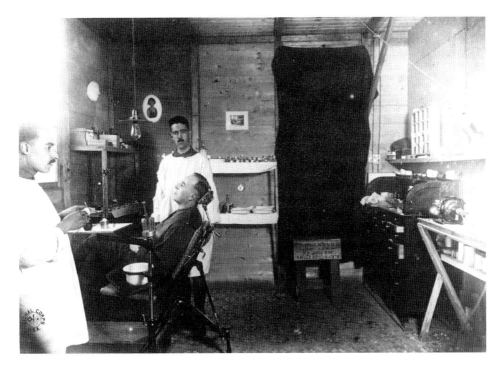

Dental Office at Camp Hospital No. 26, 1st Depot Division, Saint Aignan, France.
Photograph: Courtesy of the National Library of Medicine.

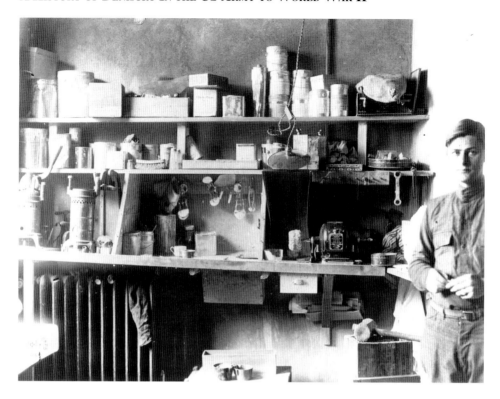

A technician in the dental laboratory at Base Hospital No. 69, Savenay, France. 1918.
Photograph: Courtesy of the National Library of Medicine.

nitrate solution, tincture of iodine (4%), or trichloracetic acid. Fowler's solution was given internally in some cases, and intravenous injections of novo-arsenoben-zol was used in one or two cases, but was not considered efficacious.[33]

At Saint Aignan, Walker found 54 cases had been diagnosed out of 18,000 troops in the past 2 months. The men were largely transients and probably arrived with the disease already developed. In general, those from the front lines were slightly more likely to be infected. Walker concluded that the two most important factors were "a mouth condition originally bad," and "a lack of oral hygiene (toothbrush)." He also surmised that "over smoking" and the "quality of the food" played a role. In addition, he concluded that there was "no evidence of the transmission of the condition from case to case." He recommended "greater insistence upon the use of the tooth brush, even under war conditions" and "thorough cleaning up of all mouths." One possible solution to the problem was "training enlisted men to remove calculus, and to make applications to the gums, thus reserving the time of the dentist for extractions and fillings."[33]

In December 1918 Captain William W Irving, Dental Corps (DC), supervising dental surgeon at Hospital Center, Savenay, recommended to Colonel Wibb E Cooper, MC, the commanding officer, that medical and dental officers "cooperate" in the treatment of Vincent's, and that the cases be isolated and obliged to "use their own or special mess kits."[34]

In his account of Vincent's Angina in the official history of the Army Medical Department, Lieutenant Colonel Joseph F Siler, MC, probably the Medical Department's leading medical researcher of the time and head of the AEF's Division of Laboratories and Infectious Diseases at Dijon, identified a total of 3,080 cases of Vincent's Angina and four deaths from 1917 through 1919, resulting in the loss of 35,440 days.[30] As to possible preventive and therapeutics measures, he concluded the following:

> No specific preventive measures were known before the war and none developed during that period. It has been established that the disease is an infection; however, the method of transmission is unknown. The organisms of Vincent are constantly present where Vincent's disease exists, but are also normal inhabitants of the mouth. The important factor seems to be in the prevention of lowered local and constitutional resistance. The best results are accomplished by proper oral hygiene. . . . It has been said that a good dentist is the best therapeutic measure. Filthy mouths must be cleaned up, and gingivitis and pyorrhea alveolaris must be adequately treated, if satisfactory improvement is to be expected. Local application of drugs, curettement, and intravenous therapy are merely adjuncts.[30]

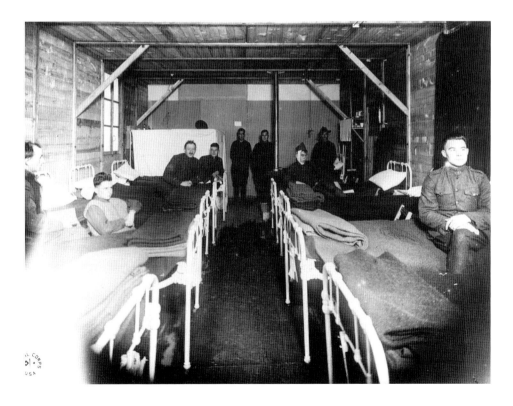

Dental patients' ward at Camp Hospital No. 26,
1st Depot Division, Saint Aignan, France.
Photograph: Courtesy of the National Library of Medicine.

Syphilis

Syphilis was always a major concern in the Army (Exhibit 14-1). After Hugh Young's first briefings on the voyage to France, Pershing successfully directed a vigorous program to repress the incidence of venereal disease in the AEF. However, syphilis remained a concern and danger to dentists because the oral cavity presents "an exceptionally fine field for syphilitic infection" and the extensive mucous surface and moisture present are "favorable to the life of the spirochaete."[35,36] In addition, there is always "mechanical irritation during mastication," which produces abrasions sufficient for the entrance of the spirochaete. The toothbrush, kissing, unsterilized dental instruments, knives, forks, spoons, cups, glasses, and common use of pipes and cigars can all transmit the disease. Chancres can appear most frequently on the lips (usually the lower lip); the tip, dorsum or sides of the tongue; the tonsils; or even in the pharynx. The sores are usually round or oval, slightly elevated, and sharply outlined. They are not painful, but there is always bilateral lymph node enlargement. Thus, no class of professional men was "more subjected to accidental infection than the dentist."[35] Several of the early contract dental surgeons became infected "innocently"; others, not so innocently. In 1913 one contract dental surgeon's contract was annulled because of absence from duty caused by secondary syphilis "contracted not in line of duty." He was treated with salvarsan. When the case came up for review, the surgeon general, Brigadier General Torney, stated that "it is a well known fact in medical practice that many of the lesions of syphilis are highly infectious and the syphilitic individual is capable of infecting persons by many routes. The conveyance of the disease by dental instruments has occurred more than once." Furthermore, he said "to permit a syphilitic dentist to continue in the practice of his profession in the Army would be to subject the officers and enlisted men who come under his treatment to the constant risk of acquiring syphilis." He recommended immediate annulment of the contract.[37] Another dentist was diagnosed in July 1913 as having secondary syphilis following a positive Wasserman examination. It was believed he acquired it as a result of a "puncture wound inflicted with dental instrument in line of duty." He never had any symptoms of the disease and served until he retired in 1932.[38]

Dental assistants became infected too. The case of a dental assistant at the 8th Infantry Infirmary, Camp Frémont, California, was recorded in the Army's syphilitic register: "The lesion occurred on the left thumb at the outer nail margin and was contracted while working on a patient's mouth. The initial lesion was followed in six weeks by marked secondaries and a double plus Wasserman reaction."[39] The "propriety of using rubber gloves when handling infected material" was stressed, as was instrument sterilization by boiling or autoclaving.[39]

In 1917 the US Army turned to Dr Hugh Hampton Young of the Johns Hopkins Hospital, Baltimore, Maryland, and Base Hospital No. 18 to head the Urological Service for the American Expeditionary Forces in France. Young had described the problems of venereal disease to Pershing and his staff onboard the *Baltic*, and Pershing already knew that venereal disease was one of the "most important problems confronting the Medical Corps" and had adopted

---

EXHIBIT 14-1

SYPHILIS IN THE US ARMY

According to LF Kishler,

> syphilis is an ancient disease, reportedly introduced into Europe in 1493 by the sailors returning with Columbus. It is peculiar to mankind and there is no disease with so great a variety of manifestations, nor none with a more insidious, deceptive and persistent course. There is no age, sex or physical condition which precludes the ravages of syphilis, and no tissue nor organ that is immune to its attack.

The known history of syphilis may be summarized as follows:

- 1903: Metchnikoff and Roux demonstrated animal inoculation with syphilitic tissue.
- 1905: Schaudin and Hoffman discovered the organism specific to syphilis, the Spirochaete Pallida.
- 1906–1907: Wasserman, Neisser, and Bruck developed the blood test for syphilis, the Wasserman test.
- 1910: Ehrlich discovered salvarsan or 606, the drug specific for the treatment of syphilis.
- 1911: Noguchi, at the Rockefeller Institute in New York, artificially cultivated the Spirochaete Pallida.

In 1919 the Surgeon General was deeply concerned about the high prevalence of venereal disease among US Army draftees and its effect on the civilian population. Congress passed the Chamberlain-Kahn Act, which charged the public health service with the "responsibility of organizing an effective campaign for the control of venereal diseases." The country's 45,000 dentists were enlisted in the fight, and a conference was held in Washington, DC, under the auspices of the National Capital Dental Society of the District of Columbia.

Data sources: (1) Kishler LF. The handling of syphilitic cases. *J Assoc Milit Dent Surg USA.* 1918;2:53–59. (2) Quetel C. *History of syphilis.* Baltimore, Md: Johns Hopkins University Press; 1992: 33–49. (3) Hirschfeld M. *The Sexual History of the World War.* New York, NY: Falstaff Press, Inc; 1937. (4) Blue R. Campaign to enlist the co-operation of the dental profession in the fight against venereal diseases. *Dental Cosmos.* 1919;61:1132.

"extraordinary measures to prevent venereal infection among his troops," both in the Philippines and Mexico. He fully expected Colonel Young to implement an aggressive approach for the AEF.[39]

Syphilis was not as common in the AEF as it was in the stateside Army. There were 12,680 primary admissions in the former and 51,528 in the latter.[30] In the American Army, the contraction of syphilis was an offense punishable by deprivation of pay and limitation of freedom until the malady was cured. For failure to report the disease and seek medical attention, a soldier was "hauled before a military court, and in case he had infected others, was sentenced to prison."[40,41]

Dr Vilray P Blair and Maxillofacial Surgery

Soon after the United States entered the war, the surgeon general's office examined the challenging issue of injuries to the face and jaw that were particularly
troublesome problems for the Allies and the Germans after 1914. In July 1917 Surgeon General Major General William Gorgas concluded that the Medical Department lacked the "number of general and dental surgeons sufficiently experienced
in plastic and oral surgery to take care of the cases of maxillofacial injuries that
we were likely to encounter." Gorgas set about securing the services of the surgeons and dental surgeons needed for this new maxillofacial service and to give
all of them additional training in plastic and oral surgery (see "War-Related Dental
Training on Civilian Campuses," Chapter 12). "These surgeons and dentists were
to work and be trained together so that units, to be composed of a surgeon and a
dental surgeon, could be formed which would give to the patients to be treated the
skill of the two professions."[42]

Gorgas formed the section of plastic and oral (maxillofacial) surgery in the
new division of surgery of the head to oversee the maxillofacial service, prepare
the training, and develop the policy for the treatment of such wounds among
American soldiers in France. Apparently on the recommendation of Dr William
Mayo of the Mayo Clinic, in late July 1917 Gorgas chose Major (later Lieutenant
Colonel) Vilray P Blair (1871–1955) of the Medical Officers' Reserve Corps, then at
the medical officers' training camp at Fort Oglethorpe, Georgia, to head up this effort as the chief of the section of plastic and oral (maxillofacial) surgery, and to act
as the consultant to the surgeon general for maxillofacial surgery. Blair was then a
leading maxillofacial, plastic, and reconstructive surgeon at the Washington University School of Medicine in Saint Louis, Missouri. In August Captain Robert H
Ivy (1881–1974), Medical Officers' Reserve Corps, holder of a DDS (1902) and MD
(1907) from the University of Pennsylvania, became his assistant. Working closely
with then Major William HG Logan, who had just become chief of the surgeon
general's new dental section in August 1917 and was himself a well-known oral
and plastic surgeon, Blair and Ivy handled the selection and specialized training
program for surgeons and dental surgeons in maxillofacial surgery first at Washington University on October 15, 1917, and later at the University of Pennsylvania
and Northwestern University. That same year, Blair added a chapter on trauma
to his already classic *Surgery and Diseases of the Mouth and Jaws: a Practical Treatise
on the Surgery and Diseases of the Mouth and Allied Subjects*,[43] and this third edition was adopted as the manual for care of military maxillofacial cases. From the
very beginning, Blair's deep personal and professional involvement in this work
shaped it both in the United States and later the AEF. In the postwar years, Blair
and Ivy became founders of modern American plastic and reconstructive surgery.
Blair was also a driving force in the establishment of the American Board of Plastic
Surgery in 1937.[42–49]

Blair's policy for the maxillofacial service was based on two "fundamental
principles": "the close cooperation of surgeons and dental surgeons"; and "the
early institution and the continuous and systematic conduct of treatment."[44] To
achieve this, Blair laid out three requirements:

. . . first, a sufficiently large personnel to be available at every advanced and at all intermediate and base hospitals; second, a definite general plan of treatment which, instituted in the advanced hospitals, would be carried out without radical change in each of the hospitals to which the wounded would be subsequently evacuated, and thirdly, and not unimportant, suitable equipment.[50]

Blair pointed out that the "proper treatment of maxillofacial injuries rests on the same surgical principles as that of wounds in any other part of the body."[50] However, this work required the special skills of the dental surgeon to be successful:

. . . because the proper splinting of a fractured jaw requires dental splints, or splints with dental attachment, and because few surgeons have familiarized themselves with the physiology and the special pathology of the oral structures, to do the work efficiently requires, as a rule, the cooperation of a surgeon with a dental surgeon who has made a special study of the subject.[50]

He later added:

except for intermaxillary wiring, only the dental surgeon is equipped to splint a fractured jaw and it is the latter who will ultimately carry the major part of the burden in the greater number of cases, but intelligent cooperation is essential throughout the whole treatment.[51]

Speaking at the October 24, 1917, meeting of the Clinical Congress of Surgeons of North America (now the American College of Surgeons) in Chicago, Blair described the structure, training, and practice of the Army's new maxillofacial service.[52] He stressed the cooperation of surgeons and dental surgeons as essential to success, and called for an end to their old antagonisms:

Of not uncommon occurrence in the present war are those distressing wounds of the face and jaw which have attracted particular attention, not only on account of the disfigurement which they cause, but even more so from the difficulty that was at first encountered in dealing with them. This difficulty is the logical outcome of an attitude that regarded dentistry and surgery as two distinct and separate professions. As long as this theory was allowed to dominate practice, a man who had an extensive injury of the face and jaw-bone had about as much chance of an ideal result as had the man with an open fracture of a limb in the days when the physician and the bone-setter could find no common ground upon which to meet. The bone-setter, and the physician who refused to recognize the surgeon, are of the past, but the surgeon and the dentist in their relation to each other only too frequently perpetuate the agnosticism of those older practitioners.[52]

Drawing heavily on the existing wartime experience of Varaztad H Kazanjian, George B Hayes, William S Davenport, and others, Blair, Ivy, and Logan planned to assign what Blair called "units," a surgeon and dentist qualified in maxillofacial surgery who had trained and worked together, to each evacuation and base hospital in France, "so that from the very first each of the patients will receive the best that surgery has to offer." In addition, Blair was to take another group of units to France to study French and British techniques and conduct "special work." By the time the training was completed in the United States in March 1918, 164 surgeons and 123 dental officers had taken the courses, but 40 of them were never assigned to either maxillofacial work or to the AEF.[49,52,53]

The American Expeditionary Force's Maxillofacial Surgery Service

While the maxillofacial medical and dental personnel were selected and trained in the United States, the AEF confronted the immediate need to treat jaw wounds and injuries. Oliver and the chief surgeon's office considered selecting a limited number of base hospitals that would be designated "jaw centers" and be provided with the trained personnel and special equipment needed to handle maxillofacial cases. Six hospitals were tentatively selected and then held in reserve for the most severe cases requiring evacuation to the United States: Base Hospital No. 18, Bazoilles (the Johns Hopkins Hospital Unit, Baltimore, Maryland); Base Hospital No. 15, Chaumont (Roosevelt Hospital Unit, New York City); Base Hospital No. 21, Dijon (Washington University School of Medicine Unit, Saint Louis); Base Hospital No. 26, Angers (University of Minnesota Unit, Minneapolis, Minnesota); Base Hospital No. 6, Bordeaux (Massachusetts General Hospital Unit, Boston); and Base Hospital No. 8, Savenay (Post-Graduate Hospital Unit, New York City).[54–56]

When the Army Sanitary School opened at Langres in December 1917, the dental section's curriculum included instruction in war dentistry and "a practical knowledge of face and jaw surgery." Much of latter instruction fell to First Lieutenant William H Potter, an experienced former professor of oral surgery at Harvard Dental School who also knew British and French practice. However, it became clear that more advanced training in "oral, plastic and prosthetic surgery" would be needed once American forces were fully engaged in combat operations and face and jaw wounds became more numerous. Thus, the American Red Cross Military Hospital No. 1 (formerly the American Ambulance) at Neuilly, was again selected as the training site for the postgraduate course because its staff, with George B Hayes and William S Davenport, had extensive experience treating such injuries since 1914 (for more information, see "The European War: The American Ambulance, Neuilly, Paris, France, 1914–1916" and "Opportunities and Missed Opportunities" in Chapter 11). A qualified faculty was easily identified and a full curriculum developed. The opening of the school was initially set for January 1918, but was then deferred until April 1. The massive German offensive against the British in Flanders that began on March 21, 1918, forced the indefinite postponement of the school's opening because all hospitals in the Paris region and forward were overwhelmed with Allied casualties. Continuing German operations that spring reached the Marne in late May and prevented the school from ever opening. By then, the arrival at Brest, France, on April 18 of Blair and his carefully selected oral and plastic surgery unit of 18 surgeons and 15 dental surgeons, all specialists in maxillofacial surgery, greatly diminished the need for the school at Neuilly.[54,57,58]

In the interim, however, various initiatives were undertaken on both sides of the Atlantic to train additional Medical and Dental corps officers in oral and plastic surgery. Apparently, Blair, Ivy, and Logan carefully reviewed those personnel passing through the maxillofacial training programs and identified the best

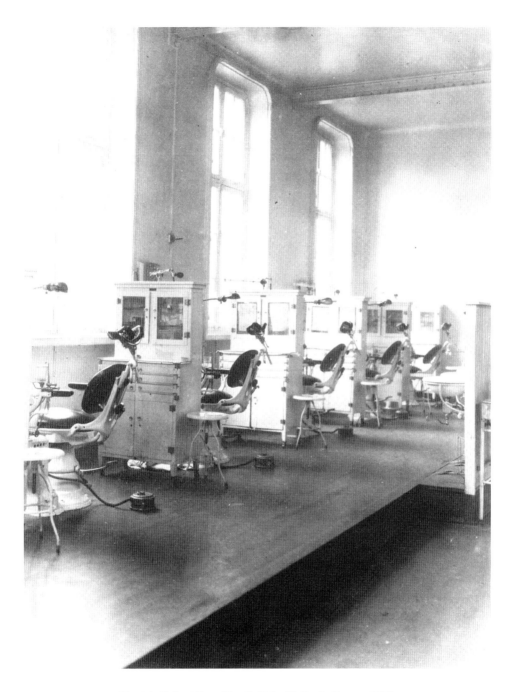

Dental clinic at Base Hospital No. 57, Paris, France, 1918.
Photograph: Courtesy of the National Library of Medicine.

candidates for continuing involvement once they had moved to France. In at least one instance, Lieutenant Colonel Walter R Parker, chief of the section of surgery of the head in the Office of The Surgeon General, informed the commander of Base Hospital No. 3 (Mount Sinai Hospital Unit, New York City) at Vauclaire, France, in Base Section No. 2, that Captain Robert T Frank, Medical Officers' Reserve Corps, the staff surgeon in oral and plastic surgery, and First Lieutenant Jacob Asch, DRC, dental surgeon, had been "nominated to do the oral and plastic surgery" for his hospital. Parker said that "it is suggested that it would be desirable, if possible, to give these men an opportunity to see some of the plastic and oral surgery that is now being done abroad." He suggested that they be allowed to visit one of the special British or French hospitals, "if only for a few days," so that they would be better able to care for such cases.[59] While Asch had attended the special training at Washington University during October 1917, there was no indication of any such training in Captain Frank's case. However, the other dental surgeon of Base Hospital No. 3, First Lieutenant Leo Stern, DRC, had also completed a 2-week special maxillofacial surgery course at the University of Pennsylvania in December 1917 before being ordered to active duty. Both Asch and Stern later attended the Army Sanitary School during April and June 1918, respectively, and received additional special training in plastic and oral surgery. Dr Frank was detached and sent for temporary duty to Base Hospital No. 15 at Chaumont, where he remained until December 1918. Asch and Stern served as the dental surgeons on duty at Base Hospital No. 3 until the hospital closed down in February 1919, after which they returned to the United States.[60–63]

Soon after his arrival in France, Blair was named AEF senior consultant in maxillofacial service and was provided with special orders from General Pershing, the AEF commander, "which swept away any difficulties I might otherwise have had."[487] Following a period as casuals observing French and British field hospitals, the members of Blair's unit spent an intensive 10-week period in England devoted to training in the reconstruction of head and face wounds. After the training, the men returned to France and were assigned to AEF hospitals. As Blair originally envisioned, one maxillofacial unit composed of a surgeon, surgical assistant, and dental surgeon was to be positioned in each evacuation hospital to initiate the early treatment that was seen as critical. A unit was also sent to each base hospital each base hospital for continuing care, but no such teams were planned for the mobile and American Red Cross military hospitals. The AEF's early plans for specialized maxillofacial service at selected base hospitals also soon disappeared under the stress of operational requirements. Careful planning gave way to a system of personal arrangements agreed to among Blair, Colonel William Keller (1874–1959), the dean of the Medical Corps' surgeons and the surgical consultant to the AEF, Colonel Oliver, and the individual hospital commanders who selected the best-qualified and most-interested personnel from their staffs for maxillofacial work. At the same time, Oliver assigned qualified dental surgeons to each base and evacuation hospital "to care for prosthetic and splint work," but they were also often diverted to other duties.[49,52,54,64]

After reaching an agreement with Keller and Oliver in a June 11, 1918, memorandum, Blair further fleshed out this concept with a set of recommendations on early treatment and evacuation policy, as well the placement and selection of surgeons and dental surgeons for the AEF's maxillofacial service. This included "specially qualified teams" located in all evacuation hospitals and in 17 base hospitals and hospital centers throughout the advance, intermediate, and base sections of the services of supply and a "reconstruction center" at Vichy with the specialized Base Hospital No. 115 that was coming from the United States.[54,64,65] One of the reasons that Vichy was selected was that French Maxillofacial Hospital No. 45 was also located there. Captain Fernand LeMaitre of the French Medical Corps, the surgical chief of at Hospital No. 45, had extensive experience in caring for facial wound cases and had developed new techniques and appliances. LeMaitre was willing to share his knowledge and cooperate with American dentisits.[66]

On June 26 Blair followed up his recommendations of June 11 with another memorandum to the chief surgeon outlining the treatment and evacuation policy to be adopted for specific cases, focusing treatment of the most serious cases at Base Hospital No. 115 at Vichy. Again, he emphasized that "these cases shall be attended by the surgeon and the dental surgeon jointly."[67]

In 1919 Blair reflected on how the new AEF maxillofacial service eventually developed:

Shortly after we arrived in France, a senior consultant for maxillofacial surgery for the American Expeditionary Forces was appointed [Blair], and a policy for the care of these cases outlined, which differed little from the plan contemplated by the Surgeon General. Information as to the general plan for evacuation and treatment of these patients was sent out. France was divided into seven parts, to each of which a local or area consultant for maxillofacial surgery was appointed. In each American hospital center the cases were concentrated as far as practicable in one hospital, where they were attended by a local consultant for the center, in cooperation with special selected dental surgeons.[50(p326)]

However, it took considerable time and effort and some changes in the original plans for this to come to fruition. The urgent need for surgeons to treat the surge of casualties generated in the heavy defensive fighting around Château-Thierry and along the Marne River (which blunted the German offensive toward Paris), and the subsequent Allied summer offensives, often required that the surgeons be diverted for more general surgical work.[50(p326)] Blair explained:

The atmosphere of war, in spite of intense concentration, is one of distraction. All plans of specialization are more or less ideal, and it takes time to put any subordinate plan into operation, especially if it is far-reaching in its application. Each hospital organized in the Surgeon-General's Office had attached to it a surgeon and a dental surgeon designated for this work; but in the earlier part of the severe fighting, all specialization was overshadowed by more vital problems. It is no secret that, owing to the lack of transportation, we were short of surgeons and dental surgeons in the American Expeditionary Forces, and that at Chateau Thierry most of the surgical consultants were ordered to form general operating teams, and they stood twelve hour shifts at the table at any hospital where they could find space; while the dental surgeons were often giving anesthetics, carrying stretchers or giving first aid treatment.[50(p326)]

Blair later added that circumstances overwhelmed his plans but not his personnel:

> . . . failure of realization to the fullest extent was not due to want of cooperation of the medical or dental professions, either in civilian life or in the Army, but to the exigencies of the war. Where the plans actually fell short, disaster was averted by the splendid spirit of the personnel who at any time and anywhere made ingenuity and enthusiasm compensate for material and conveniences when either or both of the latter were lacking.[51(p379)]

A member of Blair's group, First Lieutenant Arthur Lankford, DRC, was stationed at American Red Cross Military Hospital No. 1 at Neuilly and provided a graphic description of the role of the dentist as an anesthetist during the battle of Château-Thierry in 1918. Lankford states that the dentists were "giving the anesthetics and there were all kinds of wounds," not just jaw wounds:

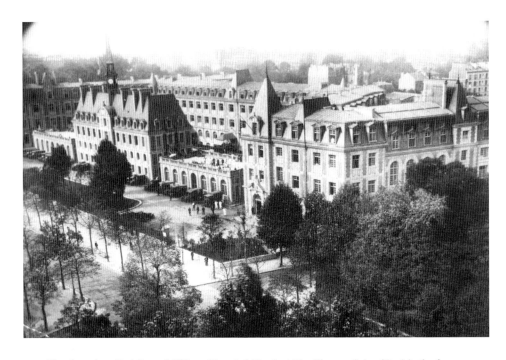

The American Red Cross Military Hospital No. 1 at Neuilly-sur-Seine (Paris), the former American Ambulance (American Hospital), came under Army Medical Department leadership from 1917 through 1919 and supported the American Expeditionary Forces. Here, in 1914, Doctors George Hayes and William Davenport first established their maxillofacial dental clinic to treat wounded French soldiers and in 1918, along with Army plastic and dental surgeons, treated American soldiers with maxillofacial injuries. Photograph: Courtesy of Dr Arthur Lankford.

I think it was eight tables in our operating room . . . and they were lined up like this with wires running across the top. They'd cut off a leg or an arm to be put in a thing on this wire, and give it a push and push it over, and by the time we had been there for two or three days, blood was an inch or so deep all over the tile floor. . . . We had stretcher bearers coming in, great big strong men. When they came to that door to bring a pa-tient in and saw the arms and legs hanging up on these wires, and the blood all over the floor, walking through it, some of them just fainted, just keeled right over . . . .

When they first came in, I took over and took care of the bone. You see, you can't build unless you've got something to build on. I would get the bones set in the proper posi-tion, get the splints made. I had to design all kinds of new kinds of splints, we had never seen anything like it before, and get the jaw stabilized, and then when the time came, we worked in pairs, the general surgeon and dental. Then when I got that all fixed, the framework of the bone for the jaw, then the surgeon would take over and I would be the assistant, and we would do the plastic work.

I would go to sleep just sitting up there. I just couldn't stand it any longer. Then by that time some team would come in from someplace and take over. I would go back to my room, bed, and I would just fall on the bed with my clothes on, and too sleepy and tired to get them off. And I would lay there maybe for a day and a night without waking up, just like I was dead. And then I would have to get up, take a bath, and wash and come on back to the operating room and start over again. That was how busy we were at that time.[68]

After the war, Dr Lankford, a 1912 graduate of the Baltimore College of Dental Surgery, resumed his dental practice in Baltimore until his retirement in the mid 1960s. He died in November 1984, at the age of 96.[69]

The experiences of trench warfare, with the "wholesale destruction of tissue by an infinite variety of projectiles and the ever-present dangers from battlefields planted with pyrogenic microorganisms through centuries of fertilization with manure," had changed the routine treatment of wounds previously found to be satisfactory. The majority of wounds caused by pieces of shell and shrapnel were infected, and even rifle wounds were "rarely aseptic." Accordingly, all wounds were treated with antiseptics with "Listerian rigor," as if all were infected. Dakin's solution (an aqueous solution of 0.5% sodium hyperchlorite) was used to irrigate the wounds. The free use of antitetanic serum largely prevented the "horrors of tetanus."[70] The antitetanus vaccine was given intramuscularly as quickly as pos-sible after the receipt of a wound. The usual British dose was 500 units, and each British soldier was given a "field card" as part of his equipment, noting the fact that he had received the injection. When the patient was evacuated to a base hospi-tal, he received a second injection of 500 units 7 days after the first, to be repeated every 7 days until 2,000 units had been given.[71]

Due to continuing heavy demands resulting from the summer's defensive and offensive operations, it took longer than originally intended to get the maxillofacial service up and running. The service had begun its work in evacuation and base hospitals, as per original plan, and where possible, teams were added to the 12 far-forward mobile hospitals (mobile hospitals nos. 1–11 and 39) that were shifted along the front to sectors of the greatest demand. If possible, a team consisting of a surgeon, surgical assistant, and dental surgeon were assigned to each evacuation hospital, with the surgeon in charge of the team. The dentist did the splinting or wiring of the jaw fractures, working in cooperation with the surgeon. However, the plan soon proved impractical because not enough teams could be formed in the United States for deployment to France, and the necessary specialized equipment that was required was either lacking or never reached the advanced hospitals. Many of the jaw wounds were also not properly classified in the forward triage; consequently patients were not sent to the waiting teams at the designated specialty base hospitals. Moreover, as the official history of maxillofacial surgery emphasized, the basic function of the advanced mobile hospitals close to the front lines was:

> to prepare patients for evacuation to the rear, it was rarely possible to make either a segregation or a selection of types of cases. Early treatment of a special character by those qualified to administer it was not subordinated, likewise, to this prime military necessity.[44,72–74]

Blair and Oliver took much of the responsibility for getting the right personnel in the right places before the maxillofacial service could really become effective. In late June Blair resurrected the concept of a special 2-month training course "to provide facilities for instructing certain dental officers in the technique of the dental part of maxillo-facial surgery" at American Red Cross Military Hospital No. 1. Although this training scheme was approved and apparently started by July 17, Blair informed Oliver that "at present, Paris looks difficult as an instruction center."[75–78]

Following his inspection tour to many of the base, camp, and evacuation hospitals then in operation, as well as to Mobile Operating Unit No. 1 and No. 39 and Field Hospital No. 23, 2nd Division, Blair forwarded a "future work plan of the Maxillo-Facial Service" to Brigadier General Ireland, the chief surgeon, on July 18, 1918. The policy agreed to by Oliver and Keller was that "provisions have been or will be made to treat these cases in every hospital to which they first come or to which they are evacuated, so that early and continuous treatment will be assured."[79] To support this promise, Oliver and Blair agreed on coordinating the assignments of the most qualified individual dental surgeons to base hospitals and to mobile hospital and surgical units. There they would be available for jaw splinting and emergency dental work, and they could be used as anesthetists when not so engaged. This often proved to be demanding duty. Most times the dentist was on call 24 hours a day, frequently working without breaks. The care of the soft parts and the general supervision of a case were the domain of the general surgeon, who had no special training in plastic work. Although not ideal, this system produced some very good results and was the best that could be done under the circumstances.[72,78–82]

Based on his inspection visits to numerous base hospitals, and perhaps also due to troubles with his training plan at Neuilly, Blair noted in a July 18 letter to the chief surgeon that many of the resident dental surgeons had serious professional weaknesses in maxillofacial procedures and care. He recommended that dental surgeons currently lacking the necessary professional skills in the maxillofacial service be assigned for temporary training at those hospitals with surgeons who were already skilled at handling such cases:

At certain Base Hospitals that have been in service in this country for a long time, the dental surgeon is not, either for want of experience, inclination or special training, at present fitted to do the dental part of the Maxillo-facial service in the most desirable manner. It is not desirable, if it can be avoided, to absolutely displace those men who have endured the waiting period, with the expectation or hope that some of this work would eventually come to their care. . . . It is believed that any discontent that might arise from such a move might be avoided by assigning those dental surgeons who have suitable academic qualifications temporarily to one of the special hospitals of the Maxillo-facial service, to later be returned to their stations when it is adjudged that they are fitted to care for the dental part of the Maxillo-facial service.[80]

After he had been in France for several months and had completed his inspections, Blair developed standard guidelines for surgeons and dental surgeons handling maxillofacial cases that were issued in bulletins and circulars of the chief surgeon. The guidance laid out eight essential principles to be followed:

1. All maxillofacial wounds shall undergo thorough mechanical cleansing.

2. There shall be no or only minimal debridement of face injuries.

3. No bone fragment having any soft tissue attachment shall be removed.

4. Immediate steps shall be taken to arrest hemorrhage, and to prevent secondary hemorrhage.

5. There shall be immediate fixation of all jaw fractures.

6. Adequate inferior drainage shall be established in all fracture cases.

7. As much primary suture of face tissues shall be done as is consistent with good surgical principles.

8. Cases shall be evacuated to the base hospitals as quickly as possible.[65,72,83]

In its guidelines on debridement and primary suture, the directives ran counter to the surgical principles used in the AEF, but for good reason. Major George C Schaeffer, MC, the maxillofacial area consultant for the hospitals at Toul, Bazoilles, Vittal, Chaumont, Rimaucourt, and Langres, a surgeon at the Justice Hospital Center at Toul, and Blair's assistant, pointed out why:

In the handling of face cases there were two reasons why we should not follow these general rules: In the first place, thorough debridement of all face injuries would have meant the sacrifice of an immense amount of facial tissue which never could have been adequately replaced, and which, if removed, would have necessitated a great amount of unsatisfactory secondary plastic surgery. In the second place, it was shown that there was practically no danger from gas infection in face wounds, no case to my knowledge having been reported.[72]

On August 21, 1918, Blair recommended that all face and jaw injuries reaching the Hospital Center at Bazoilles, France, be concentrated in a ward at Base Hospital No. 42 of that center, where Captain Hugh W Brent, Medical Reserve Corps, was in charge of the surgical care. Captain Brent had received his orders on March

30, 1918, to join Major Blair in Hoboken, New Jersey, for transportation to France "for duty at special English or French hospitals to study methods preparatory for future assignments," and was one of Blair's original team members. He completed 3 months' work in the British Jaw and Plastic Hospital at Sidcup, England, "a special course" in the United States, and was "sympathetic with and conversant with the aims of this service." [84,85] In addition, Blair put First Lieutenant B Lucien Brun, DRC, stationed at Base Hospital No. 18 (The Johns Hopkins Hospital unit), in charge of the "splinting of these cases" in cooperation with Brent. Brun had "special qualifications" for this work and had observed its application in Allied jaw hospitals in May and June. Blair believed that this arrangement would "simplify the problem of equipment and of dental mechanic" and would add greatly to the "efficiency of the Maxillo-Facial Service of that Center."[86] Working under Brent, Brun circulated among base hospitals 18, 42, 46, and 116 in the Hospital Center, Bazoilles, which treated maxillofacial cases. His more modern dental clinic and laboratory apparently fabricated all of the special splints that Brun then applied (see "Dental Work in a Base Hospital" above).[23] In his endorsement to Blair's memo, Colonel James D Glennan, MC, in the chief surgeon's office, made it clear that the commanding officers of the hospital centers could transfer personnel among the center's various hospital units and organize these "more or less specialized" units "as they see fit."[87] In other words, they were not required to establish wards and assign staff only to treat specific cases.

Maxillofacial cases evacuated to the Paris District were treated at the American Red Cross Military Hospital No. 1 at Neuilly, which had specialized in these cases since 1914 under Doctors George B Hayes and William S Davenport. The hospital, which had been under the supervision of the AEF chief surgeon since July 1917, now had both Army surgeons and dental surgeons on the staff to work under Hayes and Davenport. Other cases that could not be treated in the hospital in which they were initially admitted could be evacuated to a base hospital of a hospital center where there was a maxillofacial surgeon, or to Base Hospital No. 115 at the Vichy Hospital Center (which theater medical and dental personnel were operating pending the arrival of the unit from the United States in August or September 1918). Maxillofacial cases requiring only "occasional surgical or dental supervision" were sent from the base hospitals to convalescent camps to await further examination or operation.[88–90]

Oliver and Blair took advantage of the lull in American operations in late August and early September, prior to the Saint Mihiel offensive, to adjust the service to support the upcoming operations. Blair later commented that "after August 20, there was a breathing spell, during which this service really got on its feet; and from the Battle of the Argonne, September 25, it was on the job and delivering the goods at all stations."[50]

After months of effort, Blair finally obtained approval for the formal appointment of seven local, or area, consultants for maxillofacial service, who would be responsible for overseeing the maxillofacial surgery in the assigned hospital centers and base hospitals, as well as for handling surgical cases themselves.[50,91] On September 20 Blair appointed the seven consultants, each stationed at a hospital center, and a practicing surgeon, to oversee maxillofacial cases in the advance, intermediate, and base sections of the services of supply and the Paris region.[91]

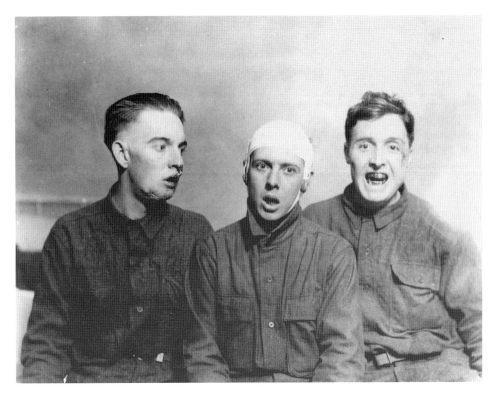

Three soldiers with splints, Base Hospital No. 6, Bordeaux, France.
Photograph: Courtesy of the National Library of Medicine.

Four days later, he sent each of the area consultants a more detailed letter laying out their responsibilities for "facilitating the coordination of the dental and surgical work in this service, and this service as a whole to other surgical services; by doing this to bring this service to its greatest efficiency."[92] Major George C Schaeffer, MC, maxillofacial consultant for the zone of the advance, advance section of the services of supply, and the Toul Hospital Center, described the obstacles that he had to overcome to develop a functioning maxillofacial service:

> . . . it was my duty to organize our forces and resources for the accomplishment of our aims. Our forces in surgeons and dentists were meager, and our resources in materials were still less. On my first visit to the advance hospitals I found practically no plastic surgeons, only a limited number of dentists, and no equipment for caring for face cases. It was necessary to secure dentists to supply the hospitals that were without them. This was done through the chief dental surgeon of the A.E.F. [Oliver]. Directors of surgery and commanding officers of hospitals had to be shown the necessity of having some systematized plan for handling our cases. They had to be convinced of the wisdom of the maxillofacial rules of treatment, and as these differed so essentially from those governing other cases, this was no mean task. It was only with difficulty that many of them were induced to consent to calling in the dentist to help splint jaw cases, but it was very gratifying on later visits to find dentists and surgeons working in close cooperation.[72(pp859–860)]

563

On the same day that he secured the appointment of the local consultants, Blair wrote to Colonel Walter Parker in the surgeon general's office to update him on the progress of the AEF's maxillofacial program. "If I were a committee I would report progress," he opened, "you know what that means." He noted some of the problems affecting the program, especially in the area of evacuation, and lamented that "they have recently changed the general evacuation order so that cases cannot be kept over three months."[93] Blair remained optimistic about his work and rejected ideas about returning to the United States:

> I believe that if we can get the service established on the basis of the present recommendations that we can retain 75% of these cases here for active duty, and save a large amount of recovery time on all. It was the hope of doing this that made me consent to come over.[91]

On October 4, 1918, the AEF Office of the Chief Surgeon issued Circular No. 50, which laid out the basic policies for handling maxillofacial cases:

> Cases evacuated to the Paris District will be treated at the American Red Cross Military Hospital No. 1. Other cases that cannot be treated in the hospital in which they are situated may, on request of the local or senior Consultant in Maxillo-facial Surgery, be evacuated to a base hospital or hospital center where there is a maxillo-facial service, or to Base Hospital No. 115, Vichy.
>
> Maxillo-facial cases requiring only occasional surgical or dental supervision may be sent from base hospitals to convalescent camps to await further examination or operation.
>
> No Maxillo-facial case should be evacuated to the United States until the patient can open his mouth sufficiently and has the pharyngeal muscle control necessary to obviate the danger of aspiration during sea sickness.
>
> Cases that have been recently repaired should be retained in hospital until the sutured wound is safely healed.[88]

All of the work done by Blair and Oliver eventually paid off. After completing a 4-day tour of advanced hospitals in the First and Second US Armies, Blair, now a lieutenant colonel, wrote to Oliver on October 26:

> I was extremely well pleased with what I found and believe that I can safely say that this service is established there and is a success. With very few exceptions the Surgeons and Dental Surgeons are working in hearty cooperation and the cases are coming back splinted, drained and with what repairs of the soft parts which at the time were indicated.[95]

The next day he wrote to the chief surgeon of the AEF, saying that existing instructions already called for early care of maxillofacial cases "by a surgeon and a dental surgeon jointly." Blair noted that "wherever this plan is in operation this service is being conducted on a very high plane of efficiency and it is believed that this efficiency cannot be accomplished in any other manner."[96] Wartime experience confirmed Blair's two "fundamental principles" of early and consistent treatment by a surgeon and dental surgeon team.

Of the 2,000 to 2,500 cases of jaw and face injuries among the American wounded in France, Oliver estimated that two thirds were treated in hospitals in France and returned to duty. Only the most severe cases that required extensive reconstructive surgery, had a recovery time exceeding 4 months, and were deemed unfit for additional duty were to be evacuated to the United States beginning in October 1918. In all, a total of 694 patients were transferred by the time the last evacuees arrived in 1919. At first they went to General Hospital No. 11 at Cape May, New Jersey, for specialized maxillofacial care. When that hospital could no longer handle all the cases, maxillofacial centers were also set up at Walter Reed General Hospital (under Lieutenant Colonel VP Blair and Robert H Ivy upon their return from France in 1919); General Hospital No. 2 at Fort McHenry, Baltimore, Maryland (under Major George C Schaeffer, MC, from the Justice Hospital Center at Toul, upon his return in 1919); and General Hospital No. 40 at Saint Louis, Missouri.[44,65,67,97–104] Blair also later worked with maxillofacial patients and as a consultant at the station hospital at Jefferson Barracks near Saint Louis, which took over patient care when General Hospital No. 40 closed.[48]

In addition to a lack of personnel and the press of operational demands, the AEF's maxillofacial service suffered severely from the need of special equipment, of which little ever arrived in France and was delivered to the teams. Blair realized that "shells and food take precedence over other things," which forced his surgeons and dentists to use "their wits."[50]

> To the credit of our dental surgeons, they used their wits, and by piecing out our own supplies with what the chief dental surgeon could obtain from the French; by beating two franc pieces into splints; by robbing the shell-cut telephone wires, and by cutting meat tins into splints, from the beginning of the Argonne there were few patients who reached the base hospitals unsplinted.[50(p326)]

Major George C Schaeffer, MC, one of the area maxillofacial surgical consultants, fully agreed:

> The ingenuity of the American dentist is such that he can be trusted to find some way out of almost any difficulty, and the lack of equipment and materials never daunted him. In the preparation for another war, should such a misfortune befall us, I have no doubt that some standardized method of procedure will be adopted and carried out; but should we ever be caught again as unprepared as we were this time, it is very comforting to know that we have dental men who can be depended on to meet the emergency as efficiently as they did in France during the later months of the war.[69(pp858–859)]

Base Hospital No. 115: the Special Head Hospital

Base Hospital No. 115 was originally organized in February 1918 as part of General Hospital No. 11 at Cape May, New Jersey. It was under the direction of the surgeon general as a "Special Head Hospital" intended to care for eye, ear, nose, throat, brain, and maxillofacial cases. The hospital was staffed with specialists and equipped as a base hospital, but was provided with all the additional equipment and supplies required for its special work. The AEF called the hospital to France in May 1918, but it shipped to England and France in a piecemeal fashion and did not reach France until August and Vichy until early September. At Vichy, Base Hospital No. 115 joined Base Hospital No. 1 (Bellevue Hospital, New York) and No. 19 (Rochester, New York) and Auxiliary Hospital Unit D (Louisville, Kentucky) in the Hospital Center. No. 115 took over the Hotel Ruhl, a 9-story concrete building then reputed to be the tallest building in France, with a maximum capacity of 1,657 beds (which also made it the largest hospital under one roof in the world).[105(pp618,621,732,733)106,107]

Awaiting the arrival of Base Hospital No. 115, Blair and Oliver assigned Major Stewart D Ruggles, DC, and Captain Thomas M Terry, DC, both from Blair's original group, to Base Hospital No. 1 and the dental department at the Hotel Ruhl beginning July 19. During an inspection in August, Colonel Henry C Fisher, the AEF's general medical inspector, reported that Ruggles had started a dental department in the hotel "using some of his own instruments and those of Base Hospital No. 1" and that "a great deal of jaw surgery is being done." On August 30 Blair recommended that the surgical part of the maxillofacial service in Base Hospital

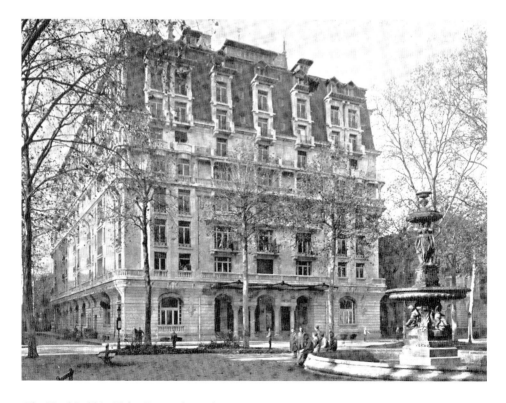

The Hotel Ruhl in Vichy, France, housed Base Hospital No. 115, the Medical Department's special head and maxillofacial hospital unit, from September 1918 until February 1919 when it closed. Reproduced from: Clarke CW. A History of U.S.A. Base Hospital No. 115, A.P.O. 781, A.E.F., Vichy, Allier, France. Memphis, Tenn: Toof; 1919.

No. 115 be under Captain Henry Dunning, MC, assisted by Captains Justin W Waugh and Harry B Huver of the Medical Officers' Reserve Corps, who were members of his original team like Ruggles and Thomas.[90] By the time the full 115th reached Vichy, Ruggles and Terry already had a significant dental and maxillofacial practice in progress.[106,108,109] On September 20 the effectiveness of the maxillofacial care at Vichy was greatly enhanced when Major Robert H Ivy, Blair's assistant in the United States who finally arrived in France, was assigned to the Hospital Center as the area maxillofacial consultant and a resident surgeon stationed at Base Hospital No. 115.[91,107]

Operational necessity soon took precedence over long-laid plans for the maxillofacial rehabilitation center. The influx of wounded soldiers resulting from the Meuse-Argonne offensive, combined with the arrival of only 10% of the needed specialized equipment and supplies, soon ended any thoughts that Base Hospital No. 115 would be able to focus solely on the care of head and maxillofacial cases.[49,105(p733),106] The outcome was lamented in the base hospital's history:

> . . . it soon became evident to the staff of the hospital that the institution would not fulfil the purposes for which it was intended, namely to function as a special head hospital. The large majority of head cases coming to the Center were sent to No. 115, but the bulk of patients admitted were the usual variety of medical and surgical cases. Very good eye and ear, nose and throat clinics were built up in the hospital, and a very active maxillo-facial service was maintained, thanks to the interest of Lieutenant Colonel V.P. Blair, the Chief Consultant in Maxillo-Facial Surgery for the A.E.F., but for a variety of reasons, preventable and otherwise, special cases were not routed to No. 115 from other hospitals in the A.E.F. in any considerable numbers. It is a source of satisfaction to the organization that it was able to handle efficiently the large number of cases of a character different from that which its personnel was specially qualified to treat.[106(p23)]

A dental surgeon's experience at a hospital such as Base Hospital No. 115 differed mostly in the severity of cases. Major Ruggles, DC, a 1896 graduate of Northwestern University Dental School, worked with jaw injuries at the hospital and recalled that longer, more complex care was required to assure that the best work possible was done on maxillofacial cases. In the month of September 1918, he treated 135 cases, including 50 fractured jaws and 60 gunshot wounds of the mouth. Unlike his British colleagues, he felt no pressure to return the soldiers to duty as fast as possible. Rather, he took the time necessary to do the most thorough and cosmetic job possible while trying to enhance patient morale, which he thought could be accomplished by the hospital facilities and the "earnest and capable men" engaged in the work.[26,97,98]

Ruggles described how the typical case was handled:

> Each case was taken up in accord with the plan devised by the section of maxillo-facial surgery. The routine work of records, X-ray and diagnosis followed as soon after the patient's arrival as was consistent with his condition. The case was gone over with the surgical staff, and any surgical work such as curettements, extractions, removal of foreign bodies was done under ether before the splinting was undertaken. All teeth in the line of fracture, or so injured as to cause trouble later were removed except when it was imperative to retain them for a temporary purpose. This applied to unattached

bone. Then free drainage was established at the most dependent point. Hemorrhage was not a serious factor, except in badly infected cases. Pneumonia developed in but two instances. Both of these favorable conditions were attributed to the rigid mouth requirements of our army, and a regular hygiene insisted upon from the beginning of the treatment. Just as the patient was able to endure the ordeal, impressions were made in modeling compound, each section separately, then assembled anatomically. From these, wax impressions were made, the splints cast in maxilor [sic], a silver-copper alloy, used by the French.[49(pp997–998)]

Feeding maxillofacial patients was also a major consideration, and Ruggles explained how it was done at Vichy:

Upon entrance all fracture cases were placed on a liquid diet consisting of soup, porridge, cocoa, eggnog, grape juice, and milk when obtainable. Five feedings a day were given. All patients with jaws closed were kept on liquids, though many appliances permitted of semi-solids for which we were glad. The dietician received regular daily reports and prepared meals according to it. A special meat grinder was installed for preparing semi-solids, thus allowing vegetables and meats to be added to the diet list. At first a loss of weight was quite apparent, but after the third week the gain was marked.[49(p999)]

The Hospital Center at Vichy and Base Hospital No. 115 treated 505 maxillofacial cases between September 12, 1918, and January 18, 1919, when the last case was ready for evacuation. Of these cases, 145 were of the soft tissues only, and 159 involved maxilla, mandible, or both and the malar bone. During this same period, Base Hospital No. 115 performed 137 operations on maxillofacial patients, 72 of which were for curettement and drainage of jaw fractures.[110]

Treatment of Jaw Fractures: Kazanjian's Technique

In June 1918 Major William C Speakman, DC, a well-known oral surgeon, traveled to Base Hospital No. 20 (Harvard Unit; British Expeditionary Forces General Hospital No. 22) at Etaples, France, to observe Dr Varaztad H Kazanjian's (1879–1974) technique for treating jaw fractures. Upon his return, Speakman described Kazanjian's pioneering work in detail. A small percentage of facial wounds could be immediately sutured (eg, those that were not complicated by the fracture of the underlying bone and were seen immediately after the injury). Kazanjian's usual treatment was first to allow the patient to recover from the shock, permitting the tissues to drain themselves. Then he removed all teeth and roots in the line of fracture and brought the fractured portions into normal apposition by means of splints specially designed to suit each case. In cases where there was considerable bone loss, Kazanjian substituted the missing portion, at least temporarily, with a vulcanite appliance. Where the bone loss was great and a plastic operation was necessary to supply muscular tissue, he made the vulcanite appliance somewhat larger than the portion actually lost in order to compensate for the contraction of the scar tissue later on. He performed his plastic operations with these enlarged vulcanite appliances in the mouth, permitting them to remain while repair was taking place. He made the appliances in two or three sections, which could be removed one at a time without interfering with the repair of the tissues. Their re-moval made it possible for the mouth to be cleaned periodically.[111]

For maxillary jaw fractures, Kazanjin devised a head cap made of gutta-per-cha, molding it across the forehead and down each side of the face in front of the ears. To the head cap, he fastened an arch bar by means of thumb screws in line with the maxillae, and in the median line or at the sides (depending on the case) of the arch bar, he fastened a fixture to support the fractured portion of the jaw. Kazanjian also believed in having his patients sit outside in reclining chairs in the "fresh air and sunshine" and leaving the wounds uncovered. The facial cases had their own ward and a special recreation lounge room. Kazanjian preferred to work under local anesthesia because patients with extensive facial wounds were espe-cially susceptible to pneumonia following general anesthesia.[111]

Treatment of Fractures

Many types of appliances for treating facial injuries evolved during the war, primarily designed by the resourceful dental surgeons called upon to handle these cases. The continuing "lack of proper equipment for this type of work" handi-capped dental officers in France, who were compelled to use "all means at hand" to treat the cases they received. However, the dental officers were able to attain amazing results.[112]

Because wounded soldiers with fractured jaws frequently suffered from shock, the immediate treatment was to stabilize them and place the jaw back in its proper position, holding it there temporarily. The early splint had to be capable of a quick release in case of emesis and of rapid replacement when that danger passed. All bone fragments that were "totally detached from their periosteum" had to be re-moved, and those attached to their periosteum retained. Teeth "in line of fracture" or teeth that were "hopelessly broken or septic" had to be removed as soon as the patient's condition allowed.[113]

Tracheotomy was avoided if possible, and free drainage was established at the lower border of the jaw because the wounds were always septic. Clotted blood, dirt, grease, powder burns, and beard hair made these wounds difficult to clean. Ether or gasoline was used to cleanse the skin as soon as the patient was anesthetized. All foreign bodies, detached tissue, broken bridges, and loose crowns and teeth were removed, and drainage was established. The first step was "to save life" and the second to "save tissue." Simple wounds were closed at once, but if the case was more complicated, the tissue was preserved until a more complete operation could be performed. After the osseous structures were taken care of, the injured mucous membrane was sutured in its proper place. Chromocized catgut was used for deep-ly buried wounds, but for the skin or mucous membrane, silkworm gut, silk, linen, and horsehair were preferred. Compound tincture of benzoin was painted on as a dressing and sterile gauze was placed over the wound. Potassium-permanganate alternated with saline was used as a mouthwash. Argyrol was used to irrigate the wound.[113]

According to Dr Kazanjian, the following facial and oral deformities influ-enced the construction of an artificial restoration:

1. The destruction of the teeth.

2. The obliteration of the alveolar ridges, with accompanying fibrous adhesions.

3. Distortion of the alveolar arches.

4. Scar tissue which limits the elasticity of the lips and cheeks.

5. The interruption of the bony continuity of the mandible by fibrous tissue.

6. Destruction of a part or whole of the maxilla, resulting in communication between the nasal and oral cavities.[114(pp69–70)]

The ultimate condition of the oral cavity for the reception of dentures had to be kept in mind when treating gunshot wounds of the face and jaw. Once adhesions and thick facial scars developed, they were hard to overcome. Plastic operations had to be planned to harmonize with the final prosthetic needs of the patient.[114(p71)]

The hardest step in the construction of prosthetic devices was taking the impression. Scar tissue, tension of the muscular tissue, partial ankylosis of the jaw, and mobility of the remaining bony parts caused "difficulty in keeping the proper 'relations.'"[114(p84)] Only plaster was available for taking an impression because hydrocolloid had not yet been invented. Vulcanite remained the denture base material of choice.

By November 1918 enough jaw fractures had been treated to indicate that wiring should not only be used as a temporary measure for battle casualties, but also as a permanent device for immobilizing the fractured parts in lieu of waiting for the different types of permanent dental splints to be fabricated at the base hospitals. Wiring immobilized the fracture, yet allowed the desired slight mobility of the joint, and in many cases it prevented a temporary ankylosis. Chewing gum was recommended for trismus, as were wedge-shaped pieces of wood operated by the patient at short intervals during the day. Special attention was to be given to cleaning the tongue by scraping it with a suitable instrument and rubbing it with a pledget of absorbent cotton loaded with pumice and hydrogen peroxide.[115]

For many years, the intermaxillary wiring technique for treating jaw fractures had been commonly referred to as "Ivy loops," named after Robert H Ivy.[45,47,104] In 1970, however, Dr Ivy set the record straight when he published the following letter in the *Journal of Plastic and Reconstructive Surgery*:

I have had a regrettable experience, myself, with the award of unfounded credit for originating a technical method of treatment. In a book just off the press, I have noticed a reference to the use of "Ivy" loops in wiring the teeth in treatment of jaw fractures. These should be known as "Oliver loops" that being the surname of the man from whom I adopted them. I gave full credit for originating this method to Colonel Robert T. Oliver, Dental Corps, U.S. Army, in my first published description in 1921, but my name has been erroneously connected with the method for almost fifty years![116]

Evaluating the Maxillofacial Service

After the war, Blair evaluated his initial plans and commented on what he would do differently in another war:

If I had the planning for the care of these injuries in another war, I would not change the general plans projected in the Office of the Surgeon General in but one particular and that would be to have each surgeon and each dental surgeon, selected to be entrusted with this work, carry his emergency equipment with him as his personal baggage with the understanding that his final assignment to this work would depend upon his ability to keep this available. . . .Transportation is the greatest problem in war and everyone participating who has any grasp of the situation is primarily concerned with getting his paraphernalia to its seat of operation. . . . We learned to our bitter sorrow that having the most complete equipment the nation and government cooperating could provide, buried in some base was no help to those who were caring for the wounded. Those concerned with the greater problems regard, first, men, next munitions, then food, all other considerations being secondary. . . . A few pounds of essentials stowed in his personal baggage would have been worth infinitely more to the dentist or the general surgeon than the several hundred pounds allotted that in time would have become available.[51(p380)]

In their official account of maxillofacial surgery in World War I, Drs Robert Ivy and Joseph Eby assessed the work of the maxillofacial surgeons and dental surgeons of the AEF and its lasting importance:

Very few new principles as regards maxillofacial surgery were developed during the war, but the large number of wounds of this character encountered as compared to their frequency in civil life afforded unprecedented opportunities for demonstrating the advantages and faults of the various operative procedures which had been devised. Based on the experience of surgeons of the allied forces, and from our own observations during our earlier engagements, our maxillofacial surgeons were enabled to draw certain conclusions which proved of the greatest value in treatment of wounds of the face and mouth.[44(p396)]

Blair himself agreed with this assessment of the wartime work and its contributions to the postwar development of maxillofacial surgery:

Very few new principles in regard to maxillo-facial surgery were developed in this war that do not apply to every type of surgery, but concentration of thought and the clinical opportunities developed special skill. In saying that there have been very few new principles evolved does not imply that there has been no improvement in the execution of the work. Much of the work now done in special hospitals bears about the same relation to the general run of pre-war plastic surgery as would a modern bungalow to a sod hut. The test of use demonstrated the superiority of some methods and the faults of others in a much more authoritative manner than would have been possible in ordinary civilian practice. The men doing this work attained much greater skill and confidence through opportunities that had never before been utilized. Our experience, among other things, emphasized the following: The utility of early continuous treatment; not that we were able to carry it out even in the majority of cases, but the contrast between those cases in which it was done and those in which it was not, was very great.[51(p382)]

Blair concluded after the war that "our service had some success in its work. In my own mind I am very enthusiastic about its accomplishments."[50(p326)] The teamwork that Oliver, Logan, Blair, and Ivy stressed between maxillofacial surgeons and dental surgeons for the good of the patient in the AEF helped shape the concept of group medicine that Surgeon General Merritte Ireland emphasized during his tenure. In 1921 Ireland directly attributed the close working relationship between the medical and dental services in the Army to the shared successes of the maxillofacial service:

> The brilliant record of professional accomplishments made by members of the dental profession in the treatment of maxilla-facial conditions, both at home and abroad during the World War, and the close affiliation brought about through comradeship in the military service, has had a far-reaching effect in developing a mutual understanding and closer relationship between members of the medical and dental professions.[117(p134)]

Getting Them Ready to Go Home

The armistice of November 11, 1918, did not end the war and did not mean that the American troops could return home immediately. On the contrary, until a peace settlement was reached and treaties signed, the war was not over. Germany could resume hostilities at any moment, although this was highly unlikely. Allied forces had to remain in Europe and in occupation of German territory until the peace was definitely achieved.

This situation provided the opportunity for all dental officers in the AEF to set up offices, unlimber their dental engines, open their chests, and get to work catching up on all of the dental work that had been postponed or that was impossible to do while the fighting was going on. Oliver pointed out in his AEF report on the dental service that following the end of hostilities,

> a bone-fide practice of high class dentistry had been seriously and consistently carried on, wherein tooth conservation, repairative and reconstructive dentistry, and the long arduous treatments for tooth reclamation are every day achievements and that masticatory restoration through various methods of prosthesis is being afforded those officers and men who have lost teeth through the enforced dental negligence of battle activities.[57(p411)]

Compared to the difficult treatment conditions prior to November 11, he noted "the marked contrast" in the quality and quantity of the dental work being done thereafter and "the pleasing resumption of magnificent professional activity, that is commendable in the highest degree." [57(p411)]

In the armies in the zone of advance (see "Quality Dental Work Resumes," Chapter 15) and the services of supply, dental officers and their assistants now had the time, equipment, and necessary supplies to provide dental care of a much higher order. Tooth conservation was stressed with permanent fillings, restorations, and "the construction of crowns, bridges, and dentures."[101(p120)] The dental work completed in Base Section No. 2, headquartered in Bordeaux, France, which had an average of 100 dentists on duty monthly, can be taken as representative of the dental service in the base sections in France after the armistice. The consolidated dental reports for January 1919 through May 1919 indicated that dental officers

TABLE 14-1

PATIENTS, SITTINGS, AND SELECTED DENTAL TREATMENTS AND
OPERATIONS AT BASE SECTION NO. 2, SERVICE OF SUPPLY,
BORDEAUX, FRANCE, JANUARY 1919–MAY 1919

	January	February	March	April	May	Total
Patients	10,482	9,043	11,021	12,367	7,394	50,307
Sittings	18,146	14,719	19,361	21,731	13,112	87,069
Dental caries	12,420	11,313	17,985	20,905	12,416	75,039
Dento-alveolar abscess	1,958	1,596	1,675	2,151	1,254	8,634
Fillings	12,117	10,405	16,150	18,270	11,125	68,067
Teeth extracted	2,591	2,655	3,320	3,889	2,258	14,713
Teeth treated	3,321	2,770	2,967	3,607	1,725	14,390
Calculus removed	1,336	1,490	2,760	3,331	3,101	12,018
Crown and bridgework	577	501	522	603	370	2,573

Data sources: (1) National Archives and Records Administration. Record Group 120. Form 57, Dental
Work at Base Section No. 2, services of supply, American Expeditionary Forces, APO 705; Colonel SD
Boak, supervising dental surgeon, January and January supplemental, February, and March 1919. File,
Dental Reports, Office of the Surgeon, Base Section No. 2. Box 2788. Entry 2400. (2) National Archives
and Records Administration. Record Group 120. Form 57, Dental Work at Base Section No. 2, services
of supply, American Expeditionary Forces, APO 705; Colonel Robert F Patterson, supervising dental
surgeon, April 1919. File, Dental Reports, Office of the Surgeon, Base Section No. 2. Box 2788. Entry
2400. (3) National Archives and Records Administration. Record Group 120. Form 57, Dental Work at
Base Section No. 2, services of supply, American Expeditionary Forces, APO 705; Colonel Robert H
Mills, supervising dental surgeon, May 1919. File, Dental Reports, Office of the Surgeon, Base Section
No. 2. Box 2788. Entry 2400.

cared for 50,307 patients in 87,069 sittings, and provided a wide variety of dental
and oral treatments and operations (Table 14-1).[118–120]
For the entire AEF, the number of soldiers treated in March 1919 was triple
those treated in September 1918 during a high point in active operations.[101(pp120–121)]
In February 1919 a total of 119,792 patients were treated with 183,031 dental
operations. When viewed in the context of totality of dental work in the AEF, the
statistics for February 1919 clearly indicated that the volume of dental work after
November 1918 was very significant (Table 14-2). Work done that month alone
represented 8.5% of the total number of patients treated and 9% of the operations
in the AEF completed between July 1917 to May 1919.[101(pp120–121)] In stressing the
importance of this work, Oliver's objective and that of the AEF dental service
was simple: "to put the teeth of the men in first-class condition, prior to their
return to the United States and release from service."[101(p120)] The emphasis the
AEF placed on sound personal dental and oral hygiene and preventive dentistry
must have left a lasting impression that millions of American soldiers carried
into their peacetime lives.

TABLE 14-2

DENTAL SERVICE IN THE AMERICAN EXPEDITIONARY FORCES,
JULY 1917–MAY 1919

Patients treated	1,396,957
Sittings	2,636,368
Medicinal treatments	497,948
Operations performed	
Fillings	1,605,424
Extractions	384,427
Total	2,013,580
Crown and bridge construction	60,387
Denture construction and repair	13,140

Data source: Ford JH. *Administration, American Expeditionary Forces*. Vol 2. In Lynch C, Ford JH, Weed FW, eds. *The Medical Department of the United States Army in the World War*. Washington, DC: Government Printing Office; 1927: 121.

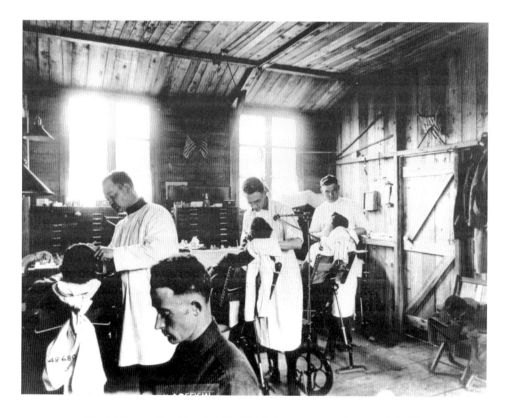

Dental Room, Base Hospital No. 65, Kerhuon, France, January 6, 1919.
Photograph: Courtesy of US Army Military History Institute. SC 48680.

The Dental Service in the American Expeditionary Forces in France

Only Part of the Story

Despite numerous obstacles and shortcomings, the AEF's dental service under Colonel Robert Oliver provided an unprecedented level of dental care to the American soldier that not only preserved oral and dental health, but also treated the most grievous war injuries. While much of the work was completed in the more peaceful surroundings of the AEF's base and camp hospitals and dental clinics, and although many patients were treated after November 11, 1918, the dental officers and assistants assigned to the front line divisions were no less responsible for maintaining the soldiers' dental health.

References

1. National Archives and Records Administration. Record Group 120. McCain to commanding general, eastern department, Governors Island, New York, Base Hospital No. 18, 6 June 1917. Letter. Box 263. Entry 2130.

2. National Archives and Records Administration. Record Group 120. Captain Walter A Baetjer, Medical Officers' Reserve Corps, Brief history of U.S. Army Hospital No. 2 from time of occupation of present quarters to-date, 20 September 1917. Letter. Box 263. Entry 2130.

3. National Archives and Records Administration. Record Group 120. Benj Alvord, adjutant general, American Expeditionary Forces, commanding general, 1st Division, AEF, Designation of United States Army Hospitals in France, 28 July 1917. Memo. Box 263. Entry 2130.

4. National Archives and Records Administration. Record Group 120. Benj Alvord, adjutant general, American Expeditionary Forces, to commanding general, 1st Division, AEF, Naming of Hospitals, 21 September 1917. Memo. Box 263. Entry 2130.

5. Base Hospital No. 18. In: Ford JH. *Administration, American Expeditionary Forces*. Vol 2. In: *The Medical Department of the United States Army in the World War*. Washington, DC: US Government Printing Office; 1927: 644–645.

6. Base Hospital 18 Association. *History of Base Hospital No. 18 American Expeditionary Forces (Johns Hopkins Unit)*. Baltimore, Md: Base Hospital 18 Association; 1919: 40.

7. Hyson JM, Jr. Dental Service Base Hospital No. 18, Johns Hopkins Hospital 1917–1919. *J Hist Dent*. 2003;51:115–116.

8. National Archives and Records Administration. Record Group 112. Winford H Smith, MD, superintendent, the Johns Hopkins Hospital, to Major Robert E Noble, Medical Corps, Office of The Surgeon General, 22 March 1917. Letter, with list, Professional personnel Base Hospital #18. File no. 166923. Box 1189. Entry 26.

9. National Archives and Records Administration. Record Group 120. Form 57, First Lieutenant B Lucien Brun, Dental Reserve Corps, Report of dental work at U.S. Army Hospital #2, Bazoilles sur Meuse, month of August 1917. Box 264. Entry 2130.

10. National Archives and Records Administration. Record Group 120. Colonel Henry C Fisher, Medical Corps, general sanitation inspector, American Expeditionary Forces, report of inspection 28 February, 1918, 5 March 1918. In: "Base Hospital No. 18". Entry 2130.

11. National Archives and Records Administration. Record Group 120. Form 57, First Lieutenant B Lucien Brun, Dental Reserve Corps, Report of dental work at base hospital No. 18, bazoilles sur meuse, month of march 1918. Box 264. Entry 2130.

12. Moffatt RT, Rice W, Miner LMS. In memoriam: William Henry Potter. *Dent Items Interest*. 1929;51:157–58.

13.   National Archives and Records Administration. Record Group 120. History of the dental section of the Army Sanitary School, Army schools, American Expeditionary Forces, France, December 19, 1917 to December 10, 1918. In: "Dental Section, Army Sanitary School." Chap IV. Box 1780. Entry 395.

14.   National Archives and Records Administration. Record Group 120. Colonel SD Boak, director, dental section, Army Sanitary School, to commandant, Army schools, American Expeditionary Forces, 18 November 1918. Memo. Folder 2. Box 1780. Entry 395.

15.   National Archives and Records Administration. Record Group 120. Form 57, First Lieutenant B Lucien Brun, Dental Reserve Corps, Report of dental work at Base Hospital No. 18, Bazoilles sur Meuse, Month of May 1918 [through August 1918]. Box 264. Entry 2130.

16.   National Archives and Records Administration. Record Group 120. Colonel Henry C Fisher, Medical Corps, report of inspection, 20 June 1918. Report. Entry 2130. Box 263.

17.   National Archives and Records Administration. Record Group 120. Return of medical officers, etc, serving at Base Hospital No. 18, American Expeditionary Forces, France, on the last day of June 1918. Box 263. Entry 2130.

18.   National Archives and Records Administration. Record Group 120. Colonel Robert T Oliver, chief dental surgeon, American Expeditionary Forces, to Major Vilray P Blair, chief consultant, maxillofacial surgery, AEF, 27 June 1918. Letter. In: "Surgery, Advance Section, Correspondence, Headquarters Medical and Surgical Consultants." File No. 710. Box 3150. Entry 2917.

19.   National Archives and Records Administration. Record Group 120. Form 57, First Lieutenant B Lucien Brun, Dental Reserve Corps, Report of dental work at Base Hospital No. 18, Bazoilles sur Meuse, month of July 1918. Box 264. Entry 2130.

20.   National Archives and Records Administration. Record Group 120. Form 57, First Lieutenant B Lucien Brun, Dental Reserve Corps, Report of dental work at base hospital No. 18, Bazoilles sur Mmeuse, month of September 1918." Box 264. Entry 2130.

21.   National Archives and Records Administration. Record Group 120. Base Hospital No. 18. Box 263. Entry 2130.

22.   National Archives and Records Administration. Record Group 120. Return of medical officers, etc, serving at Base Hospital No. 18, American Expeditionary Forces, France, on the last day of August 1918. Box 263. Entry 2130.

23.   Personal diary of B Lucian Brun, June 7, 1917–December 8, 1918. In: Biographical file of B Lucien Brun, Research Collections, Office of Medical History, OTSG/MEDCOM, Falls Church, Virginia.

24.   National Archives and Records Administration. Record Group 120. Report of dental work at Base Hospital No. 18, Bazoilles sur Meuse, month of September 1917 [through] December 1918. In: Dental reports Base Hospital 18. Box 264. Entry 2130.

25. Boehler GM. Letters from France. *J Nat Dent Assoc.* 1918;5:1090–1091.

26. Polk RL. *Polk's Dental Register and Directory of the United States and Dominion of Canada.* 14th ed. Detroit, Mich: R.L. Polk & Co; 1928: 431.

27. Symanski TV. Dental service in the first replacement depot, A.E.F., France. *Mil Surg.* 1928;63:46–47.

28. National Archives and Records Administration. Record Group 120. Report of dental work at US Navy Base Hospital No. 1 in Brest, France, month of February 1–28, 1918. Box 195. Entry 2133.

29. McKernon JF. Otolaryngology (American Expeditionary Forces). In: *Surgery, Part II.* Vol 11. In: Lynch C, Weed FW, McAfee L, eds. *The Medical Department of the United States Army in the World War.* Washington, DC: Government Printing Office; 1924: 801.

30. Siler JF. Vincent's disease. In: Siler JF. *Communicable and Other Diseases.* Vol 9. In: Lynch C, Weed FW, McAfee L, eds. *The Medical Department of the United States Army in the World War.* Washington, DC: Government Printing Office; 1928.

31. Taylor FE, McKinstry WH. The relation of peridental gingivitis to Vincent's Angina. *Br Med J.* 1917;1:421.

32. National Archives and Records Administration. Record Group 120. 1st Division American Expeditionary Forces, Staudt, Germany, First Lieutenant Myers Brownstone, Dental Corps, 14 May 1919. Memo. No. 1. Box 3399. Entry 2144.

33. National Archives and Records Administration. Record Group 120. First Lieutenant John E Walker, Medical Corps, to chief surgeon, American Expeditionary Forces, 15 May 1918. Memo. File No. 703. Folder 18. Box 5149. Entry 2065.

34. National Archives and Records Administration. Record Group 120. Captain William W Irving, Dental Corp, supervising dental surgeon, Hospital Center, Savenay, to commanding officer, Hospital Center, Savenay. Memo. No. 703. Box 2776. Entry 2348.

35. Kishler LF. The handling of syphilitic cases. *J Assoc Milit Dent Surg US.* 1918;2:53–59.

36. Quetel C. *History of syphilis.* Baltimore, Md: Johns Hopkins University Press; 1992: 33–49.

37. National Archives and Records Administration. Record Group 94. Second endorsement, Brigadier General George H Torney, surgeon general, to adjutant general of the Army, 18 September 1913. No. 1976269. Box 7064. Entry 25.

38. National Archives and Records Administration. Record Group 94. Physical examination for appointment, promotion, or retirement, Fort Sam Houston, Texas, 16 November 1916. No. 526185. Box 3655. Entry 25.

39. Lambie JS. The prevention of extra-genital chancres in the Army, based on a study of syphilitic registers on file at the Army medical schools. *Milit Surg.* 1922;50:264–274.

40. Hirschfeld M. *The Sexual History of the World War*. New York, NY: Falstaff Press, Inc; 1937.

41. Blue R. Campaign to enlist the co-operation of the dental profession in the fight against venereal diseases. *Dental Cosmos*. 1919;61:1132.

42. Bispham WN. *Training*. Vol 7. In: Lynch C, Weed FW, McAfee L, eds. *The Medical Department of the United States Army in the World War*. Washington, DC: Government Printing Office; 1927: 531–532.

43. Blair VP. *Surgery and Diseases of the Mouth and Jaws: a Practical Treatise on the Surgery and Diseases of the Mouth and Allied Subjects*. St Louis, Mo: Mosby; 1912.

44. Ivy RH, Eby JD. Maxillofacial surgery. In: *Surgery, Part 2*. Vol 11. In: Lynch C, Weed FW, McAfee L, eds. *The Medical Department of the United States Army in the World War*. Washington, DC: Government Printing Office; 1924.

45. Stelnicki EJ, Young VL, Francel T, Randall P. Vilray P. Blair, his surgical descendents, and their roles in plastic surgical development. *Plast Reconstr Surg*. 1999;103:1991.

46. Cannon B, Murray JE. The influence of the St. Louis quadrumvirate on plastic surgery. *Plast Reconstr Surg*. 1995;95:1118–1122.

47. Hallock GG. The plastic surgeon of the 20th century. *Plast Reconstr Surg*. 2001;107:1014–1024.

48. Webster JP. In memoriam, Vilray Papin Blair, 1871–1955. *Plast Reconstr Surg*. 1956;18:87.

49. Ruggles SD. America's maxillo-facial service in the World War. *Dental Summary*. 1920;40:995–997.

50. Blair VP. The maxillofacial service of the American Army in the war. *JAMA*. 1919;73:325–326.

51. Blair VP. Some observations on our war experiences with face and jaw injuries. *Milit Surg*. 1920;47:379–382.

52. Blair VP. The aims of the subsection of plastic and oral surgery. *Dental Cosmos*. 1918;40:125–127.

53. Lynch C, Ford JH, Weed FW. *The Surgeon General's Office*. Vol 1. In: Lynch C, Weed FW, McAfee L, eds. *The Medical Department of the United States Army in the World War*. Washington, DC: Government Printing Office; 1923: 460.

54. Ford JH. *Administration, American Expeditionary Forces*. Vol 2. In: Lynch C, Weed FW, McAfee L, eds. *The Medical Department of the United States Army in the World War*. Washington, DC: Government Printing Office; 1927.

55. National Archives and Records Administration. Record Group 120. Colonel JD Glennan, to Lieutenant Colonel William L Keller, director of professional services, General Headquarters, American Expeditionary Forces, "Treatment of ambulatory jaw cases, 24 April 1918. File 703," Dental Treatment (Dental Service). Box 5149. Entry 2065.

56. National Archives and Records Administration. Record Group 120. First endorsement, Keller to chief surgeon, 27 April 1918. File 703, "Dental treatment (dental service)." Box 5149. Entry 2065.

57. Oliver RT. History of the Dental Service, A.E.F. In: *Activities of the Chief Surgeon's Office*. In: *Reports of the Commander-in-Chief, Staff Sections and Services, in United States Army in the World War 1917–1919*. Vol 15. Washington, DC: US Army Center of Military History; 1991.

58. National Archives and Records Administration. Record Group 120. Base Section No. 5, services of supply, special orders no. 103, 17 April 1918. File No. 210, "Officers, Advance Section, Headquarters Medical and Surgical Consultants, 1917–May 31, 1918." Box 3148. Entry 2917.

59. National Archives and Records Administration. Record Group 120. Lieutenant Colonel Walter R Parker, Medical Corps, in charge of the section of surgery of the head, Office of The Surgeon General, US Army, to commanding officer, Base Hospital No. 3, American Expeditionary Forces, through chief surgeon, AEF, Officers assigned to plastic and oral surgery, 25 February 1918. Memo. File No. 210. Box 206. Entry 2130.

60. National Archives and Records Administration. Record Group 120. Major MA Dailey, Medical Corps, Return of medical officers serving at US Base Hospital #3, A.E.F., France, on the last day of April, May, June, July, August, September, October, November, and December 1918. File, "Returns of Medical Officers," Base Hospital No. 3. Box 203. Entry 2130.

61. National Archives and Records Administration. Record Group 120. Base Hospital No. 3, American Expeditionary Forces, Officers Medical Reserve Corps, Base Section No. 2. Memo. File no. 210. Box 206. Entry 2130.

62. National Archives and Records Administration. Record Group 120. Major MA Dailey, Medical Corps, Base Hospital No. 3, to department surgeon, Governor's Island, NY; Relative rank of First Lieutenants Asch and Stern, Dental Reserve Corps, 29 January 1918. Memo. File no. 210, Box 206. Entry 2130.

63. National Archives and Records Administration. Record Group 120. Major George Baehr, Medical Corps, commanding officer, Base Hospital No. 3, to chief surgeon, American Expeditionary Forces, Final return, officers, Base Hospital No 3, 15 February 1919. Memo. File no. 210. Box 206. Entry 2130.

64. Smith IE. The treatment of war injuries of the face and jaws in the base hospitals in France. *Dental Summary*. 1919;39:572–573.

65. National Archives and Records Administration. Record Group 120. Major VP Blair, to director of professional services, American Expeditionary Forces, Maxillofacial service: organization, disposition of cases, 11 June 1918. Memo. File no. 710, "Maxillo-Facial Surgery, Advance Section, Correspondence, Headquarters Medical and Surgical Consultants." Box 3150. Entry 2917.

66. National Archives and Records Administration. Record Group 120. Colonel Seibert D Boak, director, dental section, Army Sanitary School, to Colonel MAW Shockley, G-5, 2 July 1918. Letter. No. 3603-539. Box 1309. Entry 11.

67. National Archives and Records Administration. Record Group 120. Major Vilray P Blair, senior consultant, maxillofacial surgery, to chief surgeon, Treatment and evacuation of maxillofacial injuries in the AEF, 26 June 1918. Memo. File no. 710, "Maxillo-Facial Surgery, Advance Section, Correspondence, Headquarters Medical and Surgical Consultants." Box 3150. Entry 2917.

68. Lankford A. Dentist, Baltimore, Maryland. Interview with John M Hyson, Jr, October 28, 1979.

69. Dr Arthur Lankford, dentist here 50 years, dies at age 96. *The Baltimore Sun*. November 12, 1984.

70. Brown GVI. *The Surgery of Oral Diseases and Malformations: Their Diagnosis and Treatment*. Philadelphia, Pa: Lea & Febiger; 1918.

71. Brun L. *Reference Book Written by Dr. B. Lucien Brun, World War 1—1917–1919, Sanitary School United States Army, France*. Located at: National Museum of Dentistry Archives, Baltimore, Maryland.

72. Schaeffer GC. Experience of an area consultant in the zone of the advance. *Dental Summary*. 1919;39:856–860.

73. Schaeffer GC. Experience of an area consultant in facial surgery: in the zone of advance. *JAMA*. 1919;73:1335–1336.

74. Lynch C, Ford JH, Weed FW. *Field Operations*. Vol 8. In: Lynch C, Ford JH, Weed FW, eds. *The Medical Department of the United States Army in the World War*. Washington, DC: Government Printing Office; 1925:185–188;

75. National Archives and Records Administration. Record Group 120. Major Vilray P Blair, to chief surgeon, American Expeditionary Forces, establishment of school of instruction for dental officers, 23 June 1918. File no. 710, "Maxillo-Facial Surgery, Advance Section, Correspondence, Headquarters Medical and Surgical Consultants." Memo. Box 3150. Entry 2917.

76. National Archives and Records Administration. Record Group 120. First endorsement, Major William A Fisher, Jr, for the chief consultant, 24 June 1918. File no. 710, "Maxillo-Facial Surgery, Advance Section, Correspondence, Headquarters Medical and Surgical Consultants." Memo. Box 3150. Entry 2917.

77. National Archives and Records Administration. Record Group 120. Unidentified, to Colonel Oliver, 1 July 1918. Letter. File no. 710, "Maxillofacial Surgery, Advance Section, Correspondence, Headquarters Medical and Surgical Consultants." Memo. Box 3150. Entry 2917.

78. National Archives and Records Administration. Record Group 120. Major Vilray P Blair to Colonel Robert Oliver, 17 July 1918. Letter. File no. 710, "Maxillo-Facial Surgery, Advance Section, Correspondence, Headquarters Medical and Surgical Consultants." Memo. Box 3150. Entry 2917.

79. National Archives and Records Administration. Record Group 120. Major VP Blair, to chief surgeon, Report on maxillofacial service, 18 July 1918. Memo. File no. 710, "Maxillo-Surgery, Advance Section, Correspondence, Headquarters Medical and Surgical Consultants." Box 3150. Entry 2917.

80. McGee RP. The maxillofacial surgeon in the front line hospital. *Dental Summary*. 1919;39:834.

81. National Archives and Records Administration. Record Group 120. Major VP Blair, Medical Reserve Corps, to chief dental surgeon [Oliver], 18 July 1918. Memo. File no. 710, "Maxillo-Surgery, Advance Section, Correspondence, Headquarters Medical and Surgical Consultants." Box 3150. Entry 2917.

82. National Archives and Records Administration. Record Group 120. Major VP Blair, Medical Reserve Corps, to chief dental surgeon [Oliver], Assignment of dental surgeons, 17 July 1918. File no. 210, "Officers, Headquarters Medical and Surgical Consultants, Advance Section." Box 3148. Entry 2917.

83. National Archives and Records Administration. Record Group 120. Treatment of maxillo-facial injuries, nd. File no. 710, "Maxillo-Facial Surgery, Advance Section, Correspondence, Headquarters Medical and Surgical Consultants." Box 3150. Entry 2917.

84. National Archives and Records Administration. Record Group 120. War Department, order no. 75, 30 March 1918, Medical Department, Advanced Section. Box 3148. Entry 2917.

85. National Archives and Records Administration. Record Group 120. Major HS Osborne, Medical Corps, adjutant, headquarters, Hospital Center, Bazoilles, 4 September 1918. Memo. No. 50. "File, Memos, Circulars, Etc., Base Hospital No. 42." Box 337. Entry 2130.

86. National Archives and Records Administration. Record Group 120. Major Vilray P Blair, Medical Reserve Corps, senior consultant, maxillofacial service, American Expeditionary Forces, to chief surgeon, AEF, maxillofacial service at Bazoilles, 21 August 1918. Memo. File no. 730. Box 3161. Entry 2812.

87. National Archives and Records Administration. Record Group 120. Second endorsement, Colonel JD Glennan, Medical Corps, Office of the Chief of Staff, American Expeditionary Forces, to director of professional services, General Headquarters, AEF, 27 August 1918, to memo, Major Vilray P Blair, Medical Reserve Corps, senior consultant, maxillofacial Service, AEF, to chief surgeon, AEF, maxillofacial service at Bazoilles, 21 August 1918. File no. 730. Box 3161. Entry 2812.

88. National Archives and Records Administration. Record Group 112. Circular no. 50, American Expeditionary Forces, Major General MW Ireland, Medical Corps, chief surgeon, Instructions regarding hospitalization and evacuation of patients with disease or injury of the eye, ear, nose, throat, and maxillofacial region, 4 October 1918. File, "Chief Surgeon's Office, AEF, Circular Letters." Box 7. Entry 1011.

89. National Archives and Records Administration. Record Group 120. Major Vilray P Blair to director of museum units, Photographer. Memo. File no. 710, "Maxillofacial Surgery, Advance Section, Correspondence, Headquarters Medical and Surgical Consultants." Box 3150. Entry 2917.

90. National Archives and Records Administration. Record Group 120. Major Vilray P Blair to chief surgeon, American Expeditionary Forces, maxillofacial service at Mars Centre, 30 August 1918. Memo. File no. 710, "Maxillo-Facial Surgery, Advance Section, Correspondence, Headquarters Medical and Surgical Consultants." Box 3150. Entry 2917.

91. National Archives and Records Administration. Record Group 120. Major Vilray P Blair, to chief surgeon, American Expeditionary Forces, through chief consultant, surgical service, Local consultants in maxillofacial surgery, 20 September 1918. Memo. File no. 710, "Maxillo-Facial Surgery, Headquarters Medical and Surgical Consultants, Advance Section." Box 3150. Entry 2917.

92. National Archives and Records Administration. Record Group 120. Senior consultant in maxillofacial surgery, American Expeditionary Forces, to the local consultant in maxillofacial surgery, Information. Memo. File no. 710, "Maxillo-Facial Surgery, Headquarters Medical and Surgical Consultants, Advance Section." Box 3150. Entry 2917.

93. National Archives and Records Administration. Record Group 120. Major Vilray P Blair to Colonel Walter Parker, Office of The Surgeon General, 20 September 1918. Letter. File no. 710, "Maxillo-Facial Surgery, Headquarters Medical and Surgical Consultants, Advance Section." Box 3150. Entry 2917.

94. National Archives and Records Administration. Record Group 112. Circular no. 50, Major General MW Ireland, chief surgeon, American Expeditionary Forces, 4 October 1918. File, "Chief Surgeon, AEF, Circular Letters." Box 7. Entry 1011.

95. National Archives and Records Administration. Record Group 120. Lieutenant Colonel Vilray P Blair to chief dental surgeon, maxillofacial service, 26 October 1918. Memo. File no. 710, "Maxillo-Facial Surgery, Advance Section, Correspondence, Headquarters Medical and Surgical Consultants." Box 3150. Entry 2917.

96. National Archives and Records Administration. Record Group 120. Lieutenant Colonel Vilray P Blair, senior consultant in maxillfacial surgery, to chief surgeon, American Expeditionary Forces, maxillofacial service, 27 October 1918. Memo. File no. 710, "Maxillo-Facial Surgery, Advance Section, Correspondence, Headquarters Medical and Surgical Consultants." Box 3150. Entry 2917.

97. Ruggles SD. Experiences of the dental surgeon in a base hospital in the base section, Vichy, France. *Dental Summary*. 1919;39:855–857.

98. National Archives and Records Administration. Record Group 120. Report of dental work at US Base Hospital No. 115, American Expeditionary Forces, Vichy, France, month of September 1918, Major SD Ruggles. Box 500. Entry 2130.

99. National Archives and Records Administration. Record Group 120. Major VP Blair to chief surgeon, Treatment and evacuation of maxillofacial injuries in the A.E.F., 14 September 1918. Memo. File no. 710, "Maxillo-Facial Surgery, Advance Section, Correspondence, Headquarters Medical and Surgical Consultants". Box 3150. Entry 2917.

100. Office of The Surgeon General. *Annual Report of the Surgeon General*. Vol 2.Washington, DC: OTSG; 1919.

101. The Dental Section. In: Ford JH. *Administration, American Expeditionary Forces*. Vol 2. In Lynch C, Ford JH, Weed FW, eds. *The Medical Department of the United States Army in the World War*. Washington, DC: Government Printing Office; 1927: 122.

102. Stelnicki EJ, Young VL, Francel T, Randall P. Vilray P. Blair, his surgical descendents, and their roles in plastic surgical development. *Plast Reconstr Surg*. 1999;103:1992.

103. Hallock GG. The plastic surgeon of the 20th century. *Plast Reconstr Surg*. 2001;107;1017.

104. *Who Was Who in America, 1977–1981*. Vol 7. Chicago, Ill: Marquis Who's Who; 1981: 296.

105. Ford JH. *Administration, American Expeditionary Forces*. Vol 2. In Lynch C, Ford JH, Weed FW, eds. *The Medical Department of the United States Army in the World War*. Washington, DC: Government Printing Office; 1927.

106. National Archives and Records Administration. Record Group 120. A history of USA Base Hospital No. 115, APO 781 American Expeditionary Forces (Vichy, France: [1919]). Box 1. Entry 3142.

107. National Archives and Records Administration. Record Group 120. The history of Vichy Hospital Center, Vichy, Allier. American Expeditionary Forces. File, History of Hospital Center Vichy, Intermediate Section. Box 1. Entry 3142.

108. National Archives and Records Administration. Record Group 120. Special order no. 3, First Lieutenant RE Hare, adjutant, headquarters, Base Hospital No. 1, 19 July 1918. File, "Special orders no. 1-37, 1918, Headquarters, Hospital Center, Vichy, Intermediate Section." Box 3129. Entry 3144.

109. National Archives and Records Administration. Record Group 120. Colonel Henry C Fisher, Medical Corps, general medical inspector, American Expeditionary Forces, report of inspection, 13–14 August 1918. File, "Historical Data, Hospital Center, Vichy, Intermediate Section." Box 1. Entry 3142.

110. National Archives and Records Administration. Record Group 120. Major Robert H Ivy, Medical Corps, to chief surgeon, American Expeditionary Forces, Report of maxillofacial cases, 18 January 1919. Memo. File, "Historical Data, Hospital Center Vichy, Intermediate Section." Box 1. Entry 3142.

111. National Archives and Records Administration. Record Group 120. Major William C Speakman, Dental Corps, to Major George C Schaeffer, Office of the Chief Consultant, division of maxillofacial surgery. Memo. No. 710. Box 3150. Entry 2917.

112. Bodine RL. Standardization of splints for maxillary fractures. *Milit Dent J*. 1921;4:196.

113. McGee RP. The treatment of maxillo-facial wounds, in the zone of advance. *Milit Dent J*. 1921;4:193–195.

114. Kazanjian VH. Problems of prosthetic restoration following injuries of the face and jaw. *Milit Dent J*. 1922;5:69–84.

115. National Archives and Records Administration. Record Group 120. Colonel SD Boak, director, dental section, Army Sanitary School, to Major George C Schaeffer, Medical Corps, maxillofacial department, medical consultants' office, APO 731, 15 November 1918. Letter. Folder 2. Box 1780. Entry 395.

116. Ivy RH. Oliver, not Ivy, Loops. *J Oral Surg*. 1971;29:279.

117. General Ireland's Address. *Milit Dent J*. 1921;4:134.

118. National Archives and Records Administration. Record Group 120. Form 57, Dental work at base section No. 2, services of supply, American Expeditionary Forces, APO 705; Colonel SD Boak, supervising dental surgeon, January and January supplemental, February, and March 1919. File, "Dental Reports, Office of the Surgeon, Base Section No. 2." Box 2788. Entry 2400.

119. National Archives and Records Administration. Record Group 120. Form 57, Dental work at Base Section No. 2, services of supply, American Expeditionary Forces, APO 705; Colonel Robert F Patterson, supervising dental surgeon, April 1919. File, Dental Reports, Office of the Surgeon, Base Section No. 2. Box 2788. Entry 2400.

120. National Archives and Records Administration. Record Group 120. Form 57, Dental work at Base Section No. 2, services of supply, American Expeditionary Forces, APO 705; Colonel Robert H Mills, supervising dental surgeon, May 1919. File, Dental Reports, Office of the Surgeon, Base Section No. 2. Box 2788. Entry 2400.

Chapter XV

The Dental Service in the American Expeditionary Forces in France, 1917–1919: Combat

Introduction

The dental service that Robert Oliver and his colleagues built in France experienced its most difficult test with the combat divisions of the American Expeditionary Forces (AEF). Never before in the history of the Army or its medical department had dental officers gone directly into battle as part of a combat unit. Thanks to Oliver's efforts and those of many others in the Dental Corps, the AEF had dental officers and assistants attached to all of its front line divisions, including infantry and engineer battalions in the trenches and field artillery batteries. Without the experience of any army in history to guide it, the AEF integrated the dentists into the fabric of the division in a variety of ways. While they were sometimes assigned collateral duties with little regard for their professional backgrounds, they were more often employed as auxiliary medical officers to assist the battalion and regimental surgeons and medical detachments on the battlefield. Regardless of their assignments, the dental officers and their assistants served their fellow soldiers in times of trial, a number of them winning awards for gallantry on the battlefield and others sacrificing their lives. Their performance ultimately won the soldiers' respect and the honored place in the Army Medical Department that dentists had so long sought.

Dental Officers at the Front

While hundreds of the AEF's dental officers and their assistants were caring for both the wounded and for soldiers in need of dental work in the rear area hospitals and clinics, those in combat divisions faced situations that were not only more demanding and varied but also much more dangerous. At the front, the dental officers' responsibilities usually shifted from "dento-oral care" to assisting the Medical Corps' officers in the emergency treatment and evacuation of the sick and wounded. They often replaced unit surgeons who were killed, wounded, or gassed until replacements arrived. Dental officers were also frequently employed as surgical assistants and anesthetists in battalion and regimental aid stations and divisional field hospitals. For example, from October 4 through October 18, 1918, First Lieutenant George C McMullen with the 302nd Sanitary Train, 77th Division, served as the evacuation officer in the triage station. During the Meuse-Argonne offensive, First Lieutenant Bernard L Riley of the Dental Reserve Corps (DRC), then

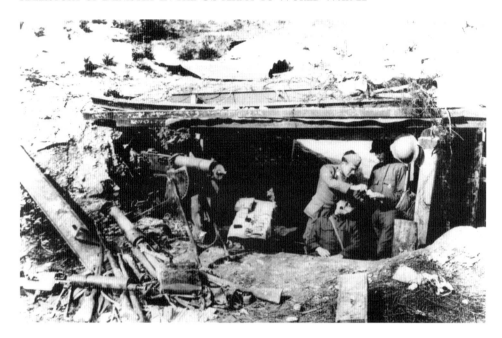

Lieutenant ER Latham, dental surgeon, 305th Field Signal Battalion, 80th Division, in a dugout working under difficult conditions. Bethincourt, Meuse, France. October 5, 1918. Photograph: Courtesy of US Army Military History Institute. SC 24888.

assigned to the First Army but formerly with the 2nd Supply Train, 2nd Division, "acted as surgical assistant in operating teams at hospital for seriously wounded" at Field Hospitals No. 15 and No. 23 of his former division. From November 1 through November 12, he was directly involved in operations on over 500 seriously wounded soldiers. During more peaceful times, division dental officers took over a wide variety of jobs, such as transportation, supply, or billeting officer, sanitary inspector, censor, or town major. In the 78th Division, for instance, two dental officers were responsible for the divisional ration dump and the operation of all of its trucks, and another acted as the adjutant of the 303rd Sanitary Train.[1-13]

Although the AEF's division surgeons sometimes varied in how they organized and used their dental officers, most of them employed their dentists as auxiliary medical officers when their units were in the trenches. Dental work was exceedingly complicated due to the conditions on the front lines and the difficulty of getting even the stripped-down portable outfits near the trenches. Most dental officers had to rely on emergency kits to reduce pain and suffering from dental or oral problems. In the trenches, the soldiers' concerns were more clearly focused on combat and survival than on dental care. The dental officers were most valuable in assisting the medical officers with the wounded.

The dental service of the front line divisions varied greatly based on whether the unit was in a training area, rest zone, or the trenches. In the rear training areas, the division's dentists could set up their portable outfits in battalion or regimental infirmaries or clinics and conduct "high-class tooth conservation service, with

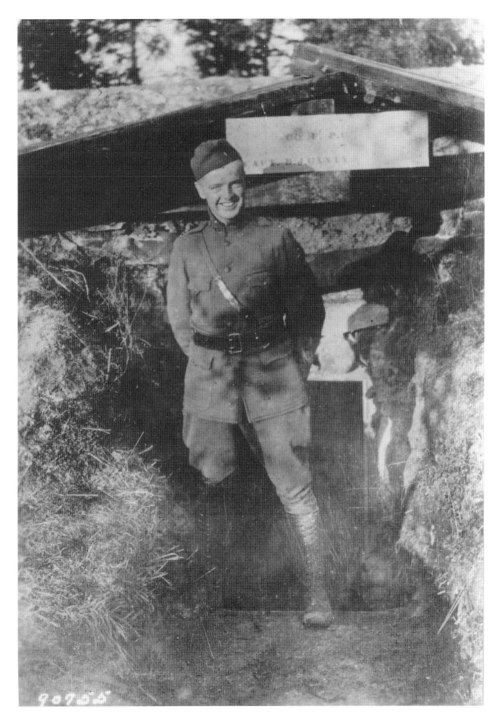

First Lieutenant Bernard L Riley, Dental Officers' Reserve Corps, 2nd Division.
Photograph: Courtesy of National Archives and Records Administration. SC 90755.

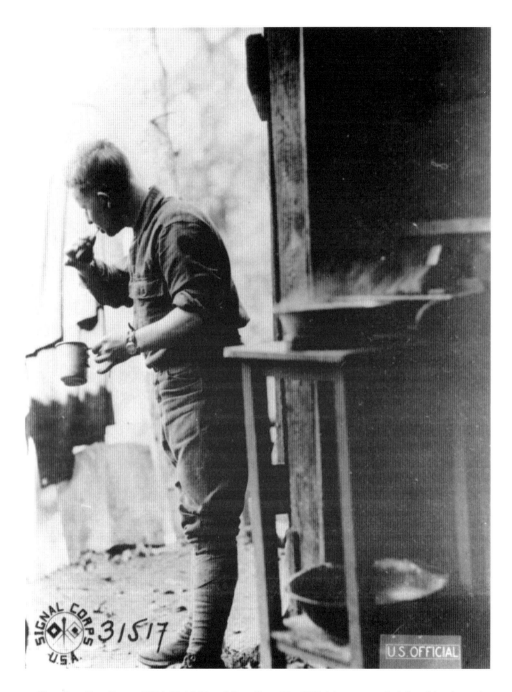

Chauffeur Sam Egger, 307th Field Signal Battalion, 82nd Division, uses witch hazel in place of toothpaste , which is very scarce. Argonne Forest, Meuse, France, October 29, 1918. Photograph: Courtesy of US Army Military History Institute. SC 31517.

a view to rendering all men dentally fit" for upcoming operations. Officers and soldiers could be surveyed, and dental records were prepared to guide priorities for follow-up treatment. Most major oral or dental health matters affecting a soldier could be addressed, and the division dental laboratory or camp hospital was usually available for more sophisticated work. When the divisions moved into combat zones, dentists' equipment and supplies were reduced to the minimum, so they could only provide emergency treatment to relieve pain and complete very simple dental service. Dental officers and their assistants carried emergency kits with them while on march and in the field to provide simple, immediate treatment that would allow soldiers to return to the front line without loss of time. However, some of the more enterprising dental officers actually moved their portable outfits into dugouts and bunkers in the support trenches and set up their "offices" to provide routine dental services for their units. Once the unit was pulled from the front lines and sent to a rest area, a fuller dental service once again resumed, but never to the extent that was possible in the training areas.[14]

On December 7, 1918, Colonel Philip W Huntington, Medical Corps (MC), who was division surgeon of the 79th Division, explained to students at the Army Sanitary School how he had organized and used his dental officers:

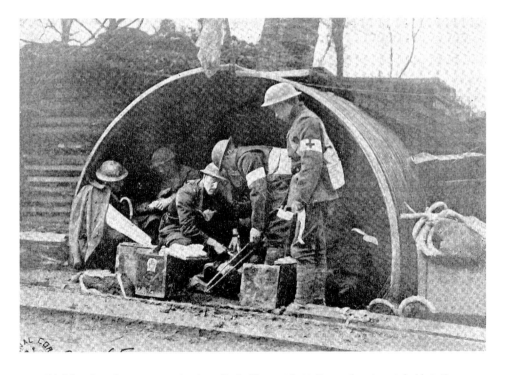

Division dental surgeons assisted medical officers at battalion and regimental aid stations during combat operations. Here wounded from the 115th Infantry Regiment, 29th Division, are treated in the Bois de Consenvoye during the Meuse-Argonne offensive, October 1918. Reproduced from: Reynolds, FC, McLaughlin, William F. 115th Infantry USA in the World War. Baltimore, Md: Read-Taylor; 1920.

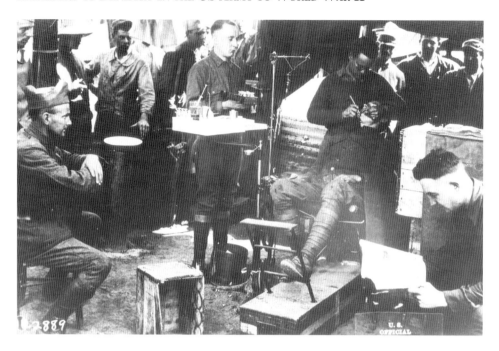

First Lieutenant John Mann, Jr, of the Dental Officer Reserve Corps, 302nd Supply Train, 77th Division, performing his daily duty in dentistry. The French soldiers look on.
On the left is Mr CA Sampson, YMCA, a noted provider of all sorts of games for American soldiers at the front. Near Fere en Tardenois, France, September 5, 1918.
Photograph: Courtesy of the US Army Military History Institute. SC22889.

> . . . what I have to say is mostly in regard to the medical work of the division in combat, but I think it will have considerable value in connection with the Dental Corps because—at least in my division—the dental officers during combat performed exactly the same duties as the medical officers. In the 79th Division the dental officers during combat serve as auxiliary medical officers. They were attached to the battalions and they went forward with the battalions and functioned in the battalion aid posts, regimental aid posts—or wherever their services might be needed—and performed exactly the same duties as medical officers, and I might say, as I told Colonel Boak, they performed very satisfactorily, very creditably, very well. I have been division surgeon ever since the Seventy-ninth was organized and am still, and the work of the dental surgeons has not been confined to dental work entirely. They were used in a military medical sense; I had that idea from the very beginning. . . .[15(p1127)]

Captain John M Hughes, Dental Corps (DC), division dental surgeon for the 29th Division, later wrote in his report to the chief surgeon of the AEF about the work of his dental officers and their assistants:

> From the time of departure from Haute Alsace 23 September to return to rest area after 29 October very little dental work was accomplished by dental surgeons with

592

the combat troops. Those who were with organizations in the rear were able to accomplish much good along this line. From the beginning of the drive on 8 October till the Division was relieved on 29 October dental surgeons with combat troops ceased to functionate [*sic*] as dental surgeons and automatically became medical officers and as such rendered untold service to wounded soldiers, and won for themselves splendid credit. They worked hard and long and on numbers of occasions attracted the attention of their fellow officers by their heroic deeds. Due credit must be given to the dental assistant, also, for they merged themselves with the sanitary detachments and rendered much assistance to the wounded.[6]

On August 31, 1918, Major Elbert Rushing, DC, the divisional dental surgeon for the 1st Division, expressed his views on dental service for a combat division in a letter to Lieutenant Colonel Rex H Rhoades, the First US Army's dental surgeon at the time. Rushing pointed out that:

Dentistry is almost an impossibility with the regiments when a Division is in action, as all the dressing stations, etc., are in dugouts, and practically no lights except candle and it is quite impossible to do Dental work. So in my opinion the only place, and as was experienced in the last fight, for Dental work was in the Field hospitals and very little done there as the hospitals were mobile and they were continuously under fire. However the Division had Dental Surgeons that did quite a bit of relief work with the Emergency Kits, but only at times, as they were doing first aid work and any and every little thing that would help. I had quite a few compliments paid the Dental Surgeons in this Division for their aid and it was very much appreciated. In fact a circular letter from Colonel Stark, Chief Surgeon, First Army, to this office complimented the Dental Surgeons for their work.[16]

In this same letter to Rhoades, Rushing also expressed his personal thoughts:

When I joined this Division, I found everything pretty rotten and disgusting. I got the cold shoulder all the way around. But I sat tight and am now carrying on pretty well. I was determined to do good or burst and I am not going to burst. I am beginning to get a little backing and am gradually winning friends and confidence and after a while I am going to have the full quota of Dental Surgeons in this division and more equipment. I am told at present, I can't have thirty-one Dental Surgeons but I'll get them all soon, it will take me a little time but I'll get them, if Col. Oliver will let me have the men. And he will, because he is behind us all, and we are for him.[16]

The division's dental officers were generally with the troops for emergency treatment, so no time was lost in sending soldiers to the rear for care. When a division moved, the dental surgeons accompanied the command and dental service was usually always available, even if for no more than pain relief. Cases were rarely evacuated to the rear, and in those instances, the cause was usually a complication requiring surgical attention. The field emergency kits that the dentists and their assistants carried consisted of the two Hospital Corps pouches, with a few selected instruments and appliances and a limited amount of supplies. In addition, the dentists and their assistants carried a cased dental engine, which weighed about 40 pounds. With this equipment, almost any treatment could be performed. The exact location of the dental surgeon was "determined by condi-

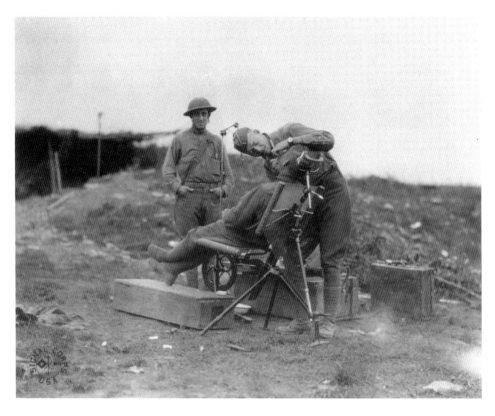

*First Lieutenant RM McNulty, dental surgeon, 309th Field Artillery Regiment, 78th Division,
with assistant Private JJ Cleveland, operates on a patient just back from the lines,
Fey-en-Haye, Meurthe et Moselle, France. September 22, 1918.
Photograph: Courtesy of US Army Military History Institute. SC 33390.*

tions and accommodations."[17]

The dental officer of each organization usually accompanied his battalion to the front line trenches and located himself at the battalion aid station, where he performed "all emergency and semi-permanent dental work necessary."[18] Troops in the trenches experienced a high percentage of alveolar abscesses and pulpitis, so it was advisable to have a dental surgeon available forward at all times. At the same time, the soldiers were little inclined to be concerned about dental work because they had, as Captain John Hughes, 29th Division dental surgeon noted, "more important things to think about." Once the divisions entered active combat operations at the front, the battalion dental surgeons were unable to do much dental work. Instead, they assisted the surgeons in caring for the wounded in the battalion and regimental aid stations and supervised their evacuation and transportation. When units suffered many casualties or lost their medical officers, the dental officers took over the medical duty, often for days at a time. The dental officers in the reserve area were located at the infirmary of the battalion headquarters and were also attached to the field hospitals (but not ambulance companies) assigned to the division's sanitary train. At field hospitals, dental officers were used principally to administer anesthetics, but they also did some dental treatment in quiet periods and in rest areas. After AEF General Headquarters issued General Order No. 99 on June 19, 1918, one of those field hospitals also housed a complete dental laboratory supporting the division's dental service. All the dental work was completed before patients were discharged from the field hospitals, including oral surgery when necessary.[5,18,19]

While working at aid stations at the front, the dental officers and their assistants were under constant threat of German artillery fire. Captain Walter E Lotz, DC, initially with the 310th Infantry Regiment and later division dental surgeon of the 78th Division, related how quickly disaster could strike:

> While on duty in an aid station near Jaulny Oct. 3rd, Capt. J.L. Remsen and his assistant, John Becker, assigned to the 308th Machine Gun Bn. along with twelve others were severely gassed. A mustard gas shell hit the door of the dugout in which the aid station had been established and caused much havoc.[20]

The dental officer's most trying time came during combat operations and the frequent shifts into and out of the lines and movement between sectors. As American forces transitioned from defensive operations to the offensive in the Aisne-Marne sector, the Saint Mihiel area, and finally the Meuse-Argonne operations of late September to early November 1918, the life of dental officers in the combat zones became much more complicated. First Lieutenant Guy A Karr, DC, 129th Infantry Regiment, 33rd Division, described what this all meant for the dental surgeon and his patients:

> From May 24th to October 25th, some 150 days, we moved 28 distinct times, marching 230 kilometers and spent 74 days in the front line trenches, making two hopovers. During this time I treated 600 patients. Of the 74 days that the regiment has been in the front line trenches I have spent 55 days at the Battalion aid station, 10 days at the transport lines four kilometers back of the front and 9 days at regimental headquarters. In my opinion one dental surgeon should always go forward with an Infantry regiment with an emergency equipment for combat use, and at least one dental surgeon should remain behind to treat the men from the transport and men who the dental surgeon in the forward area sends back. When all the dental surgeons stay behind the men who are doing the fighting must suffer.[21]

Echoing similar sentiments, First Lieutenant Howard I Denio, DC, who served with the 23rd Infantry Regiment, 2nd Division, from November 1917 to September 1918, and then with the 2nd Ammunition Train until the division returned to the United States in the summer of 1919, summed up his experience in the combat zone in the fall of 1918:

> In looking back I find that I have in a little over a year been stationed in about 45 different towns, in some for only a night, others for a week or two. I have slept in palaces and pup tents, in downy feathers and thorny briars, and many nights were spent on the road with a pack on my back. I have jumped from a cowshed to a castle and landed next day in a devastated town. Such are the fortunes of war—particularly this war. I have treated Frenchmen, Algerians, Belgians. Luxembergers [sic] and

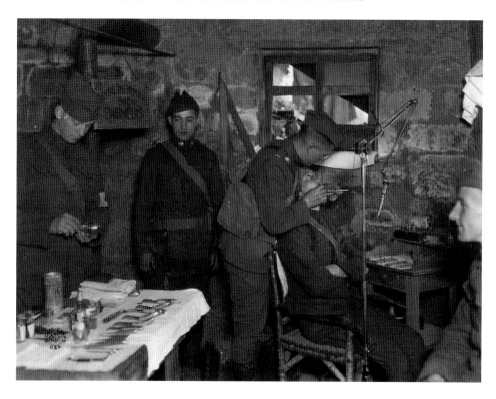

The dental infirmary of First Lieutenant Ralph F Krueger, dental surgeon, 302nd Engineers, 77th Division, near Abri du Crochet, Argonne Forest, France. October 29, 1918. Photograph: Courtesy of US Army Military History Institute. SC 42751.

Germans.[22(p121)]

In his short history of the 26th Division's dental service, Major Charles W Lewis, DC, the division dental surgeon, described his introduction to dental care in the division and his visit to the front line "office" of Lieutenant George Long, dental surgeon with the 104th Infantry Regiment (for more on Lieutenant Long, see "In Their Own Words" below):

When I reported for duty with the 26th. Division, the Headquarters and Division Surgeon's Office were located at Couvrelles. I at once proceeded to acquaint myself with conditions especially regarding dental officers and their equipment. My greatest hardship was the lack of personal transportation, however I managed to make some inspections by accompanying the Division Sanitary Inspector. The dental officers were located throughout the area with their several organizations. Some were on duty with Camp Infirmaries, while others were located in Battalion Aid Stations. Lieut. Long, 104th. Infantry was serving with his portable outfit at a Battalion Aid Station in the trenches. His office was not far from Chemin-des-Dames. Lieut. Long's office in the reserve trenches was particularly well located in a dugout in these well built trenches. He was in a position to do considerable dental work at this place and visited

596

the other battalions with his emergency outfit. This office was an exception. Most officers with the portable outfit were located with Camp Infirmaries and Field Hospitals.[7]

In his job as division dental surgeon, Major Lewis had difficulty getting around to all of his dental officers, especially those with front line units, to check on their work, assess their working conditions and problems, and to assist them, if possible. Often "the courtesy of other officers" allowed him to obtain transportation and get to the front. There he found his dental officers fully involved in every aspect of front line medical work and often overburdened with other duties:

Many of the dental officers were stationed at battalion aid and dressing stations and assisted with the evacuating of the wounded and dressing and applying splints. The dental officers serving with the 102nd. Infantry did very good work attending the wounded at the Battle of Seicheprey [20-21 April 1918]. . . .The first of July found the Division in the Chateau Thierry Sector to take part in the second battle of the Marne. The division relieved the Second Division who had very severe fighting at Belleau Woods. The dental personnel of the division performed many duties foreign to dentistry in this sector. The 103d Field Hospital was located at La Ferté and functioned as a hospital for seriously wounded. Lieut.

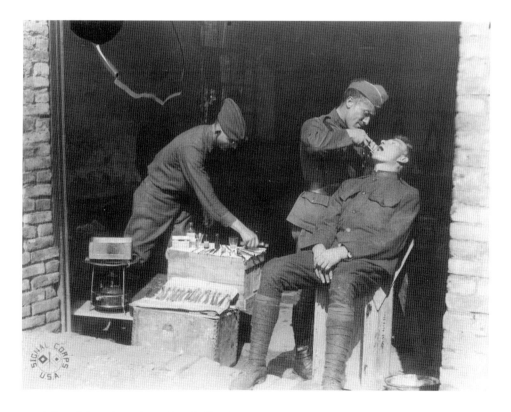

A French barn is used as a dental office by First Lieutenant Ernest R Latham, Dental Corps, 305th Field Signal Battalion, 80th Division. He and his dental assistant freeze and loosen the tooth of Sergeant McHugh before extracting it. Latham's regulation trench dental outfit is laid out for use. Beauval, France, July 31, 1918.
Photograph: Courtesy of US Army Military History Institute. SC 21591.

597

[Clifford W] Renth, the dental surgeon serving with this hospital was on duty as dental surgeon, anesthetist, supply and mess officer for the hospital. He worked valiantly, night and day as anesthetist in order to relieve surgeons and performed his own duties as well.[7]

C Franklin MacDonald, DRC, who served with the 11th Engineer Regiment (Railway), which was heavily committed in both the British and American sectors from November 1917 on, pointed out after the war that dental surgeons could do a considerable amount of useful dental work at the front, provided they were experienced, had good light and shelter, and good assistants.

As to actual dental work, a great deal of constructive dental work can be done and ought to be done in the combat zone. Amalgam, cement and gutta-percha fillings can be placed, teeth can be cleaned and gums treated. As a general rule, teeth with exposed pulps or abscessed conditions should be extracted. Root canal treatments or root fillings should rarely be attempted. Fractures of the jaws from whatever cause should never be treated by the ordinary dental officer in the combat zone. Temporary wiring, splinting or bandaging is all that is necessary. The patient should be promptly evacuated to a proper unit equipped to care for such conditions. . . .The fact that dental work is being done under adverse or difficult conditions is no excuse for poor dental work. Work may proceed more slowly and equipment may not be ideal, but decay can be completely removed, cavity margins carefully prepared, fillings well placed and properly dressed down so that there are no overhanging margins, contour and occlusion made correct, and a general finish produced worthy of inspection.[23(p1243)]

MacDonald cautioned that what could get done in the combat zone was entirely dependent upon "the capacity of the individual dental officer," who had to rely on his own resources and solve his own problems. Dental work in the combat zone required "men of some years of professional experience." Recent graduates and inexperienced dentists were far better assigned to rear areas, base hospitals, or training camps. "In the field, where conditions are not favorable and equipment often incomplete, the man of experience is needed, one who can get along with little, has confidence, skill, speed and sound judgment, the result of practice."[23]

As to the assistant, MacDonald stressed the importance of a carefully selected enlisted dental assistant in the combat zone.

The right type and temperament will prove of incalculable value under many different situations. A man who can find a wooden flooring when wood is not available, who can get a heating apparatus when stoves are not procurable, who can get coal or wood when such is not to be had, etc., is a gem. The wise dental officer also is he who asks no questions.[23(p1243)]

MacDonald concluded:

It is obvious that little in the way of rules for procedures can be laid down for the officer called on to do dental work in the combat zone. He will, for the most part, be obliged to formulate his own methods. As situations change, he must be able to change with them, adopting himself to new and, many times, unpleasant conditions. No matter how difficult the situations seem to be, dental officers who have the will and the desire to do so, will find that they can accomplish much in their small sphere of duty, toward sustaining the health, comfort and efficiency of the fighting men.[23(p1247)]

However, not all division dental surgeons believed that having the dental officers forward in the combat zone or the trenches was the best approach to take, regardless of their years of experience or maturity. For example, Major (later Colonel) Lee S Fountain, DC, division dental surgeon of the 77th Division, concluded:

The division went into action immediately on the Vesle. Here, we were up against an entirely different proposition. The activities were so intense that it was impossible to establish dental infirmaries very far in advance. After a few days something like twelve dental officers were able to operate part of the time. The others with their emergency kits were extracting a tooth or sealing in a treatment that might pass their way. From observations on the various fronts the conclusion is naturally made–no dental surgeon should ever accompany a battalion into action. The dental service required does not warrant this. Well do I recall a conversation I had with a British medical officer shortly after our arrival in France. When I explained that there were three dental surgeons to each regiment of infantry, he remarked "What a sacrifice of life that will be". Thus far, dame fortune has treated us kindly, although many have had close calls. Even tho the lives are spared, the loss in misdirected energy cannot be measured. In the Argonne sector it was a similar experience.[3]

On November 1, 1918, in a lengthy memo to Colonel Boak at the Army Sanitary School, Captain John M Hughes, DC, division dental surgeon, 29th Division, supported Fountain's position, a view that he subsequently altered in his "Dental History, 29th Division" of January 27, 1919:

The question of distribution of dental surgeons within a division during action at the front is one which has given me a great deal of concern since I have had opportunity to observe the condition associated therewith. The questions arising are whether dental surgeons will function as (a) dental officers (b) medical officers or (c) as surplus officers to do whatever is found convenient for them to do. At the front during action a dental surgeon cannot functionate [sic] except as a medical officer. If the intention is to convert dental officers into medical officers and put them in charge of dressing stations in the front lines where it is impossible to do other than the most urgent first aid work, to put them in charge of litter squads or to put them on any duty where they can serve in a capacity whereby medical and other officers are released for other duty, the intention is being carried out under the existing conditions. If dental officers are to remain dental officers, function as dental officers, restore and repair the masticatory apparatus of military personnel, and perform operations credit for which is given by the dental corps in its various branches and not by another corps, then, it is my opinion, that some modification or flexible arrangement by which this can be accomplished should be instituted. This is quite a problem.[5,6]

Despite the protests of Fountain and Hughes, the valuable contributions of the dental officers and their assistants in the rear and under fire at the front was not lost on many of their commanders and Medical Corps superiors. In his medical history report of November 27, 1918, to the division commander, Major Frederick W O'Donnell, MC, division surgeon, 89th Division, wrote of the work of the dental surgeons during the Meuse-Argonne operations:

> Owing to the fact that the Division went into action short 16 Medical Officers, shortly increased by casualties to 23, it was necessary to use the Dental Surgeons in the battalion. To say they did their duty well is putting it mildly, and nothing but appreciation has been heard of their work under conditions in which, up to this time, they had had no experience.[24]

Major Fountain looked at the entire experience in a different way:

> Without question the duty of the Dental Corps is to dentally equip each soldier as near as practicable and keep his mouth in such a condition that will render him a fighting man at all times. . . . Has the Dental Surgeon fulfilled his mission? Yes, and no. Yes, in that no body of men could have accomplished more than has been done under like circumstances. Time and again have I found a dental infirmary established where it seemed the impossible thing to do. As a concrete example, one dental surgeon's entire outfit suffered the effects of a direct hit from two Boche H.E. [high explosive] shells. The equipment was immediately replaced and he continued to function as usual. No, because only a small portion of his time has been utilized in the discharge of his professional duties, then under the most adverse circumstances where he could not do justice to the patient or himself. True, it may be said you were a jolly good lot of fellows. When we need an officer to take charge of a transport and bring supplies— you did it well. "After all is said and done, what did you do as Dental Surgeons to help win the war."[3]

In his division's dental history, Major Charles F Huber, DC, division dental surgeon for the 88th Division, concluded that despite all the hardships and difficulties, the Army dental service had achieved the recognition that dental officers had sought.

> . . . it must be said that our experience has shown the most disagreeable features of the army life of a Dental Surgeon to be those in connection with the frequent moving that is always incidental to a Division on active duty at the front. The "breaking up" office, the packing up, moving, and the tedious and most always difficult task of locating a suitable place for "setting up" when once the move has been accomplished. In the smaller French towns it is almost impossible to find a room with light suitable for Dental Operations and our Dental Surgeons have often in this respect worked under conditions truly pitiful. . . . Thus considered, the quality and quantity of the work which they have done, and the spirit in which they have accomplished it should most certainly win them the approval of our entire military institution.[25]

With the 1st Division, 1917–1918

Life at the front for a dental officer was a mixture of routine dental work and hectic periods of hazardous duty under German fire in the trenches. In a long letter of November 10, 1918, to his former colleagues of the Dallas County [Texas] Dental Society, Captain Allen N Kearby, DRC, detailed his experiences with the 18th Infantry Regiment, 1st Division, in France. He had reported for duty in late June 1917 and been sent directly to France, where he was assigned to his regiment at Haudelaincourt. There he was the only dental surgeon assigned to care for the regimental headquarters, supply company, and 1st and 3rd battalions—nearly 3,000 soldiers. Kearby was assigned an assistant, who he said "was a green man, but learned very quickly, so that now I am sure I am able to do 100% more work than I could possibly accomplish without him." Their work was ample but simple:

> The work consists of amalgam, cement and gutta percha fillings, treatment of putrescent root canals and consequent filling; devitalizing and extirpation of pulps; and filling of canals; removing salivary deposits; treatment of gingivitis and pyorrhea, extraction of teeth—(no plates, crowns, bridges or inlays)—as these cases are taken care of at the base hospitals, provided they are absolutely necessary.[26(p9)]

In January 1918 the 1st Division entered the front lines in the Toul sector.

> On Jan. 16, 1918 our Regt. left Haudelaincourt—left for the front, going to the Toul sector, the Medical Officers being on the Colonel's staff and mounted, the "doughboys" marching afoot. After two days march we reached Mansonville (Brigade Headquarters) where we stayed until the night of Jan. 19th, when we marched six kilometers to Beaumont (Regimental Headquarters) where we had out Regimental Aid Station in a dugout. Two battalions of "doughboys" continued their march to the front trenches two hundred yards beyond Seicheprey (Battalion Headquarters). I took with me nothing but extracting forceps, two excavators, a pair of dressing pliers and oil of cloves, as most of my work consisted of helping Medical Officers doing a little "first aid," and a great deal of sanitary inspection of the villages, trenches, food, [canteens], kitchens, billets and mess kits.[26(p9)]

In March the 18th Infantry was pulled from the trenches and Kearby was able to obtain leave and visit Nice for 7 days. Upon returning, he was transferred to the 2nd Battalion, 18th Infantry, at Saint Joie. The 2nd Battalion went back to the front and entered the trenches at Villers-Tournelle, opposite the Germans at Cantigny, on April 21, 1918. The regimental and battalion aid stations there were located in cellars, and the battalion received a great deal of attention from the Germans.[26(pp9–10)]

> . . . the village was industriously shelled by the d____ Boches. It was here that I was rather badly gassed on the night of May 3rd, the Boches having put 15,000 shells over (estimated by the Intelligence Department) in four hours. There were seven officers billeted in our cellar, including the two battalion (2nd) surgeons, and the following night but two of us were left, the other five including the two medical officers having been evacuated to hospitals; and as other medical officers were not sent up until May 5th, I was the only medical with the Battalion for 24 hours.[26(p10)]

When the 2nd battalion was relieved on May 12, Kearby learned that the division surgeon, Lieutenant Colonel (later Colonel) Herbert G Shaw, MC, had ordered that no dental officers would go to the front with the troops. When his battalion reentered the lines a week later, Kearby remained behind at Maisoncelle working with patients from the 16th and 28th infantry regiments "with an emergency outfit consisting of alloy, cement, etc., but a hand engine instead of a foot engine, and no chair." While there, Kearby also saw training for upcoming attacks: "I saw them rehearse the attack back at Maisoncelle, one day without tanks, and the next day with tanks—tanks were used in the real attack."[26]

On June 5 Kearby rejoined the 18th Infantry at Poillart, 14 kilometers behind Villers-Tournelle. By July 14, the 2nd Battalion had moved up to the Compiegne forest in preparation for offensive operations.[26(p11)] During July and August 1918 the 2st Division was engaged in heavy fighting around Soissons as part of the Allied offensive against German forces in the Marne salient, and Kearby and the 2nd Battalion were deeply involved.

> Began marching at 7 p.m. July 17th, and at 5 a.m. July 18th, after marching all night, we went into the attack at Conevres. At this place we established a Regimental Aid Station where I with the Major [and] the commanding officer of the Medical Detachment [Major Hiram E Ross, MC], stayed until 5 a.m. July 19th. We were kept so busy caring for the wounded (in a dugout) that we had no sleep at all and but little to eat. We turned over this station to another Division and moved forward to catch up with our own Regiment; walked eight kilometers over the battle ground, covered with every conceivable article of equipment from canteens to broken and abandoned Boche cannon, dead horses, mules, Boches, and alas—our own brave lads, reaching Chandun, a small village just in advance of our Regimental P.C. (Headquarters). Found a cellar, stuck out our Red Cross and again began caring for wounded. Here we stayed until 6 a.m. July 20th, at which time we turned our station over to an Ambulance Dressing Station, and moved forward as our "doughboys" had continued to push the Boches. This time we did not go but four kilometers, where we found a nice cliff between us and the Boches' shells, so here we hung out the flag which the wounded soldier hails with joy, because after reaching this he feels his troubles are over.
>
> Our two Battalion surgeons who were with me, soon pushed forward to get in touch with the other four Battalion surgeons of our Regiment, but ere long came back with some wounded, and it was here that Drs. [Captain David R] Morgan and Seigel [First Lieutenant HA Seigall] were wounded; the three of us at the time being engaged in cutting a wounded soldier's clothing in order to dress his wounds. In the afternoon of this the 20th of July, our Regimental Surgeon received notice that two more Captains, [Sidney A] McCurdy and [Albert W] Lindberg, had been wounded and sent to hospitals, so but four of us were left. We were relieved by Scottish troops the night of July 22, the relief to be completed before daylight of the 23rd. The Medical detachment did not get out until long after daylight (5:30 a.m.) as we had two wounded men 2 ½ kilometers from the nearest point to which the ambulances came, and we had to get them down; so at midnight I took two sergeants and the only five men we had left (the others had been killed, wounded and gassed) and started out for them. A medical officer and a sergeant were with these wounded so the ten of us brought them back, reaching the ambulance evacuation point at 4 a.m. and believe me, carrying one fourth the weight of a man on a litter is the hardest work I have ever done. Our assembling point for the Regiment was at a distance of about 15 kilometers, which we footed, and after six days, with no sleep, and eating at irregular times, most of the food consisting of corned Willie and hard tack, taken from the packs of dead and wounded—that walk was a bit tiresome.[26–28]

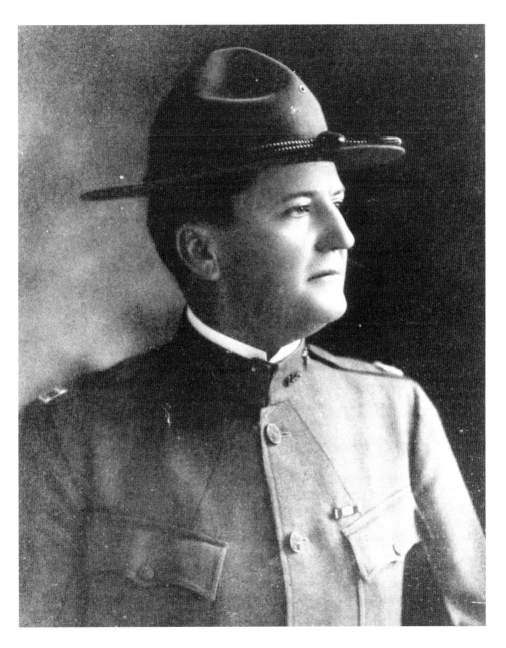

Colonel Robert T Oliver, American Expeditionary Forces, 1918.
Photograph: Courtesy of the National Library of Medicine.

On July 31 Kearby was ordered to the 1st Division's Field Hospital No. 3, which supported the 18th Infantry and where he could work steadily, "as I found there a complete portable outfit."[26(p13)] Promoted to captain in August, Kearby soon moved to the IV Corps and then II Corps Artillery Park.

A Dentist's Experience with the 2nd Division

During September 1918 Colonel Oliver instructed all dental surgeons to write down accounts of their wartime experiences for preservation and potential use in a Dental Corps history of the World War. Oliver wrote:

> It is very desirous that the Dental Corps keep a record of their work during this war. Though it may not seem important at this time to gather such information, yet in days to come it will be a wonderful asset to our profession, hence it behooves all of us to help in this matter. Therefore each dental surgeon will write an account of his experiences in the form of a history from the time of arrival in France to the present time and send in additions each month.[29,30]

In response to Oliver's directive, on October 19, 1918, First Lieutenant George E Staats, DC, 2nd Division, then at Ferme de Suippe, prepared a detailed report of his experiences with the division. After arriving in France in the fall of 1917, he was ordered to the 2nd Division Headquarters at Bourmont, which he reached by train "on a cold and stormy November night" after a few days "stop over to 'see Paris.'" He was assigned to the 5th Regiment, US Marine Corps, which had its headquarters at Brouvannes, and formed the division's 4th Infantry Brigade along with the 6th Regiment, US Marine Corps. At the post dental office Staats met Alexander G Lyle, US Navy dental surgeon, described by Staats as "a royal good fellow," who he assisted while waiting for his requisition for a "complete portable dental outfit" to be filled. He commented:

> It surely was a remarkable sight to see the lads lined up outside the door of the office awaiting treatment, while inside three dentists were working their heads off; one with his patient in the chair; another, calling an improvised chair into service; and the third with his patient on the floor (or deck as the Marines call it), mouth wide open, and head between the operators legs having a lower molar, broken beyond repair, extracted.[31]

The companies of Marines were lined up on the street and given complete dental examinations. They were then divided into the following classes:

- Class A: requiring immediate treatment with extractions or exposed pulps;
- Class B: not as urgent but in poor condition;
- Class C: good condition; and
- Class D: perfect.

Staats had still not received his dental equipment but continued to assist Dr Lyle until he was reassigned.[31]

Staats recalled one Thanksgiving at Brouvannes:

> One event during my sojourn with the Marines is noteworthy and that the Thanks-

giving dinner we had on that day. The same being served to both officers and men. Uncle Sam saw to it that his boys in France should have turkey with stuffing, cranberry sauce, sweet corn (very seldom seen over here), pumpkin pie, and all the usual "fixin's" which practically every American is accustomed to on that day. Believe me it surely was some feast and enjoyed and appreciated by all.[31]

On December 17, 1917, Staats was ordered to headquarters at Bourmont to assist Lieutenant Colonel Rex H Rhoades, the division dental surgeon, who had an infected finger. He described his experience with the future chief of the Dental Corps:

I, having no equipment and Col. Rhoades having a sore hand, did what I could to help out; but was always in extreme fear that I would either do something to displease him or injure his equipment. He had a very nice office, there, on the top floor of the school house and we did considerable work. However, there was one difficulty and that was in securing fuel to keep the place warm. We had to continually request the Q.M., and almost beg him for the very smallest allowance.[31]

On January 2, 1918, Staats received orders to report to the dental section of the Army Sanitary School at Langres to attend the school's second class. When class began the next morning, it was so cold the students had to keep their overcoats on. Staats remarked that Langres was a "cold, cold Place in the winter time with nary a place to warm up." He returned to Bourmont on January 15 and was assigned to Camp Hospital No. 3. His portable outfit finally arrived, and he was assigned a room in the "clinic building," which had been planned for "Dental and Oral Surgery." The engineers had not yet completed the plumbing. Staats wrote:

What a mess that clinic building was, with a trench thru which the pipes were to run where the hall and waiting room were planned and all the rooms filled with earth taken from the ditch. It was rather difficult to hustle those engineers to finish the job and I suppose they really thought I didn't mean business until they found out otherwise, but I got them to lay sufficient pipe in order that the ditch could be filled in front of the door of what was to be my operating room, thus giving me access to the room and getting all of the earth out of that room. Hastening to set up the equipment and starting to operate, apparently caused the engineers to think that I did mean business and they hustled up their work so that within a few days I had running water in the room. I had a bench, table, desk, and bookshelf built and a stove set up. This made a very comfortable office, operating room and laboratory and one in which I could do all kinds of work except vulcanite. The vulcanizer took rather a long time to arrive and only reached me after moving to several other areas.[31]

Staats took "great pride in the office" he had established. "That little room proved to be the busiest place in the whole hospital and we performed all kinds of dental operations. I pointedly said 'we' because Col. Rhoades assigned an assistant to me who assisted me remarkably well in establishing and maintaining the work there." He immediately began ordering supplies from C Ash & Sons in Paris (gold, solder, facings, and porcelain crowns), even though they were not on the government list. He telegraphed in the orders and they arrived by post in a few days, allowing him to render a "distinctive service," (eg, repairs to crowns and bridges, inlays, cast gold and porcelain crowns).[31]

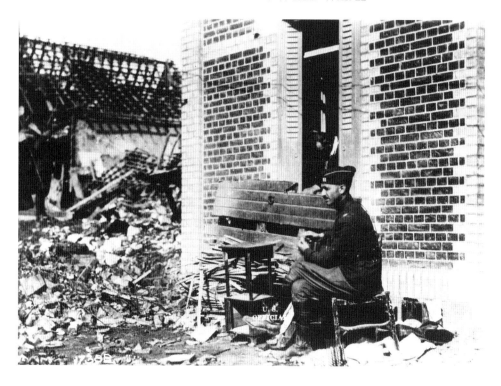

Captain Robert H Luce. Dental Officer Reserve Corps, dental surgeon, 305th Engineers,
80th Division, who was billeted in the building adjacent to those destroyed by aerial torpedo.
His own room was completely demolished. Beauval, France, July 18, 1918.
Photograph: Courtesy of US Army Military History Institute. SC 17388.

When the division moved to Ancemont, Staats's office was set up in the "Petit Chateau" and later moved to the "Grande Chateau," which had a waiting room that doubled as his bedroom, an operating room, and a laboratory. Here he also endured his first enemy attack when the medical staff came under bombardment and the house next to the "Petit Chateau" (from which they had just moved) was destroyed.[31]

The division was relieved and moved to Robert Espagne not far from Bar-le-Duc. The dental office was established in an uncompleted chateau. The division moved to Chaumont-en-Vexin next and set up a dental office. During the stay at Chaumont-en-Vexin, the vulcanizer at last arrived. The division then moved to Meaux, where Staats had "stormy and historic days in the line and little attention was given dental troubles unless very acute and severe."

> Being somewhat off the regular lines of evacuation the Division Surgeon was confronted with the problem of not having an evacuation hospital but successfully solved the problem by securing the Hôpital du Colleg de Juilly at Juilly, but not having sufficient force there, surgical teams were organized from the division and sent there. When there I served as anaesthetist on Captain Eichenberry's team [and] as Admissions and evacuation officer until Platts relieved me, Also wired a considerable number of

cases of fracture of the mandible and maxilla. There it was that I realized the purport of the courses in bandaging, and oral surgery given us at the Sanitary School. Talk about busy, why, the whole bunch were certainly kept on the jump, forty-two hours was my first round of duty without any sleep. . . . The boys effectually stopped Fritz on his "march to Paris" and were driving him back in the Bois Belleau, Boureschs and Vaux so we were all sent to La Ferte to establish and operate a hospital for seriously wounded with F.H. #23, as a nucleus. Many surgical teams from the Base Hospitals had previously arrived at Juilly to relieve us. At La Ferte Curry and Brann also joined us. My assistant effectively took care of my equipment during this period and had it transported under orders from Col. Graham [2nd Division dental surgeon replacing Lieutenant Colonel Rhoades] with the Medical Supply Depot property from Meaux to La Ferte. At that hospital my duties were principally as an anaesthetist but when Captain Brennan's operating assistant left him I assisted him in that capacity for several days until another arrived. Also wired a number of Jaw fractures.[31]

As the 26th Division relieved the 2nd Division, a 26th Division field hospital relieved Staats's group. The 2nd's Field Hospital No. 23 moved up to Mery and while there Staats and Lieutenant Cole examined and began treating the hospital staff. The next stop was Taillefontaine, where the dentists again worked at "receiving patients, giving T.S. [tetanus serum, also called ATS, anti-tetanus serum] and bandaging." After moving to Nanteuil, Staats was transferred to Field Hospital No. 16 and assisted Lieutenant Saunders for a few days. He was later transferred to the 5th Machine Gun Battalion stationed at Bregy, where he worked as the battalion dentist. The next move was to Nancy, where the battalion conducted practice. The division went back into the line after leaving Nancy and Staats went to Ville-au-Val where he procured toothbrushes from the Red Cross representative and issued them to the troops who did not have one (because of the shortage of brushes, the supply officer had previously issued only one brush for each squad). Staats considered this to be the "most equitable way of distribution." He worked on the companies rotated in the sector and held sick call in a dugout near Pont-à-Mousson, going up to the line every morning as the division prepared for the Saint Mihiel offensive. He was ordered to Field Hospital No. 15, but after only 2 days the division moved forward to Thiaucourt. Things seemed to be quiet there until Staats and two other officers were walking up the road to get their shaving gear from the trucks.

"Whizz-bangs" started coming over but landed quite a distance away and they thought the Germans were firing at one of the Allied batteries at the edge of the adjacent woods. Then about the fourth or fifth came over, (whizz-bang) exploding about 10 feet from us wounding Hilton slightly and severely wounding a lad from the 9th Infantry up the road. While Harper and myself were lifted from our feet and thrown into the ditch. Crawling up the ditch found ourselves among a battalion, dug-in on the roadside in the support position. After the wounded lad was dressed to stop the blood, Harper got an ambulance to take them to the hospital in the town. That evening the Germans started to throw big ones into the town and we were forced to operate in a dugout which was wonderfully adapted for the purpose being formed into an operating room and ward.[31]

After being relieved by the 78th Division, Staats pitched an officer's wall tent and again resumed dental practice until the division moved to Champagne, where it set up a hospital at La Vouve. This in turn was ripped down and reestablished near Suippes where the dental equipment was set up in the admissions tent so that emergency work could be provided quickly. While there, Staats also functioned as an anesthetist on one of the surgical teams. The next stop was at Sommepy, where the hospital was established about 3 or 4 kilometers behind the front lines, near seven cross roads, a bridge, ammunition dump, artillery camp, and artillery positions, all of which were targets for German gunners. During one of the frequent shellings, a round came through one of the ward tents and another broke one of the guy ropes of a tent nearby. Both were "duds." Staats recalled:

> Many splinters, of course, of those which didn't; and quite so close were heard "whizzing" thru the air. It sure was strange working and giving anesthetics, under canvas, while the shells came "whizzing" over. Unconsciously every one around the operating table would stoop as we heard the shells "whizzing" over. It surely was working under trying conditions having come out of the line I have again resumed dental practice under canvas.[31]

Lieutenant Colonel George D Graham: Division Dental Surgeon, 2nd Division

Division dental surgeons strove to maintain the highest level of dental service possible, despite the constant movements into and out of the line. On March 10, 1918, Lieutenant Colonel George D Graham, DC, became the 2nd Division's dental surgeon, replacing Lieutenant Colonel Rex Rhoades, who was appointed supervising dental surgeon for the advance section of the services of supply. Graham, one of the original Dental Corps officers from 1911 who retired as a colonel in August 1945, is one of the few division dental surgeons who left a personal account of his tenure rather than a dental history of his division. His comments provide a unique look at the problems confronting a division dental surgeon in a heavily engaged combat division.[22,32,33]

The 2nd Division was unique in the AEF, as well as in the history of the US Army, because it was a mixed (today referred to as "joint") division of US Army and US Marine Corps units, under Army and later Marine Corps command. As a result, dental support for the Marine Corps elements of the 4th Infantry Brigade (5th and 6th Marine regiments and the Marine's 6th Machine Gun Battalion) was a blend of Army and Navy Dental Corps officers, with Army dental officers working in Marine units from the first days of the division's arrival in France in 1917. When Graham arrived, the division had 16 Army and 3 Navy dentists assigned, and those numbers fluctuated throughout the war as dental officers became casualties, fell sick, or were transferred. All dentists "were equipped for field service" and a dental laboratory provided support. According to Graham, the mission of the dental officers in the division was twofold: (1) to prevent to evacuation of the trained military personnel for oral and dental reasons, and (2) "to accomplish such less urgent and more elaborate service as conditions and equipment permit."[22,34]

From late March through November 1918, the 2nd Division was actively involved in major operations on the Verdun defensive sector (March–May), the critical Aisne-Château–Thierry defensive operations and Aisne-Marne Offensive around Soissons (June–July) that stopped the German offensive and threw it back, and later operations in the Saint Mihiel and Meuse-Argonne offensives (September–November).[22,34] 2nd Division infantry typically deployed a battalion of each regiment to the trenches and the others to the reserve positions to the rear. Dental officers with the advanced elements had only emergency dental kits, consisting of four cloth rolls of equipment, medicines, and supplies in two pouches (see Chapter 13: The Dental Service in the American Expeditionary Forces in France, 1917–1919: Organization, Administration, Personnel, Training, and Supply), but the kits were always in short supply and easily lost during combat operations. Those dentists with the reserves in more tranquil settings used the modified portable field dental outfits, although not all dentists or organizations had the authorized equipment.[22,35] Once the 2nd Division began mobile offensive operations in the summer of 1918, the dentists faced a more fluid situation.

> Dental officers were installed in towns, in which troops were temporarily billeted, in dugouts, in tents and occasionally by the roadside, wherever their organizations happened to be, often under shell fire. The character of the service rendered and the equipment used was determined entirely by local conditions, and these changed from day to day, and week to week, through the course of the campaign, and it was therefore rarely possible to anticipate what tomorrow's problem in this respect would be. There was no sharp demarcation.[22(pp116–117)]

Dental officers in the 2nd Division were actively involved in all aspects of the division's medical operations. Graham later commented:

> A particularly gratifying feature of the service of the dental personnel through the different engagements of the Division was its utilization in the various functions of the Medical Department. Dental officers were not confined strictly to dental service, but when combat conditions precluded their functioning as dental surgeons, they were immediately available and were employed as utility officers of the Medical Department, where their services were of considerable practical value, and they therefore, to the credit of the dental service with combat troops, were not held in abeyance until the troops were withdrawn from the front line. They were a constant and practical part of the Medical Department personnel with their respective organizations, and were present at all times to render their own special service or to be employed otherwise as occasion required.[22(p117)]

During operations at Château-Thierry, the division added eight surgical teams to its Field Hospital No. 23 then at La Ferté-sous-Jouarre, where it received the most seriously wounded directly from division triage at Field Hospital No. 1. Each of these teams had a dental surgeon as an anesthetist. One dental surgeon, First Lieutenant Charles H Cole, DC, recently assigned to the field hospital from duty with the 5th Marines, administered anesthetics for 18 straight hours. Thereafter, dental officers were assigned to the field hospital as anesthetists in ensuing operations.[22]

Dental officers in the rear area of the division with the ammunition, supply, and sanitary trains, especially the field hospitals and dental laboratory, provided important but often unnoticed services to conserve the division's fighting strength. They gave uninterrupted dental care to soldiers and thus kept many troops with oral and dental problems from being evacuated out of the division as non-effectives. Graham wrote that "it was not the quantity of service accomplished at these times that was of most importance. . . . It was the fact that it was always available when required, and therefore saved from evacuation effectives that were urgently needed." In this respect, the dental laboratory was particularly important for the divisional dental service. The dental laboratory was first assigned to one of the field hospitals of the 2nd Sanitary Train, but was later moved to the division headquarters where it was in the center of activity and more easily reached.[22] Graham believed that the dental laboratory was critical because it:

> . . . functioned during the entire tour of the Division in the combat area and not only repeatedly saved both commissioned and enlisted personnel from evacuation, but cared for replacements that came to the Division, and who could otherwise not have been retained. A number of vulcanite dentures were made for the purpose of mastication and in a number of cases enable men to wear gas masks. These men would otherwise have been evacuated.[22(p120)]

In a memo issued on September 10, 1918, Graham urged the dental surgeons to "make every effort to accomplish dental service wherever possible." In camp, dental surgeons were expected to render treatment quickly because portable dental equipment could be "unpacked or packed within an hour." Even on marches when units were halted for only 24 hours, the dental surgeons had to be ready to work as needs arose. Under no circumstances should "an officer or soldier ever be dismissed without necessary attention." Such responsiveness was the dental surgeon's "duty and obligation," and was to be "carefully observed." If temporarily absent from their units, the dental surgeons directed their assistants to tell patients when they would return and be able to render emergency treatment.[36] Soldier care was an ever-present concern not only of the division dental surgeon but also of each dental officer with the troops in the combat zone. Graham proudly noted that the Army and Navy dental officers of the division were highly decorated for bravery and included two Navy Medal of Honor recipients (see "Awards for Heroism" below).

In Their Own Words: Personal Experiences of Dental Officers at the Front

A number of dental officers prepared accounts of varying length and detail on their experiences in France and along the western front in response to Colonel Oliver's request. However, the pressures of daily duty, constant movements, and combat operations were much more critical for most front line dental officers, and compliance with Oliver's request was limited. Thus, the number of memoirs eventually received and now preserved in the National Archives was small compared with the number of dental officers serving in France. The personal recollections that follow come from a handful of divisions that apparently stressed the comple-

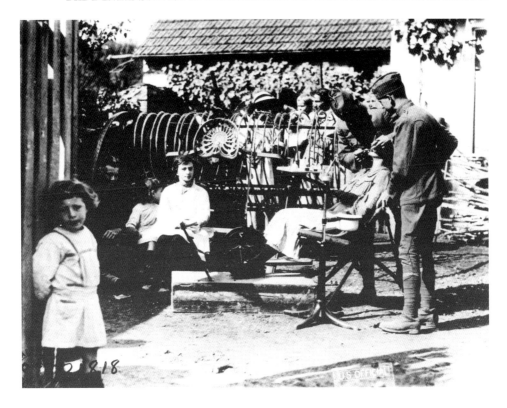

First Lieutenant PE Gilley, 4th Division Train, Dental Officer Reserve Corps, giving free treatment to a French civilian in a small town where there are no French doctors left. Rimacourt, France, August 20, 1918. Photograph: Courtesy of US Army Military History Institute. SC 21818.

tion of these narrative accounts—the 26th, 29th, 78th, and 82nd divisions. In the following excerpts, AEF divisional dental officers vividly relate their stories "in their own words," often recorded within weeks of the events.

First Lieutenant Herbert W Huff, 2nd Battalion, 114th Infantry Regiment; 114th Field Hospital, 104th Sanitary Train; and 3rd Battalion, 115th Infantry Regiment, 26th Division

After being located here [Courcelles, France] for about three weeks we again hiked to Vaux where we entrained and rode all night and reached Morvillers where we left the train and hiked about four miles to a small town called Meziere. This place afforded a very good location for a dental office and I put up my outfit on the second floor of a large school-house. The light was very good here and I accomplished quite a bit here also. After remaining here for about two weeks we left one evening about nine o'clock with the battalion [3rd] and hiked quite a distance to a rather good sized village called Montreau Chateau and here located in a building the French had used for an infirmary before we arrived. At this place we had a very good location for our office, light very good and plenty of room. While here I treated a number of civilians and finished work on a number of our men. From Montreau Chateau we had a long hike leaving about nine P.M. and arriving at Ritzwiller about three A.M. and went into barracks which the French had used for their infirmary. This building evidently had not been put up with expectations of a dentist locating there as the windows were made of paper material and very little light came through. On account of this we put our equipment in the yard under a large tree in clear weather and when it rained put it in the building, but could do only emergency work here as it was too dark. After leaving here we hiked through Dannemarie into Hagenbach which was counted as the third line at that time. Reaching there at nine-thirty and I was assigned to a dressing station in the trenches at Englengen, arriving there with my assistant and four bandsmen as litter bearers at about ten-thirty P.M. Of course, we could only do emergency work of a dental nature here as the dugout was very dark and dental outfit had been left at the battalion infirmary at Hagenbach. The emergency outfit was only carried with us into the trenches. After spending three or four days here I was relieved by a lst Lieut. of the Medical Corps and reported to the infirmary in Hagenbach where we put up our equipment and did good work. After staying here for about ten days we were relieved and hiked back to Manspach. After camping here all day we left at night and hiked into Montreau Chateau and put up our outfits in the same office as we had had before.[6]

First Lieutenant Bernard R Thornton, 327th Infantry Regiment, 82nd Division

[September 14, 1918] An order came for two companies to get in contact with the enemy at five P.M. Each company must have one Medical Officer with four medical men within twenty paces of the rear. They were to go over behind a smoke screen. I was sleeping until five when the Major came in with the order. He said that he had only one Medical Officer to send and I volunteered to be the second. In five minutes we were going down the road behind the companies and the beautiful smoke screen began to rise from our shells. In a couple of minutes the German artillery put down a barrage just behind and in the smoked screen and caught our boys in the act. They most heroically advanced and when we reached our first trench the wounded began to come in in quantities. The first chap was a clean cut fellow from New York City and had his arm shot away at the shoulder joint and you could see at least four ribs. He was not bleeding at all as some one had wrapped his shoulder with a leather string. He was bright and cheerful. We found a piece of corrugated iron to get under and work and with blankets stopped the cracks so that it was light proof. We worked here as fast as possible until twelve o'clock. Had every kind of wound to treat that shrapnel and bullets could make. I did my part of this work and the Battalion Commander came and stayed three hours with us. After he watched us work a couple of hours he suddenly said to me "Boy, you are a dentist, I did not know that you could do this kind of work." I afterwards heard that he boosted me up at Regimental Headquarters and my status changed from that day on in my battalion from a figure head to that of necessity. The lieutenants that were always throwing GUFF changed their attitudes at once. Some of them got a sample of my work and said that the Dental Corps was with them until the end. . . . [September 30, 1918] Just at daybreak the boys began moving around and pretty soon the Germans put a terrific shell fire over on us. Shells killed men on all sides of me, and I went down to the foot of the hill and found some elegant iron huts and found so many had been wounded a battalion surgeon established an aid station, and for two days and nights we were busy with the dead and wounded from the front. The Germans were most desperate in their resistance and it was a nasty job for our boys. Many of our officers were wounded here. Our battalion was ordered over the top one afternoon from Château Chéhéry [Châtel-Chéhéry] and we followed them into the town and established an aid station at the edge of the town next to the line. We reached this place at dark and had work just as soon as we were ready. We put 240 men badly wounded through our station by ten o'clock the next day, and not only the dentists worked to their utmost but also the chaplain and Y.M.C.A. man done a full size man's job. We had some very bad wounds to treat at this place and there is no time to sleep these busy days. . . . I saw many machine gun emplacements that were elbow to elbow and many of the gunners were killed on the job. I saw a number of our boys, all were lying where they fell, apparently on the run for the Germans. There were wounded everywhere and a fellow could not get any place for giving first aid to the boys in the way it should be given. . . . I met my assistant on this road, he had been lost from me, and we worked a while on the wounded. Then I learned . . . our battalion aid station was back behind a hill and we looked them up. The days that followed were busy. The most disastrous that I ever dreamed of. At one time there was only one of our line officers left for duty in our battalion and reports say only 34 men. I would not dare quote those figures, but it was nothing but bloody work from October 6th until the 26th, then it subsided. . . . Our medical detachment has received much praise for its work and the Dentists have been given an equal share of it all. In the recent emergency they proved to be the most valuable part of the Medical Department as they demonstrated their ability to do anything the doctors did and to do dental work besides. . . . I have the honor at present of being the only officer that has been on every hike and every move and every place that my battalion has made since it has been in the A.E.F.[37]

Captain Walter E Lotz, Division Dental Surgeon, 78th Division

On Sept. 12th the great drive began. The first dental aid station was established by Lieut. S.B. Crasson in the Bois de Mort above Limey. A field chair and chest were opened and a covering was made of shelter halves. A few days later Lieut, G.L. Haman established an office in a dugout in the same woods and operated until the division was relieved Oct. 5th. . . . Not far away Lieut, B.J. Connolly found a convenient German dug-out suitable for operating. Using a big old fashioned plush chair, he was able to relieve many cases, especially the men coming out. . . . Lieut. H.W. Lester, advancing with the infantry, discovered a German outfit in an abandoned German hospital at Jaulny. He immediately set to work, dug it out, cleared out a room and was on duty within a kilometer of the German lines. . . . Each dental officer, with equipment, established as best he could, but dental services were of short duration. Medical officers were being lost and first aid work fell upon the dentists. . . . Mention must be made of the work of Lieut, Robert Millington. His work in a dressing station near Grand Pre was favorably commented on by the regimental surgeon and regimental commander in a letter recommending a decoration. Exposed under shell fire, Lieut, Millington remained on duty 72 hours and was willing to continue longer when relief arrived.[20]

First Lieutenant BJ Connolly, 303rd Field Signal Battalion, 78th Division

After leaving here [Menil Park Farm], we came to the town of Chattel, where we settled down for a few weeks stay. Our medical detachment got real ambitious and cleaned up a shack in great shape and I again set up the outfit and was open to all comers, and comers came from all organizations, balloon service, ammunition trains, signal, infantry, etc. It was at this place that on the hills close by time bombs had been concealed and at intervals would explode with a terrifying noise. After about ten of these explosions and numerous shells within fifty feet of our shack, it seemed to me to be a queer place for a peaceful dentist to be plying his trade, but I was getting

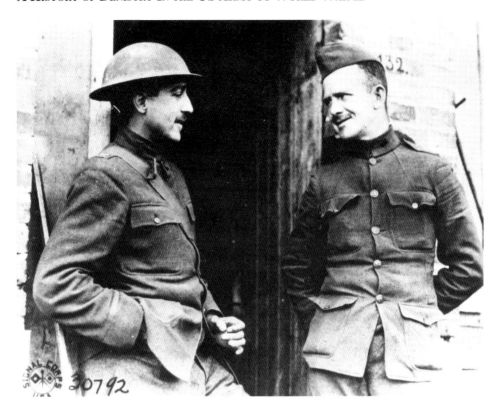

*Captain HA Granelli (right, wearing cap), Medical Corps, surgeon for the
303rd Field Signal Battalion, 78th Division, and First Lieutenant BJ Connolly,
Dental Corps (left, wearing helmet), dental surgeon, 303rd Field Signal Battalion,
at Châtel Chéhéry, Ardennes, France, October 27,1918.
Photograph: Courtesy of US Army Military History Institute. SC 30792.*

hardened to war by now and air fights and burning balloons became common and
only received a casual glance. Three weeks of intermittent work was our record here,
and it then became necessary to follow in the wake of the infantry in the last big push
that cleared out the Huns in this section of France. . . . [with the armistice he was
billeted in French countryside and turned to] doing conscientious and satisfying permanent dental work on the deserving boys of the 78th Division, endeavoring to send
them dentally fit, back to the good old U.S.A.[38]

First Lieutenant J Iredell Wyckoff, 2nd Battalion, 309th Infantry Regiment, 78th Division

When we arrived in the Bois de Rupt [September 15, 1918, in the Saint Mihiel sector],
after being shelled a little, it was very dark and no one seemed to know very much
about the place so finding a small building here I took the men with me and decided to
stay in here until it got light enough to see where we were. A short time after we got in
here the Huns shelled the woods and one shell hit the end of our building and blew it
off but did not hurt any one. . . . A short time after this someone called for the Medical

614

Detachment and on going out found a number of wounded men in a dugout so turned it into an aid station and after dressing their wounds went out to find the ambulance collecting station. The woods [were] shelled every little while and we had to duck quite often but I finally located the place and at two o'clock in the afternoon had all the cases evacuated. By the time we got them off in the ambulance we had twelve cases. . . . When we got back in the Reserve I got a shack built and finding an old chair near by set up a dental office where I was kept busy until the Division was relieved and then acted as Battalion Surgeon until another Medical Officer could be sent to us.[39]

First Lieutenant Clautus L Cope, 1st Battalion, 327th Infantry Regiment, 82nd Division

At 6.00 P.M. [October 6, 1918] we were marched to the front line position near la Forge and [were] ready to go "Over The Top" that night. Several were wounded and on one occasion I was sent for an ambulance, but failed to get one and returned. Patients were carried on litters to the nearest station. Another Medical man and myself layed [*sic*] out in the mud under heavy shelling machine gun fire. The next morning at 5.30 o'clock my battalion went "Over The Top." The battalion Surgeon and myself went forward and established a dressing station which was in an old brick building with no cellar and consequently no protection whatever. At 8.00 o'clock no ambulances had arrived so I volunteered to go see if I could get an ambulance and to replenish our exhausted supplies of dressing. The road was being shelled incessantly with high explosive shells and was by machine gun bullets. I reached the regimental aid station but could not get an ambulance to go up this road under such shelling, but did manage to get a few bandages. . . . About 4.00 o'clock three shells hit out dressing station, killing one man who was being dressed and wounded several others. The shelling was so incessant until we had to move someplace else. There was no dugout near so we moved to the place that such work could be done with a degree of safety which was back near regimental aid station. The next day the battalion Surgeon and I went out and established another dressing station in an advanced position in a dugout where we worked two days. . . . [October 12, 1918] On Thursday I was told to report to the 2nd Battalion and by doing so I learned that they were getting ready to advance. In the afternoon the 2nd Battalion went forward past a village called Fleville and "dug in" the banks of the road side for the night. The next morning at 3.00 o'clock we went forward after hiking three kilometers. The medical men were told to drop out. We "fell out" on one side of the road. I never realized that we were so close to the Germans as it was dark. We soon found out that we were sitting in "No Man's Land"; the Germans on one side of the road and the Americans on the other. The German snipers were so close that all we could do was to sit there as quietly as we could. We captured five snipers about 9.00 A.M. . . . The air was full of gas and I got enough to make me feel sick for several hours. The next day I worked at regimental aid station, and continued to administer first aid until the regimental aid station moved out. . . . For a few days I worked in an Ambulance dressing station at Fléville. After it moved out I did first aid work at regimental aid station and also took care of many dental cases which reported for treatment, using the emergency dental kit which I had carried through the above described drive.[40]

First Lieutenant Junius F Emerson, 2nd Battalion, 328th Infantry Regiment, 82nd Division

We were ordered to follow the Infantry over the top that night, the order was luck for me it read at the top—Friday, Sept 13th, 13 o'clock, order No 13. That night we established our aid station at Orangeries which is a little patch of woods where one of the Companies [*sic*] P.C. [command post] was, it was during the day our men went over and at daybreak to the town of Norroy under shell fire. . . . Just before getting into Norroy the earth opened up before me and I felt a swathing on my right leg, a runner on my left broke his leg and another man on my right got a flesh wound. My wound was only a flesh case but the runner we got him into a passing ambulance. My walking stick was ten feet away, it had a hole in the handle and only scratched my hand, in my belt over my abdomen I had a Boche canteen that I had found the day before, a piece of shrapnel bent it double but saved me from what night have been a serious wound. The ambulance came up O.K. but minus Lerner, he had been hit in the back while dressing a wounded man. That night they put over shells with gas for four hours, and we remained in town with our masks on for four hours. Several men were overcome. We had several wounded and I helped what I could. They shelled all night long, later we learned that they were coming from the outer fortifications of Metz.[41]

First Lieutenant William N Crowl, 2nd Battalion, 325th Infantry Regiment, 82nd Division

On leaving our position [near Varennes] on the night of October 9th, we were advanced up the railroad tracks, south of Châtel-Chéhéry, to the position we were to attack from the next morning, and all the way up we were shelled very heavily with gas, high explosives and shrapnel. Many casualties inflicted and one of our battalion doctors being injured. I took charge of a part of our Medical Detachment, and dressed the wounds as we followed behind the battalion. This was a very difficult task to do on account of the darkness and working most of the time in a high concentration of gas, also shellfire. That morning I was ordered by the battalion surgeon to go to assist in the aid station in Châtel-Chéhéry, and that night went on up to rejoin the 2nd Battalion. . . . [October 11, 1918] In the morning our battalion moved forward and the Medical Detachment followed with it, finally establishing with the 1st Battalion Sanitary Detachment, in the aid station a few hundred yards behind the front lines, where we all worked without stopping hardly for the next few days and nights. We had very little protection and were under almost constant shell fire and machine gun fire, and also had no shelter from the weather. The casualties were very heavy and I was unable to be of much assistance in dressing them, our battalion having now only one doctor. We were shelled very heavily the night of October 13th, and had 12 casualties among our own Sanitary Detachment including my dental assistant. . . . The regiment having advanced further our dressing station was moved forward also, where we had to work under still greater handicaps, having no shelter from the rain, and mud, and dressing the wounded at night in the darkness as best we could. I continued to help in the dressing and evacuating of the wounded until October 18th, when I was sent to the hospital. . . . Evacuated to the hospital too sick and exhausted to do duty.[42]

Captain William E Paul, 2nd Battalion, 327th Infantry Regiment, 82nd Division

[May 1918] My work here [Frenlue, France] was my first work as a battalion Dental Surgeon, for all of our regiment had worked together while in the States, and had taken the patients just as they came from all three battalions. There at Frenlue I found that I had more enthusiasm regarding my dental work than I had while at Camp Gordon, for since I had examined the whole battalion here in France, I was anxious to get each company completed of its needed dental work. I thought that some day I might get all the work completed and then would have only the emergency to look after. But the longer the work the more I realized that such was an impossibility, for to take care of the mouths of 1000 men was a job for more than one dental officer. For me the task of putting the mouths of a company into a first call condition was an endless task. . . . [July 1918] While stationed at Annienville, I received my first baptism of shell fire. Quite a few shells fell in the village every day. The first shell I heard while working, I dropped handpiece and mouth mirror, and the patient I was working on and I had a race for the nearest dug-out. After several days of this work and run schedule, I came to the conclusion that little or no dental work could be accomplished if we tried to hide from all the shells. Quite a few shells fell near us during the stay there but we did not run to a dug-out, but kept on working. We were not always successful in keeping the patient in the dental chair. . . . [September 29, 1918] About one mile before we reached Beurney we received a heavy shelling from the Boche, which caused us heavy casualties, one man in every ten being left on the field either killed or wounded. With the two Medical Officers with our battalion, we were on the extreme left. We thought we saw a near cut, so left the troops, and started running across the field. We had gone only a few yards when we found that the Boche gunners were making a supreme effort to get us with their artillery. The Officer just ahead of me got struck in the head with a piece of shrapnel, but luck was with him and he was not seriously hurt. After climbing through three stretches of wire, and at the same time dodging shells, we reached a ravine and took cover under a bank with some men of the 35th Division. These men were lying in small fox holes which offered little protection from the shrapnel. In making the near cut across the field, we became lost from the rest of our battalion. After waiting in these holes for a few minutes I saw one of our companies advancing over a hill just ahead of us, so we started to overtake them. We could see numerous men fall as they were struck with shrapnel and machine gun bullets, but we kept on. It was while going up this hill trying to overtake this company that I wondered what they intended to use a dentist for going over the top with the men. I was of no use whatever, either as a dentist or Medical Officer for my emergency outfit had been thrown away a few minutes before, and there was not a bandage or drug of any kind nearer than two miles. I had just come to the conclusion that the Dental Section of the Army Sanitary School would soon have an occasion to add another name to their honor roll, when the General sent word to the company ahead of us from advancing further. We were all told to take cover, for the attack had been called off.[43]

First Lieutenant Thomas N Page, 3rd Battalion, 326th Infantry Regiment, 82nd Division

[June 18, 1918] I was ordered away to the Army Sanitary School (I know not where) and did not get to do any work at Chaudeney. After one day travel I found the school which was at Langres, and remained there until July 6th, listening to the Birds of the S.O.S. [services of supply] tell their experiences doing squads right and left and getting lectures from able lecturers which has been a great help to me. Of course while there I learned to evacuate patients and everything I had never dreamed would be the duty of a dentist. . . . [July 7, 1918] I left the school and joined my battalion, or rather started to join when I reported to the Regimental Commander and he ordered me to set up my hardtack box at his station as there was no need of a dentist being up at the front just to get shot up. My orders had been previously issued by The Division Dental Surgeon that I would join my battalion at the front where (Whizzbangs) come and go, but I was very easily persuaded by the Colonel to stay at this P.C. [command post] which I knew must be safe as the Chaplain, Personnel Officer, and one French Captain had also established themselves there (. . . Brigade Headquarters was near). I set up and began work when it was decided that a dentist would make one more at the front if nothing else and we were to go up with as much of our equipment as we could get up. . . . [August 18, 1918] The next day were backed into a little town on a beautiful river which was named Belleville. This river being the Moselle. . . . This proved to be a quiet sector for the time being and I set my complete outfit up out in the open near the entrance of a shell proof dugout, where I could seek refuge in case old Jerry should put over a little. There was little to do at this time as the men were not thinking of teeth trouble they were writing letters, reading some worn out magazines and listening to the rats run around. . . . [October 4, 1918] We set out marching (as usual) to get into the fight, and for two days we trotted along, I taking with me only my engine and emergency kit (which was known to all dentists as the fatigue kit). On the second day we passed into the territory which had been held since 1914 by the Boche and it was a sight to look at entanglements, of what had been entanglements and see so much destruction, but we were going to be introduced to the real thing the next few days. We stopped for orders just west of Varennes, near Apri de St. Louis (A famous German dug-out). On the night of October 7th, we plodded forward in the rain and mud almost to the knee and came to Montblainville, where we stopped for dark again, as it was necessary to march under cover of darkness now. [October 8, 1918] We went into the line (or front) to relieve the 28th. Division. Of course, the fighting Battalion was selected to go in first and we hit the train, going it seemed into the very jaws of death. About 11.00 P.M. we were ordered to fall out behind the hill and little did I know that just beyond that hill was German galer, and the first thing I know I was knocked down by the explosion by a whizzbang, but unhurt, although frightened to death. This shell got one man although it did not kill him. Never was I so excited in my born days, I lay down on the wet grass with Lt. Weatherford and Mr. Harrison a Y.M.C.A. man and shells poured all around all night. We did not sleep as we were wet and cold and only two blankets for three of us. Next morning I was told that there was a little village nearby, in which we could establish a dressing station and I was surely glad to know there was a house left in that dismal forest, but when we came into the town it was not houses, but half houses and a few walls, although they were high enough to hide behind to dodge the shells. I was with Capt. Hays, M.C., Battalion Surgeon, when we made our way into the little shattered village of Châtel-Chéhéry, on the morning of October 9th, when our battalion attacked the Boche at 5.00 P.M. we established our dressing station in an old cellar where the Surgeon of the 28th. Division, had his and was ready for emergency, and they began to come in from all angles, as the machine guns of the Boche were hidden so much that the men fell fast before them. On this date I had the only fractured jaw I have had. It was a machine gun bullet through the maxille on the right side and tearing it completely in two pieces. I could only give first aid, which I did and evacuated the man. While here we had many casualties and worked hard. In the afternoon I found a little cellar in which I could get a few hours sleep and I was almost all in, when I awoke it was next morning as this was the first night that I had opportunity of sleep for four or five days and I did not mind shelling or the many dead bodies that were within ten yards of men (both American and Boche). We had no food so some one told me that the ration dump was only about a mile away and that we might get some canned goods there so I set out to find it with an enlisted man and the shelling was pretty fast and machine gun bullets whizzed by, but we went on, finally finding our reward only to be coffee, sugar, and bully beef. I was wise and only took the coffee and sugar, as I had my Pip burner along and could steal gasoline off an ambulance if one happened along. Everything worked well and we had hot coffee that afternoon and several afternoons. . . . [October 10, 1918] We left Châtel-Chéhéry and advanced with our battalion which had pushed away ahead. We dug in on a little bank with no shelling except a good way off and let us sleep on the ground and fortunately it was not raining that night. Next day was a busy day as the second [2nd Battalion] advanced and tried to take St. Juvine [*sic*], but was compelled to withdraw with heavy casualties. This was the memorable 11th of October and I cannot forget it as in the evening about 7 P.M. we were ordered to march to the river Aire and ford it under heavy shell fire. I was in the middle of the river freezing, so I thought, waiting for the men to pull up ahead on the opposite side. I had been forced to leave my engine behind with the regimental infirmary or dressing station and helped lug the litters carrying the first aid dressing splints and my emergency equipment, with a few blankets we could find off dead men or from the discarded packs. We marched a few hundred yards to a ravine and it was raining a little when we went into this ditch and almost to our knees, some times water knee deep. We were told to go to sleep (just like a man can sleep in a living hell of shells and machine gun bullets). I spread out a litter and put up for the remainder of the night, so I thought, when along four whizzbangs which didn't miss me more than an inch I thought, and I took to the banks where some men were busy digging in, and I borrowed a shovel and within five minutes I thought I was safe when in reality as I discovered the next morning I was only in a nice place to be put under cover by a shell, but thanks to a higher power none came within ten feet of me. At six A.M. old Jerry let loose on us with renewed energy, for he knew the third battalion of the 326th was in that very ditch, and that I was along and he thought he knew just where I was but missed my hiding place just a few steps and killed several men in one of the companies beside me, and wounded many.[44]

First Lieutenant George L Long, 104th Infantry Regiment, 26th Division

On or about the first of May [1918] we were sent over to the right to relieve another regiment. This place was not near so satisfactory for dental work as we were situated between the first and second lines and received very heavy bombardments daily. At this place we remained until the middle of June at which time we were relieved by another regiment and sent well back of the lines for a short repose. On June 16th 1918 we received a heavy shelling, killing many men and wounding several. At this time I was able to assist the surgeons in dressing the wounded as there were many facial wounds. . . . On August 25th 1918 we were ordered to entrain at Châtillons. After a short trip we detrained in the vicinity of Bar le duc and started on a long hike—marching by night and remaining hidden in the woods by day. Finally arrived at some woods facing the St. Mihiel Salient. On Sept. 11th 1918 we advanced to the Regt. Aid Station and on Sept. 12th we handled a large number of wounded men. This station was in advance of the aid station established by the battalion in reserve and so we received the brunt of the work. During the day we made several expeditions between our station and the front lines searching for and bringing in the wounded. The following day following close to the retreating boche we arrived at the town of St. Maurice which had been evacuated by the Germans only a short time before. At this place we established an aid station and took care of the wounded both Americans and boche. From there we held the sector to the left and was there able to accomplish some fair satisfactory dental work. We remained in that sector until ordered to take up a part of the Verdun Sector. We proceeded in the night marches for eight or ten days during which time it was impossible to do any dental work other than to temporarily relieve some soldier suffering from tooth ache. On the 14th of October 1918 we were placed in the trenches some two hundred yards from the front line at which place we received many wounded as this station was advanced beyond the two battalion stations not in the lines and was well known as it was Regt. Aid Station. We remained in this sector ten days and

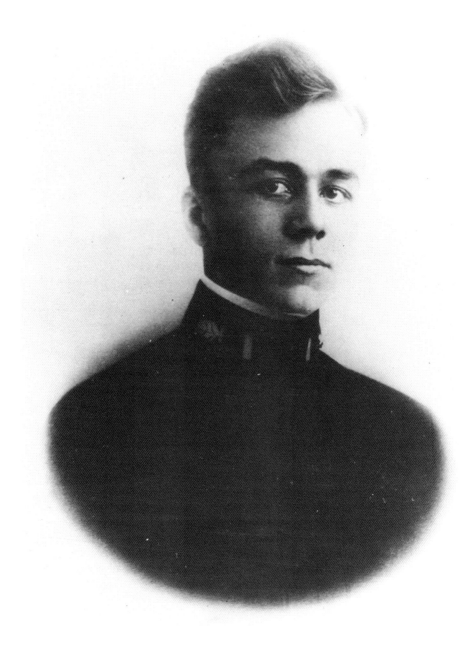

Lieutenant (junior grade) Weedon E Osborne, Dental Corps, US Navy,
was awarded a posthumous Navy Medal of Honor for his heroism while assigned to the
US Marines of the 2nd Division on June 6, 1918.
Photograph: Courtesy of National Archives and Records Administration. SC 90759.

EXHIBIT 15-1

WEEDEN E OSBORNE: MEDAL OF HONOR AND DISTINGUISHED SERVICE CROSS RECIPIENT

Weeden E Osborne was born in Chicago, Illinois, on November 13, 1892, and graduated from Northwestern University Dental School in 1915. On May 8, 1917, he was appointed a dental surgeon in the US Navy with rank of lieutenant (junior grade). He was detailed to duty with the 6th Regiment, US Marines, on March 26, 1918, and joined them on May 14, 1918, at Doucey (Marne), France. He was posthumously awarded the Medal of Honor and the Distinguished Service Cross for heroism in combat with the enemy during the advance on Bouresches, France. Although his profession gave him every justification for remaining in the rear, he volunteered for general rescue work and aided the wounded. While carrying an injured officer to safety, he was struck by a shell and killed instantly. He was the first commissioned officer of the US Navy to be killed in action during land fighting overseas.

Data sources: (1) General order no. 518, 1920, Navy Department. (2) US Navy Bureau of Medicine and Surgery. *The Medical Department of the United States Navy with the Army and Marine Corps in France in World War I: its Functions and Employment.* Washington, DC: Bureau of Medicine and Surgery, USN; 1947: 203.

---

during this time we were continually shelled and gassed and it was useless to think of attempting even emergency dental work. We were relieved for a short repose of a few days and then sent to the left of our former sector. There we remained for days at which place there was very little to do. We were relieved and moved back a short distance only to be ordered back into the lines above Bois Haumont about November 9th, 1918. Here an aid station was established and on the morning of November 11th, 1918 we advanced under considerable shelling by the boche to the town of Beaumont where at 11 o'clock the most welcome news reached us that the armistice had been signed, and that all hostilities were over. We soon realized it was true when at 11 o'clock every gun of the whole front stopped firing.[45]

Awards for Heroism

Often working under extremely hazardous and trying combat conditions, many dental officers were cited for their courage in battle and dedication.

Medal of Honor

In the 2nd Division, the Marines of the 4th Infantry Brigade came with assigned US Navy medical and dental officers and enlisted corpsmen.[22] Two US Navy dentists serving with the 2nd Division received the Navy Medal of Honor. Lieutenant (junior grade) Weeden E Osborne, DC, US Navy, 6th Marines, was cited "for extraordinary heroism in actual conflict with the enemy under fire, during the advance on Bouresches (France), on June 6th 1918, in helping to carry the wounded to a place of safety. While engaged in this heroic duty he was killed. He was at the time attached to the 6th Regiment, U.S. Marines."[46–48] Osborne was also awarded the US Army Distinguished Service Cross for his actions,[48] as well as two citation stars for the Victory Medal (redesignated the Silver Star Medal in 1932, with an oak leaf cluster for a second award) from the US Army. The citations for his awards are as follows.

- Lieutenant (junior grade) Weeden E Osborne, DC, US Navy, 6th Marines.

  Risked his life to aid the wounded when the advance upon the enemy of June 6th (1918) was temporarily checked by a hail of machine-gun fire. He helped carry Capt. Donald C. Duncan, to a place of safety when that officer was wounded and had almost reached it when a shell killed both. Having joined the regiment but a few days before its entry onto the line and, being new to the service, he displayed a heroism worthy of its best traditions. This on June 6, 1918.[48]

  For extraordinary heroism in stemming the German advance in this region and in thrusting it back from every position occupied by the Fourth Brigade from June 2d to 11th inclusive. This northeast of Chateau Thierry (France), June 2-11, 1918.[48]

On December 29, 1919, the Torpedo Boat Destroyer, Osborne, was launched at Bethlehem Shipbuilding Company in Squantum, Massachusetts, and named in his memory.[48]

The second Navy Medal of Honor was awarded to Lieutenant (junior grade) Alexander G Lyle, DC, US Navy, 5th Marines. Lyle also received a citation star (Silver Star Medal), US Army, for the action.

- Lieutenant (junior grade) Alexander G Lyle, DC, US Navy, 5th Marines.

  For extraordinary heroism and devotion to duty while serving with the 5th Regiment, U.S. Marines. Under heavy shell fire on April 23rd 1918, he rushed to the assistance of Corporal Regan, who was seriously wounded and administered such effective surgical aid while bombardment was still continuing as to save the life of Corporal Regan.[48(p200)]

  Did, under heavy shell fire, on April 23, 1918, rush to the assistance of Cpl. Thomas Regan, 5th Regiment, U.S. Marines, who was severely wounded, effectively controlling hemorrhage from the femoral artery before bombardment had finished and at the very peril of his own life, saving that of Cpl. Regan. This in the Verdun Sector, April 23, 1918.[48]

He received a second citation star for "gallantry in action against the enemy in the Soissons Sector."[48] Lyle became the first flag officer in the Navy's Dental Corps when he was promoted to rear admiral in 1943, and served as the chief of the US Navy Dental Corps from 1945–1946. Upon his retirement in 1948, Lyle was promoted to vice admiral and became the only military dental officer ever to reach three-star rank.[49]

Another Navy dentist, Lieutenant Commander (later Rear Admiral) Cornelius H Mack of the 6th Marines received the Navy Cross. Mack also received six US Army citation stars (Silver Star Medal and oak leaf clusters) for heroism in various actions in June and July at Château-Thierry and Soissons. In addition, Mack had the unique distinction of serving as the division dental surgeon of the 2nd Division

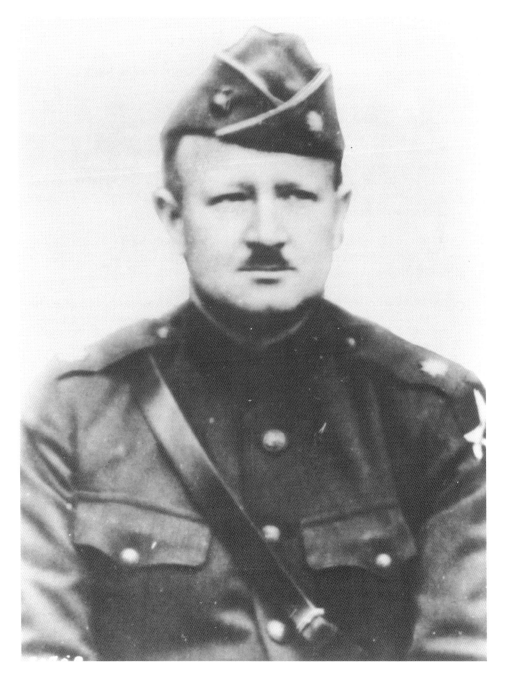

Lieutenant Commander Cornelius H Mack, Dental Corps, US Navy, served with the 2nd Division in France during World War I and received the Navy Cross for valor. Photograph: Courtesy of National Archives and Records Administration. SC 90758.

from November 1918 until the summer of 1919.[22] This was the only time in Army or US Marine Corps history that Army and Marine units were combined into a single division, commanded eventually by a Marine Corps major general.

- Lieutenant Commander (later Rear Admiral) Cornelius H Mack of the 6th Marines.

  For extraordinary heroism and devotion to duty with the 6th Regiment, U.S. Marines. In the action at the Bois de Belleau, (France), on June 12, 1918, when his dressing station was subject to a heavy gas bombardment, he remained on duty and carried on the evacuation of the wounded, refusing to leave until all wounded and Hospital Corps men had been removed to a place of safety; as a result he was severely gassed. In the action at Vierzy (France), on July 19, 1918, he accompanied the advance and was exposed for fifteen hours to the fire of machine guns and artillery, performing his duties with marked coolness and precision.[48(pp200–201)]

On October 15, 1918, Mack wrote a short letter to Lieutenant Colonel Graham, the 2nd Division's dental surgeon, for Oliver's dental history. The letter described his activities during these months:

On June 1st. 1918 my battalion entered the town of Lucy-la-Bocage taking lines in front of the Bois de Belleau at which front our regiment was more or less continually engaged actively until July 4th 1918. During this time I was engaged in dressing station work, one week in Lucy at the Battalion Dressing Station, one week at the culvert dressing station and the remaining time at advanced battalion dressing stations. All of these stations were practically at all times under violent enemy artillery fire. On June 12th the station was heavily bombarded with gas shells during a time we were evacuating many wounded and it was necessary to work without a gas mask on account of the long period over which the gas attack extended. It was necessary to evacuate the Battalion Surgeon and all the hospital corps men as they had all succumbed to the gas. . . . From the 4th July until July 16th the regiment occupied support trenches back of Montreuil and Bezu and on the latter date we left in camions for the Soissons front entering the lines on the 19th beyond Vierzy where we had a very heavy day's action, and suffered extremely high numbers of casualties. During this engagement I established the advanced dressing station of my battalion. . . . On July 20th after our relief I was evacuated for influenza and the effects of gas inhalations received during the day of June 14th.[50]

Distinguished Service Cross

In the divisions of the AEF, six Army dentists and one enlisted assistant were awarded the Distinguished Service Cross for extraordinary valor. The complete citations of their actions follow:

- William L Davidson, Captain, Dental Corps, 1st Battalion, 114th Infantry Regiment, 29th Division.

  For extraordinary heroism in action north of Verdun, France, October 12, 1918, Captain Davidson, while attending wounded under heavy fire, was himself wounded by several pieces of shell fragments. Regardless of his own wounds he continued in his care of the wounded, refusing to be treated until his regiment was relieved from the line, when several pieces of shell were removed from his head and shoulders.[51]

- Lee M English, First Lieutenant, Dental Corps, 314th Infantry Regiment, 79th Division.

  For extraordinary heroism in action near Montfaucon, France, September 29, 1918. Although he had received a very painful wound two days previous, he remained on duty at an aid station under heavy shell fire until it was completely destroyed and many of the inmates and attendants killed and wounded. He assisted in caring for these wounded and directing their evacuation and then dressed the wounded on the field until an aid station could be located farther to the rear.[52]

- Otto LH Hine, Captain, Dental Corps, 2nd Battalion, 139th Infantry Regiment, 35th Division.

  For extraordinary heroism in action near Chaudron Farm, France, September 29–30, 1918. Upon his own initiative, Captain Hine (then first lieutenant) went to a dressing station in advance of the line, after the infantry had withdrawn, and worked under heavy bombardment of gas and high explosive shells, dressing the patients and directing their evacuation. That night he returned to our lines through heavy artillery and machine-gun fire to arrange for ambulances and litters. Later he made another trip to the rear for the purpose of securing an artillery barrage to protect his dressing station. Through his exceptional courage and energy all the wounded men were safely evacuated.[53]

- Robert E Motley, First Lieutenant, Dental Corps, 125th Infantry Regiment, 32nd Division.

  For extraordinary heroism in action near Chateau-Thierry, France, July 31–August 7, near Verdun, France, October 14–16, 1918. Realizing the need for medical attention at the front, Lieutenant Motley went beyond the scope of his duties as dentist by advancing with the Infantry and establishing and maintaining dressing station with the leading elements of his command. For seven days, from July 31 to August 7, he safely evacuated many patients by his prompt and fearless action. He again volunteered and went forward in the attack of October 14–16, and on the later date, carried a message back to the supply officer, requesting food for the men. Although wounded and badly gassed, he accomplished his mission, refusing evacuation until the food was started for the lines.[54]

- Robert O Smith, First Lieutenant, Dental Corps, 356th Infantry Regiment, 89th Division.

  For extraordinary heroism in action near the Meuse River, France, November 6–11, 1918. After all the medical officers of the battalion had been wounded, Lieut. Smith for six days efficiently performed the duties of a medical officer, repeatedly moving his first-aid station forward, and administering to the wounded under perilous shell fire. After caring for the wounded, he personally searched the field of action for further casualties.[55]

- Richard J Walsh, First Lieutenant, Dental Corps, 303rd Engineer Regiment, 78th Division.

  For extraordinary heroism in action near Marcg, France, October 18, 1918. Voluntarily acting as battalion medical officer, Lieut. Walsh, although severely gassed, administered first aid to injured men under heavy shell fire. He worked constantly until all the wounded were removed to place of safety. Philadelphia, Pennsylvania.[56]

625

- Frederick Yannantuono (posthumous). Private First Class, Dental Assistant, Medical Detachment, 13th Machine Gun Battalion, 5th Division.

    For extraordinary heroism in action near Cunel, France, October 14, 1918. Private Yannantuono voluntarily went forward and administered first aid to wounded Infantry soldiers under heavy shell and machine-gun fire, in plain view of the enemy, being killed in the performance of this self-sacrificing mission.[57]

US Army award citations usually provide few details of the action for which the award was given. In the cases of Captains William Lee Davidson and Otto LH Hine, additional details are available that provide significant insight into their actions—on Davidson from his personal recollection and on Hine in the official report of First Lieutenant John F Coffman, Jr, battalion surgeon of the 2nd Battalion, 139th Infantry Regiment.

William Lee Davidson, who remained in the Dental Officers' Reserve Corps after the war, was the only Distinguished Service Cross recipient to describe his experiences as a dental officer in France and in the action for which he was recognized:

My trip from the States was uneventful, but a very delightful one, and I landed at Brest as a "casual" with my assistant, Private Harry M. Damon, (who is a graduated dentist). We landed on 6 August 1918, with thirty-eight other dental surgeons and their assistants and were quartered in the historic Ponlaneizer [Pontanezen] Barracks. One week later we were ordered to St. Aigon Noyers, and all officers reported twice daily, hoping to receive orders assigning them to their future berths. . . . On 28 August 1918, I was ordered to report to the Commanding General, 29th Division for duty and started the following day for Montreau Chateau. I reported 2 September 1918 and was assigned to the 1st Battalion, 114th Infantry. . . . From Montreau Chateau, on the night of 7 September, we left for Manspach, only to march the next night into the trenches.

. . . . And at this stage of the game, a dental surgeon wither ceases to be a dentist, or becomes both—a dentist and a physician—giving first aid and help wherever his services are needed. The object of a dental surgeon is not only to relieve pain in his line, but to keep the teeth of his men in such condition that the smallest percentage of them will be kept out of the trenches—where they are most needed–on account of dental diseases, etc. . . .

Since leaving the trenches it was impossible to do any dental work other than to relieve pain. On 30 September we were ordered to Nubercourt, only to leave there the next night for a woods, known as Vadelaincourt and we camped there for four days, going to Bois-de-Sartellie, only to leave the next night for Bois Burros. Our next move was the next night for Cumeires, where we camped for two nights. At Cote-de-Roches on 11 October we received our first real baptism of shell fire, only to march into Bois-de-Ormont on the same night and go "over the top" the following morning.

All Red Cross men and officers had their hands full from the night of 11 October. We were relieved in the 30th inst. We started to work on the wounded that first night and I had no sleep for seventy-two hours following. On 12 October it was my good fortune to give assistance I could in the way of first aid to our boys who were wounded and for five hours I was in my first barrage. And at some time that morning I was hit by shrapnel. I was fortunate enough to get the men I had dressed to a place of safety without any serious mishaps to any of them. For at this time the enemy was flooding our area with gas.

For six days our dressing station was under constant and heavy shell fire, but we lost only six patients after they reached the dressing station. Our battalion was ordered to Ravine Malville on the 20th, where we stayed until relieved. Our dressing station being in the front line there also. . . . From 11 October to the day we arrived at Bussy-la-Cote no patients presented themselves for dental treatment, which shows what the Dental Corps has done in the way of preparedness.

We were billeted in the last named village for fifteen days and once more I went back to dentistry and was able to accomplish a little along that time. (Some bits of shrapnel were removed from my wounds here). We marched to the village of Varincourt on 15 November, staying there three days, then going to Guerport where it was my pleasure to receive a Divisional citation from the commanding general. Our next move was the twentieth—going to Nancois where we entrained for Passavant, detraining of the twenty-first, marching at once to Chatillon-sur-Saone where officers and men have received the advantages of dentistry once more.[6]

On November 28, 1918, Captain John J Halnan, MC, 114th Infantry, wrote to Captain John M Hughes, DC, the division dental surgeon, about Captain Davidson's heroism on October 12:

On said date he voluntarily remained for five hours under a heavy barrage of high explosives dressing and caring for the wounded, with utter disregard for his own life. . . . During this barrage he was wounded but refused to go to a place of safety until all wounded had been evacuated. . . . He remained on duty in the first aid dressing station until his regiment was relieved, working for seventy-two hours without rest or sleep and only allowing his wounds to be thoroughly treated after his regiment was relieved.[58]

On January 5, 1919, First Lieutenant John F Coffman, Jr, MC, battalion surgeon for the 2nd Battalion, 139th Infantry Regiment, 35th Division, to which Otto LH Hine was assigned as dental surgeon, submitted his report of the battalion's operations from September 25 to October 2, 1918, in the Meuse-Argonne offensive. The battalion's objective on September 26 was Vaquois Hill and the vicinity, resulting in a large number of casualties who were treated in the battalion's battlefield aid stations.[59] He wrote:

This work was performed under an almost continual artillery and machine gun fire. 2B [aid station] was established in a trench which had been widened out and made fairly comfortable by Bosche prisoners and the supervision of our Dentist, Lt. Hine, and his assistant [Private William C Myers]. He also used German prisoners as litter bearers and from here evacuated 19 casualties. One hour prior to establishing this Aid Station Lt. Hine was on the North side of Vaquois Hill and, after following the board walks past large, well constructed concrete caves and dug-outs, he noticed a crowd of men through the fog about 30 meters ahead of him. Not being able to distinguish who they were, he turned to his assistant, Private Wm. C. Myers, who was following him, and asked him if he thought they were Bosche. As the assistant affirmed his suspicions, Lt. Hine held up his revolver which he had in his hand, and while trying to make up his mind as to exactly what course to pursue, the Germans

saw him and all held up their hands and started toward him. There were some
steps leading up to the trench that led back over the knoll between Lt. Hine and the
Germans, so he waved to them to go up the steps and counted 32 of them. Falling
in behind them he took them across the valley and up into the trenches from where
he had started that morning, turning them over to guards who were returning with
other prisoners.[59(p162)]

Operations continued over the next several days, and the sanitary detachment
kept pushing its aid stations forward with infantry until, by the 29th, they had
passed Saint Quentin and reached Baulny.

At 9:00 A.M. Lt. Hine established Aid Station 9B at Baulny, from here evacuating
16 casualties and then returned to St. Quenteen. At 10:30 A.M. Herbert Stoffle, one
of our personnel, who had been detailed with G Company and was serving with
them on the front line, and was afterwards captured by the Germans, came in and
said that he knew where there was a dressing station with lots of wounded, but
they were being taken care of; but as there were quite a few of these men, thinking that he could be of assistance, Lt. Hine with his assistant accompanying him to
Chaudron Farm, where he established Aid Station No. 10, evacuating altogether
80 casualties. There, after going into a room which was about half full of wounded
men and asking if there were any who had not been dressed and receiving the
reply that none of them had been dressed since coming from the field, he began
to work. The first two or three he dressed and tagged, then to speed up with the
dressing, he quit tagging, but soon the litter bearers brought them in so fast and as
he was the only medical officer there at that time, he could only devote his time to
placing them. That room, which was about 75 feet long and 20 feet wide, was filled
and another room of the same dimensions and yet another and then the sheds and
the barn received their portion. During this time heavy shelling was going on and
the report that the line was falling back necessitated the withdrawal of several officers and men. By this means Lt. Hine sent back word of his plight with the urgent
request for help and for means of evacuation. Two gas attacks were also put over,
which necessitated the adjustment of gas masks for the wounded that had them or
could be supplied.[59(p163)]

Only with great difficulty was Hine able to locate enough litter bearers to remove the wounded from his aid station at Chaudron Farm. His task was complicated by the withdrawal of the American forward line, of which he learned only
when Captain Randall Wilson of the infantry company holding the line in front of
him told him at about 10:00 PM: "Hell, Doc, you have got to get these men out of
here by daylight. There are only 25 men between you and the Bosche. The main
line has fallen back to the top of the hill about a half mile behind you." At midnight, "after deciding that there was no help coming and that something had to
be done, Lt. Hine got on a mule, which was in the barn of the farm, bare backed
and with a rope halter, started back to get help or protection, and if possible both."
After a frenetic night of riding from unit to unit and headquarters to headquarters,
Hine succeeded in obtaining litter bearers and troops to protect the aid station. By
5:00 PM on the 30th, Hine reported that the American and German casualties had
been evacuated from the aid station.[59] Coffman continued:

"Then came a three day march from the lines, and being nearly overcome from dysentery, bronchitis, diarrhoea [sic] and a slight attack of gas, Lt. Hine was evacuated to a hospital."[59(p164)]

Citation Stars (later Silver Star Medals)

On July 9, 1918, Congress authorized Army personnel to wear a small silver star (3/16 of an inch in diameter) on the service ribbon of a campaign medal to indicate "a citation for gallantry in action, published in orders issued from headquarters of a general officer, not warranting the award of a Medal of Honor or Distinguished Service Cross." Originally designated as citation stars, one of these silver stars was soon authorized for wear on the World War I war service medal, the Victory Medal, as well as on service ribbons of campaign medals for each citation. The citation star awards were often called Silver Star Citations, although that term had no apparent official approval. On August 8, 1932, Congress authorized the Silver Star Medal for Army personnel to replace the former citation star for all holders of the award.[60–62] At least 16 Army dental personnel received citation stars "for gallantry in action" during World War I. So far, 14 Dental Corps officers and two dental assistants have been identified as having received citation stars.

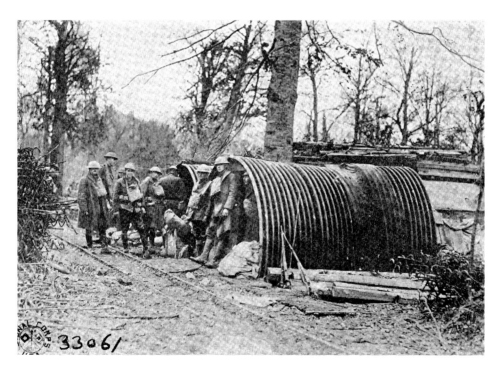

115th Infantry Regiment, 29th Division First Aid Station, Consenvoye Woods (World War I).
Reproduced from: Reynolds FC. 115th Infantry U.S.A. in the World War.
Baltimore, Md: Read-Taylor Company; 1920.

Apparently, neither the AEF chief surgeon nor the chief dental surgeon maintained a central list of the recipients of citation stars from the Army Medical Department, because none has been found in the records of the AEF in the National Archives. General Headquarters, AEF, issued citation stars in citation orders in 1919–1920, and after General Headquarters disappeared, the War Department issued citation stars in its general orders. In addition, any commanding general officer could award citation stars for gallantry in divisional and brigade general orders, which vastly multiplied the problem of identifying recipients, especially among the enlisted personnel. Moreover, while Dental Corps officers were usually identified by branch in such orders, that was not always the case. Dental assistants were listed only as members of the medical or sanitary detachment of a divisional unit. Without meticulous and time-consuming analysis of divisional rosters of dental assistants, if such documents even exist, it is almost impossible to identify citation star recipients even in the published General Headquarters, AEF, citation orders. Only Private Abel W Emmonds, a dental assistant in the Sanitary Detachment, 316th Infantry Regiment, 79th Division, and Private First Class William C Myers, 139th Infantry, 35th Division, have been clearly identified as citation star recipients.

The dental personnel identified as citation star recipients and their citations are as follows:

- Captain George N Abbott, Dental Corps, US Army, 371st Infantry Regiment, 93rd Division.

  For gallantry in action on Sept. 30, 1918, in Champagne Sector, in aiding the wounded under heavy enemy fire.[63]

- Captain Waldo J Adams, Dental Corps, US Army, 364th Infantry Regiment, 91st Division.

  For gallantry in action near Very, France, 26 September 1918, in caring for the wounded.[63]

- Captain Daniel Bratton, Dental Corps, US Army, 115th Infantry Regiment, 29th Division (2 awards).

  For gallantry in action near Bois de Consenvoye, Brabant, France, October 10–25, 1918. Having found a battalion first-aid station without medical officers, due to casualties, he voluntarily took charge and upon several occasions went out in the face of severe enemy artillery and machine-gun fire and brought back badly wounded men.[64]

  For gallantry in action at Bois de Consenovye, France, October 12, 1918. Acting as regimental gas officer upon the evacuation of both surgeons attached to the 1st Battalion, 115th Infantry, then in the assault position, he volunteered for duty as surgeon and cared for the wounded of the command. He displayed rare courage and devotion to the sick and wounded, thereby greatly contributing to the successful operations of the regiment.[65]

- First Lieutenant Harry W Burns, Dental Corps, US Army, 30th Infantry Regiment, 3rd Division.

  For gallantry in action at Crezancy, France, 15 July, 1918, in caring for the wounded under heavy enemy fire. General Headquarters AEF, Citation Orders No. 1, 3 June 1919.[66]

- First Lieutenant Frank J Canning, Dental Corps, US Army, 320th Infantry Regiment, 80th Division.

  For gallantry in action at Bois des Ogons, France, 9 October, 1918, in administering first aid to the wounded under severe shelling.[66]

- First Lieutenant John C Curry, Dental Corps, US Army, Second Ammunition Train, 2nd Division.

  At all times paid the strictest attention to his duties, and has rendered valuable service to this organization in his professional capacity. During a recent campaign, upon the death of a line officer, Lieutenant Curry executed the duties of a line officer with efficiency.[67(254)]

- Private Abel W Emmonds, Sanitary Detachment, 316th Infantry Regiment, 79th Division.

  For gallantry in action at Montfaucon, France, September 26 to October 1, 1918, in carrying messages under heavy shell fire.[68]

- First Lieutenant Owen P Gillick, Dental Corps, US Army, Medical Detachment, 23rd Infantry Regiment, 2nd Division (2 awards).

  For gallantry in action during the advance from Côte de Châtillon to L'Tanne, 8 October, 1918, in promptly giving first aid.[68]

  Attached to the Third Battalion, 23rd Infantry, accompanied the battalion in all attacks and under heavy machine gun and artillery fire operated in conjunction with the battalion surgeons an aid station on the front lines. Through his personal efforts many wounded were promptly given first aid and evacuated. This during the advance from Côte de Châtillon to L'Etanne.[67(pp231–232)]

- First Lieutenant John J Heverin, Dental Corps, US Army, Medical Detachment, 9th Infantry Regiment, 2nd Division (2 awards).

  For gallantry in action in the vicinity of Nouart, 2 November, 1918, in administering to the wounded under heavy shell fire.[68]

  Accompanied an advanced party through the German lines in the vicinity of NOUART on the night of November 2, 1918, and displayed great courage and disregard of personal safety in rendering assistance and administering first aid treatment to the wounded while under violent machine gun and artillery fire.[67(p225)]

- Captain Creighton L Lane, Dental Corps, US Army, 7th Infantry Regiment, 3rd Division.

  For gallantry in action near Le Rocq Farm, France, July 14, 15, and 25, 1918, while attending the wounded under fire.[69]

- First Lieutenant Robert EF Millington, Dental Corps, US Army, Medical Detachment, 311th Infantry Regiment, 78th Division.

  For gallantry in action during the Meuse-Argonne Offensive, France, 14 October 1918, in voluntarily rendering first aid to the wounded under heavy shell fire. General Headquarters AEF, Citation Orders No. 3, 3 June 1919.[70]

- First Lieutenant Clyde R Modie, Dental Corps, US Army, 126th Infantry Regiment, 32nd Division.

  For gallantry in action near Château-Thierry, France, 31 July, 1918, in going to the assistance of three wounded soldiers under heavy shell fire.[70]

- First Lieutenant Charles A Musgrave, Dental Corps, US Army, Medical Detachment, 314th Infantry Regiment, 79th Division (2 awards).

  For gallantry in action near Moirey, France, 1–11 November, 1918, in voluntarily caring for the wounded under heavy machine-gun and artillery fire.[70]

  For gallantry in action at Fayel Farm, Montfaucon, France, September 29, 1918. With a total disregard for his own personal danger and under heavy enemy shell fire Lieutenant Musgrave went to the assistance of a wounded soldier who had crawled into a shell hole and was calling for help. Lieutenant Musgrave remained with the wounded man, under fire, giving him first-aid treatment until with the assistance of another soldier he carried the wounded man out of the line of fire in order that better medical attention could be given. Lieutenant Musgrave later placed the wounded man on a truck and sent him to the rear.[71]

- Private First Class William C Myers, Medical Detachment, 2nd Battalion, 139th Infantry Regiment, 35th Division.

  The Division Commander takes great pleasure in citing in General Orders the following Officers and Enlisted Men, for gallantry in action during the six days' battle from September 26th to October 1st. . . . Displayed wonderful determination and courage in rescuing the wounded under heavy shell fire, rendered great assistance in dressing and evacuating the wounded, securing litters and litter bearers over difficult terrain, where it was impossible for ambulances to operate.[62]

- Captain William T Roberts, Dental Corps, US Army, attached to 5th Marine Regiment, 2nd Division.

  For gallantry in action against the enemy in the Champagne Sector.[47,72]

- Captain John A Sites, Dental Corps, US Army, 148th Infantry Regiment, 37th Division.

  For gallantry in action October 31, 1918. Voluntarily accompanying the Medical Detachment of the 148th Infantry throughout an engagement with enemy forces, he displayed great courage and devotion to duty, rendering first aid to wounded men under intense enemy fire. He was poisoned by enemy gas and evacuated to hospital.[65]

- First Lieutenant Robert P Stickley, Dental Corps, US Army, 2nd Battalion, 116th Infantry Regiment, 29th Division.

  For gallantry in action at Molleville Farm, France, 10 October 1918, in administering first aid to the wounded under heavy shell fire.[73]

Stickley's personal narrative provides more details on his experience and the actions underpinning his citation star:

Upon our arrival at Revigny, we entered the Verdun Sector, in which we undertook the greatest of our operations in France. After detraining we spent a half day in the woods and then hiked twenty-five kilometers to Seigneulles, arriving at midnight of the 24 September. . . . During the operations and movements of the battalion the position of the dental surgeon was not definite, except as to the work expected of him. It was his problem to see that his outfit was transported, and open ready for business when the battalion rested. It was also expected that dental attention be administered along the route, and this attention was given. The dental surgeons hiked and carried his pack and his sole purpose was to be with his battalion at all times. . . . On the morning of the 8 October at 5 o'clock, the zero hour, the troops advanced. Our battalion being in reserve, and advancing behind support. For the first hour the enemy responded very little with their artillery and only the advancing battalion received the brunt of their resistance. They enemy then laid down a barrage in which our battalion was caught. I advanced through the barrage and established an aid station in a partially protected shell hole. From this station I received and evacuated many wounded, being assisted by my dental assistant and four sanitary men. From this time forth, I gave up all thought of administering dental treatment and devoted my efforts to first aid work. During the first day it rained nearly all day, only letting up to hail. . . .The next day I advanced one kilometer and established another aid station, evacuating my patients from this location. On the third day I advanced two kilometers and spent the night with battalion headquarters and on the following morning went forward and established an aid station 300 yards behind the front lines. The medical officers who had also advanced with me and had established an aid station joined me and we formed a battalion aid station. . . . From this time on, myself and assistant, remained constantly with the battalion surgeon, aiding him in every way to the best of our ability. . . . We went over the top three times in the advance, the last time being with our battalion headquarters, who reached the objective with the front line of the battalion. . . . On the night we were to be relieved, by some mischance, we did not make connections with the battalion and had to spend the night in a very small dugout. The Germans threw gas shells all around us, and we were all gassed, five of the twelve in our detachment having to go to the hospital, although not going until we were relieved from the front.[6]

Croix de Guerre

The British, French, and Belgian governments also often cited dental officers and enlisted personnel with various classes of their national awards, including the French Croix de Guerre (War Cross) for heroism. No unified list of these awards for Army Medical Department personnel has been located, so it is not known how many dental officers and assistants received them. However, in its official history of the Navy Medical Department in France in World War I, the Bureau of Medicine and Surgery, US Navy, provided information on three Army Dental Corps officers in the 2nd Division who had received the France's Croix de Guerre. Their names and citations are as follows:

- First Lieutenant Mortimer J O'Hara, Dental Corps US Army, attached to 6th Machine Gun Battalion, US Marine Corps.

  He volunteered for several perilous missions under an intense bombardment. Order No. 13,505-D, Croix de Guerre (Silver Star).[72]

- Captain William T Roberts, Dental Corps, US Army, attached to 5th Regiment, US Marine Corps (also recipient of a citation star).

  From October 2-6, 1918, near St. Etienne-à-Arnes, he worked without respite under a violent bombardment bandaging the wounded and effecting their evacuation. His assistant having been sent to the rear, he displayed remarkable coolness and bravery. Order No. 13,562-D, Croix de Guerre (Silver Star).[72(p310)]

- First Lieutenant Hugo M Vollmeke, Dental Corps, US Army, 4th Machine Gun Battalion.

  On October 7, 1918, at Blanc Mont, heedless of his personal safety, he took care of the wounded and evacuated them to the rear under a violent fire of the enemy artillery and machine guns. He remained at his post without shelter in order to continue his work. Order No. 12,514-D, Croix de Guerre (Gilt Star).[47,72(pp315–316)]

Not all self-sacrificing actions were recognized with awards for gallantry under fire. On November 3, 1918, Lieutenant Colonel RC Turck, MC, division surgeon for the 35th Division, wrote to the division commander recommending citations for medical personnel who "did their duty and in many instances more than their duty, but they do not talk much about what they did. Without exception, the medical officers and men, particularly of the infantry and machine gun battalions, worked closely up with their troops, under all the fire the troops received, frequently without rest day or night." From the 137th Infantry Regiment, he singled out "The Dental Surgeons, Drs. [First Lieutenant Waller W] Harrell and [First Lieutenant Arthur J] Buff, assisted at whatever they could and established independent aid stations wherever the need for such was urgent. Their work was well performed and their willingness to do their part constantly apparent. . . . Dr. W. Harrell was gassed and obliged to go to the rear, where he was of valuable service at the hospital."[74] For "an exceptionally fine performance of duty under fire," Turck also noted:

  Private Errett P Scrivner, dental assistant, Sanitary Detachment, 137th Infantry, for exceptional gallantry in action on the engagement of September 26th to October 1st, 1918 when he was counted missing in action. Private Scrivner repeatedly went out under heavy shell fire and machine gun fire in the area immediately behind the advancing front line and administered first aid, assisted men to the dressing stations. On the morning of October 1st, 1918, he did not return from a call and has since been counted missing in action.[74]

There is no record of these 35th Division personnel, other than Private First Class William C Myers, receiving citation stars from the AEF.

The Distinguished Service Medal

Two Dental Corps officers and one civilian dentist in France received awards for distinguished service from the War Department. Colonels Robert Oliver and Seibert Boak were awarded the Distinguished Service Medal for their work in getting the AEF Dental Corps effectively organized and trained.[75]

EXHIBIT 15-2

DENTAL CORPS OFFICERS KILLED IN ACTION

- First Lieutenant Lisle P Ambelang, Dental Corps, 125th Infantry Regiment, 32nd Division. Killed August 6, 1918 by a direct hit on the battalion aid station in the vicinity of Saint Giles, France, during the Château-Thierry campaign. In recommending him for the Croix de Guerre, First Lieutenant Clyde R Modie, Dental Corps, acting division dental surgeon, described him as "always displaying calm, cool courage and excellent judgment under great stress."
- First Lieutenant Walter P Desmond, Dental Corps, regimental dental surgeon, 18th Field Artillery Regiment, 3rd Division. Killed October 6, 1918, near Montfaucon, France. Desmond had originally been commissioned in the Canadian Army Dental Corps and transferred to the US Army Dental Corps upon successful examination in 1918.
- First Lieutenant Howard M Morrissey, Dental Corps, 3rd Battalion, 360th Infantry Regiment, 90th Division. Killed November 1, 1918, by enemy artillery fire northwest of Bantheville, France, during the Meuse-Argonne offensive operations.
- First Lieutenant Joseph L Parsons, Dental Corps, 313th Machine Gun Battalion, 80th Division. Killed October 4, 1918.
- First Lieutenant Lester A Stone, Dental Corps, 103rd Infantry Regiment, 26th Division. Killed October 17, 1918, by enemy shell while in his dugout in the vicinity of Bras, France. Major Charles W Lewis, Dental Corps, the division dental surgeon, noted that "Lieut. Stone was an accomplished dental officer and had served untiringly with the division since its arrival in France."

The loss of another Dental Corps officer on October 9, 1918, Captain Melvin M Augenstein, then with the 313th Infantry Regiment, 79th Division, in the vicinity of Rupt-en-Woevre, France, resulted from an accident and was described in *The History of the Seventy-Ninth Division, AEF, during the World War, 1917–1919*:

> A tragic accident marked the first day of the 313th Infantry in its new sector. Two officers, Captain Timothy L. Barber, Medical Corps, and Captain Melvin M. Augenstein, Dental Corps, were reconnoitering some old German mine galleries near the Second Battalion P.C. [command post], in search of a location for a first-aid station. Captain Barber accidentally dropped a match which set fire to a large quantity of flares and other pyrotechnics left behind by the enemy, and both officers were so badly burned that they died a few days later.

Data sources: (1) National Archives and Records Administration. Record Group 120. First Lieutenant Clyde R Modie, Dental Corps, acting division dental surgeon, to commanding general, 32nd Division, January 5, 1919. File 210.5, Commendations, Surgeon, 32nd Division. Box 3685. Entry 2144. (2) Wythe G. *A History of the 90th Division (1920)*. Whitefish, Mont: Kessinger Publishing; 2005. (3) National Archives and Records Administration. Record Group 120. Casualty card, Lieutenant Joseph Parsons. Box 4. Entry 31. (4) National Archives and Records Administration. Record Group 120. Casualty card, Lieutenant Lester A Stone. Box 5. Entry 31. (5) National Archives and Records Administration. Record Group 120. Major Charles W Lewis, Dental Corps; "History of the Dental Service 26th Division." Medical Dept. 26th Division. Box 3585. Entry 2144. (6) *History of the Seventy-Ninth Division A.E.F. during the World War: 1917–1919*. Lancaster, Pa: Steinman and Steinman; 1919: 186.

EXHIBIT 15-3

ENLISTED DENTAL ASSISTANTS KILLED IN ACTION

- Private Oscar Schroeder, 79th Division. No information on date or location of death.
- Private Phillip J O'Connell, 39th Infantry Regiment, 4th Division. Killed August 1, 1918.[1]
- Private First Class Henry E Williams, 3rd Battalion, 326th Regiment, 82nd Division. Killed October 14, 1918.[*2]
- Private Anthony Bayarski, 3rd Battalion, 326th Infantry Regiment, 82nd Division. Killed October 14, 1918.
- Private Linten W Brush, Medical Detachment, 325th Infantry Regiment, 82nd Division. Killed October 28, 1918.[3]
- Private Frederick Yannantuono, 13th Machine Gun Battalion, 5th Division. Killed October 14, 1918. Awarded Distinguished Service Cross posthumously.
- Private James C Peak, 167th Infantry Regiment, 42d Division. Killed July 17, 1918.[‡4,5]
- Private Harry P Morrison, Medical Detachment, 114th Infantry Regiment, 29th Division. Wounded by artillery fire, October 12, 1918, died of his wounds, October 13, 1918.[6]
- Private Samuel W Gaddy, Medical Detachment, 60th Infantry Regiment, 5th Division.[7,8] No information on date or location of death.

---

[*]In his personal recollection, First Lieutenant Thomas M Page, Dental Corps, provided the following information on the death of the 31-year-old Williams:
Imagine me under shell fire with an emergency dental kit and a 45 caliber revolver in my pocket with the Boche coming or rather trying to come. I cast aside my kit and loaded my 45 ready for action with the [dough]boys whom I must help but about this time the battalion Adjutant came along and said some men needed attention as they had been wounded, so I gave up my 45 to a soldier and went to them. I learned from him that the 325th Infantry had a dressing station about 300 yards away up the ravine so I jumped up out of the ditch, hailed a man and put a wounded man on a stretcher and went along up the bank carrying him under machine gun fire, but fortunately we were not wounded. From that time on I was very busy doing first aid work and evacuating the wounded, and we had to remain in this ravine until the morning of the 14th of October, when we made an attack on old Jerry, and lost many men killed and wounded but drove him back. I did not have any dental work to do as the men were not weak enough to give into the teeth ache, so my emergency kit did me no good, except being around to make me keep nearer the ground. . . . My assistant [Henry Earl Williams] was killed by shell fire [as] he was being evacuated to the hospital for treatment of shell shock. I remained at the front till October 20th when I was evacuated to the 325th Field Hospital being exhausted.[9]
[†]In his personal report, First Lieutenant William E Paul, Dental Corps, provided additional information on the death of Private Bayarski, his dental assistant, in the vicinity of Saint Juvin, France, during the Meuse-Argonne Offensive:
It took several hours to evacuate our wounded, as there [were] so many of them. Our dressing station had several narrow escapes from shells that morning while the patients were being loaded. It was while assisting in loading the ambulances that my assistant, Anthony Bayarski, was struck by a shell and instantly killed. The shelling never ceased during that day, and they fell so near our dugout that we would not permit any of our men to attempt to move the body of my assistant. Several other men were struck and killed just in front of our dressing station. Quite a few of the wounded arrived at our station with gas masks that had been ruined by getting wet, for the

(**Exhibit 15-3** *continues*)

Exhibit 15-3 *continued*

majority of the wounded had to be carried to the river. We supplied these men with masks taken from the dead that lay near the dressing station. . . .We experienced some hardships while in this dressing station. Our first was that we had no rations. For two days the only rations we could obtain were those that we took from the packs of the dead. Our second hardship was that we [had] little or no chance to sleep on account of the wounded arriving hourly, day and night.[10,11]

‡Records indicate that the dental assistant to First Lieutenant Luther C Whitlock, 42nd Division, 167th Infantry Regiment, was killed in action on July 17, 1918, but he was not identified by name. Based on available information, it was likely that he was Private James C Peak.[4,5]

Data sources: (1) National Archives and Records Administration. Record Group 120. Casualty card, Private Philip J O'Connell. Box 4. Entry 31. (2) National Archives and Records Administration. Record Group 120. Casualty card, Private Henry E Williams. Box 11. Entry 31. (3) National Archives and Records Administration. Record Group 120. Casualty card, Private Linten W Brush. Box 1. Entry 31.(4) *Annual Report of The Surgeon General, 1919*. Vol. 2. Washington, DC: Government Printing Office; 1919. (5) Amerine WH. Alabama's Own in France. New York, NY: Eaton & Gettinger; 1919. (6) National Archives and Records Administration. Record Group 120. Captain John M Hughes, Dental Corps; "Gains and Losses of Dental Personnel, 29th Division, American EF, France (from July 1st 1918 to November 16th 1918)." Memo. In: Returns, Personnel, Dental Surgeon, 29th Division. Box 3645. Entry 2144. (7) National Archives and Records Administration. Record Group 120. Major LB Schrader, division dental surgeon; "History of the Dental Corps of Fifth Division from May 8th to October 25th 1918." In: Folder 6, Medical History of the Dental Corps, Dental Surgeon, 5th Division. Box 3475. Entry 2144. (8) National Archives and Records Administration. Record Group 120. Major LB Schrader, division dental surgeon; "History of the Dental Corps of Fifth Division from October 25th to December 31st 1918, March 27, 1919." In: Folder 6, Medical History of the Dental Corps, Dental Surgeon, 5th Division. Box 3475. Entry 2144. (9) National Archives and Records Administration. Record Group 120. First Lieutenant Thomas M Page; "Dental Corps." [Report]. Folder 11, Narrative Reports, Dental Corps, Medical Department, 82nd Division. Box 3897. Entry 2144. (10) National Archives and Records Administration. Record Group 120. Captain William E Paul; "Dental Corps." [Report]. Folder 11, Narrative Reports, Dental Corps, Medical Department, 82nd Division. Box 3897. Entry 2144. (11) Buxton GE. *Official History of 82nd Division American Expeditionary Forces: "All American" Division, 1917–1919*. Indianapolis, Ind: The Bobbs-Merrill Company; 1919: 148–150.

- Colonel Robert T Oliver, Dental Corps.

  For exceptionally meritorious and distinguished services. As chief dental surgeon he displayed remarkable ability in the performance of his numerous and exacting duties. He directed the personnel, equipment, and operations of his department with sound judgment, showing resourcefulness in solving new problems which confronted him.[76]

- Seibert D Boak, Colonel, Dental Corps, United States Army.

  For exceptionally meritorious and distinguished services in a position of great responsibility. As director of the dental section of the Army sanitary school at Langres, France, from January to December 1918, he displayed organizing and training ability and accomplishments of the highest order, in successfully directing the classification and training of dental officers for field service, thereby rendering services of great value to the American Expeditionary Forces.[65]

In an unusual but highly appropriate recognition of his contributions to the dental service of the AEF and to many wounded American soldiers, the War Department also awarded Dr George Byron Hayes, who pioneered the maxillofacial service at the American Ambulance (later American Red Cross Military Hospital No. 1) in Neuilly, Paris, a Distinguished Service Medal on December 6, 1920. Prior to the American entry into the war, he had contributed his considerable talents to aiding wounded French soldiers (see Chapter 11: From a New Corps to a World War, 1911–1917). After the arrival of Pershing and his staff in the summer of 1917, the American Red Cross Military Hospital No. 1 was taken over by the Army, but Hayes remained as head of the dental service and supervised the work of five to seven dental officers assigned to him for the remainder of the war.[77] His citation read:

> Dr. George Byron Hayes. For exceptionally meritorious and conspicuous services. An eminent dental surgeon who placed freely the advantages of his professional attainments and the full facilities of his complete clinic at Paris at the services of the American medical personnel. By the markedly distinguished record made by him in jaw and facial surgery among the wounded of the American Expeditionary Forces, and his able directorate of the school for instruction of dental personnel in maxillo facial and prosthetic surgery, he has rendered services of preeminent worth.[78]

Casualties Among Dental Personnel

During the AEF's months in the trenches, the Medical Department lost 3,954 officers and enlisted personnel killed in action, died of wounds, wounded, gassed, and disabled due to hostile action and battle-related injuries.[79] Among them were five dental officers and seven dental assistants killed in action and two dental assistants who died of wounds resulting from hostile action. A number of other dental officers and assistants were wounded in action and gassed, often seriously enough to prevent them from returning to front-line duty. The *Annual Report of The Surgeon General* for 1919 listed 36 officers and four enlisted dental assistants as wounded in combat operations. However, it seems no accurate record was maintained, so the exact numbers and names cannot be determined (Exhibit 15-2).[80–85] The enlisted dental assistants shared the hazards of front line combat service with their dental officers, resulting in a number of soldiers who were killed in action and died of wounds (Exhibit 15-3).[43,44,86–94]

Combat was not the only claimant on the lives of Dental Corps officers, either in France or the United States. Disease, accidents, and other causes claimed the lives of another 56 dental officers, 11 in France and 45 in the United States, including 8 commissioned officers in the Dental Reserve Corps who were waiting to be called up to active duty. Of these, at least 31 were victims of influenza and its complication, pneumonia, during the influenza pandemic of 1918–1919.[95–99] No known accounting exists for the names and number of enlisted dental assistants who died from disease, accidents, or other causes (Appendix 1).

Quality Dental Work Resumes

The months following the armistice were productive times for the dentists in the AEF's divisions. Freed from combat, the dental officers were able to provide the full range of dental care that front-line conditions had made impossible. As the Third US Army prepared to move into the American occupation zone in Germany, the First and Second armies settled down to wait for fighting to resume or for the end of the war. During these months, the dental officers continued performing quality dental work and prepared the soldiers to return home in accordance with Oliver's objective "to put the teeth of the men in first-class condition, prior to their return to the United States and release from service."[100(p120)]

As the newly activated Third US Army moved into the Rhineland on occupation duty in November and December 1918, the First and Second armies in France, Belgium, and Luxembourg, along with the remaining combat divisions, settled into quarters. In both armies, dental work picked up in November as the troops trained, took leave, and awaited further developments, and reached a high in February 1919 before the divisions began returning to the United States in the spring. The armies were largely able to maintain sufficient numbers of dental officers, assistants, and equipment throughout the period prior to their inactivations in April 1919 and the shipment of the divisions from France. The Second US Army retained enough dental personnel and equipment to remain at or near the authorized levels (Tables 15-1 and 15-2), allowing the dental officers to accomplish a considerable amount of oral and dental work during their remaining months in Europe (Table 15-3). The dental officers in the individual divisions were kept gainfully employed as long as the divisions remained in Europe, were in the ports of debarkation, or were on the troop transports as

TABLE 15-1

DENTAL PERSONNEL AND EQUIPMENT, SECOND US ARMY, END OF MONTH, NOVEMBER 1918–FEBRUARY 1919[*]

	November 1918	December 1918	January 1919	February 1919
Divisions	7	8	7	5
Dental officers	199	206	227	185
Dental assistants	186	211	242	188
Dental equipment				
Portable outfits	50	54	93	87
Modified outfits	89	117	127	91
Field outfits	6	7	0	0
Emergency outfits	20	32	1	0
Total	165	210	221	178
Dental laboratories	NR	4	7	9

[*]The March 1919 report has no information on dental personnel or equipment because not all Form 57 reports of dental work had been received when American Expeditionary Forces General Headquarters closed the Second US Army headquarters early in April 1919.
Data sources: (1) National Archives and Records Administration. Record Group 120. Form 57, Dental work at Second Army, American E.F., Lieutenant Colonel GH Casaday, supervising dental surgeon, November and December 1918. In: Second Army Consolidated Dental Reports. Box 3295. Entry 924.
(2) National Archives and Records Administration. Record Group 120. Form 57, Dental work at Second Army, American E.F., Lieutenant Colonel Rex H Rhoades, chief dental surgeon, January, February, and March 1919. In: Second Army Consolidated Dental Reports. Box 3295. Entry 924.

they returned across the Atlantic. For example, the dentists of the 33rd Division, a National Guard division from Illinois, shifted from France to Luxembourg in December 1918, and then moved to the French port of Brest in April before returning to the United States. During the period from November 1918 through April 1919, the division's dental officers spent countless hours at their chairs getting the soldiers ready for their homecoming (Table 15-4).[101,102] It was efforts such as these, clearly reflected in the reports of the 33rd Division and the Second Army, that led Oliver in early 1919 to commend the "the pleasing resumption of magnificent professional activity."[103–105]

Dentistry's Contributions to the War and the War's Contributions to Dentistry

The front line combat service of dental officers and assistants, sharing the privations, dangers, and losses of trench warfare and modern combat with the soldiers, line officers, and also officers of the Medical Corps, finally won for the Dental Corps the long-sought recognition of its value to and role in the Army Medical Department and Army. First Lieutenant Robert P Stickley, dental surgeon with the 2nd Battalion, 116th Infantry Regiment, 29th Division, who received a citation star for his heroism in action at Molleville Farm, France, on October 10, 1918, perhaps

TABLE 15-2

DENTAL OFFICERS PER DIVISION, SECOND US ARMY TROOPS NOVEMBER 26, 1918–MARCH 22, 1919

Organization	November 26, 1918	December 28, 1918	January 25, 1919	February 22, 1919	March 22, 1919
5th Division	X	28	26	32	31
7th Division	18	20	21	28	28
28th Division	21	21	21	21	X
33d Division	29	23	28	29	30
35th Division	22	29	29	X	X
79th Division	X	16	32	31	31
85th Division	17	7	X	X	X
88th Division	25	21	28	29	28
92nd Division	29	X	X	X	X
VI Corps	9	12	8	2	2
IX Corps	X	9	8	3	3
Second Army	10	19	22	27	24
Total	**180**	**205**	**223**	**202**	**177**

Data sources: (1) National Archives and Records Administration. Record Group 120. Colonel GH Casaday, Dental Corps; "Dental personnel and equipment, Second Army, November 26, 1918, and January 1, 1919." Box 3295. Entry 924. (2) National Archives and Records Administration. Record Group 120. Lieutenant Colonel Rex H Rhoades, chief dental surgeon; "Dental Personnel and Equipment, Second Army, January 31, 1919, February 25, 1919, and March 24, 1919." Report. File, Dental Personnel, Dental Surgeon, Second Army. Box 3295. Entry 924.

best summarized the numerous contributions of the AEF's dental officers and assistants to the war effort when he wrote:

> In conclusion, I would add, that the privilege of alleviating pain and suffering for the soldier, before the conflict, and in going through the conflict with him, and being at his side to dress his wounds, is worthy of the aspirations of any profession, and I claim this honor for the dental profession of the American Expeditionary Forces in France.[6]

As early as December 1918, the American dental press was already placing a much larger emphasis on the entire dental profession's contributions to the war. In the December 1918 edition of *Dental Register*, editor Nelville S Hoff outlined dentistry's many contributions to the war effort, followed by his views on what the war had done for dentistry.[104,105] Hoff believed that the war had proven the righteousness of the dental profession's long struggle for professional recognition and acceptance that was intertwined with the quest for dental services in the US Army and Navy:

> Perhaps one of the most pronounced benefits our profession has acquired during the war is the legal acknowledgment of the claims our profession has made for many

TABLE 15-3

PATIENTS, SITTINGS, AND SELECTED DENTAL TREATMENTS AND OPERATIONS, SECOND US ARMY, NOVEMBER 1918–MARCH 1919[*]

	November 1918	December 1918	January 1919	February 1919	March 1919	Total
Patients	13,707	17,219	20,784	14,117	8,484	74,311
Sittings	18,303	24,084	33,210	24,252	14,189	114,038
Dental caries	13,661	18,694	26,295	21,438	14,765	94,853
Dento-alveolar abscess	1,758	3,345	3,530	2,406	1,362	12,401
Fillings	11,778	13,911	25,279	21,477	14,962	77,407
Teeth extracted	3,510	4,781	5,330	4,151	2,190	16,802
Teeth treated	3,213	5,425	8,872	6,148	X	23,658[†]
Calculus removed	2,503	3,483	3,706	3,446	1,535	14,673
Crown and bridgework	718	835	1,042	722	535	3,852

[*]Not all dental officers had submitted their Form 57 reports when American Expeditionary Forces General Headquarters closed Second US Army headquarters early in April 1919.
[†]November 1918–February 1919 only.
Data sources: (1) National Archives and Records Administration. Record Group 120. Form 57, Dental work at Second Army, American E.F., Lieutenant Colonel GH Casaday, supervising dental surgeon, November and December 1918. In: Second Army Consolidated Dental Reports. Box 3295. Entry 924.
(2) National Archives and Records Administration. Record Group 120. Form 57, Dental work at Second Army, American E.F., Lieutenant Colonel Rex H Rhoades, chief dental surgeon, January, February, and March 1919. In: Second Army Consolidated Dental Reports. Box 3295. Entry 924.

TABLE 15-4

PATIENTS, SITTINGS, AND SELECTED DENTAL TREATMENTS AND
OPERATIONS, 33RD DIVISION, SECOND US ARMY,
NOVEMBER 1918–APRIL 1919

	November 1918	December 1918	January 1919	February 1919	March 1919	April 1919	Total
Patients	3,300	1,867	3,394	3,040	2,771	1,408	15,780
Sittings	4,688	2,268	5,339	4,970	4,504	2,286	24,055
Dental caries	3,417	1,678	3,237	3,625	3,790	1,848	17,595
Dento-alveolar abscess	377	174	403	462	365	178	1,959
Fillings	3,026	1,506	3,403	3,653	3,777	1,818	17,183
Teeth extracted	553	248	449	550	470	262	2,532
Teeth treated	1,445	844	1,758	1,263	1,230	425	6,965
Calculus removed	709	269	897	779	791	437	3,882
Crown and bridgework	193	97	181	148	151	102	872

Data sources: (1) National Archives and Records Administration. Record Group 120. Form 57, Consolidated Report of Dental Work at 33rd Division, American E.F., Major RW Pearson, Dental Corps, division dental surgeon, November and December 1918, January, February, March, and April 1919. File, Daily Reports, Dental Work, Dental Surgeon, 33 Division. Box 3705. Entry 2144. (2) National Archives and Records Administration. Record Group 120. Form 57, Consolidated Report of Dental Work at 33rd Division, American E.F., Major John M Evey, Dental Corps, division dental surgeon, April 1919. File, Daily Reports, Dental Work, Dental Surgeon, 33 Division. Box 3705. Entry 2144.

years for an equitable recognition of its professional standing by the United States Government. For years we have been humiliated because Congress refused to give our profession a dignified rank in the army and navy. The war emergency so clearly demonstrated the professional standing of dentistry that we easily acquired what before had seemed like a distant probability. From these most obvious facts we, as a profession, can feel that while the war has been a great calamity it has brought our profession considerable advantages which otherwise would not have materialized so promptly.[107(pp553–554)]

Hoff also enumerated what dentistry, as a profession, gained from the war, emphasizing the dentists' practical, professional experiences and the benefits of working more closely with their medical colleagues:

First we can acknowledge our obligation for the wonderful opportunity the war gave us to demonstrate to the world the value of dentistry as an equipment for a good soldier. We have had the chance to show how much better fighting man is the soldier with good teeth. Incidentally we have had a chance to convince our medical associates of the fact that a well man is more largely dependent on good teeth than they have generally believed. The war has given our dentists a chance to acquire unusual skill in surgical and prosthetic treatments and restorations that do not offer in civil practice in ordinary peace times. The experience and training some of our dentists have had opportunity to secure in the field hospitals in association with medical practitioners has been wonderfully rare and beneficial to them. It has brought the medical and dental men into intimate and profitable relations with each other and we are sure that dentists who have been privileged to have an extended experience of this kind will be better prepared for civil practice.[107(p553)]

In a March 1919 editorial, Otto U King, editor of the *Journal of the National Dental Association*, wrote of the importance of dentists in conserving fighting strength for the Army:

When the history of this war shall have been adequately written, with all the ramifications of the activities connected therewith, the fact will be apparent that dentistry has played no small part in keeping the men fit for the fighting lines. At the outbreak of the war, very many men were made eligible for military duty by reason of the work done for them by dentists—men whose services would have been lost to the army had it not been for this work.[108(p275)]

Referring back to the long, arduous, and obviously unforgotten struggle to gain dental service and commissioned status for dentists in the Army and Navy that stretched back to the Civil War, King welcomed the changes that the war had brought about:

The fact that the Government recognizes and appreciates what has been done by the profession, is clearly evident in the changed attitude of Government officials toward matters pertaining to dentistry since the war broke out. Today, they are cordially receptive to any advance suggested by the profession, where previously to this, it had been a slow, tedious process to obtain any appreciable or tangible reform. . . . The fact must be apparent to even the most casual observer that the status of dentistry has undergone a complete change in this brief period.[108(p276–277)]

APPENDIX 1

US ARMY DENTAL CORPS OFFICERS KILLED IN ACTION AND DIED OF DISEASE, ACCIDENT, AND OTHER CAUSES APRIL 1, 1917–JUNE 30, 1920

Name, Place of Origin	Assigned to	Location of Death	Date of Death
Killed in Action			
First Lieutenant Lisle P Ambelang Cascade, Wisconsin	125th Infantry Regiment 32nd Division, AEF, France	Vicinity of Saint Giles, France	August 6, 1918
First Lieutenant Walter P Desmond Medford, Massachusetts	18th Field Artillery Regiment 3rd Division, AEF, France	Vicinity of Montfaucon, France	October 6, 1918
First Lieutenant Harold S Morrissey Kenosha, Wisconsin	360th Infantry Regiment 90th Division, AEF, France	Vicinity of Bantheville, France	November 1, 1918
First Lieutenant Joseph H Parsons Erie, Pennsylvania	313th Machine Gun Battalion 80th Division, AEF, France	NR	October 4, 1918
First Lieutenant Lester A Stone Pittsfield, Massachusetts	103rd Infantry Regiment 26th Division, AEF, France	Vicinity of Bras, France	October 17, 1918
Died of Disease, Accident, and Other Causes			
Captain Melvin M Augenstein Hagerstown, Maryland	313th Infantry Regiment 79th Division, AEF, France	Vicinity of Rupt-en-Woevre, France	October 16, 1918
First Lieutenant Charles J Balbach Millville, Pennsylvania	NR	AEF, France	March 10, 1919
First Lieutenant Frederic A Ballachey Buffalo, New York	NR	Camp Dix, New Jersey	September 26, 1918
First Lieutenant Alexander D Baris Brooklyn, New York	317th Labor Battalion	AEF, France	February 28, 1919
First Lieutenant Horace A Birdsong Lulu, Mississippi	NR	Camp Mills, New York	May 10, 1918

Name	Place		Date
First Lieutenant Vance W Bliss, Santa Cruz, California	AEF, France	NR	October 12, 1918
First Lieutenant Francis E Boazman, Chappells, South Carolina	Camp Sherman, Ohio	NR	October 19, 1918
First Lieutenant Charles H Boisseau, Smithton, Pennsylvania	Camp Upton, Long Island, New York	NR	October 12, 1918
Captain James E Cox, Charlestown, Massachusetts	Columbus, Ohio	NR	April 11, 1920
First Lieutenant Oliver W Davies, Los Angeles, California	Hoboken, New Jersey	NR	November 3, 1918
First Lieutenant Joseph R Earley, New Castle, Pennsylvania	Camp Stewart, Virginia	NR	October 8, 1918
First Lieutenant Ralph H Fickes, Vandergrift, Pennsylvania	Fort Oglethorpe, Georgia	NR	October 18, 1918
First Lieutenant Lionel G Fleming, Saint Martinsville, Louisiana	Camp Lee, Virginia	NR	October 4, 1918
First Lieutenant Ronald E Fletcher, Mount Vernon, New York	Fort Oglethorpe, Georgia	NR	December 21, 1918
First Lieutenant Gale Friday, Fremont, Indiana	Camp Sheridan, Alabama	NR	November 14, 1918
First Lieutenant Roy S Glass, Frackville, Pennsylvania	Frackville, Pennsylvania	NR	October 19, 1918
Captain Walter Grandage, Bridgeport, Connecticut	Camp Devens, Massachusetts	NR	October 7, 1918
First Lieutenant Clark B Hannah, Los Angeles, California	Camp Fremont, California	NR	October 18, 1918
First Lieutenant Winfred E Henshaw, Peru, Illinois	Chicago, Illinois	NR	September 28, 1918
First Lieutenant Wade H Hoffman, Oil City, Pennsylvania	Camp Upton, Long Island, New York	NR	October 14, 1918

Name	Unit	Place	Date
First Lieutenant Alexander H Jones Youngstown, Ohio	Field Artillery Training School	Saumur, AEF, France	October 1, 1918
Captain Earl P Jones Mansfield, Ohio	16th Engineer Regiment	AEF, France	October 17, 1918
First Lieutenant Albert L Kreitman New York, New York	NR	Camp Meade, Maryland	October 4, 1918
Captain Harry B Laird Tecumseh, Oklahoma	NR	Fort Sill, Oklahoma	May 5, 1919
First Lieutenant Frank S Leonard Indianapolis, Indiana	NR	American Red Cross Hospital No. 1 Neuilly, Paris, AEF, France	January 13, 1919
First Lieutenant William M Lubitz Brooklyn, New York	NR	Camp Dix, New Jersey	October 11, 1918
First Lieutenant Frank E McNett LaCrosse, Wisconsin	NR	Fort Oglethorpe, Georgia	December 18, 1918
First Lieutenant George W Mattox Elberton, Georgia	122nd Infantry Regiment 31st Division	AEF, France	October 15, 1918
First Lieutenant Samuel F Moffett Cottello, Texas	NR	Fort Bliss, Texas	January 16, 1919
First Lieutenant Adrian L Morin San Francisco, California	NR	Camp Fremont, California	October 18, 1918
First Lieutenant Max Neal Pittsburgh, Pennsylvania	Base Hospital No. 27, AEF	Angers, France	March 16, 1919
First Lieutenant Will C Niles Newton, Massachusetts	NR	Boston, Massachusetts	October 4, 1918
First Lieutenant Loy A Patterson Hennessey, Oklahoma	NR	Camp Beauregard, Louisiana	July 19, 1918
First Lieutenant Walter F Peterson Minneapolis, Minnesota	NR	Camp Custer, Michigan	September 6, 1918

Name		Location	Date
Major Merton M Postle, Chicago, Illinois	NR	Camp Zachary Taylor, Kentucky	October 15, 1918
First Lieutenant Walter O Reinhard, Rio, Wisconsin	NR	Camp Custer, Michigan	October 3, 1918
Lieutenant Colonel Mortimer Sanderson, Philadelphia, Pennsylvania	NR	Camp Cody, New Mexico	July 30, 1918
First Lieutenant Francis R Simm, Pierre, South Dakota	NR	Fort Oglethorpe, Georgia	October 7, 1918
First Lieutenant John S Simons, Henderson, Minnesota	NR	Camp Tobyhanna, Pennsylvania	October 2, 1918
First Lieutenant Cecil C Smith, Violet Hill, Arkansas	NR	Camp Travis, Texas	October 18, 1918
First Lieutenant Bernard F Staples, Boston, Massachusetts	NR	Camp Devens, Massachusetts	September 24, 1918
First Lieutenant Delmar H Stocker, Tunkhannock, Pennsylvania	Camp Hospital No. 21, AEF	Bourbonne-les-Bains, France	October 3, 1918
First Lieutenant Alfred G Wald, Huntington, Pennsylvania	NR	Camp Jackson, South Carolina	October 15, 1918
First Lieutenant Raymond A Walker, New Haven, Connecticut	NR	Camp Devens, Massachusetts	September 28, 1918
Captain Harrison B Wall, Cleveland, Ohio	NR	Camp Custer, Michigan	March 28, 1918
First Lieutenant George E Wilcox, Minonck, Illinois	332nd Machine Gun Battalion 86th Division	Southampton, England	September 28, 1918
Captain Fielding M Wilhite, Parents, Kansas	NR	Fort Riley, Kansas	April 24, 1919
First Lieutenant Edwin B Zwink, Eustis, Nebraska	NR	Camp Cody, New Mexico	November 7, 1918

Dental Reserve Corps Officers Who Died Prior to Entering Active Service

First Lieutenant Lester J Allison	N/A	Iowa City, Iowa	April 20, 1918
First Lieutenant Ernst L Casselman	N/A	Effingham, Illinois	November 5, 1918
First Lieutenant Harry E Duwe	N/A	Arlington, Iowa	October 28, 1918
First Lieutenant Roy E Hanson	N/A	Cambridge Springs, Pennsylvania	November 25, 1918
First Lieutenant Carl R Henry	N/A	Cuba, Illinois	September 4, 1918
First Lieutenant John C Higgins	N/A	McAdoo, Pennsylvania	October 18, 1918
First Lieutenant Lloyd A Osborne	N/A	Fremont, Iowa	July 24, 1918
First Lieutenant Raymond M Weidert	N/A	Wilcox, Pennsylvania	November 7, 1918

AEF: American Expeditionary Forces
N/A: not applicable
NR: not reported
Data sources: (1) Medical Field Service School. *In Memoriam: The Medical Department of the United States Army in the World War.* Vol 1. In: *Supplement, Army Medical Bulletin No. 27.* Carlisle Barracks, Pennsylvania: DA; 1932: 10–26. (2) Lynch C, Weed FW, McAfee L. In memoriam. In: *The Surgeon General's Office.* In: *The Medical Department of the United States Army in the World War.* Vol 1. Washington, DC: Government Printing Office; 1923: 587–604. (3) In memoriam. *J Am Dent Assoc.* 1924;11:952–953. (4) Dental officers who died while on active duty. *J Nat Dent Assoc.* 1919;6:287–288. (5) Office of the Surgeon General. *Annual Report of the Surgeon General.* Washington, DC: OTSG; 1919: 1309, 1435–1438.

References

1. National Archives and Records Administration. Record Group 120. History of the Dental Section of the Army Sanitary School, Army schools, American Expeditionary Forces, France, December 19, 1917 to December 10, 1918. In: Dental Section, Army Sanitary School. Box 1780. Entry 396.

2. Stone FP. Duties of a dental officer and his relation to medical officers. *Milit Dent J.* 1922;5:151.

3. National Archives and Records Administration. Record Group 120. Major LS Fountain, Dental Corps, division dental surgeon, 77th Division; Dental History 77th Division, October 18, 1918. Folder 1, Correspondence, Dental Division, Army Sanitary School (A–L). Box 1780. Entry 395.

4. National Archives and Records Administration. Record Group 120. Major LB Schrader, division dental surgeon; "History of the Dental Corps of Fifth Division from May 8th to October 25th 1918 and From October 25th to December 31st 1918," March 27, 1919. Folder 6, Medical History of the Dental Corps, Dental Surgeon, 5th Division. Box 3475. Entry 2144.

5. National Archives and Records Administration. Record Group 120. Captain John M Hughes, Dental Corps, division dental surgeon, 29th Division, to Colonel SD Boak, Dental Section, Army Sanitary School, location of dental surgeons, November 1, 1918. Memo. Folder 12, Dental History, 29th Division Surgeon. Box 3642. Entry 2144.

6. National Archives and Records Administration. Record Group 120. Captain John M Hughes, Dental Corps, division dental surgeon, to chief surgeon, American Expeditionary Forces, Dental history, 29th Division, January 27, 1919. Folder 12, Dental History, 29th Division Surgeon. Box 3642. Entry 2144.

7. National Archives and Records Administration. Record Group 120. Major Charles W Lewis, Dental Corps; "History of the dental service 26th Division." In: Medical Department 26th Division. Box 3585. Entry 2144.

8. National Archives and Records Administration. Record Group 120. Captain Walter E Lotz, Dental Corps, division dental surgeon; "Dental History, February 15, 1919." Folder 19, Medical Department 78th Division. Report. Box 3842. Entry 2144.

9. Ford JH. *Administration, American Expeditionary Forces.* Vol 2. In: Lynch C, Weed FW, McAfee L, eds. *The Medical Department of the United States Army in the World War.* Washington, DC: Government Printing Office; 1927.

10. Grissinger JW. Field service. *Milit Surg.* 1927;61:594.

11. Wunderlich FR. The medical service of the infantry division in combat-service of Medical, Dental and Veterinary Corps: Part 2. The Dental Corps. *Milit Surg.* 1927;60:666.

12. National Archives and Records Administration. Record Group 120. Form 57, First Lieutenant Bernard L Riley; "Report of Dental work at Headquarters, American First Army, November (16 to 30), 1918." Box 3279A. Entry 864.

13. National Archives and Records Administration. Record Group 120. Form 57, First Lieutenant GC McMullen; "Report of Dental Work at Headquarters, Second Army, October 1918." Box 3291. Entry 923.

14. The dental section. In: Ford JH. *Administration, American Expeditionary Forces*. Vol 2. In: Lynch C, Weed FW, McAfee L, eds. *The Medical Department of the United States Army in the World War.* Washington, DC: Government Printing Office; 1927.

15. Huntington PW. Problems of the regimental surgeon—the dental surgeon as an auxiliary medical officer, 7 December 1918, Army Sanitary School No. 171. Appendix. In: Bispham WN. *Training*. Vol 3. In: Lynch C, Weed FW, McAfee L, eds. *The Medical Department of the United States Army in the World War.* Washington, DC: Government Printing Office; 1927: 1127.

16. National Archives and Records Administration. Record Group 120. Major Elbert E Rushing, dental surgeon, 1st Division, to Lieutenant Colonel Rex H Rhoades, chief dental surgeon, First Army, August 31, 1918. Letter. Folder 13. Box 3398. Entry 2144.

17. National Archives and Records Administration. Record Group 120. Lieutenant Colonel Robert F Patterson, Dental Corps, division dental surgeon, 30th Division, American Expeditionary Forces, to division surgeon, 30th Division, August 26, 1918. Letter. Folder 19. Box 3654. Entry 2144.

18. National Archives and Records Administration. Record Group 120. First Lieutenant James A Taylor, division dental surgeon, 35th Division, American Expeditionary Forces, to division surgeon, 35th Division, July 7, 1918. Memo. File 703. Folder 18. Box 5149. Entry 2065.

19. National Archives and Records Administration. Record Group 120. Major Howard I Benedict, Dental Corps, division dental surgeon, 32nd Division, to division surgeon, 32nd Division, August 16, 1918. Memo. Folder 20. Box 3683. Entry 2144.

20. National Archives and Records Administration. Record Group 120. Captain Walter E Lotz, Dental Corps, division dental surgeon; "Dental History, February 15, 1919, 5." Report. Folder 19, Medical Department 78th Division. Box 3842. Entry 2144.

21. National Archives and Records Administration. Record Group 120. Major RW Pearson, Dental Corps, division dental surgeon, 33rd Division; "Dental History, April 18, 1919, 3." Folder 1, Medical History Surgeon 33rd Division. Box 3704. Entry 2144.

22. Graham GD. Dental history of the Second Division, A.E.F., March 10th to November 6th, 1918. *J Assoc Milit Dent Surg*. 1919;3:115–121.

23. MacDonald CF. Dental service in the combat zone. *J Am Dent Assoc*. 1927;14:1243–1247.

24. National Archives and Records Administration. Record Group 120. Major FW O'Donnell, Medical Corps, division surgeon; "Medical History of the 89th Division During Operations in the Argonne-Meuse Sector, November 27, 1918, 10"; attachment to Major FW O'Donnell, MC, division surgeon, to commanding general, 89th Division, Report, November 27, 1918. Folder 1, History 10/1/17–3/21/19, Surgeon, 89th Division. Box 3968. Entry 2144.

25. Huber CH. Dental history of the 88th Division. In: *Dental History, 88th Division, World War I*. Available at: Research Collections, Office of Medical History, Falls Church, Virginia.

26. An interesting letter from Capt. Allen N. Kearby. *Tex Dent J*. 1919;36:8–13.

27. National Archives and Records Administration. Record Group 120. Colonel Herbert G Shaw, Medical Corps, division surgeon, 1st Division; "Return of Medical Officers etc Serving in the First Division, AEF, on the Last Day of June 1918." In: Returns of Medical Officers, Surgeon, 1st Division. Box 3399. Entry 21244.

28. National Archives and Records Administration. Record Group 120. Colonel JI Mabee, Medical Corps; "Return of Medical Officers etc Serving in the First Division, AEF, on the Last Day of July 1918." In: Returns of Medical Officers, Surgeon, 1st Division. Box 3399. Entry 21244.

29. National Archives and Records Administration. Record Group 120. Lieutenant Colonel Rex H Rhoades, chief dental surgeon, First Army, to all division dental surgeons; "Dental History." In: Correspondence Dental Surgeon, Medical Department, 29th Division. Box 3645. Entry 2144.

30. National Archives and Records Administration. Record Group 120. Memo No. 5, Captain John M Hughes, Dental Corps, division dental surgeon, 29th Division, to all dental surgeons, 29th Division, American Expeditionary Forces, October 8, 1918. In: Memos, Dental Surgeon, Medical Department, 29th Division. Box 3645. Entry 2144.

31. National Archives and Records Administration. Record Group 120. First Lieutenant George E Staats, Dental Corps; "My Experiences While Serving with the Second Division, American Expeditionary Forces, October 19, 1918." Report. Folder 4. Box 3410. Entry 2144.

32. US Adjutant General's Office. *Official Army Register*. Vol 1. Washington, DC: US Government Printing Office; 1947: 1413.

33. Biographical File of Colonel Rex H Rhoades, Dental Corps. Biographical Files, Research Collections, OTSG/MEDCOM. Falls Church, Virginia.

34. American Battle Monuments Commission. *2d Division, Summary of Operations in the World War*. Washington, DC: US Government Printing Office; 1944.

35. National Archives and Records Administration. Record Group 120. Lieutenant Colonel George D Graham, Dental Corps, dental surgeon, 2nd Division, August 29, 1918, to dental officers, 2nd Division. Memo. Box 3414. Entry 2144.

36. National Archives and Records Administration. Record Group 120. Lieutenant Colonel George D Graham, Dental Corps, dental surgeon, 2nd Division, September 10, 1918, to dental officers, 2nd Division. Memo. Box 3414. Entry 2144.

37. National Archives and Records Administration. Record Group 120. First Lieutenant Bernard R Thornton; "Dental Corps." [Report]. Folder 11, Narrative Reports, Dental Corps, Medical Department, 82nd Division. Box 3897. Entry 2144.

38. National Archives and Records Administration. Record Group 120. Lieutenant BJ Connolly, 303rd Field Signal Battalion, nd. Memo. Folder 19, Medical Department 78th Division. Box 3842. Entry 2144.

39. National Archives and Records Administration. Record Group 120. First Lieutenant J Iredell Wyckoff, Dental Corps, 2nd Battalion, 309th Infantry Regiment, 78th Division. Memo. Folder 19, Medical Department 78th Division. Box 3842. Entry 2144.

40. National Archives and Records Administration. Record Group 120. First Lieutenant Clautus L Cope; "Dental Corps." [Report]. Folder 11, Narrative Reports, Dental Corps, Medical Department, 82nd Division. Box 3897. Entry 2144.

41. National Archives and Records Administration. Record Group 120. First Lieutenant Junius F Emerson; "Dental Corps." [Report]. Folder 11, Narrative Reports, Dental Corps, Medical Department, 82nd Division. Box 3897. Entry 2144.

42. National Archives and Records Administration. Record Group 120. First Lieutenant William N Crowl; "Dental Corps." [Report]. Folder 11, Narrative Reports, Dental Corps, Medical Department, 82nd Division. Box 3897. Entry 2144.

43. National Archives and Records Administration. Record Group 120. Captain William E Paul; "Dental Corps." [Report]. Folder 11, Narrative Reports, Dental Corps, Medical Department, 82nd Division. Box 3897. Entry 2144.

44. National Archives and Records Administration. Record Group 120. First Lieutenant Thomas M Page; "Dental Corps." [Report]. Folder 11, Narrative Reports, Dental Corps, Medical Department, 82nd Division. Box 3897. Entry 2144.

45. National Archives and Records Administration. Record Group 120. First Lieutenant George L Long, Dental Corps; "Dental History of Duties and Stations, January 2, 1919." Folder 4, Narrative Reports, Dental Corps, Medical Department, 26th Division. Box 3585. Entry 2144.

46. US War Department. General order no. 518, 1920. In: US Navy Bureau of Medicine and Surgery. *The Medical Department of the United States Navy with the Army and Marine Corps in France in World War I: its Functions and Employment.* Washington, DC: Bureau of Medicine and Surgery, USN; 1947.

47. US War Department. *The Medical Department of the United States Navy with the Army and Marine Corps in France in World War I: its Functions and Employment.* Washington, DC: Bureau of Medicine and Surgery, USN; 1947.

48. US War Department. General order no. 126, 1918. In: US Navy Bureau of Medicine and Surgery. *The Medical Department of the United States Navy with the Army and Marine Corps in France in World War I: its Functions and Employment.* Washington, DC: Bureau of Medicine and Surgery, USN; 1947: 203.

49. Vice Admiral Alexander G Lyle, DC, US Navy. Biographical Files, Research Collections, OTSG/MEDCOM. Falls Church, Virginia.

50. National Archives and Records Administration. Record Group 120. Lieutenant Commander Cornelius H Mack, Dental Corps, US Navy, to division dental surgeon, 2nd Division, October 15, 1918. Narrative Reports of Medical and Dental Officers of the 2nd Division, in Surgeon, 2nd Division. Box 3410. Entry 2144.

51. US War Department. General order no. 24, April 26, 1920. In: *War Department, General Orders and Bulletins 1920*. Washington, DC: Government Printing Office; 1921: 2.

52. US War Department. General order no. 37, March 11, 1919. In: *War Department, General Orders and Bulletins 1919*. Washington, DC: Government Printing Office; 1920: 49.

53. US War Department. General order no. 81, June 26, 1919. In: *War Department, General Orders and Bulletins 1919*. Washington, DC: Government Printing Office; 1920: 5.

54. US War Department. General order no. 59, May 3, 1919. In: *War Department, General Orders and Bulletins 1919*. Washington, DC: Government Printing Office; 1920: 44.

55. US War Department. General order no. 32, March 1, 1919. In: *War Department, General Orders and Bulletins 1919*. Washington, DC: Government Printing Office; 1920: 38–39.

56. US War Department. General order no. 44, April 2, 1919. In: *War Department, General Orders and Bulletins 1919*. Washington, DC: Government Printing Office; 1920: 75.

57. US War Department. General order no. 95, July 26, 1919. In: *War Department, General Orders and Bulletins 1919*. Washington, DC: Government Printing Office; 1920: 22.

58. National Archives and Records Administration. Record Group 120. Captain John J Halnan, Medical Corps, 114th Infantry, to division dental surgeon, 29th Division, 28 November 1918, in Memo, Captain John M Hughes, Dental Corps, division dental surgeon, 29th Division, to chief surgeon, American Expeditionary Forces; "Dental History, 29th Division." Memo. Folder 12, Dental History, 29th Division Surgeon. Memo. Box 3642. Entry 2144.

59. Coffman JF. History of sanitary detachment, 2nd. Bn. 139th Inf. During Argonne Meuse Battle, Sept. 25th to Oct. 2nd, 1918. In: Kenamore C. *The Story of the 139th Infantry*. Saint Louis, Missouri: Guard Publishing Co; 1920: 161–164.

60. Kerrigan EE. *American War Medals and Decorations*. New York, NY: The Viking Press; 1964: 24.

61. US War Department. Bulletin no. 43, War Department, 22 July 1918. In: *War Department, General Orders and Bulletins 1918*. Washington, DC: Government Printing Office; 1919: 43.

62. US War Department. General order no. 83, War Department, June 30, 1919. In: *War Department, General Orders and Bulletins 1918*. Washington, DC: Government Printing Office; 1919.

63. National Archives and Records Administration. Record Group 120. General headquarters, American Expeditionary Forces, Citations order no. 7, June 3, 1919. Box 5079. Entry 458.

64. US War Department. General order no. 15, April 4, 1921. In: *War Department, General Orders and Bulletins 1921*. Washington, DC: Government Printing Office; 1922: 8.

65. US War Department. General order no. 15, April 5, 1923. In: *War Department, General Orders and Bulletins* 1923. Washington, DC: Government Printing Office; 1924: 51.

66. National Archives and Records Administration. Record Group 120. General headquarters, American Expeditionary Forces, Citations order no. 1, June 3, 1919. Box 5079. Entry 458.

67. Derby R. *"Wade in, Sanitary!": the Story of a Division Surgeon in France*. New York, NY: GP Putnam's Sons; 1919: 254.

68. National Archives and Records Administration. Record Group 120. General headquarters, American Expeditionary Forces, Citations Orders No. 2, June 3, 1919. Box 5079. Entry 458.

69. National Archives and Records Administration. Record Group 120. General headquarters, American Expeditionary Forces, Citations order no. 8, March 1, 1920. Box 5079. Entry 458.

70. National Archives and Records Administration. Record Group 120. General headquarters, American Expeditionary Forces, Citations order no. 3, June 3, 1919. Box 5079. Entry 458.

71. US War Department. General order no. 3, February 1, 1929. In: *War Department, General Orders and Bulletins 1929*. Washington, DC: Government Printing Office; 1930: 6.

72. Spaulding OL, Wright JW. *The Second Division American Expeditionary Force in France, 1917–1919*. New York, NY: The Hillman Press, Inc; 1937: 310, 315–316.

73. National Archives and Records Administration. Record Group 120. General headquarters, American Expeditionary Forces, Citations order no. 4, June 3, 1919. Box 5079. Entry 458.

74. National Archives and Records Administration. Record Group 120. Lieutenant Colonel RC Turck, Medical Corps, division surgeon, to commanding general, 35th Division; "Reference Citations, November 3, 1918." Memo. In: 35th Division Commendations 1918. Box 3724. Entry 2144.

75. Hume EE. The medical book of merit. *Mil Surg*. 1925;56:259–298.

76. US War Department. General order no. 103, August 16, 1919. In: *War Department, General Orders and Bulletins 1919*. Washington, DC: Government Printing Office; 1920: 3.

77. Ring ME. The life and work of Dr. George Byron Hayes, pioneer maxillofacial surgeon. *J Hist Dent*. 1999;47:106–108.

78. US War Department. General order no. 72, December 6, 1920. In: *War Department, General Orders and Bulletins 1920*. Washington, DC: Government Printing Office; 1921.

79. Love AG. Statistics. In: Lynch C, ed. *Medical and Casualty Statistics*. Vol 15. In: *The Medical Department of the United States Army in the World War*. Washington, DC: Government Printing Office; 1925: 1028.

80. National Archives and Records Administration. Record Group 120. First Lieutenant Clyde R Modie, Dental Corps, acting division dental surgeon, to commanding general, 32nd Division, January 5, 1919. File 210.5, Commendations, Surgeon, 32 Division. Box 3685. Entry 2144.

81. Wythe G. *A History of the 90th Division (1920)*. Whitefish, Mont: Kessinger Publishing; 2005.

82. National Archives and Records Administration. Record Group 120. Casualty card, Lieutenant Joseph Parsons. Box 4. Entry 31.

83. National Archives and Records Administration. Record Group 120. Casualty card, Lieutenant Lester A Stone. Box 5. Entry 31.

84. National Archives and Records Administration. Record Group 120. Major Charles W Lewis, Dental Corps; "History of the Dental Service 26th Division." Medical Dept. 26th Division. Box 3585. Entry 2144.

85. *History of the Seventy-Ninth Division A.E.F. during the World War: 1917–1919*. Lancaster, Pa: Steinman and Steinman; 1919: 186.

86. National Archives and Records Administration. Record Group 120. Casualty card, Private Philip J O'Connell. Box 4. Entry 31.

87. National Archives and Records Administration. Record Group 120. Casualty card, Private Henry E Williams. Box 11. Entry 31.

88. National Archives and Records Administration. Record Group 120. Casualty card, Private Linten W Brush. Box 1. Entry 31.

89. *Annual Report of The Surgeon General, 1919*. Vol 2. Washington, DC: Government Printing Office; 1919.

90. Amerine WH. *Alabama's Own in France*. New York, NY: Eaton & Gettinger; 1919: 341, 413.

91. National Archives and Records Administration. Record Group 120. Captain John M Hughes, Dental Corps; "Gains and Losses of Dental Personnel, 29th Division, American E.F., France (from July 1st 1918 to November 16th 1918)." Memo. In: Returns, Personnel, Dental Surgeon, 29th Division. Box 3645. Entry 2144.

92. National Archives and Records Administration. Record Group 120. Major LB Schrader, division dental surgeon; "History of the Dental Corps of Fifth Division from May 8th to October 25th 1918." In: Folder 6, Medical History of the Dental Corps, Dental Surgeon, 5th Division. Box 3475. Entry 2144.

93. National Archives and Records Administration. Record Group 120. Major LB Schrader, division dental surgeon; "History of the Dental Corps of Fifth Division from October 25th to December 31st 1918, March 27, 1919." In: Folder 6, Medical History of the Dental Corps, Dental Surgeon, 5th Division. Box 3475. Entry 2144.

94. Buxton GE. *Official History of 82nd Division American Expeditionary Forces: "All American" Division, 1917–1919*. Indianapolis, Ind: The Bobbs-Merrill Company; 1919: 148–150.

95. Medical Field Service School. In memoriam: the Medical Department of the United States Army in the World War, Vol 1. *The Army Medical Bulletin*. 1932;27(Suppl):10–26.

96. Lynch C, Weed FW, McAfee L. In memoriam. In: *The Surgeon General's Office*. Vol 1. In: Weed F, ed. *The Medical Department of the United States Army in the World War*. Washington, DC: Government Printing Office; 1923: 587–604.

97. Casualties in the Dental Department, U.S.A. *J Assoc Milit Dent Surg*. 1919;3:104–105.

98. In memoriam. *J Am Dent Assoc*. 1924;11: 952–953.

99. Dental officers who died while on active duty. *J Nat Dent Assoc*. 1919;6:287–288.

100. Ford JH. The dental section. In: *Administration, American Expeditionary Forces*. Vol 2. In: Weed F, ed. *The Medical Department of the United States Army in the World War*. Washington, DC: US Government Printing Office; 1927: 120.

101. National Archives and Records Administration. Record Group 120. Form 57, Consolidated Report of Dental Work at 33rd Division, American E.F., Major RW Pearson, Dental Corps, division dental surgeon, November and December 1918, January, February, March, and April 1919. File, Daily Reports, Dental Work, Dental Surgeon, 33 Division. Box 3705. Entry 2144.

102. National Archives and Records Administration. Record Group 120. Form 57, Consolidated Report of Dental Work at 33rd Division, American E.F., Major John M Evey, Dental Corps, division dental surgeon, April 1919. File, Daily Reports, Dental Work, Dental Surgeon, 33rd Division. Box 3705. Entry 2144.

103. Oliver R. History of the dental service, A.E.F. In: Activities of the Chief Surgeon's Office. In: *Reports of the Commander-in-Chief, Staff Sections and Services*. Vol 15. In: *United States Army in the World War 1917–1919*. Washington, DC: US Army Center of Military History; 1991; 411.

104. National Archives and Records Administration. Record Group 120. Form 57, Dental work at Second Army, American E.F., Lieutenant Colonel GH Casaday, supervising dental surgeon, November and December 1918. In: Second Army Consolidated Dental Reports. Box 3295. Entry 924.

105. National Archives and Records Administration. Record Group 120. Form 57, Dental work at Second Army, American E.F., Lieutenant Colonel Rex H Rhoades, chief dental surgeon, January, February, and March 1919. In: Second Army Consolidated Dental Reports. Box 3295. Entry 924.

106. Hoff NS. Dentistry's contribution to the war. *Dent Reg*. 1918;72:552–553,

107. Hoff NS. What has the war done for dentistry. *Dental Reg*. 1918;72:553–554.

108. King OU. Dentistry's contribution to the war. *J Nat Dent Assoc*. 1919;6:275–277.

Chapter XVI

INTERVENTION AND OCCUPATION: FOREIGN EXCURSIONS IN THE WAKE OF THE WORLD WAR, 1918–1923

Introduction

In the aftermath of World War I, American military forces remained engaged in active operations against Russian Bolshevik forces in northern Russia and Siberia as part of what was known as the "Allied Intervention." At the same time, troops from the American Expeditionary Forces (AEF) in France moved into parts of western Germany to assure compliance with the terms of the November 11, 1918, armistice and any peace treaties that would end the war. Dental surgeons accompanied the troops dispatched to Russia to counter Vladimir Lenin's Red Army and into Germany to guarantee the armistice.

As the war drew to a close and the guns fell silent over the western front, American forces still found themselves in dangerous places. The collapse of the tsar's government in Russia and the seizure of power in 1917 by Vladimir Lenin's Bolsheviks led to the eventual outbreak throughout the former Russian Empire of a vicious civil war between Lenin's Bolsheviks and their "Red" Army and a variety of anti-communist opposing factions that came to be known as the "Whites." The Bolshevik withdrawal from the war in the Treaty of Brest-Litovsk in March 1918 allowed the German high command to concentrate its forces on the western front in the spring of 1918 for what it hoped would be the war-winning offensive. The Allies need to reopen the Russian front became desperate as a result of this German offensive, and President Woodrow Wilson reluctantly yielded to Allied pressure and authorized the use of American troops in expeditions to northwestern Russia and Siberia. In addition, the Allies were concerned about the fate of those forces friendly to the west still in Russia, especially the so-called "Czech Legion" composed of Czech and Slovak former Austro-Hungarian army prisoners of war in Russia, and especially about the possible Bolshevik seizure and use of the huge stocks of war material originally sent to aid the tsarist regime.[1]

Northwestern Russia and Siberia were selected because they contained the only Russian ports to which the Allies had access at all seasons, Murmansk and Archangel in the north and Vladivostok in far eastern Siberia. Distrustful of the Bolsheviks' attempts to spread the communist revolution to a war-weary Europe, the western Allies wanted to secure the vast amounts of stores that had accumulated around their docks. Although Wilson tried to remain neutral over internal Russian affairs, his allies hoped that intervention would contribute to Bolsheviks' eventual collapse.[2,3]

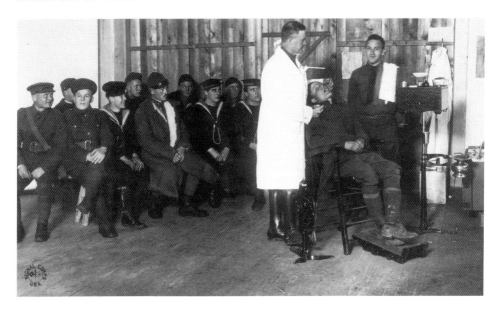

First Lieutenant Will L Jones, Dental Reserve Corps, working on a patient in his dental office
in the Young Men's Christian Association (YMCA) building at Archangel, Russia,
on October 17, 1918, with a room full of Allied soldiers and sailors awaiting dental treatment.
Photograph: Courtesy of US Army Military History Institute. SC 34639.

Although theoretically the two US expeditions were elements of a single scheme, the lack of clear objectives and the vast distance between them made their experiences completely different. Americans in northwestern Russia functioned as a major combat element of a mixed Allied force. Those in Siberia tried to carry out neutral security missions, but more often were caught in violent confrontations between Bolsheviks, anti-Bolshevik White forces, and the Japanese members of the Allied expedition who had their own imperial objectives in eastern Siberia.

North Russia Expedition

The North Russia Expedition, under the command of Colonel George E Stewart, left Newcastle, England, on August 26, 1918. It consisted of elements of the 85th Division—the 339th Infantry Regiment; 1st Battalion, 310th Engineer Regiment; and Detachment, 310th Sanitary Train. The total strength of the expedition was 4,770 officers and soldiers. The medical organizations were the 337th Ambulance Company and 337th Field Hospital, 310th Sanitary Train, and the medical detachments of the 339th Infantry and 1st Battalion, 310th Engineers, for a total strength of 27 officers and 269 soldiers. The troops embarked on three transports and arrived in Archangel on September 5, 1918.[4]

The immediate problem facing the Medical Department was the proper distribution of personnel, including dental, for the 400-mile front that encircled Archangel on three sides, from Pinega on the east, Ust Padenga on the south, and Onega on the west. Pinega was 112 miles from Archangel, Ust Padenga was 234 miles, and Onega was 145 miles, scattered in an area of 15,000 square miles of complete wilderness. Under the circumstances, it was impossible to keep the medical organizations intact. The 27 medical officers and 269 enlisted soldiers were "pooled" and sent in groups of as little as two to as many as 35 to the various fronts. The Medical Department headquarters was established under Major Jonas R Longley, Medical Corps (MC), in the Convalescent Hospital Building on Nabersnaya Street in Archangel. The hospitals, dressing stations, and first aid posts outside of Archangel cared for all the sick and wounded Allied troops, regardless of nationality.[4]

In September 1918 the expedition's four dental officers were assigned as follows: Captain Howard W Geiger, Dental Reserve Corps (DRC),[5,6,7] a 1913 graduate of the University of Michigan, College of Dental Surgery, at Ann Arbor, was with the Railroad Force (Force A), Casualty Clearing Hospital, at Obozerskaya;

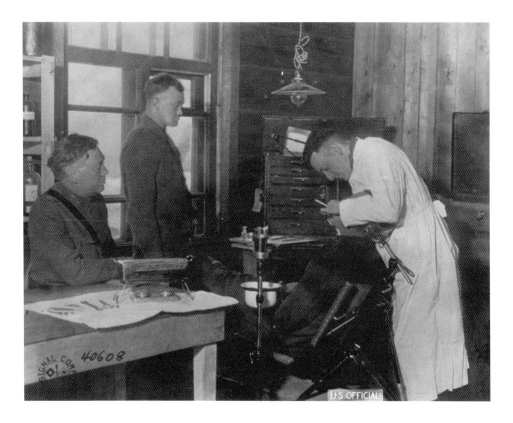

*In the office of the medical detachment of Company B, 310th Engineer Regiment,
from left to right, Lieutenant RW Springer, Medical Corps, and Private Irvin Wingerter,
watch as First Lieutenant Walter E Roe, Dental Reserve Corps, cares for
Corporal John E Craft at Bakharitza, Russia, on November 18, 1918.
Photograph: Courtesy of US Army Military History Institute. SC 40608.*

661

First Lieutenant Walter E Roe, DRC,[5,6,8] with the Medical Detachment, 310th Engineers and 339th Infantry, 337th Field Hospital Casualty Clearing Station (Force C), at Bakharitza; First Lieutenant Nines Simmons, DRC,[5,6,9,10] at the American Red Cross Hospital, Archangel; and First Lieutenant Will L Jones, DRC,[5,6,11] at the dental office, Allied Young Men's Christian Association (YMCA), Archangel.[12,13]

Another dentist was added to the dental staff in October 1918, when Private First Class and surgeon's assistant James H Howell, DDS,[5] was placed on duty (assigned as acting dental surgeon) at Field Hospital No. 337, Detachment A, Force C, Beresniki. In 1914–1915 Howell, a 1913 graduate of the University of Michigan, College of Dental Surgery, Ann Arbor, had been an instructor in physiology at the Detroit College of Medicine and Surgery. On April 20, 1919, Private Howell moved to the 337th's Detachment B, at Ossinova.[14–16]

In April 1919 a new dental officer, First Lieutenant Joseph L Rahm, DDS arrived.[5] Rahm was a 1916 graduate of the Louisville College of Dentistry (Dental Department of the Central University of Kentucky) at Louisville, Kentucky. After the war, he practiced in Shively, Kentucky. He was assigned for duty to Companies No. 167 and No. 168, North Russian Transportation Corps, at Camp Nissen, Murmansk, and on the USS Yankton. In June 1919 he shifted to Soroks, Russia, with the Transportation Corps, treating Russian army and navy, Canadian army (First Depot Battalion), British Supply Mission, and Russian civilian patients.[17]

Captain Geiger's movements from October 1918 to June 1919 indicate the itinerant nature of the dental work in North Russia. In October 1918 he was transferred to the infirmary at Olga Barracks, Archangel. In January 1919 he was reported sick after a hernia operation in the American Red Cross Hospital, Archangel. The next month he was back at work part time in the infirmary, Olga Barracks. In May 1919 he was with the medical detachment, 339th Infantry, Economie. In June 1919 Geiger was on "special duty," by verbal authority of the commanding general, at Economie, Russia.[14–16]

The American forces were engaged in heavy fighting throughout the winter under the most severe Arctic conditions. Supported by a highly efficient Canadian field artillery battery, they became the mainstay of the Allied combat effort. In the United States, President Wilson came under growing pressure after the armistice to withdraw the troops from their increasingly pointless mission. As a result, in February 1919 the secretary of war announced plans to withdraw US forces as soon as ice conditions permitted. A small staff under Brigadier General Wilds P Richardson arrived to supervise the withdrawal and by July 1919, a smooth evacuation was completed. One of the last officers to leave was First Lieutenant Walter E Roe, who was providing care to embassy, consulate, Red Cross, and YMCA personnel.[18,19]

From September 5, 1918, to June 20, 1919, the few dental surgeons with the expedition cared for 4,102 military and 227 other patients. They treated a total of 4,591 cases of dental caries, four oral wounds, and six jaw fractures; extracted 1,514 teeth; and completed 4,806 fillings of all types. Considering the conditions under which they worked, the dental surgeons were most productive.[20]

In his report of June 20, 1919, Lieutenant Colonel Erastus Corning, MC, chief surgeon of the North Russian Expeditionary Force, stated:

In general it is believed that the distribution of personnel and the hospital facilities provided have been fully adequate to meet the needs of the situation. The character of the terrain, the distances to be traversed, the primitive means of transportation and the severe and prolonged winter, made certain difficulties and hardships inherent in the situation, but no complaints were made of failure to provide prompt and adequate medical care or attention, and no cases came under observation where the condition of the patient was attributable to neglect or improper treatment.[21]

Siberia

US forces arrived at Vladivostok, Siberia, somewhat better organized than their north Russia counterparts, but equally unclear as to their mission. On August 6, 1918, War Department orders alerted the 31st and the 27th Infantry Regiments on duty in the Philippines to move to Russia. Their advance parties were on the ground by the 15th, and within days American units were supporting Japanese attacks on Bolshevik strongholds along the railroad north of the port. These actions halted with the arrival in September of Major General William S Graves, the force commander. He understood his mission to be that of a neutral security role. Accordingly, American forces were pulled out of combat and stationed at key sites along the railroad, at coal mines, and at power plants to safeguard them. This meant that the troops were scattered in small groups as far away as Lake Baikal, a month's journey by slow rail.[2,18,22]

Medical support for the force consisted of the two regimental medical detachments, Field Hospital No. 4, Evacuation Hospital No. 17, Ambulance Company No. 4, and a small laboratory. Major (later Colonel) Frederick R Wunderlich, Dental Corps (DC), deployed with the expedition as its sole dentist. Accompanied by his assistant, Private First Class Grover C Mullins, and a portable dental kit, he began work in a dirty portside warehouse on August 21. Hygiene in the building was so bad that he performed only emergency care until he found a better office nearby, which he occupied until October 1918. He was joined by First Lieutenants Vernon L Lane, DRC, and Lynn D Blandford, DRC, on September 2.[23]

The two new dentists arrived with only their portable kits and no stock of expendable materials. The same held for an additional eight dental officers who arrived on September 29. Dental work was hampered by shortages until January 1919, when adequate supplies finally became available. In the meantime, Wunderlich assigned Lane to support the 31st Infantry and Blanchard to support the 27th Infantry. The other dentists scattered to various semi-permanent clinics attached to hospitals in towns along the railroad. One of the new dentists, Major Bruce H Roberts, reported a deplorable situation at his post in Khabarovsk:

There were, on my arrival at this station, three dental surgeons operating in one room, in the military hospital, about eighteen by ten feet in dimension. This same room also served as a waiting room for patients, thus making six men of the dental corps, medical department, and at least two or three patients in the room at one time, such condition not being conducive to efficient reports and cleanliness of the office. There was at the time however two rooms in another building being prepared for occupancy by the dental surgeons which will serve to a much better purpose. . . .There was no water, steam or hot air sterilizer for dental instruments in the dental operating room but one on a stove in the kitchen, sometimes; and when in use necessitated the dental assistants passing thru several doors, going and coming from the dental office. . . . There was one w.e [white enamel] basin for six men to keep their hands in a cleanly condition while about patients and one G.I. bucket for the purpose of carrying water for the same reason for these six men and supply the needs at the chair.[24]

Roberts recommended he remain at Khabarovsk where his rank might help improve the situation, as he could deal better with hospital officials than more junior officers. He eventually succeeded in upgrading conditions.[25,26]

During this time, dental work was mostly routine because the troops were engaged in normal duties with little exposure to combat. No major oral surgery was ever performed. An unusually large number of Vincent's Angina cases occurred during the first 10 months in country, which Wunderlich attributed to poor oral hygiene prior to arrival and the recent recruitment of men "in a deplorable state as far as their teeth and mouths are concerned." Although the Angina cases declined after June 1919, dentists were still overwhelmed because of oral problems of new replacements coming from the United States. This showed the need for complete treatment in the United States, where better facilities, personnel, and supplies were available, before sending a soldier overseas. Wunderlich noted that completing a recruit's dental work in the recruit depot "would save much time and relieve dental surgeons in the field from much of the routine work. A dental surgeon in the field is very busy with emergency cases and his equipment is not such as to permit all the necessary dental work for men who have received no previous attention."[26]

In his final report, Wunderlich also commented that the huge distances and unit dispersion eventually required that all the eight or nine dentists in the command scatter more and work at different offices on their own. This increased the need for more supplies than the approved issue. The inefficiency of transportation also meant a lot more time wasted traveling between posts. Under these conditions, Wunderlich concluded that a ratio of one dentist to 1,000 soldiers "is inadequate" and that a ratio of one to five hundred troops "is essential to provide adequate dental service to troops in the field."

The need for highly competent dental assistants was also made apparent by the Siberian conditions. Wunderlich recommended that assistants be given greater rank and proficiency pay so that more would remain in the service. He also identified nine enlisted dental assistants currently serving in Siberia who were graduate dentists and sought permission to establish an examining board to qualify them for commissions in the DRC. Although additional dentists were badly needed in Siberia, the surgeon general's office denied this request in September 1919.[26,27]

Regarding their dental equipment, Wunderlich reached the same conclusion that Oliver and his colleagues had in France:

The portable dental equipment provided for dental surgeons in the field is far too large and bulky to be readily portable under field conditions. There are frequent occasions where there is no rail transportation and very limited wagon transportation, and for such occasions there should be provided one small chest that should contain the necessary instruments and materials to treat emergency cases in the field.[26]

Another problem was encountered in providing care for Allied forces and prisoners of war. Except for a small Canadian detachment, none of the other Allied contingents had a dental service. US dentists were constantly being pressed by all others for help, unexpectedly consuming time and supplies. In addition, large numbers of German and Austrian prisoners of war had been in the area for as long as 4 years and had received no dental care from the Russians. Under US supervision, German, Austrian, and Hungarian physicians and dentists were identified and assisted with care. Prisoners with special skills worked at the Vladivostok Base Hospital laboratory to produce dental plates for their fellow prisoners. When these prisoners began to be repatriated in late 1919, prisoner-dentists were sufficiently equipped to provide shipboard care.[28,29]

By the autumn of 1919 it was apparent that the presence of the United States was serving little useful purpose and congressional pressure mounted to get the troops out of Siberia. The British and French withdrew their token forces in September and General Graves announced intentions for the United States to follow suit. The first group of soldiers embarked in January 1920, and the last Americans left Vladivostok on April 1, 1920, taking the Medical Department with them. In his final report, Wunderlich reported that in Siberia, his dentists had seen 11,194 patients in a force averaging a little under 8,000 men, had 23,361 sittings, completed 10,903 fillings, and extracted 2,628 teeth. By the time the expedition left Siberia, the War Department and Congress were already engaged in creating a postwar force that reflected America's new global role while continuing to occupy a large slice of western Germany. [3,26]

The Occupation of Germany

The armistice included provisions for an Allied occupation force on the west bank of the Rhine River along with several bridgeheads on the east bank. As a result, US forces were committed to occupation duty in Germany at least until a formal peace treaty was signed, and, as it turned out, for several years beyond that. For the most part, the US zone consisted of a strip of the Rhineland between Luxembourg and the city of Coblenz on the Rhine River. On November 15, 1918, General Pershing activated the Third Army, commanded by Major General Joseph Dickman, to control the occupation forces. The same day, Dickman began directing the movement of his III, IV, and VII Corps eastward into Germany.[30]

The new field army controlled over 240,000 troops during this early phase, and all were accompanied by the requisite medical and dental support. While the III Corps with three divisions moved east of the Rhine, the IV and VII Corps, with five divisions, occupied the Moselle Valley from Coblenz to Luxembourg along the line of communications. By December 15 the Third Army headquarters was in place at Coblenz, a major German administrative center. US forces throughout the zone were well established by Christmas, and the entire command was brought up to full strength with soldiers from units being disbanded in France.[31]

The forces were kept working at levels far beyond peacetime training activities due to both political turmoil and the possible need to use military force should peace negotiations break down. Personnel turbulence aggravated their efforts.

665

Gains and losses of units began as soon as the Third Army entered Germany, and once peace was agreed to at Versailles, France, in June 1919, losses became torrential. The surge of units homeward required the Third Army to work closely with the US Liquidation Commission to dispose of the massive amounts of material left behind, much of it being transferred to wartime allies.[32]

After the signing of the Versailles Treaty that ended World War I in June 1919, there was little chance for hostilities to be renewed. On July 2 the Third Army was inactivated, and its remaining personnel and equipment were transferred to the newly created American Forces in Germany (AFG) headquarters, which remained at Coblenz. Major General Henry T Allen, the commander of the 90th Division on the western front, became AFG commander, serving until the AFG itself was inactivated in January 1923. He supervised US military activities in that capacity everywhere in Europe except Russia.[33]

Shortage of Dentists Continues

The shortage of dental officers during the Third Army's brief existence compelled some commanders to employ civilian dentists to treat their personnel. In April 1919 Captain OJ Pederson, MC, surgeon, American Military Supply Depot, Base Section No. 9, Rotterdam, Holland, notified the base surgeon that he had been forced to "temporarily engage" the services of a civilian dentist to come to the infirmary to treat the "most urgent cases." He had requested a military dental surgeon three times without success.[34]

The next month, Pederson again complained, this time to the commanding officer of Base Section No. 9, on the "need of dental surgeons." He stated that the expected dental surgeon had not appeared and "a longer delay only causes so much more unnecessary suffering for the needy cases." A few of the patients had to go to a civilian dentist "at their own expense" because they needed immediate attention.[35] Captain Donald K Billings endorsed Pederson's memo, stating, "continual requests come to this office for dental treatment which we cannot furnish here. Condition of teeth of some men is such that an unfavorable report would be sure to follow an inspection by an Inspector General."[36] Captain Samuel D Clayton, MC, port surgeon, Base Section No. 9, agreed that a dental surgeon was indeed urgently needed because the soldiers had been going to local dentists and paying for work themselves. He estimated that half of the troops needed dental treatment.[37] On May 19, 1919, Captain Marcus F Wielage, DRC, was assigned to Rotterdam.[38] When he was reassigned for return to the United States in July 1919, Captain Pederson requested advice as to the "disposition of future dental cases occurring in this command." He was ordered to send them to Camp Hospital No. 122 in Germany.[39]

On March 6, 1919, Captain William S Mitchell, commanding the Field Remount Squadron No. 306, had the misfortune of being kicked in the face by a horse. He stated that his "left front upper tooth, and the two teeth back of it were broken off, and the jaw partly broken." The dental officer of the IV Corps Artillery Park at Mayence, who treated Mitchell, did not have the laboratory equipment for constructing the necessary bridgework. Mitchell successfully requested that he be sent to a Coblenz clinic where the prosthesis could be made.[40]

US Military Mission Berlin, 1919

A few weeks after the signing of the armistice in November 1918, the Interallied Commission on the Repatriation of Prisoners of War was established as a branch of the Permanent International Armistice Commission. At first it was composed of American, British, and French Missions, but later other nations were added. The commission's duty was the care and return to their homes of the Allied prisoners of War. As this work with Allied prisoners neared completion, a subsidiary commission, the Interallied Commission on the Repatriation of Russian Prisoners of War, was formed, the American section of which was named the "United States Military Mission." Its scope included Balkan prisoners of war—Romanians, Serbians, and Greeks.[41]

Because of the high proportion of medical and sanitary issues, it became evident quite early that the US Army Medical Department could play a valuable role in conveying trains of prisoners for repatriation. Twenty US detachments from the AEF, each composed of line officers, a medical officer, and enlisted personnel, were assigned to the repatriation of the Russian prisoner of war camps. The units began to arrive in the unoccupied area from February 15–22, 1919. Captain TAL Parsons, MC, was appointed the staff surgeon for the US Military Mission. His area of interest included approximately 30 prison camps containing from 300,000 to 700,000 Russian prisoners. Some prisoners were working in adjacent farms or factories. The sanitary conditions were horrible, despite the fact that the Interallied Commission employed 32 Russian doctors and 15 Russian nurses in the camps. As soon as the infectious disease problem was evaluated, additional medical officers, tuberculosis and eye specialists, and dental officers were requisitioned. Upon their arrival in Berlin on March 19, 1919, the US medical personnel were deployed to the various camps.[41]

Major Gerald G Burns served as the dental chief with offices in Berlin. He commanded 18 dental officers, who were charged with taking care of the dental needs of the US detachment's troops and with alleviating the dental problems of the Russian prisoners. Weekly dental work reports were required (Table 16-1).[41]

Under the terms of the armistice, the American Red Cross Commission in Germany participated in the return of the Russian prisoners. It sent 60 soldiers to Berlin on February 17, 1919. They furnished "medical and surgical relief, hospital equipment and diet foods and clothing" for the Russian prisoners. Their most important contribution was food and medicine from depots at Mainz and Coblenz.[41]

The dental work accomplished by the Dental Corps in Russian prisoner-of-war camps included: examination of 15,079 prisoners to ascertain if treatment was required; 5,160 diagnoses; 1,987 fillings; 85 cases of crown and bridge work; and 3,025 other operations (1,644 teeth extracted). All work was completed in 3,436 sittings.[41]

On May 20, 1919, six US medical and dental officers went to Marienburg, West Prussia, to oversee the transports convoying Russian prisoners into Russia. The prisoners were taken through the German lines to a point near the Bolshevik front, detrained, and given sufficient food for a few days. The medical and dental officers were under orders to "properly care" for the prisoners en route and see that the food was correctly distributed.[41]

TABLE 16-1

DENTAL ASSIGNMENTS IN THE MAIN CAMPS UNDER AMERICAN
CONTROL*

Dentist	Location
Captain William J Barto	Altdamm
First Lieutenant LeRoy P Hartley	Bautzen
First Lieutenant Ewing B Connell	Cassel
First Lieutenant Earle D Beacham	Cottbus
Captain Hubert F Christiansen	Frankfurt ad Oder
First Lieutenant Waldo J Adams	Gardelegen
Captain Raymond Mulcahy	Gustrow
Captain Charles B Seeley	Lamsdorf
First Lieutenant Joseph I Hartwig	Chemnitz
Captain Frank P Gormley	Heilsburg
First Lieutenant John L Burnside	Langensalza
Captain John W Kistler	Merseburg
First Lieutenant Winifried P McDaniels	PR-Holland
First Lieutenant Kenneth R Lindsay	Sagan
Captain Orin W Wallace	Stargard
First Lieutenant Herbert Muench	Quedlinburg
First Lieutenant Herman G Ebling	Ruhleben
First Lieutenant Verna R Dush	Zerbst

*Other camps were under British and Italian control.
Data source: National Archives and Records Administration. Record Group 120. History medical department, United States Military Mission, Berlin, Germany, office of the staff surgeon, US Military Mission, 10 August 1919. Box 3376. Entry 1614.

Polish Typhus Relief Expedition, 1919

A few months later, in August 1919, the Polish Typhus Relief Expedition, composed of about 25 officers and 500 enlisted troops, was ordered to Poland to organize and conduct a campaign against typhus fever. A direct appeal had been made to President Wilson at the peace conference by representatives of the Polish government, who asked for aid in fighting the typhus epidemic raging in Poland. He agreed to sell Poland approximately $3 million worth of medical supplies and send in military personnel to set up the distribution and provide instruction on how to use the supplies. The soldiers came chiefly from the divisions on their way home through Brest. A total of 1,600 railroad cars were necessary to ship the supplies. In October 1919 the expedition was placed under the control of the American commander in Germany and its strength was reduced to 15 officers and 60 enlisted troops.[42,43] Among the expedition's medical detachment (stationed in Warsaw) of five officers was one dental officer, Captain (later Colonel) Samuel J Rohde, DC.[44]

The country was in pitiful shape. Divided among Germany, Russia, and Austria-Hungary since the late 18th century, the new Poland that emerged in 1919 from the demise of those three empires had been ravaged by the fighting since 1914 and then by German military occupation since 1916. On top of that, over 2,400,000 Russian refugees from the civil war raging in Russia began streaming in from the east, bringing least 25,000 cases of typhus with them. The transmission agent was the louse, and bathing and delousing were unheard of among the refugees, causing the Polish government to mandate both before entry into the country. A chain of quarantine stations was set up with bathing and delousing plants and epidemic hospitals were established. The Americans set up an automobile repair shop at Warsaw and "flying columns" were sent to selected districts to bathe and delouse the occupants, clean up their housing, and instruct them in the rudiments of sanitation.[43]

In November 1919 Rohde reported he was responsible for the care of 200 officers and soldiers and explained a lack of productivity by noting, "with a temperature of zero and below, fuel is extremely difficult to procure, apparently. Have had fire in neither office nor quarters today, because I could get no coal or wood, and do not know when I shall get the next issue of fuel."[45]

Rohde served with the organization for approximately 10 months with only a portable dental outfit. Besides Army personnel, he also served members of the various American relief organizations, such as the Red Cross, YMCA, Young Women's Christian Association (YWCA), American Relief Administration (ARA) under future President Herbert H Hoover (also known as the Hoover Mission), the legation and consulate, and members of Allied Missions in Poland. Americans returning home after discharge from the Polish army were given dental treatment while in the quarantine camp at Grupa, Poland. They were examined, cases of gingivitis were treated, retained roots were extracted, and other emergency work was done. Because this work was too much for one dental officer to accomplish, Rohde trained three "intelligent" enlisted soldiers to help him. Also, because of the nature of the expedition, its diverse scope, and the large amount of territory covered, the dental surgeon, along with the other officers in the organization, had to assist in other duties. These included examining the quarantined men at the time of delousing, running the refugee trains at the time of the Bolshevik advance, and performing unit duties such as acting adjutant and summary court.[46]

Rohde was transferred to duty at Danzig Free City in July 1920 and then returned to the AFG on August 28, 1920, ending direct dental support in Poland.[47] Although the expedition's activities were first scheduled to cease on June 30, 1920, the War Department extended them to November 1, 1920.[42]

American Forces in Germany

When the AFG was first formed, the original instructions given to the Medical Department were to plan for a force of approximately 6,500 troops, but it soon became evident that this force would be considerably larger for some time. As the Third Army shrank in size and released its final divisions, the various evacuation hospitals and other medical field units operating with the Army also closed until the Coblenz Base Hospital, one field hospital, one evacuation ambulance company, and one hospital train alone remained.[42]

Three of the six remaining dental officers not in tactical units, along with their dental assistants, were concentrated at the attending dental surgeon's office in Coblenz. The office had full "base equipment" and a laboratory. This arrangement ensured an efficient distribution of patients and that difficult cases would be handled competently. Other dentists with field equipment worked out of the Coblenz Base Hospital, while a few could be found in units authorized dental surgeons. At first, a great deal of the dentists' time was consumed treating patients not entitled to care. Finally, the AFG surgeon decided to limit dental treatment to people authorized by Army Regulations and to perform only emergency work for all others.[42,48]

Dental Equipment

After the armistice, there was a shortage of dental equipment throughout the AFG. Permanent dental base equipment had been included in the US Army stores turned over to the French by the liquidation committee. Some pieces of dental equipment, like base chairs, fountain cuspidors, and steel cabinets, were left by the Third Army to furnish the base hospital and the attending dental surgeon's office at Coblenz. Some equipment was returned to the United States by the Advance Medical Supply Depot at Trier, Germany, when it closed. Additional base dental equipment had been requisitioned in August 1919, but because of a misunderstanding, this requisition was not forwarded. Finally in October 1920, new equipment arrived to provide all the dental officers in the AFG's four combat battalions with base dental chairs, fountain cuspidors, electric engines, electric switchboards with hot air syringes, and electric spray bottle heaters. One of the five dentists with a special brigade destined for Silesia had a base equipment chair, engine, and cabinet. Base equipment was not requested for the other dental officers attached to that organization because it was scheduled for field duty during a plebiscite to be held there. However, the Silesia brigade never deployed and its elements were integrated into the AFG.[46]

Dental Clinic, Base Hospital, Coblenz

The dental clinic at the Base Hospital, Coblenz, occupied two large, well-ventilated rooms with north light, hot and cold water, and two fountain cuspidors in the dispensary building. Although portable equipment was used first, by November 1919, the clinic was entirely equipped with two base outfits. In addition to the dental clinic, a dental ward was maintained until March 1, 1920, at which time it was deemed advisable to place dental cases in various other hospital wards. Vincent's Angina cases were moved to the ear, nose, and throat department; jaw fractures were placed under the orthopedic service; and others were reassigned according to the nature of the case. The overwhelming majority (especially from September through December 1919) of all the dental cases were Vincent's Angina, which was treated with a 5% solution of chromic acid twice a day. The jaw fractures were all of the mandible and were treated with intermaxillary wiring. Interestingly, one of the hospital rules given to syphilitic patients was "always keep clean by frequent bathing; keep teeth clean."[49]

In January 1921 Lieutenant Colonel Hugh O Scott, the AFG attending dental surgeon, recommended that all gold work be constructed in the central dental laboratory under his direction. This created uniformity in the work, eliminated the requisition of much lab equipment, and reduced paper work.[46]

An inspection by the medical officer of Provisional Guard Company No. 11 at Sinzig, Germany, in November 1919 revealed that 75% of the soldiers needed dental attention. The company commander was concerned about the "impracticability" of having the troops go to Coblenz for treatment without seriously affecting the "strength and duty" of his organization and creating an "undue shortage of personnel." He was also concerned about the "irregularity of transportation," which caused a longer absence from duty. Putting a dentist on duty until the backlog of dental care was completed would solve these problems.[50] As a result, Captain CR Hays, DC, and his dental assistant were assigned to Captain Porterfield's company.[51] The previous month, a dental survey of the 1st Field Battalion, Signal Corps, showed that 553 enlisted soldiers out of the total command of 1,039 needed dental treatment.[52]

Dental Appointments

Broken appointments became a significant problem for the Dental Corps in occupied Germany. In August 1919 Major Oscar G Skelton, attending dental surgeon, proposed that a "form letter" be sent to the commanding officer of all those who missed their appointments. Basically, the letter stated that the individual (name, rank) belonging to his organization had missed his appointment at a specified time and date. The commander was notified so that he could take "such action as you may deem necessary, also to obviate any complaint of nonreceipt of Dental treatment that may arise."[53] Colonel Earl H Bruns, chief surgeon, concurred and ordered that 300 forms be printed.[54]

The problems with broken appointments persisted for Major Skelton in 1920. On April 7, 1920, he sent a memo to the chief surgeon concerning the "loss of time as a result of Dental appointments being broken." More cooperation was needed from the organizational commanders to notify the dental surgeon in advance if an enlisted soldier could not keep his appointment. In this manner, the dental surgeon could devote his time to another patient. He urged patients to use the telephone to make appointments to save the duty time it took to make the appointment in person. If pain was a problem, emergency treatment would commence immediately in order to avoid incapacitation from duty. Officers and their families were also asked to give advance notice if they were unable to keep their appointments. Precious metals for gold work were kept on hand, but were not furnished "free of cost by the Government." The dental surgeons had to buy it at their personal expense and could only charge the cost of materials used.[55]

Furthermore, Skelton noted that at its present strength, the AFG Dental Corps could not replace any teeth missing prior to entrance into the service. However, in cases of "disfigurement or a lack of masticating surface," bridge and plate work could be provided. Unfortunately, there was only the one dental laboratory at Coblenz for the occupation force, and its capacity was limited.[55]

671

Complaints against German Dentists, 1920–1921

Meanwhile, Skelton reported that the work of the German dentists on US troops was "repeatedly found to be faulty." According to Skelton, they had no conception of dentistry, "except from a certain mechanical standpoint." Their mechanical work was fair, but they had no knowledge of the "tooth upon which the work rests." Infected teeth were frequently crowned, teeth with pulps exposed by caries were filled, and the great majority of the teeth crowned could have been filled. Major Skelton recommended "such patronage should be discouraged."[55]

Acting on Skelton's recommendation, Colonel Earl H Bruns, the chief surgeon, requested that this information be published in bulletin form.[56] Consequently, on April 12, 1920, General Allen's headquarters, AFG, issued Order No. 43, detailing the information on the German dentists and the rules for keeping dental appointments.[57]

Three days later, April 15, 1920, Skelton found out that Private Erwin Hardt, Supply Detachment, 6th Field Artillery, had paid a German dentist 3,000 marks for dental treatment. Skelton felt that the price was "excessive" and that the dentist's office should be placed "Off Limits" to the American troops and "prosecuted for overcharging."[58]

The chief surgeon's official report for the year 1919–1920 stated that "great damage" had been done to the mouths of the American soldiers by the German dentists, thus necessitating "additional work" by Army dental surgeons. The German dentists did not know the "first principles of first class dentistry." They routinely used arsenic preparations for pain relief, which they did not remove before placing crowns. They failed to seal root canals and crowned good teeth with poorly fitted gold crowns. They paid no attention to the occlusion or carrying the crown margins subgingivally when constructing crowns. For this inferior work, they charged "exorbitant" prices.[59]

By 1921 the complaints against German dentists for overcharging had increased. On February 9, 1921, a Coblenz dentist was reported for inserting a defective bridge that had violated the pulp of a live abutment tooth. Actually, the restored space (missing the lower first molar with the space closed) was so small (half the width of the tooth) that an "ethical dentist" would have recommended no restoration at all. In his report to the chief surgeon on February 9, 1921, Lieutenant Colonel Hugh O Scott, attending dental surgeon, stated:

> Cases of this kind, where crowns and bridges are poorly constructed and ill fitting have been the cause of much extra work for the Army Dental Surgeons and have been in my estimation, the primary cause of so much trench mouth or Vincent's angina, and the reason why cases do not yield readily to treatment, the microorganism being harbored under the ragged edges of crowns and lacerated gums.[60]

On February 9, 1921, Colonel Frank R Keefer, chief surgeon, remarked: "German dentists are very inferior to the Americans, in education, workmanship and ethical conduct. Some of them are making large sums out of our soldiers." He asked the AFG adjutant whether "under our own regulations or the German law, the soldier has a legal case against the dentist for malpractice."[61]

When the malpractice matter finally reached the judge advocate, Lieutenant Colonel Kyle Rucker, on February 11, 1921, he ruled:

The Commanding General has authority to place this dentist, as well as every other dentist in the city of Coblenz "off limits" to the personnel of these Forces. In this connection, attention is called to Paragraph 5, Orders #43, 12 April 1920, in which the Service was warned with reference to the character of work performed by German dentists and the patronage of same was officially discouraged. It is deemed that this sets forth the policy of the Commanding General with reference to this subject; that he did not care to place a business of this character off limits but advised the personnel not to patronize same. If, in the face of this advice the soldiers patronize these places, they do so at their own risk.

In this connection, attention is called to the attached advertisements which were taken from the *Amaroc* [the command newspaper] of February 11th, in which these dentists are openly seeking the patronage of these Forces. It is believed that advertisements of this kind should not be permitted in a Service paper if these Headquarters have advised their personnel against the patronage of these places.[62]

Furthermore, he stated:

While under the orders of the Rhineland Commission which have been published by the Commanding General, the members of these Forces can enter civil suit in the German courts, it is not believed that the Commanding General desires to encourage litigation by or against members of these Forces. For this reason a suit for malpractice is not believed desirable.[62]

A handwritten note attached to the bottom of this ruling initialed "H.T.A." (Major General Henry T Allen) states: "I am not sure that this matter should be recognized officially. If our soldiers insist in paying German dentists whilst they might be treated by our own, that is their affair." It seems General Allen may have been concerned about litigation against his own troops occupying Germany.[63]

Again, on February 14, 1921, notwithstanding the judge advocate's ruling, Lieutenant Colonel Scott called the civilian dental work "pure robbery." He noted that German dentists advertised daily in the *Amaroc News*, "Come in and let me examine your teeth free of charge" as a method of "roping in the American Soldier." Scott suggested that if the money was not returned, a malpractice suit could be instigated under German law. He also requested that some dental offices in Coblenz be put "Off Limits" to American soldiers and that those offices not be permitted to advertise in the *Amaroc News*.[64]

Because of the inferior work of the German dentists, the American commanding general's policy was to extend the courtesy of dental service to the Interallied Rhineland Commission (English, French, Belgian), welfare workers (YMCA, YWCA, Salvation Army), Allied soldiers in the area, and civilian government employees. In 1920 this amounted to 1,239 patients treated and 3,499 sittings.[46]

During 1920 the average number of dental officers on duty with the AFG was 18.67. During this period, the injuries treated and operations performed totaled 65,675. The total number of persons treated was 13,280, representing 33,262 sittings. The courtesy of the dental service continued to be extended to Allies and associated civilian agencies. A total of 3.499 sittings were given to these others.[59]

The large reduction in dental personnel in 1921 made it impossible to provide "adequate dental service" to troops distributed in so many towns in the occupied area of Germany. The further reduction of force size and troop concentration closer to Coblenz finally eased the problem. Five dental surgeons were assigned to the attending dental surgeon's office in Coblenz, one was to the base hospital in Coblenz, and two itinerant served Andernach, Mayence, Engers, and Antwerp.[65]

In his annual report, Lieutenant Colonel Scott discussed the Army's inability to retain in the service of "well trained enlisted assistants." He recommended that surplus enlisted personnel be assigned to a school for training dental assistants and that "permanent ratings according to ability" be established as an inducement to "efficient men" to reenlist.[65] He also recommended that precious metals (gold) be authorized for officers and "certain" enlisted soldiers where indicated. Doing so would "improve the physical condition of patients treated, eliminate 'cheap gold work' as done by 'Advertising Dentists,' of itself a detriment to patient's health, in most cases, and resultant unnecessary work." It would also raise the "morale" of the dental officers as well the line's opinion of the dental profession.[65]

On December 31, 1921, the strength of the AFG was 7,805 soldiers, and by the end of 1922, this shrank to a total of 1,192.[66] At the start of 1922, the AFG Medical Department consisted of only eight dental officers, 48 medical officers, three veterinary officers, three medical administrative officers, two warrant officers, 42 nurses, and 689 enlisted soldiers. By June 19, 1922, after a progressive reduction, there remained only one dental officer, six medical officers, one veterinary officer, two nurses, and 33 enlisted soldiers. On November 30, 1922, the last remaining dental surgeon left for the United States to be discharged. A German dentist was employed for the treatment of the command's emergency cases until the last American left in January 1923.[67]

Back in the United States

While American soldiers and their dental surgeons were involved in the Allied interventions in Russia and in the occupation of the Rhineland, the Army Medical Department and the leadership of the Dental Corps were working to shape a postwar Dental Corps to satisfy the demands of a vastly different peacetime US Army. This was not to be an easy task.

References

1. Bradley J. *Allied Intervention in Russia.* New York, NY: Basic Books; 1968: 31–36.

2. Manning CA. *The Siberian Fiasco.* New York, NY: Library Publishers; 1952: 109.

3. White JA. *The Siberian Intervention.* Princeton, NJ: Princeton University Press, 1950: 259–260.

4. National Archives and Records Administration. Record Group 120. Lieutenant Colonel Erastus Corning, MC, chief surgeon, American Expeditionary Forces, North Russia, to commanding general, AEF, North Russia, "Report of medical service, American E.F., North Russia," 20 June 1919. Report. Box 3250. Entry 1551.

5. Polk RL. *Polk's Dental Register and Directory of the United States and Dominion of Canada.* 14th ed. Detroit, Mich: RL Polk & Co; 1928: 357.

6. National Archives and Records Administration. Record Group 120. Chief surgeon, American Expeditionary Forces, North Russia, to base section surgeon, Base Section No. 3, Services of Supply, AEF, "Monthly distribution reports of medical officers, surgeon, archangel, American North Russian Expeditionary Forces [31 October 1918–31 May 1919]." Report. Box 3250. Entry 1551.

7. National Archives and Records Administration. Record Group 120. Lieutenant Colonel Erastus Corning, MC, chief surgeon, American Expeditionary Forces, North Russia, to adjutant, AEF, North Russia, 3 June 1919. Memo. File no. 210. Box 3251. Entry 1550.

8. National Archives and Records Administration. Record Group 120. Special orders no. 14. Major Jonas R Longley, MC, chief surgeon, American North Russian Expeditionary Forces , Archangel, Russia, 16 October 1918. Box 3251. Entry 1550.

9. National Archives and Records Administration. Record Group 120. Special orders no. 25, Major Jonas R Longley, MC, chief surgeon, American North Russian Expeditionary Forces, Archangel, Russia, 11 February 1919. Box 3251. Entry 1550.

10. National Archives and Records Administration. Record Group 120. Major John C Hall, MC, Medical Detachment, 339th Infantry Regiment, to commanding officer, 339th Infantry Detachment, Economie, Russia, 3 June 1919. Memo. File no. 200. Box 3251. Entry 1550.

11. National Archives and Records Administration. Record Group 120. "Nominal list of personnel, Medical Detachment, 339th Infantry," Lieutenant Colonel Erastus Corning, chief surgeon, headquarters, American Expeditionary Forces, North Russia, 31 May 1919. File no. 200. Box 3251. Entry 1550.

12. National Archives and Records Administration. Record Group 120. Major Jonas R Longley, MC, chief surgeon, American Expeditionary Forces, North Russia, to base section surgeon, Base Section No. 3, Services of Supply, AEF, "Distribution of medical officers' personnel Sept. 30, 1918," 30 September 1918. Report. Box 3250. Entry 1551.

13.   National Archives and Records Administration. Record Group 120. Captain Howard W Geiger, DRC, dental surgeon, American North Russian Expeditionary Forces, "Weekly dental report," 24 September 1918. Report. Box 3250. Entry 1551.

14.   National Archives and Records Administration. Record Group 120. Captain Howard W Geiger, DRC, dental surgeon, American North Russian Expeditionary Forces, "Weekly dental report," 5 October 1918. Report. Box 3250. Entry 1551.

15.   National Archives and Records Administration. Record Group 120. Private James H Howell, dental surgeon, to Major JR Longley, American North Russian Expeditionary Forces, "Dental report for month ending October 24, 1918," 24 October 1918. Report. Box 3250. Entry 1551.

16.   National Archives and Records Administration. Record Group 120. Private James H Howell, dental surgeon, 337th Field Hospital, "Report of dental work for month of April 1919." Report. Box 3250. Entry 1551.

17.   National Archives and Records Administration. First Lieutenant Joseph L Rahm, "Report of dental work at Camp Nissen, Murmansk, Russia, month of April (from the 10 to 30th) 1919," and "Report of dental work at Soroka, Russia, North Russian Transportation Corps, month of June 1919." Reports. Box 3250. Entry 1551.

18.   Silverlight J. *The Victor's Dilemma: Allied Intervention in the Russian Civil War, 1917–1920*. New York, NY: Weybright and Talley; 1970: 186-87.

19.   National Archives and Records Administration. Record Group 120. Lieutenant Colonel Erastus Corning, MC, chief surgeon, American Expeditionary Forces, North Russia, to commanding general, AEF, North Russia, Archangel, 2 June 1919. Memo. File no. 210. Box 3251. Entry 1550.

20.   National Archives and Records Administration. Record Group 120. Appendix D, "Statistical summary of dental work." In: Lieutenant Colonel Erastus Corning, MC, chief surgeon, to commanding general, American Expeditionary Forces, North Russia, 20 June 1919, File "Organizational records, medical department, North Russia Expeditionary Forces, Surgeon Archangel." Report. Box 3250. Entry 1551.

21.   National Archives and Records Administration. Record Group 120. Lieutenant Colonel Erastus Corning, MC, chief surgeon, to commanding general, American Expeditionary Forces, North Russia, 20 June 1919, File "Organizational records, medical department, North Russia Expeditionary Forces, Surgeon Archangel." Report. Box 3250. Entry 1551.

22.   National Archives and Records Administration. Record Group 395. American Expeditionary Forces Siberia surgeon general's report, April 20, 1919. Entry 5997.

23.   National Archives and Records Administration. Record Group 395. Report, location of medical officers in the American Expeditionary Forces Siberia. Box 3233. Entry 6012.

24. National Archives and Records Administration. Record Group 395. Exhibit A, Kharbarosk, Siberia. In: Report, Major BH Roberts, DC, to chief surgeon, enclosure to report, Major FR Wunderlich, DC, to surgeon general, American Expeditionary Forces, Siberia, 4 December 1918, File 703: "Dental surgeon, Vladivostok, AEF Siberia." Box 3235. Entry 6012.

25. National Archives and Records Administration. Record Group 395. Major FR Wunderlich, DC, to chief surgeon, American Expeditionary Forces Siberia (report), and Colonel James S Wilson, MC, chief surgeon (first endorsement), both 4 December 1918. Report Box 3235, Entry 6012.

26. National Archives and Records Administration. Record Group 395. Major FR Wunderlich, Dental history of American Expeditionary Forces, Siberia from August 15, 1918 to December 31, 1919. Box 3230. Entry 6018.

27. National Archives and Records Administration. Record Group 395. Major FR Wunderlich to chief surgeon, "Examinations for Dental Reserve Corps," 30 June 1919, and endorsements, file no. 221: "Dental assistants, Surgeon Vladivostok, AEF in Siberia." Box 3234. Entry 6012.

28. National Archives and Records Administration. Record Group 395. Lieutenant Colonel Toparkoff, assitant quartermaster general, Priamur Military District, to staff of American troops, 20 November 1919; and Lieutenant Colonel TW King, adjutant general reply, 22 November 1918. Letters. Box 76. Entry 5997.

29. Wunderlich FR. A glimpse of Siberia. *Milit Dent J.* 1921:4:81–82.

30. Nelson KL. *Victors Divided: America and the Allies in Germany, 1918–1923.* Berkeley, Calif: University of California Press; 1975: 26–27, 29.

31. Fraenkel E. *Military Occupation and the Rule of Law: Occupational Government in the Rhineland, 1918–1923.* New York, NY: Oxford University Press; 1944: 7.

32. National Archives and Records Administration. Record Group 120. Third Army, G-2 Report. Historical file 193-11.4. Entry 931.

33. Allen HT. *My Rhineland Journal.* Boston, Mass: Houghton Mifflin Co; 1923: 6–7.

34. National Archives and Records Administration. Record Group 120. Captain OJ Pederson, surgeon, American Military Supply Depot, Base Section No. 9, Rotterdam, Holland, to base surgeon, Base Section No. 9, Antwerp-Rotterdam, 2 April 1919. Memo. File no. 703. Box 2987. Entry 1400.

35. National Archives and Records Administration. Record Group 120. Captain OJ Pederson, surgeon, American Military Supply Depot, Base Section No. 9, Rotterdam, Holland, to base commander, Base Section No. 9, Antwerp-Rotterdam, 3 May 1919. Memo. File no. 703. Box 2987. Entry 1400.

36. National Archives and Records Administration. Record Group 120. Captain Donald K Billings, Base Section No. 9, Antwerp-Rotterdam Base, Rotterdam, 4 May 1919. Endorsement. File no. 703. Box 2987. Entry 1400.

37. National Archives and Records Administration. Record Group 120. Captain Samuel D Clayton, MC, port surgeon, Base Section No. 9, Rotterdam, Holland, 13 May 1919. Endorsement. File no. 703. Box 2987. Entry 1400.

38. National Archives and Records Administration. Record Group 120. Colonel James L Bevans, MC, office of the base surgeon, Base Section No. 9, Antwerp, Belgium, 16 May 1919. File no. 703. Box 2987. Entry 1400.

39. National Archives and Records Administration. Record Group 120. Captain OJ Pederson, MC, surgeon, Headquarters Detachment, Base Section No. 9, Rotterdam, Holland, to base surgeon, Base Section No. 9, Antwerp, Belgium, 3 July 1919. Memo. File no. 703. Box 2987. Entry 1400.

40. National Archives and Records Administration. Record Group 120. Captain William S Mitchell, Field Remount Squadron no. 306, to chief surgeon, American Expeditionary Forces, 1 April 1919. Memo. File no. 211.19. Box 60. Entry 1074.

41. National Archives and Records Administration. Record Group 120. History medical department, United States Military Mission, Berlin, Germany, office of the staff surgeon, US Military Mission, 10 August 1919. Box 3376. Entry 1614.

42. National Archives and Records Administration. Record Group 120. Major Thomas J Flynn (for Colonel Frank R Keefer, chief surgeon), American Forces in Germany, to G-2, History 1921–1923, surgeon, Coblenz, American Forces in Germany, 2 March 1922. Box 3302. Entry 1484.

43. Rohde SJ. Experiences with the American Polish Relief Expedition. *Milit Dent Surg.* 1921;4:24–25.

44. National Archives and Records Administration. Record Group 120. Major Francis M Pitts, adjutant, headquarters, American Polish Relief Expedition, US Army, to American Legation, Warsaw, Poland, "Personnel," 31 October 1919. Memo. File no. 210. Box 3. Entry 1524.

45. National Archives and Records Administration. Record Group 120. Captain SJ Rohde, American Polish Relief Expedition, to chief dental surgeon, American Forces in Germany, 19 November 1919. Memo. File no. 703. Box 3318. Entry 1482.

46. National Archives and Records Administration. Record Group 120. Lieutenant Colonel Hugh O Scott, attending dental surgeon, American Forces in Germany, to surgeon general (through surgeon, American Forces in Germany); "Report and History of Dental Service A.F. in G. 1920, 8 January 1921." Report. Box 3302. Entry 1484.

47. National Archives and Records Administration. Record Group 120. Return of medical officers, etc, serving in the American Polish Relief Expedition United States Army during the month of August 1920. Box 3258. Entry 1484.

48. National Archives and Records Administration. Record Group 120. Colonel Frank R Keefer, chief surgeon, American Forces in Germany, to surgeon general, US Army, Washington, DC; "Report of Activities of the Medical Department, AFG, for the Calendar Year, 1921, 31 January 1921." Report. Box 3302. Entry 1484.

49. National Archives and Records Administration. Record Group 120. History of the base hospital, American Forces in Germany from August 20th, 1919 to June 1st, 1920. Box 3324. Entry 1498.

50. National Archives and Records Administration. Record Group 120. Captain Charles Porterfield, Jr, commander, Provisional Guard Company No. 11, to chief surgeon, American Forces in Germany, 19 November 1919. Memo. File no. 703. Box 3318. Entry 1482.

51. National Archives and Records Administration. Record Group 120. Colonel Earl H Bruns, chief surgeon, American Forces in Germany, 21 November 1919. Endorsement. File no. 703. Box 3318. Entry 1482.

52. National Archives and Records Administration. Record Group 120. Captain George W Snyder, MC, surgeon, 1st Field Battalion, Signal Corps, Coblenz, Germany, to Colonel Frank R Keefer, chief surgeon, American Forces in Germany, 15 October 1920. Memo. File no. 703. Box 3318. Entry 1482.

53. National Archives and Records Administration. Record Group 120. Major Oscar G Skelton, attending dental surgeon, American Forces in Germany, APO 927, to colonel Earl H Bruns, chief surgeon, 29 August 1919. Memo. File no. 703. Box 3318. Entry 1482.

54. National Archives and Records Administration. Record Group 120. Colonel Earl H Bruns, chief surgeon, American Forces in Germany, 1 September 1919. Endorsement. File no. 703. Box 3318. Entry 1482.

55. National Archives and Records Administration. Record Group 120. Major Oscar G Skelton, attending dental surgeon, American Forces in Germany, Coblenz, to Colonel Earl H Bruns, chief surgeon, American Forces in Germany, 7 April 1920. Memo. File no. 703. Box 3318. Entry 1482.

56. National Archives and Records Administration. Record Group 120. Colonel Earl H Bruns, chief surgeon, American Forces in Germany, to assistant chief of staff], G-4, 8 April 1920. Memo. File no. 703. Box 3318. Entry 1482.

57. National Archives and Records Administration. Record Group 120. Major General Henry T Allen, Orders no. 43, headquarters, American Forces in Germany, Coblenz, 12 April 1920. File no. 703. Box 3318. Entry 1482.

58. National Archives and Records Administration. Record Group 120. Major Oscar G Skelton, attending dental surgeon, American Forces in Germany, to chief surgeon, American Forces in Germany, 15 April 1920. Memo. File no. 703. Box 3318. Entry 1482.

59. National Archives and Records Administration. Record Group 120. Surgeon, American Forces in Germany, Coblenz, to commanding general, American Forces in Germany, history 1919–1920, 31 December 1920. Report. Box 3302. Entry 1484.

60. National Archives and Records Administration. Record Group 120. Lieutenant Colonel Hugh O Scott, attending dental surgeon, American Forces in Germany, to chief surgeon, American Forces in Germany, 9 February 1921. Memo. File no. 703. Box 3318. Entry 1482.

61. National Archives and Records Administration. Record Group 120. Colonel Frank R Keefer, chief surgeon, American Forces in Germany, to adjutant, American Forces in Germany, 9 February 1921. Memo. File no. 703. Box 3318. Entry 1482.

62. National Archives and Records Administration. Record Group 120. Lieutenant Colonel Kyle Rucker, judge advocate, to chief of staff, American Forces in Germany, 11 February 1921. Memo. File no. 703. Box 3318. Entry 1482.

63. National Archives and Records Administration. Record Group 120. Note, Major General Henry T Allen, attached to memo of Lieutenant Colonel Kyle Rucker, judge advocate, to chief of staff, American Forces in Germany, 11 February 1921. File no. 703. Box 3318. Entry 1482.

64. National Archives and Records Administration. Record Group 120. Lieutenant Colonel Hugh O Scott, attending dental surgeon, American Forces in Germany, to chief surgeon, American Forces in Germany, 14 February 1921. Memo. File no. 703. Entry 1482. Box 3318.

65. National Archives and Records Administration. Record Group 120. Lieutenant Colonel Hugh O Scott, dental surgeon, American Forces in Germany, to surgeon general, Annual report and history of dental service 1921, 11 February 1922. Report. Box 3324. Entry 1496.

66. National Archives and Records Administration. Record Group 120. Report to surgeon general, report of activities of the Medical Department, American Forces in Germany for the calendar year 1922, 28 January 1923. Box 3324. Entry 1498.

67. National Archives and Records Administration. Record Group 120. Lieutenant Colonel RB Miller, surgeon, American Forces in Germany, to assistant chief of staff, G-2 (through AC of S, G-4), Historical report of the Medical Department, A.F.G. for 1922, 23 January 1923. Report. Box 3302. Entry 1484.

Chapter XVII

A Return to Normalcy: From the World War to the Depression, 1919–1929

Introduction

The armistice and eventual return of the American Expeditionary Force's (AEF's) dental personnel to the United States after the war marked the conclusion of an innovative effort to provide adequate dental and oral care to a massive force overseas. The growth and maturity of the Army's dental services during the war set a firm foundation for postwar organization and planning. At the same time, a cadre of war-proven Dental Corps officers with unrivaled personal experiences in command, administration, and combat were on hand to provide leadership and carry out the plans. The respect and acceptance that the front line dental officers had won from their medical colleagues, line commanders, and fellow soldiers was perhaps just as important for the future of the postwar Dental Corps. By fighting the enemy rather than each other (as they so often had since 1901), the officers of the Medical and Dental Corps of the AEF had built a highly efficient and effective system of care for sick and wounded American soldiers. A major question now was whether this spirit could be maintained as the nation tried to return to normalcy in the wake of the World War.

Colonel Logan's Farewell Letter

Upon leaving active duty on February 12, 1919, Colonel William HG Logan, chief of the dental section in the surgeon general's office, sent a 4-page letter to all members of the Dental Corps in which he summarized the wartime achievements and looked forward to the future. After dealing with the ongoing issues of personnel in the downsizing Army, he highlighted the adjutant general's action of September 30, 1918, "which established the precedent for the assignment of two Dental officers per thousand." A critical issue for the Dental Corps, though, was whether this ratio would be retained in the rapidly emerging peacetime Army.[1] Logan wrote:

> Of this I can say that it is my opinion the Powers that Be in the Surgeon General's Office, the Chief of Staff and the War Department have reached the conclusion and concur in the desire of the Dental Profession and Dental Corps that an assignment of two Dental Officers per thousand shall be allowed hereafter in any Army that represents the United States of America. . . . Newton D. Baker, Secretary of War, and General March, Chief of Staff, appeared before the Military Committee of Congress, and

approved a Bill for the reorganization of the Army, which included the quota of two per thousand of Dental Officers.[1]

Logan believed that the problems both he and Robert Oliver had with the war-time tables of organization had at last been solved. "A Table of Organization has in substance and detail been approved," he wrote, "specifying the number of Dental Officers with their grades, to be assigned at all stations."[1]

While claiming no credit for this major change from the prewar era, Logan said that Dental Corps officers "shall, at all times, in the future, be on duty in the surgeon general's office, looking after the interests of their Corps under the direction of the Surgeon General, and all this will come without a request of any member of the Dental Corps or from any member of the profession at large." Lieutenant Colonel Frank LK Laflamme (1877–1966) would temporarily take over Logan's duties, but Logan believed that a senior Dental Corps colonel would soon be placed in charge.[1] He urged the Dental Corps to have patience, writing:

> As to which one will probably be assigned, I am without an opinion, but for whoever is called upon to assume responsibilities for the Dental Corps, I ask for them your hearty cooperation and take the liberty of suggesting to all members of the Dental Corps that they do not make unusual personal requests for special detail, but shall be charitable in your conclusions before reaching the decision that important policies are not being carried forward as rapidly as would seem should be consummated by those stationed at some distances from Washington.[1]

Unlike the prewar days, Logan reassured the members of the Dental Corps that the surgeon general "fully approves the establishment of a Dental Officers' Training School in connection with the Army Medical School at Washington, D.C., in close proximity with the Walter Reed General Hospital, and in my opinion, the General Staff also concurs."[1] Logan continued, writing:

> The general plans for the building are completed, the subjects to be taught selected, the number of hours to be devoted to each, number of students to receive training in each course designated, and the rank for the seventeen teachers needed for instructive purposes approved; the building to be 50 x 150; the number of professors and assistant professors seventeen Dental Officers to be detailed for each course of instruction about ninety; duration of the course four and a half months, two courses per year; one hundred and eighty to two hundred receiving instruction annually gives a total in attendance in five years of one thousand Dental Officers, or the quota allowed for an Army of five hundred thousand.[1]

Logan had clearly learned the war's lessons about how to turn a large influx of untrained civilians into Army Dental Corps officers ready for military duties. Moreover, he understood that skills once acquired had to be regularly honed, so all Dental Corps officers were now required to attend a 2-month military training course at Camp Greenleaf, Fort Oglethorpe, Georgia (site of the largest wartime medical officers' training camp), every 5 years. Those who had not yet completed the post-graduate professional training at the new dental school would then proceed to Washington to do so.[1]

During the war the Army's existing policy on dental treatment, which provided only emergency care, had undergone a complete reversal, now allowing for full care. Logan believed that "approval has been secured from those in authority in the surgeon general's office for a change, in the immediate future, to have full Dentistry performed in the Army."[1] The consequence, he said, was quite significant: "At every Fort or Post that can properly be designated as a permanent station hereafter will be found equipment that will compare favorably with that of civilian Dentists."[1]

Logan was optimistic about these positive developments, writing:

I believe the most ambitious hopes for the future welfare of the Dental Corps will be realized inside of a year or eighteen months, at the most, for in that time, I have faith that the quota of two per thousand will be authorized by War Department approval, without any further request by members of the Dental Corps; that a post-graduate school of instruction will be established where all members of the Dental Corps will receive instruction once every five years for the duration of their service, that full Dentistry will be authorized in the Army; that complete Dental equipment will be found at all permanent stations.[1]

He concluded by providing three suggestions that he urged members of the Dental Corps to accept:

First: That discord should not be allowed to develop among the members of the Dental Corps in regard to important questions of policy;

Second: That political activities for Legislation shall not be permitted; and

Finally: The Senior Dental Officers should not endeavor to confine themselves to executive duties unless the detail fully warrants such restriction.[1]

In the April 1919 issue of the *Journal of the Association of Military Dental Surgeons of the United States*, the journal's editor, William C Fisher (1876–1932), commented on Logan's letter. Fisher, a prominent New York City dentist, had been a contract dental surgeon from 1901 to 1904, and a lieutenant colonel in the Dental Officers' Reserve Corps (DORC) during World War I (he was promoted to colonel in the 1920s). He fully endorsed Logan's views on the tables of organization for the Dental Corps, the need for a permanent presence in the surgeon general's office, and the establishment a new training school for dental officers in Washington linked to the Army Medical School. Fisher noted that "when that is an accomplished fact it will indeed be a huge stride in advance, not only for the Dental Corps but for the dental profession at large." He also fully supported Logan on the importance of postgraduate professional education.[2]

However, Fisher doubted that a ratio of two dentists per thousand troops would be approved without political pressure because the congress that had accepted General March's recommendations was now gone and the legislation would have to be resubmitted. Fisher was an able administrator and believed that Logan should have brought some senior dental officers into his office in Washington in 1917 and 1918 to build an efficient organization that could replace him when

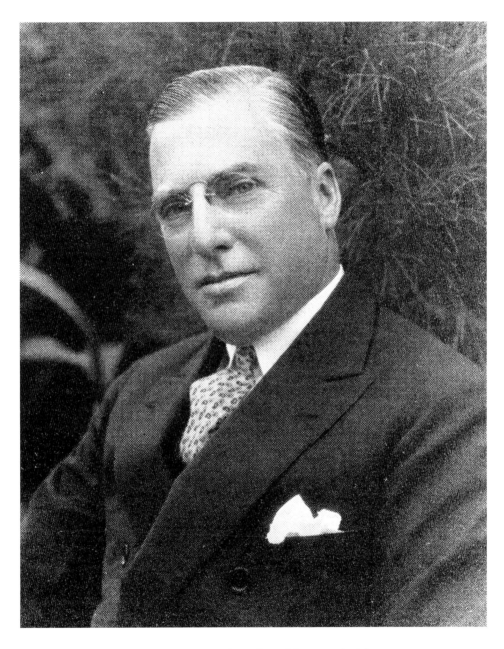

Doctor William C Fisher, editor of the Journal of the
Association of Military Dental Surgeons of the United States.
Photograph: Courtesy of the National Library of Medicine.

he returned to his civilian pursuits. "But he did not," Fisher lamented, "and it now falls to those officers to take up the work where he has laid it down without the experience that they might have gained under his administration."[2(p80)]

As to Logan's concluding three points, Fisher added an extended comment:

> In commending these three suggestions there can be no difference of opinion regarding the first; regarding the second, as to what is meant by "political activities for legislation shall not be permitted," we are unable at this time to fully conceive. If Colonel Logan means petty political activities, we certainly are in accord with him, but if he means that the Corps should not at any time interest itself in legislation improving their Corps, thus improving the dental service in the Army, then we take issue with him. For without certain dignified political activities the Corps naturally will suffer. There is an old saying that no one will look out for you as well as you will look out for yourself, which we think applies to organizations as well as to individuals. We trust that we will not be misunderstood, and in order that we are not misunderstood we will again state that petty political activities regarding personal advancement or preference should not be tolerated. . . . As to his final suggestion regarding senior dental officers, we believe that there is sufficient administrative work in the Dental Corps, especially in the next few years, to keep every colonel and lieutenant colonel, and many of the majors, busy in that particular activity.[2(pp79–80)]

The Dental Corps' Initial Adjustments to Peace

After the armistice, the Dental Corps in Europe and the United States began adjusting to the realities of peace and the requirements of a postwar Army. Temporary officers of the DORC, then on active duty, requested their releases from service, were discharged as "rapidly as the interest of the service would permit," or could apply for any vacancies in the Regular Army if they were under the age of 32. The number of reserve dentists on active duty was slashed from 4,391 in November 1918 to 2,001 on July 1, 1919. As personnel returned from France, divisions demobilized and the camps and cantonments were closed, and another 1,824 reserve officers were released from July through October. On November 1, 1919, only 176 remained on active duty. By June 30, 1920, only 126 DORC members were still on active duty, which meant that the remaining Regular Army dentists had to shoulder most of the burden of dental care. Pending the new National Defense Act, the authorizations of the Regular Army Dental Corps dropped from 218 on July 1, 1919, to 196 on June 30, 1920. At the same time, however, "the demands for dental service in general hospitals . . . required the assignment of officers in addition to the authorized quota." As a result, during 1919 and 1920, the Dental Corps was stretched to its very limits, with 60 dental officers in Germany (18), Poland (1), Panama (3), Hawaii (8), China (1), Alaska (temporary duty), the Philippines (19), Puerto Rico (2), and Siberia (8), and 256 serving in the United States. In addition, 16 other dental officers were assigned to duty with the Army Transport Service to provide professional services on the Atlantic transports returning the overseas troops and the hospitalized.[3,4]

Army Reorganization and Reality

As Logan's letter was reaching the members of the Dental Corps early in 1919, the American forces occupying their section of Germany were organizing for their stay, which would last nearly 4 more years. At this time, the War Department was already focused on demobilization and the structure of the postwar force. True to the American military tradition of hasty demobilization after wars, the War Department had already discharged over 2,000,000 soldiers by September 1919, when the last combat unit, the 1st Division, returned from France.[5] Simultaneously, the War Department began to grapple with issues of reorganization, modernization, and mobilization that would continue to be studied, debated, and remain largely unresolved for the next 20 years. The wartime changes to the National Defense Act of 1916 had been temporary, and the extent of American involvement overseas made it apparent that permanent changes were in order so that the nation would be better prepared for future conflicts than it had been in 1917. General Peyton March, the chief of staff, favored a 500,000-person force backed by a large reserve based on peacetime conscription. The political feasibility of such a large peacetime Army was another question entirely.[6]

Congress did not treat March's plan favorably. Even while it debated the size of the future force, Congress continued to reduce the active force. What finally emerged from Congress was the National Defense Act of 1920 (Public Law 66-242, June 4, 1920); the first comprehensive plan for the nation's defense ever drawn up and written into law. The first clause of the act said "that the Army of the United States shall consist of the Regular Army, the National Guard while in the service of the United States, and the organized Reserves, including the Officers' Reserve Corps and the Enlisted Reserve Corps." The small peacetime Regular Army was not to exceed an enlisted strength of 280,000 and would provide the nucleus of a larger force to be mobilized from the National Guard (limited to 435,000 strength), the Organized Reserve Corps, and conscription to build to an initial echelon of 2,375,000 soldiers in six field armies. Under this act the Dental Corps was authorized a strength of 298 officers, 102 more than currently held Regular Army commissions. More fully developed mobilization plans in 1921 required a total force of 6,558,000 within 19 months. In peacetime the Regular Army would staff a large number of divisions, corps, and field units at minimal strengths, to be filled during mobilization. Federal control over the National Guard increased in light of its role as the primary reserve for the active force. A civilian military training corps program, similar to the pre-World War I "Plattsburg Camps," was launched to sustain public participation and interest in Army affairs while providing wholesome summer training activities for young men of military age. Also authorized was an expanded Reserve Officers' Training Corps (ROTC) for university students that was to provide a main personnel source for the officers of the Organized Reserve Corps (ORC) and included medical, dental, and veterinary units.[6–12]

The act also replaced the former military departments and divided the country into nine geographic corps areas for administration, training, and reserve component affairs. In 1921 each corps area theoretically held one regular, two guard, and three ORC divisions, for a total of 54 divisions—nine regular, 18 guard, and

27 ORC divisions—and that same year 10 cavalry divisions were added, four in the National Guard and six in the ORC. All of these divisions, as well as the Army, corps, and line of communications (also called communications zone) command echelons and the nondivisional medical units had extensive requirements for Reserve Dental Corps officers.[7–9, 11–13]

The Army's new, expanded involvement with the reserve components required a large Regular Army overhead. Doing so within the limits of shrinking budgets under the parsimonious administrations of President Warren G Harding (1865–1923; president March 1921–August 1923) and his successor, Calvin Coolidge (1872–1933; president August 1923–March 1929), and growing public indifference proved impossible. Congressional budget-cutting intervention only aggravated an already serious problem. The Army Appropriations Act of June 30, 1921 (for fiscal year 1922) cut the Army from 280,000 to 150,000, and reduced the authorized strength of the Dental Corps to 180 officers. Even though General John J Pershing, the new chief of staff as of July 1921, opposed these reductions, the next Army Appropriations Act of June 30, 1922 (for fiscal year 1923) cut even farther into the Regular Army, reducing it to 137,000—125,000 enlisted and 12,000 officers—with an authorized Dental Corps of 158 officers as of January 1, 1923. However, the large mobilization force remained with its equally large requirements for National Guard and ORC personnel and had even grown under plans for a 6,558,000-person force. The 1922 reduction required dropping or forcibly retiring more than 1,000 officers and demoting another 800 who wished to remain on active duty. The shattering effects led Congress to make some minor upward strength adjustments in January 1923, but the damage had been done. Army strength was reduced more over the following years, reaching its low point of 133,949 in 1927, including 12,076 officers and 119,929 enlisted soldiers, and remained relatively constant until the end of the decade when it reached slightly more than 138,000. The reduction in Army strength and the radical modification of many of the programs envisioned in the 1920 National Defense Act strongly affected the Regular and Reserve Dental Corps, whose sizes continued to be based primarily on the old ratio of one dentist per thousand total Army strength.[6,7,9,14]

Thus, within several years of Logan's February 1919 predictions, many of the major gains he had envisioned seemed to have been lost in Congress's radical reductions. The long-sought ratio of two dentists per thousand soldiers was not approved and the official ratio returned to the ratio in effect since 1901. Two years later, the large 500,000-person Army that Logan predicted disappeared, slipping first to 280,000, then to 150,000, and finally 137,000. None of this boded well for the Dental Corps' postwar development and severely tested the Corps' leadership.

Dental Corps Leadership in the 1920s

As Logan had noted in his farewell letter, the assignment of a senior Dental Corps officer who would be both chief of the dental section at the surgeon general's office and de facto chief of the Dental Corps became permanent after the war. Lieutenant Colonel Laflamme temporarily held that position and fought the needed battles for the Dental Corps until Colonel Robert T Oliver returned from

France. In August 1919 Laflamme moved to the US Military Academy, where he remained until October 1925.[4,15]

Two of the most significant changes for the Dental Corps occurred in September and November 1919. On September 18 Colonel Robert T Oliver, the ranking colonel in the corps, assumed the duties as chief of the dental section in the personnel branch of the surgeon general's office. In view of the changed postwar responsibilities and Oliver's long relationship with Major General Ireland, the surgeon general, on November 24 the dental division replaced the dental section. The new dental division was "raised to the dignity" of a separate organization within the surgeon general's office, reporting directly to Ireland and responsible for "all professional and administrative matters pertaining to the Dental Corps." Throughout the 1920s the dental division held overall responsibility for the direction of the Army's entire dental service but remained small, with only the chief and an assistant, usually a captain, authorized and assigned.[4,16–19]

Oliver and Ireland, who had served together in France and earlier, had already established a close working relationship and shared a clear understanding of the importance of modern dentistry to health and readiness in the Army. This benefited the Dental Corps throughout Oliver's time as chief and for the duration of Ireland's tenure until his retirement in May 1931. Their friendly relationship was never more clearly seen than in Ireland's whole-hearted participation in the annual meetings of the National Dental Association (NDA) and Association of Military Dental Surgeons of the United States in Milwaukee, Wisconsin, in August 1921. At this time Oliver was president of the Association of Military Dental Surgeons as well as vice president of the NDA. At Oliver's invitation, Ireland came to address both associations on the status of the Dental Corps and dentistry in the Army, something that no previous surgeon general had ever done. In introducing Ireland to the military dentists, Oliver remarked: "I have always said with a spirit of pride and affection that the gentleman who is here with us today, although he belongs to a different corps and a different profession, is perhaps the greatest champion of modern dentistry in the United States outside of our profession." Ireland opened his address simply and directly: "The interest I have in dentistry, and the interest I may have had as to the place for dentistry in the Army is very materially due to Colonel Oliver. You all know that."[20–22]

During his nearly 5 years as chief and with Ireland's support, Oliver made many contributions to the development of the postwar Dental Corps that were perhaps even more significant in the history of Army dentistry than those he made in France. Drawing heavily on his experience in the AEF, he fully integrated Dental Corps officers for the first time into the field training and professional education programs of the Army and the Medical Department. He pursued Logan's idea of an Army dental school that provided postgraduate education and research appointments for officers and complete technical training for enlisted dental technicians. Civilian postgraduate education opportunities for Dental Corps officers were also introduced during his tenure. Oliver oversaw the addition of authorized requirements for dental officers and technicians to the official Army and Medical Department tables of organization and pushed the development and acquisition of new field dental equipment. Important new Army regulations governing the

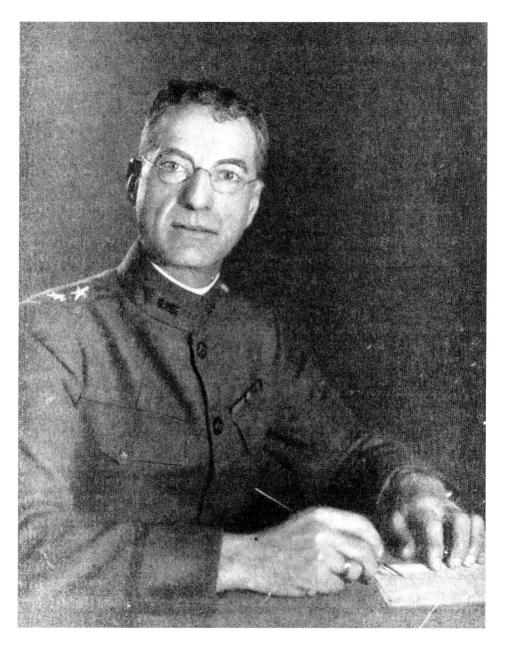

Major General Merritte W Ireland in 1919.
Photograph: Courtesy of the National Library of Medicine.

Dental Corps and dental care in the Army were written during his tour and published after his reassignment. While doing all of this, Oliver also fought to maintain a functional Army dental service in the face of heavy reductions in authorized personnel and stringent limitations on funding during the early 1920s.

On July 1, 1924, Oliver completed his tour as chief of the dental division and chief of the Dental Corps. He moved to New York City for duty at the Second Corps Area Laboratory and served as technical advisor at the New York General Intermediate Depot. In 1926 he was transferred to Philadelphia, Pennsylvania, to act as the new assistant professor of military science and tactics at the University of Pennsylvania's School of Dentistry and was in charge of one of the Army's largest dental ROTC units. While there, Oliver served as president of the American Dental Association in 1930–1931. He remained in Philadelphia until his retirement in January 1932 and died on July 11, 1937, after a long illness. During World War II, Oliver General Hospital in Augusta, Georgia, was named in his honor. Since its dedication on November 4, 1969, the Oliver Dental Clinic at Fort Jackson, South Carolina, has perpetuated his memory and many achievements in the Dental Corps and Medical Department.[17,22–24]

With Oliver's reassignment, Lieutenant Colonel Rex H Rhoades assumed the duties as chief of the dental division and the Dental Corps. Like Oliver, Rhoades brought experience in Army dentistry to the office as it struggled to maintain a quality dental service with limited personnel and resources. After being hired as a contract dental surgeon in November 1902, Rhoades had served at numerous posts in the United States and the Philippines before becoming one of the original commissioned officers of the Dental Corps on April 28, 1911. During World War I, he saw service with the 2nd Division as division dental surgeon in France from November 1917 to March 1918, and then became the supervising dental surgeon for the advance section of the services of supply from March to August 1918, and the chief dental surgeon for the First US Army from August 1918 to January 1919. For his wartime service, Rhoades received a wound chevron (Purple Heart Medal after February 22, 1932) and battle clasps for the defensive operations and the Saint Mihiel and Meuse-Argonne offensives of 1918. From 1921 to June 1924, he was assistant surgeon and chief dental surgeon at the Sixth Corps Area headquarters at Fort Sheridan, Illinois, and professor of military science and tactics for the dental ROTC unit at Northwestern University's School of Dentistry in Chicago. Upon Rhoades's departure for Washington, Lieutenant Colonel Robert H Mills, himself a future Dental Corps chief (1942–1946), assumed this post.[25–28]

Rhoades served until June 15, 1928, when Colonel Julien R Bernheim, another of the early contract dental surgeons and original member of the Dental Corps, succeeded him. Rhoades was transferred to the US Military Academy at West Point, New York, where he was the senior dental surgeon until 1932, when he was recalled to serve a second term as chief beginning exactly 4 years after he left, June 15, 1932. Rhoades was the only Dental Corps chief ever to serve two tours. He retired in September 1934 and died on September 11, 1959, at Walter Reed Army Hospital. On June 25, 1964, the new dental clinic at Fort Sam Houston, Texas, was named in his honor.[26,27]

Like Robert Oliver and Rex Rhoades, Colonel Julien R Bernheim had extensive

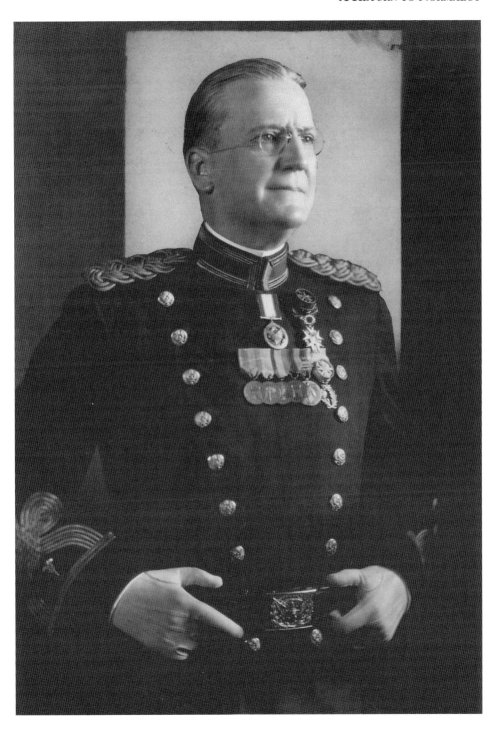

Colonel Robert T Oliver, president of the American Dental Association 1930–1931.
Photograph: Courtesy of the American Dental Association.

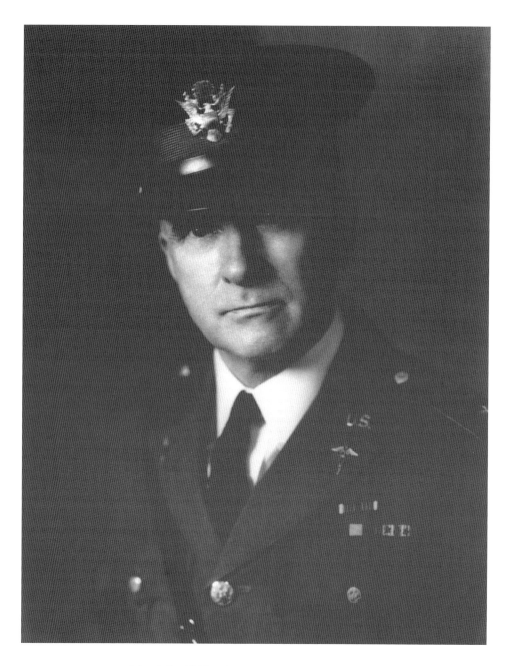

Colonel Rex H Rhoades upon retirement in July 1935.
Photograph: Courtesy of National Archives and Records Administration. US Army photo P-2445.

experience in the Medical Department dating back to his time as a contract dental surgeon (in April 1902 he was hired to replace the recently deceased Charles Petre). His foreign service included two tours in the Philippines (1902–1905 and 1908–1911) and numerous stateside assignments. Unlike Oliver and Rhoades, Bernheim never served in France or overseas during World War I. Rather he headed the dental service at the attending surgeon's office in Washington, DC, before serving in the finance and supply division in the surgeon general's office, and then in the purchase, storage, and traffic division of the War Department General Staff, until he was transferred to Letterman General Hospital to serve as the chief of the dental service in February 1919. From July 1923 through May 1928, he was the chief of the dental service at the station hospital at Fort Sam Houston, Texas, and dental advisor to Eighth Corps Area headquarters. While on this duty, he was promoted to Colonel on April 9, 1928. He served as chief from June 15, 1928, until June 15, 1932, after which he remained on duty in the Dental Corps. He served as chief of the dental service at Tripler General Hospital, Honolulu, Hawaii (August 1932–October 1934), then at the Presidio of San Francisco and Ninth Corps Area headquarters (October 1934–August 1936), before once again holding the post as chief of the dental service at Letterman until July 1940. He returned to Hawaii for another tour as chief of Tripler's dental service, and was at that post when the Japanese attacked Pearl Harbor on December 7, 1941. Returning to the United States in September 1942, Bernheim was assigned to the San Francisco Port of Embarkation, a post he held until he died at Letterman General Hospital on March 16, 1943, just prior to his scheduled retirement on March 31. The Bernheim Dental Clinic at Fort Benning, Georgia, was named for him.[29,30]

The Dental Corps, Dental Practice, and the Impact of the 1922 Army Reductions

The National Defense Act of June 4, 1920, gave the Dental Corps "all the rights, privileges, credits of service for promotion, increased service pay, and retirement heretofore authorized in part by the acts of March 3, 1911, June 3, 1916, comptroller's decision of July 22, 1916, and the act of October 6, 1917." In part trumping the general staff's plans of August 1919 to roll back the act of October 6, 1917, Congress placed the Dental Corps on "equal status as one of the integral corps of the Medical Department of the Army" but repealed the part of the 1917 law that gave Dental Corps officers "the same grades proportionally distributed among such grades as are now, or may be hereafter, provided by law for the Medical Corps." The number of dental officers authorized for the 280,000-soldier Army under the new law was 298.[4,10,31] Congress had returned to the original proportion of one dentist per thousand troops despite new commitments, the changed character of reconstructive dental operations, and the increased demands for "higher professional attention along lines of preventive dentistry and in consultation with medical officers in locating obscure pathological conditions as possible etiologic factors to systemic disease."[4]

Army policies on dental care had changed considerably during the war. With the return of peace and into 1920, the Medical Department was able to maintain a high level of dental care, partly because it retained a sufficient number of reservists on active duty to care for the large number of patients still in the general hospitals and partly due to the increased authorizations arising from the new National Defense Act.[4,32] According to the surgeon general's annual report in 1920:

> Dental activities for the year have been eminently satisfactory and the number and character of constructive operations resulting have been very gratifying. It is both pleasing and noteworthy to record the great increase in number of cases where dental officers through clinic findings and skillful radiography, have rendered able assistance to medical officers in the diagnosis and treatment of obscure lesions of dental origin—contributing factors to undermined health and efficiency.[4(p304)]

The quality of dental service at the general hospitals had reached the highest levels ever, with adequate numbers of dental officers under the direction of "experienced senior officers of recognized ability." Emergency dental cases were still the predominant type of work performed in these hospitals, but oral prophylaxis was increasingly popular with the enlisted soldiers.[4]

The most serious of the remaining dental patients were the maxillofacial cases, 694 of which had been transferred from France during 1918 and 1919. By June 1919, 320 maxillofacial patients had been discharged and the remaining 374 were concentrated at four centers in the United States—Walter Reed General Hospital in Washington, DC; General Hospital No. 2 at Fort McHenry, Baltimore, Maryland; Columbus Barracks, Ohio; and the station hospital at Jefferson Barracks, Saint Louis, Missouri. At each of these hospitals an experienced chief headed a special maxillofacial service that consisted of ward surgeons, surgical assistants, dental surgeons, and prosthetists. According to the surgeon general's 1919 annual report, "The successful treatment of these cases does not depend upon one man alone, but close cooperation and teamwork between the surgical and dental departments is absolutely essential."[3] These cases challenged the best of the Dental Corps' oral surgeons, but were also important sources for learning how to treat such injuries. For example, the surgeon general's 1920 report says:

> This has required officers of marked professional ability in the construction of splints and special appliances used in the reconstructive treatment of mutilated bones of the face and jaw and in the restoration of masticatory apparatus lost through gunshot wounds or injuries. The large amount of clinical material thus available has been taken advantage of by all dental officers on duty at these stations and careful understudy made of the surgical and dental procedures followed by these specialists. It is to be regretted that more dental officers could not have been given opportunity to obtain practical knowledge of the modern treatment of those interesting and important war injuries.[4(pp302–303)]

By 1921 the maxillofacial cases under care had dropped substantially, and the services at General Hospital No. 2 and Columbus Barracks were closed. The few remaining cases that required additional reconstructive treatment and those requiring routine replacement of prosthetic devices were cared for at Walter Reed and Jefferson Barracks.[21,32] In fiscal year 1923 the maxillofacial service at Jefferson Barracks was ended and everything was then handled at Walter Reed. Virtually all of the reconstruction treatment was completed, and only the more routine replacement of special prosthetic appliances remained the major responsibility.[33]

In the immediate postwar years, an old, prewar problem reemerged—the issue of "others entitled to treatment" under prevailing Army regulations, mainly dependents of officers and enlisted soldiers and retirees. At many locations, the numbers of such patients were large, and the 1920 surgeon general's report addressed the problem as follows:

> While this class of service is authorized "when practicable," it has become an established custom to grant to families of officers and enlisted men the same character of service usually accorded respectively to them. Thus, the dental officer spends approximately the same amount of time and effort to the case with these patients as with officers and men and the sum of the activities should justly be recorded and credited.[4(p305)]

Another matter that had been a problem since 1901 was apparently resolved when the Army changed its policy on the use of precious metals in 1920. That October the surgeon general's office issued Circular Letter No. 129, which finally added gold to the dental supplies "furnished free by the Government" for use in restorative dentistry for military personnel. Designated "special materials," precious metals were to be stocked at all stations where laboratory equipment was installed. Use was limited to trauma injuries incurred in the line of duty and special cases described in the circular, but was allowed for both officers and enlisted soldiers. Dependents were charged a fixed rate per grain, payable to the Medical Department. Surgeon General's Office Circular No. 149 of December 23, 1920, provided all the necessary accounting and expenditure controls for use of the special materials.[4] The new rules were explained as follows:

> The operation of this policy relieves the dental officer of the necessity of making a charge to brother officers or their families for special materials required in modern practice, and thus terminates an objectionable custom that has existed in the Dental Corps for the past 20 years. . . . While the system governing the expenditure and accounting for these materials is necessarily strict, it nevertheless provides means through which full modern dental service may be rendered in legitimate and meritorious cases. It is meeting with hearty approval throughout the Army.[10(p123)]

The Army Appropriations Act of June 30, 1921, allowed postwar fiscal realities to intrude adversely into the Medical Department and Dental Corps. The act cut the Army's authorized strength to 150,000 soldiers and 13,000 officers. It also reduced the Dental Corps' authorization from 298 officers to 193 on July 1, 1921, and then to 180 August 10, 1921. Despite these cutbacks, the Dental Corps section of the 1922 *Annual Report of the Surgeon General* began with this assessment: "During the past year, the Dental Corps has functioned more smoothly and efficiently than during any previous year of its existence." This result was actually attributed to an increased number of dental officers "accruing under the terms of the reorganization act, June 4, 1920, which permitted a general expansion of the dental service to meet all station requirements and a development of professional activities at general hospitals and other important clinics."[32] The annual report read:

When the Army was reduced to 150,000, the Dental Corps was found with a surplus of approximately 60 officers over and above the authorized quota of one dental officer for each thousand officers and enlisted men of the Army. This excess number being more nearly that of the ideal number required—namely, two dental officers to one thousand total strength of the Army—permitted a full and more complete development of the dental service in conjunction with the medical and surgical service at general hospitals and in several of the more important large clinics throughout the country.[32(p130)]

Although the authorized strength of the Dental Corps had dropped to 193 in July of 1921, its in-service strength was up to 250 on July 1, 1921, due to 54 surplus officers and four retirees on active duty with dental ROTC units. The in-service strength was 239 on March 31, 1922, due to 56 surplus officers and three retirees. However, the act of June 30, 1922, required a general reduction in the Army, which cut the overall strength to 125,000 men and 12,000 officers. When the Army lost approximately 1,000 of its 13,000 officers (about 8%), the Dental Corps' share was 75 of 233 officers (about 32%). In the first authorized departure from the one-dentist-per-thousand-troops ratio, the Dental Corps' strength was fixed at 158 dental officers as of January 1, 1923, allowing approximately 20 dental officers in excess of the proportion of one per thousand Army total strength.[10,32,33] The 1923 *Annual Report of the Surgeon General* commented that the Dental Corps "functioned under two widely divergent policies" during the year:

During the first six months [July–December 1922] the broad policies of the previous year remained in force. Based upon favorable conditions incident to an adequate number of dental officers and a generous appropriation, these policies had featured a general expansion of service to include the highest type of professional achievement for the military clientele at all Army stations and that important development of professional activities at general hospitals, known as group treatment, where the medical, surgical, and special services blend in harmonious cooperation in treating the sick. During the succeeding six months [January–June 1923] it became necessary to abandon almost wholly the general features of the above-cited policies and even to modify that pertaining to general hospitals on account of the crippling reduction in commissioned personnel and the great restriction in appropriations required by the provisions of the act of June 30, 1922.[33(p124)]

On February 15, 1923, the surgeon general's office sent a draft of its proposed Circular Letter No. 6 (Dental No. 1) to the Army's adjutant general for review. The letter, titled "Reorganization of the Dental Service," would establish the new policies governing the reduced dental practice in the Medical Department. It noted:

While the attached circular letter which the Surgeon General proposes to send to all Medical Department units and to each dental officer of the Army is largely technical in character it embodies certain restrictions as to treatment, especially with reference to the families of officers and men and to retired personnel, that must now be enforced because of the existing shortage of dental officers and to which exception may be taken by some of the prospective patients concerned.[34]

Two days later, the adjutant general replied that such sweeping changes were of interest to all Army officers and enlisted soldiers and requested "such instructions as are of general interest to the service be prepared and submitted to this office for necessary action." The surgeon general complied and on February 26 returned the requested information as a draft circular titled "Policies Governing Dental Attendance." On March 1 the proposed Army-wide circular was forwarded to General Pershing, chief of staff, for his approval. Both Pershing and the secretary of war approved, and on March 12, 1923, the War Department published Circular No. 20. The circular's third section, "Policies governing dental attendance," as originally proposed by the surgeon general, established the new policies that governed dental practice in the Army and limited the scope of dental treatment.[35–38]

On March 14, 1923, the surgeon general's office issued Circular Letter No. 6 (Dental No. 1), "Reorganization of the Dental Service," which outlined the professional and technical procedures for implementing the new policies in War Department Circular No. 20. Basically, the peacetime Army was interested in preventing lost duty time because of "dental diseases or deficiencies." The Corps' secondary duty was to "relieve suffering among and promote the dental comfort of all authorized garrison personnel." The new policy limited dependent care to emergency only, and restricted the use of gold to officer personnel only.[39–41]

The cuts and the new policies necessitated by them were crippling to the Army dental service—the number of dental officers available was so greatly slashed that heavy reductions were soon made in those assigned to hospitals, dispensaries, and corps areas. Circular No. 20 confirmed that it was impossible to continue the previous level of dental service for Army personnel. Among the expedients introduced was placing dentists at posts where the largest numbers of personnel were stationed in each corps area. Part-time dental service was inaugurated at those stations where dental officers had been regularly assigned in the past. The 1923 annual report labeled the reintroduction of itinerant dental service as "wholly unsatisfactory . . . an unsound, ineffectual, and unprofitable attempt to administer piecemeal profession service."[33] At a few of the smaller stations, dental service was completely abandoned. The use of civilian dental hygienists to augment the dental officers was attempted in 1924, but a lack of funding meant they could only be hired at five stations.[42] Civilian dentists were employed for emergency treatment and reimbursed by the Medical Department under the provisions of Army Regulations paragraph 1476 ½ .[39,43] Many beneficiaries did not take the cutbacks in family and retiree care very favorably, and Army dentists often suffered the consequences. The 1923 surgeon general's report read:

> From a professional standpoint it was found necessary to prescribe certain types of dental treatment that reasonably could be followed in meting out the modicum of service yet available. This required radical departure from the class of dental practice heretofore afforded the Army and caused the deprivation of dental service for wives and families and for retired officers, except emergency treatment for the relief of pain and the simple constructive procedures of first aid. . . . The imposed radical departure from the full and beneficial character of service heretofore freely afforded officers and enlisted men and that extended to the wives and families of officers and enlisted men in garrisons has caused great dissatisfaction and considerable well-warranted protest.[33(p125)]

William H Hoblitzell, a former Dental Corps captain, later observed that these changes substantially reduced job satisfaction, "the daily routine became somewhat tiresome and the incentive to accomplish things began to jade." He left the service for private practice in Cincinnati.[44]

The personnel and budget reductions forced Oliver and the Dental Corps to balance many factors of Army dental practice to meet the demands of its various missions. One of the wider impacts of these reductions and the ensuing policy changes was found in the Army's dispensaries and general and station hospitals, where the largest amount of dental work was done. Never losing sight of his primary mission to care for soldiers, Oliver kept as many dentists at their chairs as he could while limiting those in administrative, training, and educational assignments. Rhoades and Bernheim both followed Oliver's policy in this regard. Oliver also tried to maintain the practice of physicians and dentists working together to study and treat patients; a method that he and Ireland had increasingly come to support as "an established axiom."[20,33,42] This was not always easy.

Every effort was put forth to retain the facilities for group treatment in the larger hospitals, for it had been shown conclusively that the dental factor in the study of systemic disease had proven of very great value and importance in both diagnosis and treatment. Even in the face of adversity, the important primary function of the dental service prescribed in times of peace—namely, to assist in conserving the physical efficiency of military personnel and to prevent the loss of duty time through dental diseases or deficiencies—was not overlooked, nor was the duty to relieve human suffering forgotten.[33(p125)]

In a theme that was repeated for some years to come, the Dental Corps report for 1923, probably written by Oliver, pulled no punches in describing the underlying cause of the problem, the consequences of the inadequate manning, and the need for remedial action by the War Department:

> The present urgent requirement of the Army Dental Corps is an increase in personnel. It is obvious that a satisfactory type of dental treatment can not be made available to the personnel of the Army with the present quota of officers based upon an apportionment of 1 to 1,000 total strength of the Army, arbitrarily determined upon 23 years ago when the Dental Corps was first established. At that time the importance of dentistry in relation to general health was not yet understood, and modern professional procedures during the last few years and the real value of dentistry in the Military Establishment, conclusively proven during the late war, has served to demonstrate the inconsistency of attempting adequate dental service with insufficient personnel to warrant such undertaking. The only remedy is legislation. It is recommended, therefore, that request be made to the War Department for such legislation as will provide a quota of dental officers in the United States Army apportioned at the rate of not less than 2 dental officers per thousand strength of the Army. It is believed that the General Staff and The Adjutant General, as well as a majority of individuals in the Military Establishment, will heartily endorse such recommendation. Having enjoyed an excellent dental service during the past several years, and then been deprived of it during the last few months, has brought the Army personnel to a realization of the importance of military dentistry as an adjunct of the Medical Department in the conservation of health and physical efficiency and a necessary service for the relief of suffering and the preservation of human comfort among all members of the military service dependent upon the resources of a military station.[33,42,45–48]

Further complicating Oliver's already delicate juggling act were mandatory requirements that Dental Corps officers serve as instructors in various training courses, including the following: the Dental ROTC academic courses and annual summer camps; various National Guard and ORC summer camps; the citizens' military training camps (CMTCs); and the Army Dental and Medical Field Service Schools (where dental officers also had to attend mandatory training as students). Oliver also recognized the need to provide postgraduate, specialized professional training at civilian institutions for at least some selected dental officers.

The Dental Reserve Officers' Training Corps

The National Defense Act of 1920 authorized the establishment of ROTC units at medical, dental, and veterinary medicine schools as part of the overall ORC. In September 1920 the adjutant general authorized the surgeon general to organize the Medical Department's ROTC units. Oliver immediately notified the corps areas' dental surgeons about the new dental ROTC program and encouraged their involvement. At the same time, Surgeon General Ireland wrote to the deans of 10 selected Class A dental schools—those rated most highly according to the Dental Educational Council of America's standards for admission, administration, and curriculum—about establishing dental ROTC units.[32,49–52] A strong supporter of the Medical Department ROTC program, Ireland explained why ROTC was so critical at the NDA's annual meeting in Milwaukee in August 1921:

> These R.O.T.C. units will eventually constitute our principal replacement agency in keeping the reserve roster at a satisfactory level. Each graduate of the advanced military course will be given a commission in the reserve corps. If the majority of them join the reserve, it is estimated that they will provide an annual increment of sufficient size to take care of the normal replacements for both the regular and reserve corps and will more than offset our prospective losses.[53(p936)]

Most of the dental schools initially contacted were connected with universities that already had ROTC units established on campus; some even had affiliated reserve hospital units. Instruction was to commence on October 1, 1920. However, half of the 10 schools selected were unable to participate because of the late start. Therefore, the basic course was only inaugurated at Saint Louis University, Saint Louis, Missouri; North Pacific Dental College, Portland, Oregon; University of Pennsylvania, Philadelphia; University of Minnesota, Minneapolis; and Northwestern University, Chicago, Illinois (the other five schools selected were University of California, College of Dentistry, San Francisco; Harvard University Dental School, Boston; University of Michigan, College of Dentistry, Ann Arbor; University of Pittsburgh, College of Dentistry, Pittsburgh; and Vanderbilt University, School of Dentistry, Nashville, Tennessee). Because of the shortage of dental officers, medical officers were selected as professors of military science and tactics at these colleges and 468 dental students were enrolled. In 1921–1922, dental programs at three more schools were added: Ohio State University, Columbus; Creighton University, Omaha, Nebraska; and State University of Iowa, Iowa City. Five dental officers, including three already retired, attended a special basic field training and then the normal course of instruction at the Medical Field Service School in 1921 before assuming their assignments as instructors to replace the medical officers at these institutions for the fall semester. Among the new ROTC instructors were four of the original contract dental surgeons—Captain Clarence Lauderdale at Saint Louis University and Colonel Frank Wolven at University of Pennsylvania, both now retired, and Lieutenant Colonels John McAlister at Creighton University and Rex Rhoades at Northwestern University (Rhoades also acted as Sixth Corps Area dental surgeon). The instructors' experiences reflected the importance that the Medical Department and Dental Corps attached to the ROTC program.[10,32,54,55]

The ROTC cadets were to receive 90 hours of instruction per year for 4 collegiate years, divided into a basic course (first 2 years) and an advanced course (last 2 years). The Dental Corps and surgeon general believed that it was impractical for the students to wear uniforms or to engage in drills because of their busy academic schedule, so this training was deferred to the ROTC summer camp of instruction. After completing the basic course, each student was to attend a 6-week summer camp for practical training in drill and the field duties of all Medical Department officers. The dental officers assigned as professors of military science and tactics were provided with all the textbooks and War Department documents necessary to prepare the course. The courses covered subjects such as hygiene and first aid, customs of the service, field equipment, articles of war and Army Regulations, medico-military history, discipline, food preparation in the field, splinting, gas protection, and litter transportation of wounded.[54,56,57]

The course of instruction at the summer camps was similar to that given to reserve medical officers and began at 7:00AM with 2 hours of calisthenics and squad and company drills. The later periods were used for practical exercises, demonstrations, and lectures on topics like personal hygiene, water purification, first aid, field sanitation, care of the sick and wounded in the field, and handling Army equipment. In the June 1923 camp at Carlisle Barracks, the four student companies were organized into the four components of a medical regiment: regimental detachment, collecting company, ambulance company, and hospital company. They rotated at the end of each week so every student saw service in each of the different units prior to leaving the camp. The students were quartered in tents and used field equipment and mess kits. They served kitchen police in rotation. The post gymnasium, three tennis courts, two baseball diamonds, volleyball equipment, track facilities, band concerts, and trips to the Gettysburg battlefield provided recreation. That year similar but smaller medical ROTC camps were held at Fort Snelling, Minnesota; Camp Lewis, Washington; and Fort Sam Houston, Texas.[58]

Just as Ireland had predicted in 1921, the dental ROTC units were steady producers of militarily-trained dental officers for the DORC and for the Regular Army throughout the 1920s. Enrollment increased from 468 in the program's first year, 1920–1921, to a decade high of 1,365 in 1925 before falling off to 995 in 1929 as the American economy boomed and the prospects of civilian practice without military obligations lured aspiring dentists. While the exact number of graduate dentists who were commissioned through the program each year from 1921 to 1925 is not known, the cumulative total through and including 1925 was 350. In the years

TABLE 17-1

DENTAL RESERVE OFFICERS' TRAINING CORPS ENROLLMENT AND
COMMISSIONED GRADUATES, 1925–1929

	1925	1926	1927	1928	1929
Basic first year	NR	518	290	337	290
Basic second year	NR	423	516	252	307
Advanced first year	NR	189	280	240	159
Advanced second year	NR	208	212	236	239
Total enrollment	1,365	1,338	1,298	1,065	995
Graduated & commissioned in DORC	160	217	182	213	203
Cumulative graduates commissioned since 1921	350	567	749	962	1,165

NR: not reported
Data Sources: (1) Office of the Surgeon General. *Annual Report of the Surgeon General.* Washington, DC:
OTSG; 1925–1929.

from 1926 through 1929, 815 new dental officers were commissioned in the DORC,
making a cumulative total of 1,165, or 25% of the 1929 strength of 4,664 officers
(Table 17-1).[10,45–48,59]

Citizens' Military Training Camps

Another strain on the Dental Corps' limited personnel resources throughout
the decade was the CMTC, a training program for potential officers and enlisted
personnel that was introduced in the National Defense Act of 1920. Unlike the
campus-based ROTC program, the CMTC was based around summer training
camps. In the summer of 1923 Army dental officers assisted Medical Corps surgeons in completing physical surveys of each CMTC trainee and also provided all
the necessary professional services. The next summer, dental examinations were
also required during physicals. This meant a complete survey of the teeth and
mouth, with "detailed notations" on patients' dental and oral conditions. Some
30,000 trainees were examined during the camps, and all of them were informed of
their "dental and oral defects, received such emergency treatment as was required,
and were advised to seek immediate correction on their return home, [and] had
explained to them the importance of proper care of the teeth as a prophylactic
measure."[42] The dental work at the CMTCs benefited both the dental officers and
especially the trainees, who were sent home with instructions on how to care for
their dental and oral health:

It is believed the general information pertaining to the maintenance of sound teeth
and oral health thus diffused throughout each group of young men of military age

from practically every State in the Union will have beneficent effect in establishing a wholesome desire on their part in securing and maintaining dental fitness as an adjunct to physical efficiency for military service.

The CMTCs continued throughout the 1920s under the jurisdiction of the nine corps areas.[42(p183)]

The Dental Service in the Reorganized Army

The corps areas occupied critical positions and had very significant responsibilities within the Army's new institutional command structure after 1920. Oliver saw this change as an opportunity to decentralize supervision of dental work. During the war, senior dental officers were assigned to the territorial departments, where they acted as assistants to the department surgeons and played a large role in the overall improvement and standardization of the dental service. According to Oliver's instructions of September 8, 1920, the new corps area dental surgeon, who was the assistant to the surgeon, had advisory, administrative, and supervisory responsibilities for the dental activities within each region and was also in charge of the headquarters dental clinic. This plan, however, did not find favor with some of the corps area commanders, who, when later required to reduce their headquarters, saw a supervising dental surgeon "as a surplus officer." The Medical Department reassigned each of these surplus officers to be in charge of a local clinic or even a dental ROTC unit, and was able to "retain him on duty within reach of the Surgeon for such service as may be required in consultation, supervision, or special administration." By the end of the decade, these more senior dental officers in the corps areas had become advisors to the surgeons on dental matters but still retained their other assignments. As such, they contributed to the increased efficiency of the dental service, despite the uncertainty of their positions and relationships to the corps area surgeons and their staffs.[4,10,32,48,60]

When the War Department set about rebuilding the peacetime field army, it began with a new divisional structure based on the lessons of the war. The new tables of organization of October 7, 1920, for the Army infantry division yielded 19,385 officers and enlisted soldiers. Unlike its wartime ancestors, this division fully incorporated dental surgeons and technicians within its tables of organization, thus eliminating one of the Dental Corps' struggles from the war years. Robert Oliver's involvement in this reshaping is unclear, but his experiences in France most likely made him a prominent actor.[12]

The new square infantry division of 1920, with two infantry brigades of two regiments each, looked much the same as its predecessors. However, the units were significantly smaller (3,755 in the 1917 infantry regiment versus 3,041 in 1920) except for the regimental medical detachment, which now numbered 11 officers and 84 enlisted soldiers as opposed to the former 4 officers and 33 enlisted soldiers. A medical regiment of 904 officers and enlisted soldiers (later increased to 962, including those attached to the division surgeon's office) replaced the former sanitary train, but was roughly the same size as its predecessor. The medical regiment had three ambulance and three hospital companies rather than four, and added three sanitary or collecting companies of litter-bearers to help the regimental medical detachments evacuate the sick and wounded.[12,61-63] The division dental organization in Table of Organization 90W (October 28, 1925) for the infantry division's medical service authorized 22 dental officers (Table 17-2).[61,63]

The restructuring that took place throughout the 1920s was mostly an academic exercise because Congress routinely provided only about half of what the War Department asked for in its yearly budgets. The June 30, 1922 act reduced infantry divisions, which had already been cut down as part of the overall mobilization planning with a peacetime strength of 10,910 soldiers, to 9,200 people. By the mid 1920s, much of the Regular Army ceased to exist as a functional military organization capable of any sustained combat operations, and the National Guard and ORC divisions were no better off. In July 1926, Brigadier General (later Lieutenant General) Hugh A Drum (1879–1951), then commander of the 1st Division, wrote to the commander of the Second Corps Area that "it is not an exaggeration to say that the division as a unit exists only on paper."[12]

During the early 1920s, the surgeon general's office developed tables of organization for all Army medical units that the War Department General Staff then reviewed and approved. The tables for some of the tactical medical units, for instance, the medical regiment and Army-level units, included organizational equipment, such as trucks, ambulances, and mule-drawn wagons. The shifting strength of the Army from 500,000 down to 137,000, and the requirement for peacetime and wartime tables for some units meant that tables of organization were often revised. For many of the units that existed just during wartime, only wartime tables were

TABLE 17-2

DIVISION DENTAL ORGANIZATION IN TABLE OF ORGANIZATION 90W (OCTOBER 28, 1925) FOR THE INFANTRY DIVISION'S MEDICAL SERVICE

Group	Number of Units	Major (Assistant to Commander, Division Surgeon)	Captains or Lieutenants per Unit in Hospital Companies	Total Number of Officers
Medical regiment	1	1	6	7
Infantry regiment	4	0	2	8
Artillery regiments	2	0	2	4
Engineer regiment	1	0	1	1
Division train	1	0	1	1
Quartermaster Corps special troops	1	0	1	1

Data sources: (1) Table 90 W—infantry regiment, division, 25 October 1925, and table 81 W—medical regiment, 28 October 1925. In: Medical Field Service School. 1928: tables of organization medical department. *The Army Medical Bulletin.* Carlisle Barracks, Pa: Medical Field Service School;1928(no. 22). (2) Stone FP. Duties of a dental officer and his relation to medical officers. *Milit Dent J.* 1922;5:147–151.

prepared. Other units, such as the medical regiment, had both peacetime and wartime tables. By 1924 tables of organization for 29 types of army, corps, and communications zone (line of communications or services of supply) field and hospital medical units were completed.

During 1926 the ongoing changes in Army strength and plans required that all pre-1925 tables based on a 280,000 troop force had to be revised. By 1928 official peacetime and wartime tables for all medical units were published following War Department approval. Not all medical units required dentists in their tables of organization. However, for those that did, the work of the 1920s established the official organization and authorization for officers and dental technicians and also created tables of basic allowances and equipment that underpinned doctrine as well as mobilization and war planning (Table 17-3).[4,32,42,45–47,59,64]

Dental Officers in the Organized Reserves

While the Regular Army Dental Corps strained to meet its postwar obligations, the DORC retained much of its wartime strength because 2,255 DORC officers leaving active duty from January through June 1919 opted for inactive reserve status. The DORC actually increased slightly from 3,665 in June 1919 to 3,699 in June 1920, including 59 African American dental surgeons.[3,4]

With the National Defense Act of 1920, the DORC became part of the new ORC, although the term "Dental Reserve Corps" was commonly used well into the 1930s. The new mobilization planning requirements placed an enormous burden on the Regular Army to organize and support the reserve components within each corps area and on the ORC to staff these units. Although the numbers constantly changed with the changing mobilization plans, the ORC dental commitment for full mobilization normally ran between 5,000 and 6,500 officers. The Dental Corps struggled to recruit sufficient personnel to maintain those numbers during the 1920s, but it never succeeded, despite repeated efforts to entice wartime reservists back to the colors (Table 17-4). In 1922 the requirement for dental officers in the ORC was 7,825, but only 3,710 were available. Four years later, in August 1926, Rhoades noted that 4,454 of 5,188 dental officers called for in War Department plans were then in the DORC. Actually, a reduction in the number of medical units in the ORC had resulted in a lower requirement and thus this more favorable situation. A small number of African American dental surgeons remained in the ORC to support African American units that would be mobilized.[4,10,32,33,42,45–48,59,65–69]

Dental officers in the ORC were assigned to authorized organizations of the mobilization Army of the United States during peacetime, such as medical regiments, surgical, evacuation, and general hospitals (formerly designated base hospitals), and medical detachments of infantry regiments. They were placed in three different assignment groups—general, branch, or territorial—of which the latter two were most important. The surgeon general selected the personnel in the branch assignment group and assigned them to special duties within the Medical Department. The territorial assignment group was the largest and included all DORC personnel not assigned to the other two groups. Officers assigned to troop duty, usually those in the junior grades, were in this group and came under the

TABLE 17-3

DENTAL SERVICE STRENGTH IN SELECTED UNIT TABLES OF
ORGANIZATION

Table of Organization Number	Date	Type of Unit (size)	Dental Corps Officers	Dental Technicians
81W	October 28, 1925	Medical regiment, division	1 major (division dental surgeon) 3 captains 3 first lieutenants	6
81P	April 10, 1925	Medical regiment, division	1 major/captain 1 captain 1 first lieutenant	1
90W	October 25, 1925	Medical service, infantry division	1 major 10 captains 11 first lieutenants	22
90P	June 15, 1928	Medical service, infantry division	1 major/captain 8 lieutenants	9
190W	October 14, 1926	Army Corps troops	1 lieutenant colonel 13 captains 11 first lieutenants	14
281 W	August 16, 1927	Army medical service	1 colonel 2 majors 27 captain 24 first lieutenants	54
283W`	June 15, 1928	Evacuation hospital (750 beds)	1 captain 1 first lieutenant	2
284W	February 23, 1927	Surgical hospital (250 beds)	1 first lieutenant	1
285W	February 27, 1927	Convalescent hospital (3,000 patients)	1 majors 2 captains 2 first lieutenants	5
290W	August 16, 1927	Army troops	1 colonel 2 majors 42 captains 52 first lieutenants	97
689W	April 2, 1926	Auxiliary surgical group—maxillofacial surgical units	25 majors (oral surgeons)	25

W: indicates wartime
P: indicates peacetime
Data Source: Medical Field Service School. 1928: tables of organization Medical Department. *The Army Medical Bulletin*. Carlisle Barracks, Pa: Medical Field Service School;1928 (no. 22).

TABLE 17-4

DENTAL OFFICERS IN THE ORGANIZED RESERVES, 1920–1929
(AS OF JUNE 30)

Year	Total Strength	White	African American	Gross Gain/Loss	Promotions
1920	3,699	3,640	59	713/76	0
1921	3,761	NR	NR	129/67	0
1922	3,760	3,697	63	70/71	0
1923	3,241	3,194	47	326/845	35
1924	3,055	3,006	49	645/831	198
1925	3,666	3,618	48	760/149	411
1926	4,133	4,082	51	540/73	41
1927	4,464	4,407	57	427/96	27
1928	4,647	NR	NR	471/288	9
1929	4,664	NR	NR	484/467	57

NR: not reported
Data sources: (1) Vail WD. The Dental Reserve Corps. *Dent Bull.* 1936;7:21. (2) Office of the Surgeon
General. *Annual Report of the Surgeon General.* Washington, DC: OTSG; 1920–1929.

command of the corps area to which the units belonged. To maintain their skills, annual individual and unit training was required, including 14-day summer training camps, which included CMTC, ROTC, or unit camps. From 1926 through 1929, an average of 404 reserve dental officers completed 14-day training camps each year.[45–48,70–72]

During the 1920s the number of nondivisional medical units in the ORC varied from a high of 1,077 in 1923 to 753 in 1927. All of these medical units in 1927 required 16,753 Medical Department officers, but only 7,100 were then assigned in the territorial assignment group. Staffing these ORC medical units remained a high priority, but not one that could necessarily be achieved.[33,42,45,46,59]

Dental Equipment and Supplies

When the war ended, the Medical Department was left with an enormous amount of modern medical and dental equipment and supplies, vastly in excess of any possible peacetime requirements. The wartime experience, especially in France, had indicated very serious problems with the portable dental outfit that had forced Oliver to develop emergency dental kits for the dentists with the front-line troops. One clear lesson from the war was that the field dental equipment was badly in need of an extensive overhaul. On the other hand, the permanent equipment in the stateside dental clinics was relatively new, generally in good condition, and far superior to anything the prewar dental officers ever had.

The first problem the Medical Department faced was what to do with the now-surplus, permanent dental equipment located in dental clinics and the supplies on posts and in warehouses all over the United States and in France. At least part of the answer was simple—the closure of many of the temporary camps and cantonments freed this modern equipment for transfer to and use on the Army's permanent posts, while the rest was sold as surplus. In regard to the situation, the 1920 *Annual Report of the Surgeon General* read, "for the first time in the corps' history, the installation of complete operating equipment and laboratory with modern electrical appliances have [*sic*] been made in each of the dental offices at the permanent posts of the Army."[4(p304)] The equipment procured to provide complete dental service for the soldiers of the wartime Army was of a much higher quality than ever before permitted and allowed Army dentists to provide "a higher class and greater number of operations." An added advantage of this change for the Army's dental officers was that the fully equipped post dental clinics ended the former bothersome, time-consuming practice of shipping their "bulky equipment by express from station to station" while on itinerary service.[4(p304)]

In October 1919 the War Department appointed a board of dental officers to revise the dental supply tables and to standardize the portable dental equipment, which had come under heavy criticism from the field and combat unit dentists as "too heavy and bulky to be readily transportable." The board carefully examined the requirements for equipment that could be used in both peace and war, experimented to reduce the "weight and bulk of all field equipment," and pushed for "the adoption of new types that will meet the requirements of war-service conditions."[4(p303)] Reviewing the wartime experience with the different sets of dental equipment and supplies, the board outlined the basic new tables of dental equipment:

> Base equipment for general hospitals, large infirmaries, and clinics; portable equipment for station hospitals, evacuation hospitals, and stations in the zone of communications; field equipment for use with organizations of an army in the field—army troops, corps troops, and sanitary trains; division equipment for use in combat divisions and emergency kits, being the personal equipment required for each dental officer on duty with combat organizations.[4(p303)]

As for the portable dental outfit for field use, the board reduced the wartime collection of six chests weighing 475 pounds and occupying 27 cubic feet to three chests weighing 209 pounds and occupying 8.7 cubic feet. They were designated Dental Chests A (dental engine), B (portable chair), and C (instruments and supplies), and were a marked improvement over the wartime outfits.[73,74]

By 1921 sufficient progress had been made in the study and development of new equipment and supplies to permit the authorization of new dental equipment for the individual dental officer, the dispensary, and the hospital company of the medical regiment. The individual equipment consisted of two aluminum cases, A and B, carried on the belt and by shoulder strap, respectively, at all times. All dental officers below the grade of lieutenant colonel were to carry Case A (later renamed the Dental Officer's Case), and all enlisted dental technicians below the grade of technical sergeant carried Case B (later renamed the Dental Technician's Case). Based on the extemporized wartime rolls in the AEF's emergency dental kits, the cases' contents would enable dentists to render emergency first aid and dental relief anywhere on the battlefield. For the dispensary and hospital company equipment, the old portable dental outfit was slimmed down to be more easily transportable but still adequate enough to meet "the demands for simple operations of reparative dentistry" for the former and "for the construction of maxillary splints" for the latter.[10(p122)]

During 1922 the process for the development of medical and dental equipment and supplies changed significantly with the establishment of the coordination, organization, and equipment division in the surgeon general's office and with the opening of the Medical Field Service School and the Medical Department Equipment Laboratory at Carlisle Barracks under Major John P Fletcher, MC. The development of dental equipment now fell within the context of research and development that was coordinated from the surgeon general's office and closely linked to the ongoing development of tables of organization, equipment, and supply. Among its many other projects, the equipment lab turned to the development of various new field dental kits.[32,45,74,75]

After some study during the mid 1920s, the dental division determined the equipment, instruments, and supplies that were required for a new field dental operating outfit, the dental officer's and dental private's kits, a field dental laboratory, and a maxillofacial set for extended field operations. With the dental division's lists in hand, the equipment laboratory designed a light field operating set in which all of the required items neatly fit into a single, easily transportable

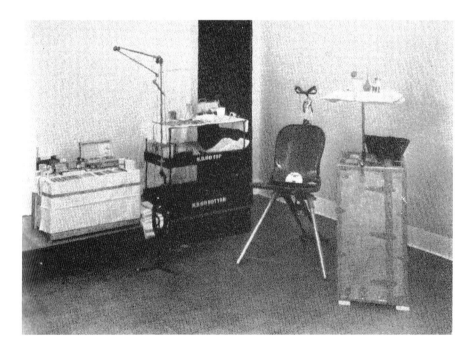

*Portable dental outfit developed at the Medical Field Service School
and used in the 1930s and World War II.
Photograph: Courtesy of the Medical Field Service School, Carlisle Barracks, Pennsylvania.*

Medical Department chest. In 1926 the lab announced the successful development of the new field dental operating set, Medical Department Chest Number 60. Along with test copies of the officer's and private's kits that the laboratory fit into newly designed canvas pouches, trial versions of Chest Number 60 were sent to the 2nd Division at Fort Sam Houston, where they were successfully tested during the Eighth Corps Area's 1927 summer maneuvers. The field dental laboratory set (Medical Department Chests numbers 61 and 62) and a special maxillofacial set (Medical Department Chest number 63) were finished and tested shortly thereafter, but in time were included, along with the three other sets, in the Medical Department's new medical supply table (AR 40-1710) published on April 23, 1928.[45–47, 73,75]

In an article titled "Research-Development of Medical Field Equipment" that appeared in the December 1929 issue of *Military Surgeon*, John Fletcher provided a fuller description of the field dental operating set:

> As the laboratory's activities have not been confined to the division area, neither have they been confined to equipment for the medical service alone. A field dental set has been produced which packs in one standard container. This is known as MD 60. Packed within the container are a table board, two trays with spacer brackets, and a folding dental chair. The old portable dental chair weighed approximately 100

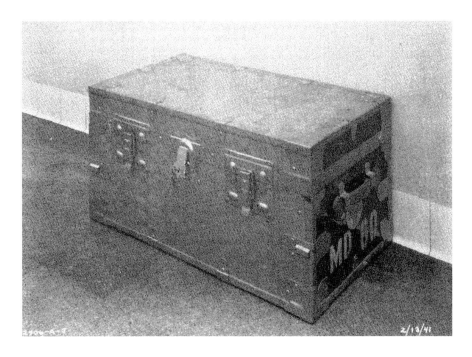

Medical Department Chest No. 60, which contains
the portable dental outfit for battalion or regimental dispensary.
Developed at the Medical Field Service School, Carlisle Barracks, Pennsylvania.
Photograph: Courtesy of the Medical Field Service School.

pounds and occupied three cubic feet of space, many of its parts were cast iron, it was easily broken and difficult to erect. The portable chair in this new set occupies just one cubic foot of space, weighs twenty-two and one-half pounds and there are no loose pieces. It can be set up ready for use in one minute. A portable dental engine of the foot-type is carried in one of the trays, the other of which carries instruments and supplies. The container when empty is stood on end and to it is attached an instrument bracket shelf so that from this one container weighing 160 pounds, can be erected a dental chair, a dental engine, an instrument table, and an instrument stand.[76(pp839–840)]

In addition to their personal dental cases, each dental officer and technician in a tactical unit also had a recently approved dental officer's kit and dental private's (later enlisted man's) kit. These kits, carried in large canvas pouches over the shoulder, were updated and remodeled versions of the emergency kits carried on the western front in 1918. The kits complemented each other and held the basic instruments, medicines, and supplies that the dental officer and dental technician would need to treat emergency cases in combat when the field dental operating outfit was not available.[74,75] With only small modifications, all of the field dental kits developed and tested at the Medical Department equipment laboratory in the 1920s saw extensive and successful worldwide service during World War II.[74]

While the development of new field dental equipment progressed, the dental division also had to deal with the stocks of dental supplies already on hand. The Army decided to use what was needed now rather than procure new supplies, store in medical depots around the country what was usable in the future, and dispose of the dated, poorer quality, and excess that was beyond reasonable future requirements. The cuts of the early 1920s only aggravated the policy of using war surplus supplies until they were largely exhausted in 1925.[10,32,42]

Supply requirements for various mobilization scenarios were studied at the surgeon general's office and Medical Field Service School as new tables of equipment, allowance, supply were prepared to support the reorganized Army of the 1920s. Once approved by the War Department, these items were procured as funds allowed. This meant large quantities of modern dental equipment and supplies had to be procured and stored in depots to meet normal requirements and to be available as war reserve stocks for possible mobilization. Unlike much of the previous wartime procurement, the supply and dental Divisions drew up much tighter technical specifications with the Bureau of Standards beginning in 1924 and worked for standardization of equipment and supplies to assure that any items procured consistently met Dental Corps and Medical Department quality standards. By 1927 tables of equipment for many of the principal tactical and communications zone medical units, which included their dental equipment and supplies, were completed and had received the War Department's approval for procurement.[33,42,45–47,59,73]

New Standard Classification of Dental Cases

Army dentistry was increasingly focused on prevention in the early 1920s. A key to success on this front and for the "health conservation" that the surgeon general encouraged was to have a better understanding of the dental and oral conditions of the Army's officers and soldiers and an accepted system for classifying their dental and oral health. On January 7, 1921, the surgeon general issued

Circular Letter No. 1, titled "Standard Classification of Dental Cases," which superseded all existing classification systems. Circular No. 1 established a "standardized classification of dental cases and a uniform method of procedure in the treatment of routine cases." Dental cases in the Army were now classified into four groups based on their need for treatment—all cases requiring treatment were in Classes I–III, which also set the order of priority of treatment, and cases requiring no treatment were in Class IV. The circular outlined a sequence of treatment, with all emergency cases to be treated first (Class I), then "all cases favorable for preventive dentistry" (Class II), and finally those needing "prolonged treatment and constructive dentistry" (Class III) (Table 17-5).[10,77]

The classification scheme was based on the "theory of furnishing the greatest amount of service to the largest clientele." As the 1921 annual report explained:

TABLE 17-5

CONDITIONS INCLUDED IN ARMY DENTAL CLASSES

Class I: Cases requiring immediate attention (emergency cases)	Class II: Cases requiring early attention (favorable cases for preventive dentistry)	Class III: Cases requiring extended attention (constructive dentistry)	Class IV: Cases not requiring attention
• Traumatic injuries • Acute infections • Extractions • Salivary calculus (extensive) • Cavities with extensive decay approaching the pulp, cavities involving the pulp • Defects not listed above, but of a nature requiring emergency treatment	• Minor filling operations • Defective fillings (except root canal fillings) • Inflammatory conditions of the soft tissues • Extractions (deferred) • Prophylactic treatments • Defects not listed above, but cases favorable for preventive dentistry, including orthodontia	• Routine filling operations and restorations • Artificial restorations required as a result of traumatic injury • Periapical infections, commonly classed as focal infections • Defective root canal fillings and tooth restorations • Extractions (resultant) • crowns, bridges, and dentures • Defects not listed above but requiring extensive treatment	N/A

Data source: Darnall CR. Office of the Surgeon General, circular letter no. 1, "Standard classification of dental cases," 7 January 1921. *Milit Dent J*. 1922;5:104–105.

> The methods and procedure outlined were the result of careful study, in which the service recommended was in direct harmony and consonance with modern methods of dental practice in civil life. The instructions issued are comprehensive and definite and provide for sufficient latitude to accommodate individual initiative in the professional treatment of cases of varying symptoms, sequelae, etc.[10]

The new classification standards were part of a larger system of examination and treatment that was designed to inspect and classify every officer and soldier in each command and record the information on Form 79, "Register of Dental Patient." Initially, the dental officer was required to complete a dental survey or inspection of his command and classify all cases according to the standards. After that, a plan of treatment could be initiated that provided the priority for treatment, beginning with patients in classes I and II.[77]

The exact origins of this new standard classification system are not clear. Various systems of classifying and reporting on dental patients had been used since 1901. During the war, each recruit passing through the recruit depot was surveyed and classified "to insure the greatest number of recruits possible being placed in a dentally fit condition prior to their assignment to organizations. This is done primarily to improve the general health of the recruit, and secondary, to lessen the duties imposed upon dental surgeons at posts or stations throughout the country."[4(p306)]

Before the recruits left the depot, they were given as much dental work as possible. The dental surgeon filled out a form detailing the administered treatment and what remained to be done, then the form was sent to the dental surgeon at the next duty station. Similar surveys were conducted on each patient that was admitted to a general hospital, either at the dental clinic or bedside, "with a view of primarily eliminating all oral or dental conditions that may have bearing upon the general pathology of the case." This process enhanced the professional cooperation of medical and dental officers and the overall care of the patients.[4(pp305–306)]

Annual Dental Surveys of Officer and Enlisted Personnel as a Preventive Dentistry Effort

The 1920s saw the implementation of more detailed annual dental examinations, the use of the standard classification system for dental cases, the collection and recording of dental and oral conditions found, and an analysis of this data as part of a preventive medicine and dentistry program. The data collection began with Army commissioned and warrant officers in 1924. That year, the data revealed "a very unfavorable condition among the officer personnel." Dental officers were "directed to make further efforts toward a better dental condition among our more permanent military personnel." In 1925 the data collected indicated improved dental conditions among officers. However, the officers represented only a small part of the total Army, so plans were developed to extend the annual examinations and data collection to enlisted personnel. The tables of organization reasoned "in this way the dental condition of military personnel will more accurately be determined and dental attendance can be directed with more beneficial results."[42,59]

The soldiers' health and readiness remained the primary concern.

As in the past, the aim of the Dental Corps continues to be preventive dentistry and dental officers have been encouraged to teach and practice prevention at every opportunity. The cooperation of medical and dental officers in the removal of all foci of infection suspected of adversely affecting the health of the patient, continues to be routine in Army hospitals. This team work in group practice of medicine constitutes no small part towards maintaining the non-effective rate at a minimum.[59]

The first dental survey examined 82,751 Army enlisted soldiers and lasted from January through June 1926. These surveys were much more cursory than the annual officer examinations and probably undercounted those in need of dental care. Unlike officer personnel who continued to show improving dental conditions after the first dental examinations in 1924, improvements among the enlisted personnel over the following years were more difficult to track because those soldiers were less permanent in the Army. The 1929 survey indicated that 45,733 enlisted soldiers (42.55%) fell into classes I and II, requiring immediate or early treatment, and showed little or no improvement over 1926 (42%), 1927 (40%), and 1928 (42.04%). Based on data collected, the 1926 annual report concluded that about 50% of Army personnel were "continually in need of dental service" and this held true for remaining years of the decade.[45,46,48]

These annual examinations and surveys were carried out throughout the remainder of the 1920s and showed steadily improved conditions for officers, with Class IV cases increasing from 42% in 1924 to 72.68% in 1929, and Class I dropping from 12% in 1924 to 3.21% in 1929. Enlisted personnel showed only slight improvements in classes I, III, and IV, but a small decline in Class II from 1926 through 1929. This data provided a clear indication of where preventive dentistry and education efforts had to be focused (Table 17-6, Table 17-7).

Army Regulations—a New Approach

After the war, the War Department changed its entire approach to Army Regulations (AR), which governed the Army's every activity. Since the 19th century, the regulations were published as individual paragraphs in general orders or changes to existing paragraphs and in an overall annual compendium of all regulations and called "Regulations for the Army of the United States" (or simply, "Army Regulations"). During World War I ARs became a tangle of frequent revisions and changes. In June 1919 the Army embarked on a new system of easily compiled and revisable loose leaf pamphlets, with different departments and subjects each receiving a specific AR number within the system. All Medical Department regulations were to be published in the AR 40 series that replaced all Medical Department paragraphs in former ARs. The new regulations were to include "all regulations, orders, circulars, etc., which are of permanent application and which relate primarily to administration of the Medical Department." They were written and coordinated during the early 1920s and began appearing in the middle of the decade.[10,33,45,59,78,79]

The new format of the ARs was part of a much larger process that also included

TABLE 17-6

DENTAL CLASSIFICATION OF ARMY PERSONNEL BASED ON ANNUAL PHYSICAL EXAMINATIONS OF OFFICER PERSONNEL (OFFICERS AND WARRANT OFFICERS), 1924–1929 (AS PERCENTAGE OF THOSE EXAMINED)

	1924	1925	1926	1927	1928	1929
Class I	12	8	7	5	4.4	3.21
Class II	30	24	22	20	20.02	16.14
Class III	14	10	8	7	5.99	7.97
Class IV	42	58	63	68	69.59	72.68

Data sources: (1) Office of the Surgeon General. *Annual Report of the Surgeon General*. Washington, DC: OTSG; 1925. (2) Office of the Surgeon General. *Annual Report of the Surgeon General*. Washington, DC: OTSG; 1929.

replacing and rescinding the *Manual of the Medical Department*, which provided everything from medical doctrine to tables of supply. Much of this revision was done at the recently opened Medical Field Service School under the direction of the surgeon general's office, often with dental officers specially assigned. With the publication of AR 40-1710, "Medical Department Supply Table and Price List, Medical Supplies," on April 23, 1928, completely new and updated lists replaced the old and often outdated medical, dental, and veterinary tables of supply and equipment in the *Manual of the Medical Department*.[59,75]

Two of the three most important dental regulations appeared on October 10, 1925, when AR 40-15, "Medical Department. Dental Corps—General Provisions," and AR 40-510, "Medical Department, Dental Attendance" were published. The third appeared on October 20 when AR 40-1010, "Medical Department. Dental Reports, Returns, and Records," was published.[80–82] The January 1922 regulation revisions pertaining to commissioning and promotion in the Dental Corps were published in the series on personnel as AR 605-15, "Commissioned Officers. Appointment in the Dental Corps, Regular Army" on November 20, 1925, and in AR 605-60, "Commissioned Officers. Subjects of Professional Examination for Promotion in the Dental Corps, Regular Army" on August 16, 1926. AR 40-15 detailed the functions and structure of the dental service, the duties of dental officers and enlisted technicians, and the responsibilities of dental clinics.[45,80–84] Under AR 40-510, dental attendance was clearly defined:

> The term "dental attendance" as used in these regulations embraces the medical, surgical, and mechanical treatment of oral diseases, injuries, and deficiencies that come with the field of dental and oral surgery as commonly practiced by the dental profession, the advice relating thereto and the oral examinations connected therewith given to persons by a dental officer or a civilian dentist. It is that phase of medical attendance which, on account of its technical nature, requires the services of a dentist.[81]

TABLE 17-7

DENTAL CLASSIFICATION OF ARMY PERSONNEL BASED ON ANNUAL
DENTAL SURVEYS OF ENLISTED PERSONNEL, 1926*–1929
(AS PERCENTAGE OF THOSE EXAMINED)

	1926	1927	1928	1929
Class I	17	16	16.27	13.83
Class II	25	24	25.77	28.72
Class III	9	8	7.54	6.22
Class IV	49	52	50.42	51.23

* Data collection began in January–June 1926 and continued each January–June thereafter.
Data sources: (1) Office of the Surgeon General. *Annual Report of the Surgeon General.* Washington, DC: OTSG; 1925. (2) Office of the Surgeon General. *Annual Report of the Surgeon General.* Washington, DC: OTSG; 1929.

This regulation included the provisions of Circular No. 1 of January 7, 1921, on dental classification as well as the fee schedule for all procedures performed by civilian dentists within the United States.[81] AR 40-1010, "Medical Department. Dental Reports, Returns, and Records," specified all of the requirements for monthly dental reports (Form 57 MD), the maintenance of the register of dental patients (Form 79 MD), and the expenditure of special materials (Form 18b MD) as well as the standard terms and authorized abbreviations for diagnosis and treatment that would be used on Form 79.[82]

Medical Field Service School

Surgeon General Merritte W Ireland believed recent wartime experience clearly demonstrated that realistic field training was essential for all Medical Department officers—including dentists and veterinarians. With that in mind, on April 28, 1920, Ireland requested that the adjutant general turn over the US military reservation at Carlisle Barracks, Pennsylvania, to be "permanently assigned to the Medical Department for use as a field school." Carlisle Barracks, which was on the site of the former Carlisle Indian School, then housed General Hospital No. 31, established in the fall of 1918 as one of the first rehabilitation hospitals to care for the sick and wounded returning from France. The hospital had reached its peak of activity in 1919 and the number of patients steadily declined thereafter. Once General Hospital No. 31 closed, Ireland's survey indicated that it would be an excellent site for the school. Many of the existing facilities from the Indian school and the general hospital were already suitable for use or could be easily converted, and Carlisle's location was convenient for field training in the nearby mountains and at Gettysburg.[85–88]

The War Department concurred and on June 30, 1920, the Army turned Carlisle Barracks over to Surgeon General Ireland to establish a school of instruction in the medical field service. On December 23, 1920, War Department Circular No. 419 officially designated the new school as the "Medical Field Service School," an Army special service school. Within the Medical Department in the years before World War II, however, it was more often called the West Point of the Medical Department. Courses stressing military responsibility and field duties were to be conducted for both officers and enlisted soldiers. The officers' courses were for Medical Department officers of the Regular Army, ORC, and National Guard. Three courses were planned: the basic course for newly commissioned officers of the Regular Army; the advanced course for the higher grade regular officers; and the field officers' course for the National Guard and ORC. Newly commissioned Dental Corps first lieutenants were to be placed on active duty status in the ORC. They were then ordered to the Medical Field Service School at Carlisle Barracks, where they received 4 months of intensive training in "field service activities of the Medical Department," with "special emphasis" on field dental service. A noncommissioned officers' course for selected enlisted soldiers of all three components was also established. During the summers from mid June through July, the faculty and staff, in coordination with the 1st Medical Regiment (also stationed at Carlisle Barracks), was fully engaged in training regimental medical detachments, sanitation units, medical regiments of the ORC, and students in medical, dental, and veterinary units of the ROTC. In addition, officers and noncommissioned officers of the National Guard and reserve and hospital units of the ORC were to come to Carlisle Barracks for their annual instruction and training. The new Medical Field Service School was given the responsibility of providing comprehensive, career-oriented military training never before entrusted to any single entity within the Medical Department in peacetime.[70,86,87,89]

Although competing for the limited faculty, facilities, equipment, space, and time at Carlisle Barracks, these training programs were part of a carefully thought-out concept for the military and professional training, education, and development of the officers of the Army Medical Department from the time of their initial entry into service. The Medical Field Service School's basic course for all incoming officers was originally intended to be the first link in a career-long chain, and it was supposed to be completed before any other schooling. The Army Medical School had been preparing Medical Corps officers for military medicine since 1893. The surgeon general now planned to add to it new Army Dental and Veterinary Schools, the Army School of Nursing (established in 1918), and Walter Reed General Hospital, all located at the Walter Reed complex in Washington, to form the Army Medical Center. When the center opened in August 1923, it was the heart of the Army Medical Department's Professional Educational System (later redesignated the medical department schools). Medical, dental, and veterinary graduates of the Medical Field Service School's basic course were to move on to these professional technical and clinical schools. Thus, within a year, the new officers completed the sequence of the basic officer's course, including field training, and their basic professional course, and were ready for their first assignments in the Army Medical Department.[20,32,33,90]

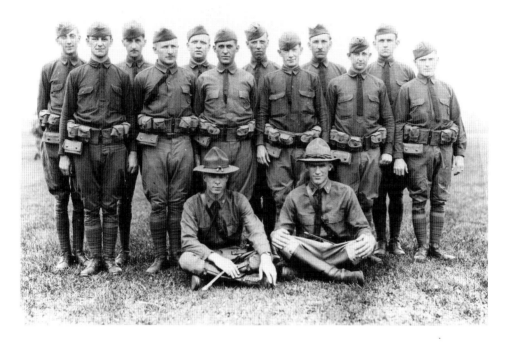

Reserve Officer Training Corps Summer Camp 1922. Saint Louis University Dental ROTC at Medical Field Service School, Carlisle Barracks, Pennsylvania. Photograph: Courtesy of the National Library of Medicine.

The first class of student officers, which consisted of 50 medical and 20 dental officers, reported for duty on May 27, 1921, and classes began on June 1, 1921.[89] The commandant, Colonel Percy M Ashburn, MC, greeted the first class with these remarks: "Bear in mind that this is a new school, that it has not yet had the shaking down which comes from practice and experience, that our schedules are yet untried and subject to revision, that with your class the course must be shortened and condensed, that the equipment is not complete, and that we are not yet what we hope to become."[91,92]

Although not obvious at first, one of the most critical positions for the Dental Corps was that of the senior dental representative assigned to the new Medical Field Service School. The first Dental Corps officer to hold this post from 1921 to 1925 was Lieutenant Colonel Frank P Stone, DC, one of the original contract dental surgeons who had extensive field and staff supervisory experience in the AEF during the war and would later serve as chief of the Dental Corps from 1934 to 1938. To better understand the training, Stone completed the special field training and basic course at the Medical Field Service School in the summer of 1921, along with the new Dental ROTC professors of military science and tactics. As the Dental Corps' mentor and advisor for all active, reserve, and National Guard dental officers who passed through the school, Stone and his successors gained a unique knowledge of the Corps' personnel and had a crucial role in shaping their careers. With his years of experience dating back to the trails of Mindanao with Jack Pershing, Stone brought a very realistic perspective to his new duties—to prepare all dental officers for possible combat in close cooperation with other members of the Medical Department, especially the medical officers. Stone was responsible for all the dental instruction at the school and in the numerous other courses offered there, including the Medical Department short basic course for reserve and National Guard officers.[10,32,92–95] In an article in the June 1923 issue of *Military Dental Journal*, Stone wrote that this course was absolutely essential to prepare reserve and National Guard dental officers for combat operations:

> My personal experience in the Army in the last 22 years convinces me that dental officers can not function to any great extent in a strictly professional capacity in an active campaign with troops, and particularly during combat. Their services are valuable when these troops are resting or are awaiting combat. They must be with the troops, so they should know how to function when the troops go into battle. Many surgeons deserve credit for using their dental personnel properly in combat during the late war, and many dental officers deserve credit for using their own initiative in helping out in an emergency, but there were many also who were censured, ridiculed, relieved from duty, and one case reported court-martialed for failure to function properly during combat. This should not happen again, and their training here at the Medical Field Service School is the remedy. Dental officers should know what to do and medical officers should know what to expect of their dental officers during active warfare, and neither should be left to their own initiative to act at so critical a time. . . . It is, therefore, the duty of dental officers who wish to serve their country in war to know something about their duties and to receive instruction to fit them for their best service.[96(p76)]

Among his many duties, Stone also set up and administered voluntary correspondence courses for all dental officers in the National Guard and ORC, which were part of the larger program of Army correspondence courses that began in 1923–1924. These courses covered military dentistry as well as a wide range of other military subjects, such as Army organization, administration, and tactics, and were designed specifically "to provide the citizen soldier with an opportunity for systematic and practical training and instruction which will fit him to perform the active duties of his branch pertaining to his present rank, and which will also prepare him for promotion to the higher grades." Major Frederick R Wunderlich, completed the basic course in 1921 prior to his Dental ROTC assignment at the University of Minnesota and later replaced Stone from 1925 to 1929. In 1927 he wrote of the importance of the National Guard and ROTC training, including the correspondence courses,[32,42,97–99] drawing a rare but crucial distinction between the dental officer and the dental surgeon:

> There is, in the final analysis, but one objective in all military training. The attainment of the efficiency standard or competency of the individual to fill the position which he holds or for which he is being trained is the end sought. . . . The maintenance of professional ideals fostered by contact with professional societies and the daily practice of his profession will assure the Army of well-qualified dental surgeons. This professional

skill, supplemented by the indicated training of a military nature, constitutes the requirements of a dental officer as distinguished from a dental surgeon. The ability of the individual dental surgeon to make available his full potential value, both professional and military, is the end sought in training and the attainment of this end marks the competent dental officer.[99(p9)]

On July 7, 1923, the Medical Field Service School began a 15-day training course for 56 reserve officers, 9 of whom were dental. The program was similar to ROTC, except the students were housed in barracks rather than tents. The group of 56 was split into four sections to simulate a regimental medical detachment, an ambulance company, a sanitary company and battalion, and a hospital company. Lectures were followed by practical demonstrations, during which students carried out the work required of these units during actual combat. During the practical exercises, the simulated wounded were brought to the battalion aid station by the litter-bearer squads of the regimental medical detachment. They were treated at the station, having splints adjusted and bandages placed, and hemorrhage and shock were put under control. Next, the patients were evacuated to the collecting station operated by the sanitary company and battalion toward the rear, transported by either the ambulances of the ambulance company or sent back as walking cases to the hospital (operated by the hospital company). From the hospital company the wounded were sent to the evacuation hospital even further removed from the front lines.[100]

In addition to this general training, the dental officers were given instruction in the organization and administration of the Dental Corps, dental field administration, and "methods employed in treating and evacuating jaw casualties." Casualty management was covered and reinforced through conferences, exercises, demonstrations, examinations, and critiques by faculty dental officers.[89,101]

It was not until the mid-1920s that the various training programs at the Medical Field Service School were brought into line with War Department guidance for Army service schools on the scheduling of the officer basic (January 2–June 30) and advanced (September 15–December 15) courses, the professional courses at the Army Medical Center's schools were coordinated with those at the Medical Field Service School, and everything was then specified in published Army Regulations. The "shaking down" that Percy Ashburn had mentioned in 1921 consumed a good deal of time and attention during the first several years. Some of the shortcomings in the instructional courses and of the instructors themselves were identified and soon corrected. Others, such as the weather in the area of Carlisle Barracks that hampered field training during the winter months, could only be remedied through major scheduling changes. Accordingly, the Medical Department requested and received the War Department's approval in May 1924 to switch the Medical Field Service School basic course to the months of February through May, aligning the training with existing ARs and allowing field training in the more favorable spring weather. This change made it necessary to realign the basic professional courses at the Army medical, dental, and veterinary schools at the Army Medical Center from January through June to September through December. As a result, in 1924 the professional basic courses were offered from September 2, 1924, to February 10, 1925, after which the graduates were ordered to the Medical Field Service School basic course beginning February 11.[88, 102–107] Thus, the original officer training sequence of 1921 was reversed, with the field training following the professional training.

When finalized, courses at the Medical Field Service School and the Army Medical Center's schools formed an interlocking, functioning system that endured until the eve of World War II. The annual programs coordinated the training, dental, and veterinary divisions at the surgeon general's office, the surgeons of the corps areas, the ORC and National Guard Bureau, the schools of the Army Medical Center, and Walter Reed General Hospital. From approximately September 1 to January 31, the new appointees and "inexperienced junior officers" of the three corps attended the professional basic courses at the Army medical, dental, and veterinary schools in Washington. They then moved to Carlisle Barracks for the Medical Field Service School basic course, which was given from approximately February 1 through May 31, a schedule that allowed realistic field training in the late spring months. Field duties during the summer training cycle of June and July for the National Guard, units of the ORC, CMTC, and ROTC then followed. For more senior officers, the advanced course at the Medical Field Service School was offered from October 15 to December 15, 1926. The advanced courses at the dental and veterinary Schools, when ready and offered, coincided with that of the Army Medical School, which were from February 1 through May 31, because they all shared the limited faculty and facilities of the medical school and Walter Reed General Hospital.[4,10,32,33,42,59,45–48,68,102–105,107]

During the 1920s a total of 84 Dental Corps officers graduated from the Medical Field Service School; 83 completed the basic course, but only one completed the advanced course (Table 17-8). That sole Dental Corps officer was Colonel Rex Rhoades, who attended from the course from October 15 through December 15, 1927.[32,33,42,45–48,59,98(p820),108]

By 1924 Oliver and the Dental Corps were already well pleased with the results of this training and reported:

> The value of this basic instruction to the dental officer can not be overestimated. It affords him a comprehensive knowledge of the Army, the mission of the Medical Department, the integral function of the Dental Corps, and tends to divorce him from the narrow sphere of professional activity to which he is inclined to gravitate in the daily routine of office practice.[42(p184)]

The Army Dental School

A new and critical link in the chain of professional development for dental officers was the more advanced, postgraduate-level Army Dental School located on the grounds of Walter Reed General Hospital in Washington, DC. William HG Logan had strongly advocated such a school in February 1919, and many leading Army dentists had thought about and discussed it since 1901. John Sayre Marshall and Robert Oliver, both dental educators, had originally conceived of an Army dental school during the initial meetings of the dental examining board in February 1901. As Oliver later related, "The primal reason actuating the original thought

TABLE 17-8

DENTAL CORPS GRADUATES OF THE MEDICAL FIELD SERVICE
SCHOOL, 1921–1929

	1921–1922	1923	1924	1925	1926	1927	1928	1929	Total per Course
Basic Course	22	13	9	6	8	7	9	9	83
Advanced Course*	N/A	N/A	N/A	N/A	0	1	0	0	1
Total per year	22	13	9	6	8	8	9	9	84

*First offered in 1926.
Data sources: Office of the Surgeon General. *Annual Report of the Surgeon General*. Washington, DC: OTSG; 1922, 1924–1930.

of these two dental educators was the manifest necessity of preparing and training young dental men, just entering the Corps, to meet the new conditions of life—physical, mental and professional—in which they were suddenly thrust."[90(p59)]

In the years after 1901, dental officers continued to discuss the need for a school as a means for "standardization of methods of conducting military dental practice at home and with troops in the field" as well as for "a standardization in the preparation of reports and returns." Oliver had established the first such school for dental officers at Fort Bliss, Texas, during the Mexican Punitive Expedition in 1916, and created similar dental training schools in the 1st, 2nd, 26th, 32nd, and 42nd Divisions of the AEF until the Army Sanitary School at Langres became operational in December 1917. The establishment of the dental school in connection with the medical officers' training camps at Fort Riley, Kansas, and Camp Greenleaf, Georgia, and the success of their graduates during the war confirmed the wisdom of a school for Dental Corps officers. Upon his return to Washington in September 1919, Oliver became the leading advocate for this new school and guided its creation through the surgeon general's office and general staff in 1920–1921.[90,107]

On January 6, 1922, the secretary of war finally authorized the new Army Dental School as a special service school of the War Department. Its mission was to:

teach newly appointed dental officers the practical application of approved methods of professional procedure in the military service, to furnish post-graduate courses in advanced military dental surgery to members of the Dental Corps, to provide an organization for the investigation, study and research of dental problems, a source of authoritative information on professional matters, and the training of enlisted personnel to meet the requirements of the dental service.[109(p18)]

Walter Reed General Hospital was selected as the site of the new school because of its large dental clinic, expert faculty, and the advanced bacteriological, pathological, and chemical laboratories of the Army Medical School, which was to be relocated from its current building in Washington to a new building on the hospital's grounds in 1923.[32]

Addressing the school's formal opening on January 9, 1922, Major General Merritte W Ireland, the surgeon general, told the students and faculty of the Army Dental School:

> I trust every officer here appreciates the importance of this hour, when the first session of the Army Dental School is begun. I predict this event is epoch-making in the future of the Dental Corps and that its importance will grow as the years go by. . . . I am sure the course here will be equal to, if not better, than any post-graduate instruction you could receive in any city in the United States. . . . You are starting a Dental Corps School which will enable you to get together every year, a liberal number of your officers will learn to know each other, will establish a community of interest and thereby develop a pride in the service which will be of inestimable value. . . . I urge upon you to make the most of this vast opportunity here for advancement, which will be of the greatest value to you through your service. And do not forget that you are a part of the medical profession. The advances made during the last few years have demonstrated your outstanding value to group practice and we all realize that we are more and more dependent upon each other. I think it most unfortunate that dentistry should have been taught for more than eighty years as a separate profession. The great opportunities for advancement in the means of relieving suffering humanity lie in coordinated activities.[109(pp19–21)]

Ireland's speech strongly endorsed not only the Army Dental School but also the role of the Dental Corps within the Army Medical Department. Speaking at the 1923 graduation, Oliver also stressed the uniqueness and potential contributions of the school:

> The Army Dental School is the first school in the world to teach the new specialty of military dentistry and is the first to incorporate in its curriculum the full courses in the basic sciences of medicine. Its teaching staff is composed equally of selected medical and dental officers of the Army. The benefits derived from the dental school shall not be confined only to the Dental Corps and its clientele in the military service, but promises to extend to the dental profession and, in a larger measure, to our great citizen body.[90(pp64–65)]

While Ireland seemed to share Oliver's opinion of the school, the tougher challenge was converting Ireland's words and Oliver's vision for the Army Dental School into reality. For that, Oliver turned to Colonel Seibert D Boak, DC, the first commandant (later designated director), who was also in charge of the dental clinic at Walter Reed General Hospital, and Colonel Raymond E Ingalls, DC, the assistant to the commandant (later executive officer) and head of the department of prostheses. Boak, one of the original contract dental surgeons of 1901, had gained significant experience in educational work when he successfully directed the dental section of the Army Sanitary School at Langres, France, for its duration from January to December 1918 (for his work, AEF General Headquarters awarded Boak a Distinguished Service Medal in 1923). The building housing the new school was a Walter Reed hospital ward remodeled to meet the needs of the school, which would be remodeled again later in the decade. It contained lecture halls, a library, a museum, conference rooms, and offices for the commandant and his assistant.[109–112]

According to the *Annual Report of the Surgeon General* for 1922, the opening of the Army Dental School corrected some of "the greatest handicaps in the development of the dental service" and was "one of the most important events in the history of the Dental Corps." Except for a brief period during World War I, the Dental Corps lacked a location and program to train newly commissioned dental officers in "their military duties and the adaptation of professional procedures to an expeditious and satisfactory military dental practice." Without this training, most newly commissioned Dental Corps officers, who had little or no familiarity with the Army, were assigned directly to stations without other Army dentists. These stations had little contact with the civilian dental community that would have permitted the new dental officers to maintain their professional dental skills. In combination with the Medical Field Service School, the new Army Dental School removed these shortcomings in professional development and education and promised "the maintenance of a highly trained commissioned personnel in the Dental Corps of the Army."[32]

The Army Dental School leadership changed three times during the remaining years of the 1920s, but each new commandant brought significant experience that improved both the school and the dental clinic at Walter Reed. In September 1923 Colonel Franklin F Wing, DC, another original contract dental surgeon, became the school's commandant and chief of the Walter Reed Dental Clinic, replacing Seibert Boak, who was reassigned to the Philippines. Lieutenant Colonel Raymond E Ingalls, DC, now reduced in rank due to the officer reductions, remained the executive officer until June 1925.[59,112,113] In the summer of 1926 Major William S Rice, DC, who Oliver dispatched to set up the initial dental school at the 1st Division in September 1917 and who later established the dental section of the Army Sanitary School at Langres in December 1917, assumed the duties as the director. Captain Clyde W Scogin, DC, was the executive officer until February 1928, when Major Oscar P Snyder, a future Dental Corps chief (1954–1956), replaced him.[45] On July 1, 1929, Lieutenant Colonel Frank LK Laflamme, who had briefly held the post of Dental Corps chief in 1919, became the director of the Army Dental School, replacing Rice when he resigned from the Army in November. Laflamme remained in that position until August 4, 1932.[114–116]

Students admitted to the basic course were primarily officers of the Dental Corps. From 1922 to 1924 those who had first satisfactorily completed the Medical Field Service School at Carlisle Barracks usually attended. That prerequisite changed when the Medical Field Service School began to follow completion of the Army Dental School. Qualified National Guard and ORC dental officers were also admitted, as were foreign dental officers by invitation of the chief of staff or under regulations prescribed by the War Department. The surgeon general selected the officers to take the course on the recommendation of the Dental Corps chief. National Guard eligibility was determined by the provisions of section 16 of the Act of January 21, 1903, as amended by the Act of May 27, 1908 (35 Stats, 402).[59,109]

According to the Army Dental School's annual report of 1928, the basic course was designed:

> as an intensive course of special training in the adaptation of professional procedures to the requirements of the military service and to qualify officers of the Dental Corps to take their places with the specialty of dental medicine in the scheme of "group medicine" as practiced in the Army. Notwithstanding the fact that recent graduates who enter the Corps are well grounded in that basic theories and technical procedures of clinical dentistry, it has been found advisable to give them, immediately a broader conception of professional dentistry as a specialty of medicine, and to this end there is included a course in preventive medicine and clinical pathology at the Army Medical School.[117]

On June 22, 1922, at the National Museum Auditorium in Washington, DC, General John J Pershing, the chief of staff, presented the diplomas to the first class of 14 Dental Corps officers who graduated alongside the students from the Army Medical School.[109]

The Army Dental School shared key faculty members with the Army Medical School, also located at Walter Reed after September 1923, which was especially strong in the areas of surgery and preventive medicine. The basic courses of instruction were in clinical dentistry; dental and oral surgical prosthesis; oral surgery and exodontia; preventative dentistry and oral hygiene; bacteriology, pathology and preventive medicine; chemistry; and oral and dental roentgenology.

TABLE 17-9

HOURS OF INSTRUCTION, ARMY DENTAL SCHOOL, BASIC COURSE, 1922–1927

Department	Lectures and Examinations	Laboratory and Clinic	Lectures and Laboratory	Total Hours
Clinical dentistry	17	99		116
Prosthesis	36	174		210
Oral surgery	39	48		87
Preventive medicine and clinical pathology			180	180
Roentgenology	11	15	27	53
Special lectures	8	9		17
Total hours	**111**	**345**	**207**	**663**

Data sources: (1) Basic course, Army Dental School, seventh annual session, September 1, 1928 to January 31, 1928. In: *A History of the Army Dental School, 1927–1928.* Located at: Research Collections, Office of Medical History, OTSG/MEDCOM, Falls Church, Va. (2) Ninth annual basic course for officers, session September 3, 1929 to January 31, 1930. In: *A History of the Army Dental School, 1 July 1929–4 August 1932.* Located at: Research Collections, Office of Medical History, OTSG/MEDCOM, Falls Church, Va.

TABLE 17-10

HOURS OF INSTRUCTION: ARMY DENTAL SCHOOL BASIC COURSE,
1928–1929

Department	Lectures and Examinations	Laboratory and Clinic	Lectures and Laboratory	Total Hours
Clinical dentistry	20	98		118
Prosthesis	36	171		207
Oral surgery	40	57		97
Preventive medicine and clinical pathology			191	191
Roentgenology	8	19	30	57
Special lectures	7	0	8	15
Total hours	**111**	**345**	**229**	**685**

Data sources: (1) Basic course, Army Dental School, seventh annual session, September 1, 1928 to January 31, 1928. In: *A History of the Army Dental School, 1927–1928*. Located at: Research Collections, Office of Medical History, OTSG/MEDCOM, Falls Church, Va. (2) Ninth annual basic course for officers, session September 3, 1929 to January 31, 1930. In: *A History of the Army Dental School, 1 July 1929–4 August 1932*. Located at: Research Collections, Office of Medical History, OTSG/MEDCOM, Falls Church, Va.

The instruction in bacteriology and pathology in the curriculum was much more intense than that required of dentists in civilian education. Until 1928 the basic students took 663 hours of instruction, 207 of those hours together with the medical school classes (Table 17-9, Table 17-10). During the 1927–1928 school year, this combined instruction was temporarily cut to 153 hours, but the following year it was pushed back up to 229 hours.[118,119]

An advanced course was initially planned for September 15 to December 15, 1923, but it was cancelled "owing to the general wide disturbance of morale due to the shortage of personnel as the reduction program for dental officers progressed." The continuing disturbance in the Dental Corps in the ensuing years meant that the inaugural advanced course did not begin until February 1, 1928, when Major Oscar Snyder reported to replace Captain Clyde W Scogin (1890–1938; DDS, Colorado College of Dental Surgery, later University of Denver, 1915), the school's executive officer and an instructor in the department of oral surgery. Scogin had served as a dental surgeon in various units of the 89th Division throughout the war in the United States and France, completed postgraduate instruction in oral surgery at several civilian schools, and had already earned a national reputation in oral surgery for his work on "nutritional support for the maxillofacial patient." Snyder's arrival freed Scogin to take the course in conjunction with the Medical Corps students attending the Army Medical School's advanced course, which ran from February 1 to May 31, 1928. While the students selected for the advanced course were to be chosen from dental officers who showed "special fitness for particular subject" they wished to pursue, no students had yet been selected nor had any advanced course been run, due to the continuing scarcity of dental officers. Apparently the time was right to establish the precedent for the new course of instruction. Scogin had demonstrated that he was capable of completing a rigorous course of study and could demonstrate the importance of the advanced course for Dental Corps officers. His course of instruction totaled 579 hours (Table 17-11). The surgical service at Walter Reed General Hospital provided 102 of the surgical hours in surgical principles and the practice of oral and maxillofacial surgery.[33,120–122]

Regarding the first advanced course, the Army Dental School's history for 1927–1928 says:

> This year also marked the beginning of the Advanced Course for officers. While only one officer was in attendance the course was very important in establishing a precedent and schedule for this instruction, as well as demonstrating the great benefit to be derived from a more intimate relation in the character of instruction given to the Dental and Medical Officers general practice. This Advance Course was made possible by a special refresher course given at the Army Medical School, which included in its schedule a great deal of material and instruction which is required by Dental Officers who are specializing in Oral Surgery. All of the instruction given by Medical Officers was taken with the Medical Class and our one student not only was able to keep up with the class but we are unofficially informed had a relatively high standing.[123]

After completing the advanced course, Captain Scogin went on to attend the basic course at the Medical Field Service School in 1928–1929. Upon graduation he was the first Dental Corps officer to receive the Skinner Award, which was pre-

TABLE 17-11

CAPTAIN CLYDE W SCOGIN'S COURSE OF INSTRUCTION AT THE ARMY MEDICAL SCHOOL

Course	Number of Hours
Clinical dentistry	56
Oral surgical prosthesis	56
Oral surgery	235.5
Preventive medicine and clinical pathology	153.5
Special roentgenology	60
Special lectures	18
Total	579

Data sources: (1) Office of the Surgeon General. *Annual Report of the Surgeon General*. Washington, DC: OTSG; 1923. (2) The Army Dental School. *Milit Dent J*. 1922;5:25–26. (3) First annual advanced course for officers, session February 1, 1928 to May 31, 1928. In: *A History of the Army Dental School, 1927–1928*. Located at: Research Collections, Office of Medical History, OTSG/MEDCOM, Falls Church, Va. (4) Major Clyde W. Scogin (1890–1938). *Dent Bull*. 1938;9:154. (5) Major Clyde W Scogin. In: Biographical Files, Research Collection, Office of Medical History, OTSG/MEDCOM, Falls Church, Va.

sented to the student with the highest standing in each basic course class. Scogin was promoted to major in November 1929 and was assigned dental surgeon for the US Army Forces in China at Tientsin, where he contracted an illness. After his return to the United States in 1932 he was hospitalized at Fitzsimons General Hospital in Denver, Colorado, but never regained his health. Clyde Scogin was retired on September 30, 1933, due to a service connected disability, and he died at Fitzsimons on April 26, 1938.[98(p1050),121,122,124,125]

In addition to recommending officers for courses at the school, the surgeon general also selected enlisted soldiers to attend courses for dental technicians (chair assistants), dental hygienists, dental mechanics, and dental radiographic technicians and to take advantage of the talented instructors and facilities available at Walter Reed.[32] The Dental Corps had realized for many years that adequately trained dental technicians were critical to successful dental and oral care in the Army, and the establishment of the new Army Dental School provided the ideal location for such an enlisted training program:

> A dental officer, assisted by a properly trained and efficient technician, is enabled to increase the quality and quantity of his service. The training of an adequate sized corps of dental technicians, as herein contemplated, is believed to be a sound and economic policy that will greatly improve the professional service of the Dental Corps.[32(p135)]

No enlisted personnel were trained in 1922 because the school's training program was being set up. An extensive training program was developed that began in 1923 and by 1928, it consisted of a 6-month course (usually January through June) with 905 hours of instruction, laboratory, and clinic for technicians in dental mechanics and a 4-month course (usually January through April) of 567 hours for technicians in dental hygiene. The first three enlisted students completed their training in 1923—two dental mechanics and one dental hygienist. They "were assigned to duty in laboratories of dental clinics, where their services were urgently needed" and were soon "valuable adjuncts in the respective dental services." From 1923 through 1929, a total of 43 enlisted soldiers were reported as trained—30 as dental mechanics and 13 as dental hygienists—but the total number was actually higher because the number of enlisted dental technicians trained in 1924 was not reported. In 1927 the opening of the Walter Reed Central Dental Laboratory allowed the dental technicians to receive an entire month of "practical instruction" in the laboratory for the first time, which handled "a greater quantity and variety of practical cases."[33,42,45–48,59,123]

During the 1920s a total of 81 Dental Corps officers completed the Army Dental School—79 in the basic course and two in the advanced course, which began with one student each in the 1928 and 1929 classes (Major John L Schock)(Table 17-12, Table 17-13).[4,10,32,33,42,45–48,59,108]

In his address to the graduates of the second Army Dental School class on June 8, 1923, Colonel Oliver laid out his vision for the school and for Army dentistry within the larger context of the development of medical science:

> Our school, with a broader conception of the profession of dentistry in conjunction with that of its older sister, medicine, appears to be the first beacon light to aid and

TABLE 17-12

OFFICER GRADUATES OF THE ARMY DENTAL SCHOOL, 1922–1929

	1922	1923	1924	1925	1926	1927	1928	1929	Total
Basic course	14	13	11	7	7	9	9	9	79
Advanced course	0	0	0	0	0	0	1	1	2
Total officers	**14**	**13**	**11**	**7**	**7**	**9**	**10**	**10**	**81**

Data sources: (1) Office of the Surgeon General. *Annual Report of the Surgeon General.* Washington, DC: OTSG; 1922–1930.

direct the return of dentistry to the fold of medicine, there to travel along the great broad highway intended for the progress of the healing art. Should it be successful in directing the mental trend of the entire profession toward a general convergence of dentistry back to medicine and surgery, from which it so abruptly departed in 1839, and should it be the means of engendering broader views relative to the importance of the specialty of dental surgery in connection with the general application of medical and surgical procedures in the treatment of mankind, it will indeed have rendered signal service to humanity.[90(p65)]

Dental Caries Research: Captain Fernando E Rodriguez

In his June 1923 speech, Oliver stressed the potential benefits of the Army Dental School and even discussed one of the first and most significant of those: the research of Captain Fernando E Rodriguez (1888–1932) on the bacteriology of dental caries. Rodriguez was born on February 24, 1888, in Puerto Rico, and received his dental degree from Georgetown University in 1913. After a short time in private practice in Washington, DC, he entered the United States Indian Medical Service. While serving as a field dentist with the Pima Indians in Arizona, he studied the stained and mottled enamel of his patients' teeth and determined that

TABLE 17-13

ENLISTED GRADUATES OF THE ARMY DENTAL SCHOOL, 1922–1929

	1922	1923	1924	1925	1926	1927	1928	1929	Total
Dental mechanics	0	2	NR	6	5	5	5	7	30
Dental hygienists	0	1	NR	2	4	3	1	2	13
Total enlisted	**0**	**3**	**NR**	**8**	**9**	**8**	**6**	**9**	**43**

Data sources: Office of the Surgeon General. *Annual Report of the Surgeon General.* Washington, DC: OTSG; 1922–1930.

drinking water had caused the condition. This discovery contributed significantly to the study of mottled enamel. On September 14, 1917, Rodriguez was appointed a first lieutenant in the Dental Reserve Corps at Camp Upton, New York. After completing the medical officer's training camp at Camp Greenleaf, Georgia, he accepted a commission in the Regular Army Dental Corps on February 15, 1918. He served in San Juan, Puerto Rico, from August 1919 until February 1921, when he reported to the Army Medical School in Washington, DC, for "duty as student and investigator of the bacteriological aspect of dental diseases." Shortly after his arrival, Rodriguez's article, titled "Oral Lesions in Tropical Diseases," was published in the March 1921 issue of *Military Dental Journal*.[126–128]

Based on his research at the Army Medical School under the direction of Major Henry J Nichols (1887–1927), MC, assistant director of laboratories, and Major James F Coupal, MC, pathologist at the Army Medical Museum and the Army Dental School, Rodriguez published his first article on the etiology of dental caries, called "Studies in the Specific Bacteriology of Dental Caries." This article appeared in the December 1922 edition of *Military Dental Journal*.[129] From his experiments, he reached the following conclusions:

1. A distinctly high-acid producing group of bacteria, morphologically distinguishable into three types, is constantly found in the deep layers of dental decay.

2. This group may be differentiated, bio-chemically, from the other acid producers of the mouth by a constant optimum H-ion concentration varying from pH 3.9 to pH 2.9.

3. These organisms, in pure culture, survive and are active in degrees of alkalinity equivalent to normal reactions of the saliva.

4. When normal previously sterilized teeth are subjected to the direct action of these bacteria, caries-like lesions are produced.

5. Histological sections of the artificial lesion present the gross clinical characteristics of the natural process and the localization of the experimental organisms in the deep tooth areas.

6. The group has been tentatively placed under Tribe V, *Lactobacillae*, Classification S.A.B., and will accordingly be designated with the group name Lactobacillus odontolyticus, Types 1, 2 and 3, respectively.[129]

Military Dental Journal wrote that Rodriguez's work was "the most valuable advance made in the etiology of dental caries since Miller's time," referring to Willoughby D Miller, DDS (1853–1907), who published a major study titled "Micro-organisms of the Human Mouth" in 1889. The journal also said that there was an "urgent need in military dentistry for an agent that will arrest or retard the progress of dental caries in recruits and others stationed where dental service is not always available or those going into combat or on field maneuvers."[51,130]

Commenting on Rodriquez's research, Oliver said:

It is with some degree of pride that we invite attention to the splendid research work recently accomplished by medical and dental officers, working side by side in the laboratories of our schools, in which absolute findings have been made and recorded of that particular bacteria which produces dental caries. Groups of this bacteria have been segregated, classified and actually put to work developing dental caries under observation. Accepting this as a literal fact, it is readily conceivable that the next real progressive step in behalf of mankind is to find the natural antidote for that class of bacteria and begin study of ways and means leading to its universal application. This will then prove to be the most important step in the history of preventive dentistry and one of but little less importance in preventive medicine. The development of such an antidote will render salient service to the medical profession in the prevention of disease and in so doing will earn for dentistry far greater appreciation as an important specialty of the healing art.[90(p65)]

In 1923 Rodriguez was honored with an appointment to the Committee of Dental Investigation of the National Research Council, a group established by the president in 1918 to coordinate scientific activity in the country.[131,132] Shortly afterward, Rodriguez became the first US government dental scientist to be elected as a fellow of the American College of Dentists and a member of the International Society for Dental Research. He received a Bachelor of Science degree in 1924 from Georgetown. As he gained national prominence, Rodriguez continued his research on dental caries into the 1930s and published articles in the *Journal of the American Dental Association*.[133,134] Promoted to major in 1929, Rodriguez died unexpectedly at Walter Reed General Hospital on October 21, 1932. He was buried in Arlington Cemetery with full military honors. On August 31, 1944, Rodriguez General Hospital at Fort Brooke in San Juan, Puerto Rico, was dedicated in his honor. The general hospital was closed in February 1949, but the outpatient clinic located at Fort Buchanan was later renamed the Rodriquez Army Health Clinic and it continues to serve the Army today.[135] Rodriguez's pioneering research became the basis for future studies of the bacteriology of dental caries and was a major milestone in the history of dentistry.

The Dental Corps Medal

When the first Army Dental School class graduated in a joint ceremony with their medical school colleagues in June 1922, participants noted that while physicians were the recipients of three achievement medals, the dentists got none. Dental officers in the audience resolved to rectify the situation by raising funds from Corps members to endow a medal for the dental honor graduate. Students at the school successfully persuaded the school commandant to solicit a pro rata assessment of all members of the Dental Corps to raise funds to pay for the design of the medal and endow its future manufacture and award.[136]

In May 1924 a medal design was approved for the Army Dental School to present to the top graduate of each class. It was to be cast by Bailey, Banks & Biddle Company of Philadelphia from a rough freehand drawing made in the dental division at the surgeon general's office. It was described as:

a 14-carat gold medal, one-eighth of an inch in thickness and one and seven-eights inches in diameter. On the obverse side around the upper segment, appear the words, THE DENTAL CORPS, and around the lower segment, the words, 'United States Army.' In the center appear a sturdy dexter hand grasping a well-defined blazing torch of knowledge, while in semi-circle above it there are five stars and to its right the emblem of the Dental Corps of the U.S.A., the caduceus with superimposed letter D. The significance of this design is allegorical and represents the strong right hand of the Dental Corps holding aloft the torch of knowledge, way up in the firmament, thus setting on high the Corps' standard of excellence as a coveted ideal for attainment, one well worthy of consistent effort. The reverse side shows a laurel wreath around the border, tied at the bottom with a bow of ribbon. The upper center contains in large letters the words "The Corps Medal" and in smaller words "awarded to (name) for highest standing Army Dental School, Washington," with blank space below for the date figures.[136(pp103–104)]

The first recipient of the new medal was Captain (later Colonel) Walter D Vail, the honor graduate for the class of 1924. Vail was born in Kansas on July 26, 1886, and graduated from the Saint Louis Dental College in 1912.[136]

Specialized Postgraduate Instruction at Civilian Institutions

The National Defense Act of 1920 authorized postgraduate instruction at civilian institutions for Army dental officers. The following year, Oliver and the surgeon general selected three field grade officers to receive this kind of instruction—Majors Neal A Harper (later Brigadier General), BC Warfield, and Leigh C Fairbank. They were detailed to the Dewey School of Orthodontia (New York University) in New York City for a full postgraduate course from June through September 1921. Upon completion, they were assigned to station and general hospitals or headquarters' clinics at corps areas where they would handle and advise other dental surgeons on orthodontic work, which had long been a major problem in Army dental care. Major Leigh C Fairbank (1889–1966) was later the first dental division chief and Dental Corps chief (March 1938 to March 1942) to hold the rank of brigadier general, and had a distinguished career as an orthodontist both in the Army and in private practice.

The dental division planned to send three or four officers to the course annually until a group of 12 orthodontists were available "for special assignment at important stations having a large child population." In 1922 the Army sent another three dental officers to the special summer course. These officers, like their predecessors, were later able to "supply a deficiency in the treatment of Army children that has long been a crying need." The personnel cuts and budget reductions of 1922–1923, however, ended this important program because neither the officers' time nor the Army's funds could be spared any longer. For the remainder of the decade, only occasional short-term training was possible, often in conjunction with local dental schools or specialty clinics put on by the American Dental Association, formerly the National Dental Association, which had readopted its 19th century name in 1922.[10,32,33,42]

This situation remained little changed through 1929, when the *Annual Report of the Surgeon General* said that once again, the heavy demands in the Army for dental service meant that no officers could be detailed to civilian schools for extended instruction. The consequences of this deficiency were quite significant and portended a long-term problem elevating the quality of specialty practice in the Dental Corps:

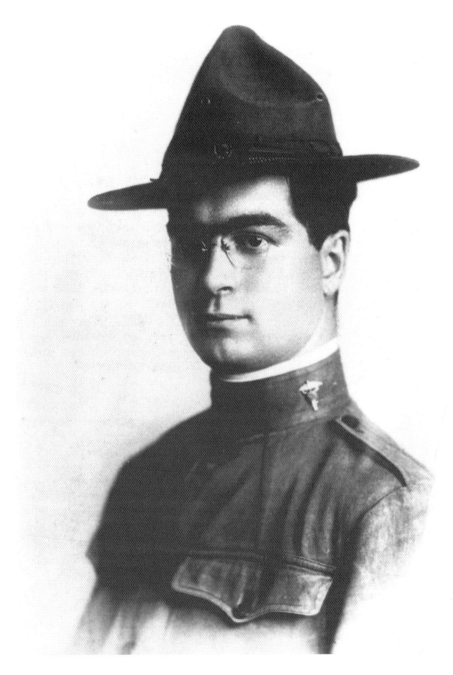

Leigh C Fairbank, first Dental Corps chief to hold the rank of brigadier general.
Photograph: Courtesy of Leigh C Fairbank's daughter, Maryalice Minor.

Many of the dental schools are conducting each year excellent postgraduate courses pertaining to the various specialties of dental practice and in order to keep dental officers abreast of the latest thought and developments in dentistry, it is highly desirable that a certain number of them be detailed for study at such institutions as soon as a sufficient number of officers become available to permit such action.[48(p237)]

The benefits to be gained by the individual dentist and the Dental Corps from such instruction were evident from Major Fairbank's experience in the early 1920s. Fairbank had no training in orthodontics, but while serving as a contract dental surgeon at Fort Sam Houston (from 1914 to 1916; before he was commissioned and sent to the Philippines until 1919), his experiences treating jaw fractures led him to correct malocclusions in children. His first formal training in orthodontia was at the Dewey School in 1921. After returning to his assigned post at Fort Leavenworth, Kansas, Fairbank wrote a short piece, titled "Orthodontia in the Military Service," which appeared in the March 1922 issue of *Military Dental Journal*. He noted that orthodontia was a dental specialty that had contributed greatly to the success of maxillofacial work during the recent war. Prior to the war, the Dental Corps had not developed such specialties, but now Fairbank concluded that orthodontia was "recognized as necessary in the progressive development of our Corps."[137,138] He wrote:

Orthodontia, carefully, earnestly and painstakingly applied, can have a very beneficial influence upon the impression of the worth of the Dental Corps. It presents an opportunity to render a lasting service to the younger members of the military service and the children of officers and enlisted men. There is also a grave and serious obligation with the work in this new field, which is not to be disregarded. A most gratifying service can be rendered, and yet, the prevention of unsightly facial disfigurement, not to mention complete loss of function of some teeth, requires diligent study and painstaking attention to detail.[137(p15)]

With more than one thousand children at the Fort Leavenworth garrison, Fairbank found many types of malocclusion to work on. For many Army parents who could not afford the great expense of taking their children to nearby specialists, the dental clinic provided a very welcome service. This result was exactly what those who had sent Fairbank to the Dewey School had planned. Fairbank found that educating the parents about orthodontic work was often more difficult than dealing with the children. He wrote, "it is a joy to see how systematic some of the little patients are in regard to brushing their teeth. One of the great benefits of orthodontic treatment is that children become systematic in the care and attention they give their teeth, a habit worthy of emulation by all of our patients."[137]

While Fairbank saw the great benefits that his work brought to his patients, he also realized that this work was practice for his potential wartime responsibilities:

The hope of the dental officers undertaking this work is to bring the advantages of this specialty to a very high state of development within the Corps; to render a lasting and beneficial service, and, when called upon in a national emergency requiring coordination of all our activities in the demands of war, to take our place in the maxillo-facial section and render an acceptable service.[137(p17)]

Central Dental Laboratories

Dental officers in the 1920s had to devote as much of their time as possible to the many patients they had to care for, leaving them little time to work in their laboratories on prosthetic appliances. It was not until fiscal year 1927 that the dental division was able to provide a new service to relieve the dentists and their technicians of this time-consuming aspect of their work. By then, the Army Dental School had produced a sufficient number of well-trained enlisted dental mechanics who could make and also oversee the manufacture of prosthetics in a dental laboratory. In 1926–1927, the dental division opened three new central dental laboratories that provided the same services to Army dentists as commercial laboratories provided to their civilian colleagues. Army dental mechanics at these labs could expertly construct and repair bridges, crowns, dentures, and inlays, which freed the operating dental officers and their technicians to spend many more hours at their chairs. The first laboratory, Walter Reed Central Dental Laboratory, was opened at Walter Reed General Hospital and served all dental officers in the First through Seventh Corps areas. It soon became an important adjunct to the training of officers and enlisted technicians at the Army Dental School. A similar laboratory at Letterman General Hospital supported the Ninth Corps Area, and another at the station hospital at Fort Sam Houston supported the Eighth Corps Area.[46]

The central dental labs quickly contributed to the increased efficiency of the dental service and took some of the load off dental officers and technicians throughout the Army. All dental officers in the continental United States could utilize the skilled dental mechanics to produce needed appliances. The labs handled 644 cases in fiscal year 1928 and 1,076 the following year as the labs ironed out their procedures and increased their capacity. Denture output increased from 149 to 269 and partial dentures from 345 to 559, and the labs became a critical component in the Army's dental service.[47,48]

The Need for Professional Information: Military Dental Journal and Dental Bulletin

Military Dental Journal, the quarterly publication of the Association of Military Dental Surgeons of the United States from 1917 through 1924 (not published in 1920), was the unofficial gazette for the dental officers of the Army, Navy, public health service, and any dentist interested in military dentistry. Each issue carried articles and items of professional and personal interest for officers of the Regular Army, Dental Officers' Reserve Corps, and National Guard, as well as the US Navy and public health service. As such, it was an important voice for the military dental community and the community's only real channel of information. At the end of 1924 the association terminated publication of the journal "for at least a year" due to insufficient membership, and it never reappeared.[139,140]

The variety of information previously provided in *Military Dental Journal* was apparently sorely missed within the Dental Corps. On January 1, 1929, the Army Dental School published the first mimeographed issue of what was supposed to be a new monthly, *Dental Bulletin*. This new, much-needed professional bulletin was sent to each dental officer in the Army as well as to corps area and department headquarters. According to the 1929 *Annual Report of the Surgeon General*,

Each issue contains professional articles prepared by officers of the Dental Corps and others, instructions and comments prepared by the dental division of this office concerning the conduct of dental service and a section devoted to news and events of interest to the personnel of the dental service. The publication of this bulletin has satisfied a definite need of the dental service and has elicited much favorable comment from various sources.[48]

"A Perfect System": The Pressures of Too Much Work, Not Enough Dental Officers, and Decaying Morale during the 1920s

While serving as Dental Corps chief, Colonels Oliver, Rhoades, and Bernheim each faced very serious problems providing professional dental services to the widely scattered Army. After the Dental Corps' strength was fixed at 158 officers on January 1, 1923, they constantly juggled their limited resources to provide administrative control at the surgeon general's office and in the corps areas where the chief dental surgeon had to double in another post, advanced military training, and postgraduate instruction opportunities. In addition, numerous posts had to be filled in the United States, Hawaii, the Panama Canal Department and Zone, Puerto Rico, the Philippines, and even in China. For many years, an Army dental officer served with the 2nd and 3rd Battalions, 15th Infantry, in Tientsin, China, when the China garrison was a part of the Philippine Department and dental surgeons were assigned from there. A dental officer was usually assigned to 1 year of China service. However, in April 1923, the China Expedition became a separate command (the US Army Forces in China) and assignments were made from the United States rather than the Philippines. The tour of duty was also increased to 3 years, placing a new dental officer in China every third year.[141]

Elsewhere in the 1920s, dental officers were still itinerants traveling the Alaskan circuit. Captain Joseph L Boyd told of his 4 months of temporary duty in Alaska in 1923, saying that he used the "engine room of the boat as an operating room, a pickle keg for a chair and the river for a cuspidor" on the boat trip to Fort Gibbon. Where there were only a few patients at remote camps, he removed only the foot engine from the truck, left the instrument case in the rear of the truck at working height, and used a common chair with a board covered with a pillow for a headrest. This field setup was quickly assembled and taken down, much easier than setting up the M 1895 SS White issue chair.[142]

In 1924 Colonel John DL Hartman told the chief signal officer the problem he was having getting dental treatment for his troops stationed in Seattle, Washington, who worked the Washington-Alaska Military Cable and Telegraph System. It seemed that the nearest Army dentist was at Fort Worden, which was inconvenient for his troops to get to. They had orders to have their dental work completed before going to Alaska, but in some cases had to pay a civilian dentist to do the work, which they could ill afford. Hartman wanted to know if they could have their work done at the Veterans' Bureau in Seattle.[143] Instead, on August 14, 1924, the surgeon general authorized Hartman to employ a civilian dentist to treat his soldiers during the fiscal year 1925. However, no bridges or crowns were authorized at public expense.[144]

To offset some of the pressure on the Dental Corps, in 1924 the surgeon general obtained the War Department's approval to call up five reserve dental officers for active duty at Army hospitals. The hospitals to which they were assigned were ones that treated beneficiaries of the US Veterans' Bureau, which accounted for 28.9% of all their patients. The bureau provided funds to cover pay and allowances for the five reservists, who were carefully selected from among those living closest to the hospitals. Walter Reed General Hospital, Washington, DC, gained one lieutenant; Fitzsimons General Hospital, Denver, Colorado, got one captain and one lieutenant (First Lieutenant James M Epperly, later chief of the Dental Corps); Letterman General Hospital, San Francisco, got one captain; and Fort Sam Houston Station Hospital, Texas, gained one lieutenant. As a result, the dental treatment available to the veterans was significantly enhanced and one of the Dental Corps' burdens was slightly reduced. In 1925 the number of DORC officers serving Veterans' Bureau beneficiaries grew to nine and remained at that strength for the remainder of the 1920s.[42,45–48,145]

The "objectionable itinerary service" reinstituted in 1923 as a result of the reductions was continued in 1924 to ensure that the smaller stations received "some sort of dental service." Many dental officers were now serving two to four stations with periodic visits, and more than 30% of the dental officers within the territorial limits of the United States served itinerantly duty during the year. The net result of this service was not only a diminished dental service across the board but also a significant decay in the morale of the dentists who were pulling this duty.[42] The 1924 *Annual Report of the Surgeon General* captured this problem in the following passage:

> Such temporary service at best is but a makeshift, unsatisfactory to local personnel and to the dental officers concerned. A limited time in which to attend the multitude of cases usually found at each station results in the accomplishment of little more than relief measures or emergency treatment for strictly military personnel. This unwholesome type of service in peace times has been conducive to lowering the morale of dental officers who become discontented and discouraged by the long absences from home and family.[42(p182)]

As the surgeon general had anticipated early in 1923, the policies restricting dental service were not well received throughout the Army. By late that year, numerous personal and official complaints had been received that the discontinuation of dental services for the families of officers and enlisted soldiers had reduced the soldiers' pay and allowances. From late 1923 into early 1924, these complaints sparked an exchange among the War Department General Staff, the adjutant general, and the surgeon general about the limited dental service, Circular No. 20, and why the Dental Corps could not provide required services like the Medical Corps did. Colonel TQ Donaldson, acting assistant chief of staff, G-1, went so far as to conclude that: "It seems suitable that the same spirit of service should govern the Dental Corps and that its officers should not be restrained by any prohibition against rendering full service within the limits of their capabilities." Similar comments and comparisons to the Medical Corps from the adjutant general caused Surgeon General Ireland to respond:

The disabilities in the dental service for the Army at present are fundamental. They are not the fault of the Medical Department nor of the Dental Corps nor of the War Department, but are believed to be the result of lack of liberality in the personnel authorized by legislation. Under the present law 158 dental officers are allowed. That is not sufficient to render dental service to the United States Army, and there is no argument or no action that will make this number sufficient to give satisfactory service to the Army at its present strength and distribution. These are facts that we must accept.[146]

Ireland stood by the restrictions in Circular No. 20 as "fundamentally correct and that its provisions should be continued in effect." He noted that the War Department had reviewed and approved these policies before they were put into effect.[146] As to comparisons between the Medical Corps and Dental Corps and contentions that dental officers could do more, Ireland drew the line:

I appreciate very thoroughly the compliment that is paid the officers of the Medical Corps . . . I trust, however, that the reputation the Medical Corps has acquired by a century of devotion to duty will not in any way be used to the detriment of the Dental Corps, which is an entirely new organization. The members of the Dental Corps were not commissioned until 1911, and in reality had no professional supervision by this office until after the World War. The dental officer therefore has not acquired the traditions from a long history of service and accomplishment that the medical officer has acquired. I have, however, been very intimately associated with the work of the dental officers since their first recognition by legislation in 1901. I believe their devotion to duty from the beginning has been most commendable and everything that could be expected, and in my opinion the officers of this Corps have acquitted themselves under the trying circumstances of their service in a most commendable way. I know from my personal contact that they appreciate thoroughly the rapid manner in which they have been accepted by the military hierarchy and recognized by legislation; also the way in which the Medical Corps has accepted them one hundred percent into its traditions and into its organization. There is no disposition on the part of the Dental Corps or the Medical Department to limit their service in so far as their numbers will permit. On the other hand every effort is being made to give the maximum amount of service that can be given with the facilities allowed by legislation. This policy is going to be continued to the fullest extent so far as this office is concerned. My own opinion is that the present number of dental surgeons is not sufficient to render efficient service to the Army, and I trust that in time, and when considered opportune, this fact will be recognized by the War Department in an appropriate recommendation for an increase in the Corps.[146]

This exchange highlighted the growing problems that the War Department had with the more restrictive provisions of Circular No. 20. Subsequent discussions resulted in the eventual rescission of that circular's third section, with the publication of War Department Circular No. 6 on February 4, 1925 (pending the completion and issue of new Army regulations covering dental care).[147] By rescinding section III and providing dental care for officers and enlisted soldiers ordered to foreign or detached service, Circular No. 6 made two simple statements:

. . . 4. Members of the Dental Corps will serve free of charge all those entitled to free medical treatment by medical officers.

5. Members of the Dental Corps will operate upon those entitled to their services. Materials issued by the Government will be expended only in operations upon those entitled to free services. Emergency work for officers and enlisted men will have precedence at all times over other work.[147]

Within 2 days of the appearance of Circular No. 6, Rhoades sent a letter to "all dental officers" to discuss the changes. He wrote:

It is expected by The Surgeon General that each dental officer will assume in the proper spirit the additional responsibility which has been placed upon you of formulating your own policy governing dental attendance under present regulations and after the rescinding of Section III, Circular 20, W.D., 1923.[148]

Rhoades supported the regulation in Circular No. 6 "to attend first the dental requirements of strictly military personnel." Then he said, if time permitted, military dentists were "permitted and expected to attend certain others. For these certain others you are authorized to use any materials supplied." The "certain others" were the families of military personnel and retirees who had received very limited dental care since early 1923.[148]

In his letter, Rhoades strongly advised all Army dentists to increase the efficiency of both their office management and their assistants. He recommended scheduling schemes that permitted swiftly filling cancelled or missed appointments with family members requiring treatment, and urged dentists to use Saturday mornings to manage their patient loads. Rhoades cautioned each dentist to "guard very carefully your professional reputation," writing:

Every operation should be the best of which you are capable. To complete more operations at the expense of finished operations will be directly disastrous to your professional reputation and indirectly disastrous to the professional reputation of our Corps. Simply because you are called upon to render much more dental service than is possible, you should never state that treatment is not necessary, unless that is the case.[148]

Rhoades concluded his letter with an appeal to the professionalism of the Army's dentists that was clearly intended to lift their morale and address their apparent anxieties about renewing treatment of families and retirees:

If the best results to the Army and to our Corps are to be obtained, each of us must develop in our heart the true professional spirit. When a patient presents, our first impulse should be "What can I do to be of most help to this patient?" We must feel towards patients exactly as the good dentist in civil life feels towards his family practice. All their requirements should be our concern. When we develop that same professional feeling towards the Army which the good dentist in civil life does towards his family practice, we will really possess that true professional spirit, and ways will be found whereby much dental attendance will become available to the others in the Army who are of so much concern to the military personnel. This will develop, and it is most desirable that there be developed in return, a real sympathetic friendship for the Dental Corps. . . . Our Corps is a selected Corps of dentists. All are capable of doing good work. With this and with each of us a professional man a heart, our Corps will have attained 100% in professional efficiency, and apprehension regarding the results to follow extending dental service to families, will soon vanish.[148]

The changes of early 1925 seemed to bring a general improvement. The 1925 *Annual Report of the Surgeon General* noted the positive results of Circular No. 6, commenting:

> During the past year more liberty of action has been granted to and responsibility placed upon dental officers in conducting the dental service. The same persons are now entitled to dental attendance under the same conditions and precedence for treatment as are entitled to medical attendance. Certain restrictions on the use of special dental materials have been removed and dental officers are authorized to use economically any materials supplied to the Army in rendering dental service to those entitled thereto. They are, however, directed to utilize the less expensive materials when good dentistry can be accomplished with such materials.[59(p234)]

Despite this slight improvement, the overall situation of the Medical Department and Army dentistry had not greatly improved due to the continuing lack of Dental Corps personnel. Accordingly, in 1926 the surgeon general attempted to resolve problems caused by the personnel shortage with a proposed amendment of section 10 of the National Defense Act based on the requirements for a 280,000-person Army. Among other things, the amendment would have increased Dental Corps personnel to 560 officers and added a brigadier general as its chief, similar to the approved wartime staffing of the dental division in the surgeon general's office. The surgeon general's concept was to replace the existing percentage basis for personnel allocation with "proposed actual numerical requirements" similar to the Army's other branches. Over the following 3 years, no legislative relief was enacted.[45–48,64,149]

The laments of 1924 were repeated in the 1928 *Annual Report of the Surgeon General*. The report added a brief but vivid glimpse of exactly what the deficiencies meant to the quality of dental care in the Army and what work was like for the average Army dentist in such "a perfect system":

> Dental attendance is of such a nature that little can be delegated to any but graduates in dentistry, which requires that it be rendered almost entirely by dental officers. The service confines one almost entirely to operating, which is most tedious. An average of six hours each day devoted to professional service is as much as can be expected if the health of the dental officer is to be maintained. . . . When days which officers do not devote to professional service are deducted, such as holidays, leaves of absence, travel time in change of station, other duties, sickness, etc., there remains but about 225 days per year devoted to operating at the dental chair. With 135 officers operating at the dental chair for 6 hours per day for 225 days per year, there is available to 135,000 military personnel an average of little more than one hour per year for each person for dental treatment. That is presuming there are no broken appointments, but continuous operating on all days—a perfect system.[47(p246)]

The severe limitations on resources compelled the Army to streamline a variety of activities. The Army made determined efforts during the 1920s to learn from the management techniques then developing in civilian society. In one form or another, the business culture and collateral economic issues influenced Dental Corps activities as well. Dental officers throughout the Army had collected statistics and data on their work since 1901, but during the 1920s the process was refined with new reporting requirements that emphasized preventive dentistry and trends in operations, the classification system, and prevalence of dental and oral diseases in accordance with new ARs. On April 12, 1928, 2 months before he was reassigned, Rex Rhoades, outgoing chief of the Dental Division and Dental Corps, consolidated the information collected over the years 1925–1927, analyzed the trends, and distributed his conclusions to all Dental Corps officers (Table 17-14).[150] Rhoades discussed what the data indicated about the nature of the Army's dental service:

> A study of the above tabulation presents most gratifying results. It indicates the trend in professional procedure in the dental service during the last three calendar years. This trend has been decidedly towards lines of prevention of chronic dental infections. The tabulation also indicates that where chronic infections have developed more extractions have been the rule and in many cases extracted teeth replaced by bridges and artificial dentures. The reduction in root canal fillings and artificial crowns indicates the extent to which the time element devoted to root canal therapy has been reduced. The decrease in temporary fillings and the increase in permanent fillings show that dental officers are now using more extensively the permanent filling materials.[150]

Rhoades identified a trend toward greater preventive dentistry and a decline in operations involving chronic problems. The lower number of root canals indicated to him "that fewer areas of infection have been sealed in vital tissue beyond root apices by root canal fillings" and that "less time has been devoted to root canal therapy and the increase of 19,583 permanent fillings in 1927 over that of 1925 indi-

TABLE 17-14

DENTAL SERVICE IN THE US ARMY, SELECTED OPERATIONS, 1925–1927

Operation	Totals			Average per Dental Officer			Increase / Decrease per Dental Officer
	1925	1926	1927	1925	1926	1927	
Prophylaxis	27.123	31,408	33,423	195	226	240	+45
Permanent fillings	97,717	102,200	117,300	703	735	844	+141
Teeth extracted	50,335	54,313	61,636	362	390	443	+81
Bridges	725	948	1,038	5	7	7	+2
Artificial dentures	2,552	3,051	3,496	18	22	25	+7
Temporary fillings	15,746	9,548	6,771	113	68	48	-65
Root canal fillings	4,794	3,728	3,087	34	27	22	-12
Artificial crowns	1,153	1,183	1,048	8	8	7	-1

Data source: National Archives and Records Administration. Record Group 112. Lieutenant Colonel Rex Rhoades, DC, to Dental Surgeons; Efficiency in the dental service, April 12, 1928. Letter. File no. 703.1. Box 105. Entry 29.

cates that much of this time has been devoted to the insertion of permanent fillings before the dental pulp has become infected from approaching caries." Periodontal problems seemed to be as great a cause of tooth loss as caries, and he urged more attention be paid to gum diseases. The record indicated that greater use could be made of the new central dental laboratories, further freeing dentists for their primary mission. Rhoades also concluded that productivity would be enhanced with better appointment and office task scheduling, as he had first urged back in February 1925, and he observed that improving the efficiency of administrative duties would also enhance the quality of work being done.[150] In his summary, Rhoades wrote that there was still much room for improvement:

> The Surgeon General is pleased with the yearly increase in efficiency which is taking place in the dental service. After reviewing the compiled individual accomplishment of each officer for the past three calendar years we know there is yet much room for improvement since some are still below the average accomplishment for all dental officers in 1925. If these officers would so arrange and manage their offices as to eliminate lost motion, if they would arrange to send for members of families who have applied for treatment when appointments are broken and military personnel cannot be obtained as patients, if they would standardize professional procedure, and if they would reduce palliative treatment to a minimum, efficiency in the dental service throughout the Army would be still further improved. . . . Under the direction of the Surgeon General we individually and collectively should continue to make the dental service a little more efficient each year to the end that it may become one of the outstanding specialties in health promotion of the general medical service of the Army.[150]

In October 1928 the short supply of dentists prompted Captain Robert C Craven, DC, to suggest that one of the dental officers on duty at the Medical Field Service School at Carlisle Barracks give a "simple lecture on the extraction of teeth" to the Medical Corps students. He had lectured on the subject to the physicians of his hospital with much interest. Craven thought such instruction might prove useful to any physicians who would be stationed at a post without a dentist and have to extract a tooth. Colonel Bernheim, the new Dental Corps chief as of June 15, 1928, passed the recommendation along to the plans and training division.[151,152]

Unlike the Dental Corps' officers, the enlisted soldiers who worked in the dental service rarely saw themselves in the spotlight. In fact, their numbers are even difficult to track down, and their achievements were little noted. In 1927 152 enlisted soldiers served in various dental positions within the Army's dental service, but many more served in the tactical units. By 1929 that number had increased to 198, including 5 staff sergeants, 14 sergeants, 2 corporals, 90 privates first class, and 87 privates. Most of the enlisted personnel were chair assistants (one for each dentist) or dental mechanics in the various dental laboratories, and their training at the Army Dental School was by this time thorough and professional. A noncommissioned officer was assigned to the larger clinics, which often employed three or more enlisted soldiers.[46,48,68]

By 1929 the gloomy picture of "a perfect system" for dental officers remained unchanged because the Army had stabilized and the number of Dental Corps officers remained fixed at 158. More than 80% of the authorized Dental Corps officers were assigned to treating patients, but that number was insufficient to prevent dental disease from getting "entirely out of control, many cases passing into chronic stages before treatment can be initiated." Their continued itinerant practice was marked by repeated temporary duty trips to posts without dental officers. With approximately 135,000 soldiers in the Army and "thousands of dependents and others entitled to treatment," the 1929 annual report concluded that "it is apparent that adequate dental attendance can not be provided with the present authorized number of dental officers."[47,48] As the soldiers' dental and oral health deteriorated, morale sank throughout the Army's frustrated dental service, which knew what had to be done to correct the situation but lacked the resources to do it. Perhaps intended to attract congressional attention and corrective action, the report noted:

> Military personnel are given a dental examination at least once each year and every effort is made by dental officers to practice prevention of chronic dental conditions, but it is utterly impossible to attain this most desirable objective without an adequate increase in the Dental Corps. The hopelessness of providing proper dental service under present conditions is demoralizing to the morale of dental officers throughout the Army, inviting as it does frequent undeserved criticism of the service.[48(p247)]

There were few signs that this situation would change for the better any time soon. The decade after 1921 was bleak for the Dental Corps in terms of new officer personnel (Table 17-15). The capping of its authorized strength at 158 on January 1, 1923, and subsequent dismissal or retirement of 75 officers by June 30, 1923, led to a period of stagnation. No new officers were appointed between 1922 and 1926, even when vacancies existed in 1924 and 1925. From 1924—1929 15 losses occurred, but only 12 new appointments were made, and those came during 1926—1928.[4,32,33,42,46,48,59]

TABLE 17-15

REGULAR ARMY DENTAL CORPS: STRENGTH, LOSSES, APPOINTMENTS, AND VACANCIES, FISCAL YEARS 1920–1929[*]

	1920	1921	1922	1923	1924	1925	1926	1927	1928	1929
Authorized strength	196[†]	193[††]	158	158	158	158	158	158	158	158
Actual strength	196	250[§]	236[¥]	159[¶]	156[¶]	154[¶]	154	158	158	155
Losses	34	25	13	75	3	2	3	2	2	3
Appointments	14	75	0	0	0	0	4	6	2	0
Vacancies	102	0	0	0	3	5	4	0	0	3

[*]As of June 30 of each fiscal year.
[†]National Defense Act of 1920 increased authorizations to 298, effective July 1, 1920.
[††]Authorizations reduced to 193, effective February 7, 1921.
[§]Includes 4 retired officers on active duty in Dental ROTC.
[¥]Includes 3 retired officers on active duty in Dental ROTC.
[¶]Includes 1 retired officer on active duty in Dental ROTC.
Data source: Office of the Surgeon General. *Annual Report of the Surgeon General.* Washington, DC: OTSG; 1920–1925, 1927, 1929.

Depression and a New Decade

The 1920s was a period of often harsh readjustment to the realities of peace for the Army and the Medical Department. The Dental Corps suffered its share of the travail, but its leadership constantly struggled to maintain a reasonable level of dental service for the officers, soldiers, and military families it cared for. While not exactly the rosy future that William HG Logan had so optimistically predicted in February 1919, the 1920s actually turned out to be a period of some significant growth for the Dental Corps. Important foundations were laid in professional education and development, authorization for dental personnel in tables of organization, research, dental supplies, and equipment development and fielding. The Medical Field Service and Army Dental Schools produced important advances, such as the integrated field training of dental officers, the development of the field dental operating sets and kits, the basic and advanced dental officers' courses, and the work of Captain Fernando Rodriguez on dental caries. Despite a decade of congressional neglect and public indifference, a great deal was achieved. However, it was far from the anticipated "return to normalcy" for the Dental Corps and dentistry in the US Army. The stock market crash in October 1929 and the government's desperate efforts to economize portended even more stringent times in the coming decade.

References

1. Colonel William HG Logan to the members of the Dental Corps, permanent organization, and all chiefs of Dental Service; "Status of the Dental Service in the United States Army," February 12, 1919. Letter. Papers of Major General Oscar P Snyder, DC, Research Collections, Office of Medical History, Office of The Surgeon General, Falls Church, Va.

2. Fisher WC. Editorial: Colonel Logan's farewell letter to the Dental Corps. *J Assoc Milit Dent Surg US*. 1919;3:78–80.

3. Office of The Surgeon General. *Annual Report of the Surgeon General*. Vol 2. Washington, DC: OTSG; 1919.

4. Office of The Surgeon General. *Annual Report of the Surgeon General*. Washington, DC: OTSG; 1920.

5. Risch E. *Quartermaster Support of the Army: a History of the Corps, 1775–1939*. Washington, DC: Quartermaster Historian's Office, Office of the Quartermaster General; 1962: 697.

6. Weigley RF. *History of the United States Army*. New York, NY: Macmillan Co.; 1967: 396.

7. Ganoe WA. *History of the United States Army*. New York, NY: D Appleton and Co.; 1924: 483.

8. Hewes JE Jr. *From Root to McNamara: Army Organization and Administration, 1900–1963*. Washington, DC: US Army Center of Military History, 1975.

9. Kreidberg MA, Henry MG. *History of Military Mobilization in the United States Army, 1775–1945*. Washington, DC: Department of the Army; 1955.

10. Office of The Surgeon General. *Annual Report of the Surgeon General*. Washington, DC: OTSG; 1921.

11. The Army of the United States. *Milit Dent J*. 1924;7:22.

12. Wilson JB. *Maneuver and Firepower: the Evolution of Divisions and Separate Brigades*. Washington, DC: US Army Center of Military History; 1998.

13. Matters of interest to reserve officers. *Milit Dent J*. 1922;3:157–160.

14. Ireland MW. Dental preparedness from medical department viewpoint. *J Nat Dent Assoc*. 1921;8:937–938.

15. Biographical file of Colonel Frank LK Laflamme. In: Biographical Files, Research Collection, Office of Medical History, OTSG/MEDCOM, Falls Church, Va.

16. Office order no. 1145, Colonel CR Darnall, executive officer, surgeon general's office, 24 November 1918. *Milit Dent J*. 1922;5:152.

17. Hyson JM, Jr. Robert T Oliver, DDS: oral surgeon, Army dental chief, president ADA. *J Hist Dent*. 2003;51:124.

18. Colonel Robert T. Oliver, retired. *Mil Surg*. 1937;81:234.

19. Tables 707P, Office of the Surgeon General, 7 June 1926. In: Medical Field Service School, 1928 tables of organization medical department. *The Army Medical Bulletin*;1928.

20. General Ireland's address. *Milit Dent J*. 1921;4:133.

21. Transactions of the Eighth Annual Convention of A.M.D.S. (extracts). *Milit Dent J*. 1921;4:165.

22. Biographical files on Major General Merritte W Ireland and Colonel Robert T Oliver. In: Biographical Files, Research Collections, Office of Medical History, OTSG/MEDCOM, Falls Church, Va.

23. Robert T. Oliver 1868–1937. *Dent Bull*. 1937;8:233–234.

24. Army general hospital named for pioneer dental officer. *Mil Surg*. 1947;101:442–443.

25. Colonel Rex H. Rhoades retires. *Dent Bull*. 1935;6:45–46.

26. Brooke Army Medical Center. Chronology of Colonel Rex Hays Rhoades (November 30, 1875–September 11, 1959). In: Biographical Files, Research Collections, Office of Medical History, OTSG/MEDCOM, Falls Church, Va.

27. Walter Reed Army Hospital. Former chief of Army Dental Corps dies at Walter Reed, September 11, 1959. In: Biographical Files, Research Collections, Office of Medical History, OTSG/MEDCOM, Falls Church, Va.

28. Major General Robert H. Mills. *Bull US Army Med Dep*. 1946;5:626.

29. Bernheim, Colonel Julien Rex. In: *Encyclopedia of American Biography*. New York, NY: The American Historical Society; 1944: 268–270.

30. Biographical file on Colonel Julien R Bernheim. In: Biographical Files, Research Collections, OTSG/MEDCOM, Falls Church, Va.

31. National Archives and Records Administration. Record Group 165. Memorandum for the chief of staff, Colonel Francis E Lacey, Jr, acting director, War Plans Division, acting assistant chief of staff, August 18, 1919. File no. 382; Dental Corps. Box 48. Entry 8.

32. Office of the Surgeon General. *Annual Report of the Surgeon General*. Washington, DC: OTSG; 1922.

33. Office of the Surgeon General. *Annual Report of the Surgeon General*. Washington, DC: OTSG; 1923.

34. National Archives and Records Administration. Record Group 407. Major AD Tuttle, Medical Corps, chief, Organization Division, surgeon general's office, to the adjutant general, February 15, 1923. Letter, with enclosure, surgeon general's office, circular letter no. 6 (dental no. 1); Reorganization of the dental service, February 1923. File no. 703 (2-15-23). Box 1092.

35. National Archives and Records Administration. Record Group 407. First endorsement, adjutant general to surgeon general, February 1923. File 703 (2-15-23). Box 1092.

36. National Archives and Records Administration. Record Group 407. Second endorsement, Major AD Tuttle, Medical Corps, chief, Organization Division, surgeon general's office, to the adjutant general, February 26, 1923, with enclosure, draft circular; Policies governing dental attendance, February 24, 1923. File 703 (2-15-23). Box 1092.

37. National Archives and Records Administration. Record Group 407. Memorandum for the chief of staff, Colonel TQ Donaldson, acting assistant chief of staff, G-1; Dental treatment, March 1, 1923, with enclosure, draft circular, March 1923. File 703 (2-15-23). Box 1092.

38. National Archives and Records Administration. Record Group 407. Circular no. 20, War Department, March 12, 1923. File 703 (2-15-23). Box 1092.

39. Reorganization of dental service. *Milit Dent J.* 1923;6:24–27.

40. National Archives and Records Administration. Record Group 112. Draft, circular letter no. 6 (dental no. 1), Lieutenant Colonel CR Reynolds, Medical Corps, executive officer, surgeon general's office; 'Reorganization of the dental service.' File 703.-1. Box 386. Entry 29.

41. National Archives and Records Administration. Record Group 112. War Department circular no. 20, John J Pershing, general of the armies, chief of staff, March 12, 1923. File 703.-1. Box 386. Entry 29.

42. Office of the Surgeon General. *Annual Report of the Surgeon General*. Washington, DC: OTSG; 1924.

43. Dental Sub-Division, OTSG. The Army and the Dental Corps. *Dental Supplement to the Army medical Bulletin*. 1936;7:145.

44. Hoblitzell WH. Service in the United States Army Dental Corps. *Dent Summ*. 1925;45:564–565.

45. Office of the Surgeon General. *Annual Report of the Surgeon General*. Washington, DC: OTSG; 1926.

46. Office of the Surgeon General. *Annual Report of the Surgeon General*. Washington, DC: OTSG; 1927.

47. Office of the Surgeon General. *Annual Report of the Surgeon General*. Washington, DC: OTSG; 1928.

48. Office of the Surgeon General. *Annual Report of the Surgeon General*. Washington, DC: OTSG; 1929.

49. National Archives and Records Administration. Record Group 112. Colonel Robert T Oliver, chief, Dental Division, surgeon general's office, to corps dental surgeon, Sixth Corps Area, September 22, 1920, and to corps dental surgeon, Third Corps Area, September 24, 1920. Memo. File 326.6-1. Box 180. Entry 29.

50. National Archives and Records Administration. Record Group 112. MW Ireland, surgeon general, to deans, Harvard University Dental School, Northwestern University Dental School, and University of Minnesota College of Dentistry, September 29, 1920. Memo. File 326.6-1. Box 180. Entry 29.

51. Asbell MB. *Dentistry: a Historical Perspective*. Bryn Mawr, Pa: Dorrance & Company, Inc; 1988: 192–193.

52. Lufkin AW. *A History of Dentistry*. Philadelphia, Pa: Lea & Febiger; 1948: 191.

53. Ireland MW. Dental preparedness from medical department viewpoint. *J Natl Dent Assoc*. 1921;8:936.

54. National Archives and Records Administration. Record Group 165. Colonel William M Cruikshank, assistant director, War Plans Division, to chief of staff, September 27, 1920. Memo. File no. 7973. Folder 7951-8000. Box 35. Entry 279.

55. Army Dental Corps. *Army & Navy Register*. Quoted in: *Dental Cosmos*. 1921;63:96.

56. National Archives and Records Administration. Record Group 112. MW Ireland, surgeon general, to deans, Harvard University Dental School, Northwestern University Dental School, and University of Minnesota College of Dentistry, September 29, 1920. Memoranda. File 326.6-1. Box 180. Entry 29.

57. National Archives and Records Administration. Record Group 165. Programme of training and instruction of Dental Corps units of the R.O.T.C. File no. 7973. Folder 7951-8000. Box 35. Entry 279.

58. US Army. The annual medical department R.O.T.C. camp Carlisle Barracks, Penn., June–July, 1923. *Milit Dent Surg*. 1923;6:133.

59. Office of the Surgeon General. *Annual Report of the Surgeon General*. Washington, DC: OTSG; 1925.

60. National Archives and Records Administration. Record Group 112. Memorandum for corps dental surgeons, Colonel Robert T Oliver, September 8, 1920. File no. 703.-1. Box 386. Entry 29.

61. Table 90 W—infantry regiment, division, 25 October 1925, and table 81 W—medical regiment, 28 October 1925. In: Medical Field Service School. 1928: tables of organization medical department. *The Army Medical Bulletin*. Carlisle Barracks, Pa: Medical Field Service School;1928(no. 22).

62. Medical Field Service School. The medical regiment. *The Army Medical Bulletin*. Carlisle Barracks, Pa: Medical Field Service School;1925(no.13).

63. Stone FP. Duties of a dental officer and his relation to medical officers. *Milit Dent J*. 1922;5:147–151.

64. US Army. 1928: Tables of organization medical department. *The Army Medical Bulletin*. 1928;22.

65. Vail WD. The Dental Reserve Corps. *Dent Bull*. 1936;7:21.

66. More Dental Reserve officers needed. *Milit Dent J*. 1923;6:16–17.

67. Appointment in Reserve Corps. *Milit Dent J*. 1924;7:212–213.

68. Rhoades RH. The dental service of the Army of the United States. *J Amer Dent Assoc*. 1928;15:259–263.

69. Matters of interest to reserve officers. *Milit Dent J*. 1922;5:159.

70. Gaynor CJ. The Organized Reserve Corps procurement, training, distribution and purpose of the medical section. *Dental Bulletin Supplement to the Army Medical Bulletin*. 1937;8:116–120.

71. Regrouping of Dental Reserve Officers. *Milit Dent J*. 1922;5:163.

72. The meaning of B.A.G. and T.A.G. *Milit Dent J*. 1924;7:210–211.

73. Smalley HE. Advancement made during the past twenty years in dental equipment and supplies and their purchase. *Dent Bull*. 1937;8:176–178.

74. Jeffcoat GF. *A History of the United States Army Dental Service in World War II*. Washington, DC: Office of the Surgeon General; 1955; 180–186.

75. US Department of the Army. *Supply Table and Price List, Medical Supplies*. Washington, DC: DA; 1928. Army Regulation 40-1710.

76. Fletcher JP. Research-Development of medical field equipment. *Mil Surg*. 1929;65:839–840.

77. Darnall CR. Office of the Surgeon General, circular letter no. 1, "Standard classification of dental cases," 7 January 1921. *Milit Dent J*. 1922;5:104–105.

78. US War Department. General orders no. 82, 28 June 1919. War Department, General Orders and Bulletins 1928. Washington, DC: Government Printing Office; 1929.

79. *Regulations of the Army of the United States, 1913*. Washington, DC: Government Printing Office; 1913.

80. US Army. AR 40-15, Medical department: Dental Corps—general provisions, 10 October 1920. In: *Army Regulations*. Research Collections, Office of Medical History, OTSG/MEDCOM, Falls Church, Va.

81. US Department of the Army. AR 40-510, Medical department: dental attendance, 10 October 1925. In: *Army Regulations*. Research Collections, Office of Medical History, OTSG/MEDCOM, Falls Church, Va.

82. US Department of the Army. AR 40-1010, Medical department: dental reports, returns, and records, 20 October 1925. In: *Army Regulations*. Research Collections, Office of Medical History, OTSG/MEDCOM, Falls Church, Va.

83. US Department of the Army. *Commissioned officers: Appointment in the Dental Corps, Regular Army*. Washington, DC: DA; 1925. Army Regulation 605-15.

84 US Department of the Army. *Commissioned officers. Subjects of professional examination for promotion in the Dental Corps, Regular Army*. Washington, DC: DA; 1926. Army Regulation 605-60.

85. Surgeon General Ireland to Adjutant General, April 28, 1920. Letter. Carlisle Papers, US Army Military History Institute, Carlisle Barracks, Pa.

86. *History of Carlisle Barracks Pennsylvania (1757–1952)*. Carlisle Barracks, Pa: Public Information Office; 1952): 20.

87. The Medical Field Service School. *The Army Medical Bulletin*. 1930;1:1–23.

88. Tousey TG. *Military History of Carlisle and Carlisle Barracks*. Richmond, Va: The Dietz Press; 1939: 360–364.

89. Schutt AM. *Origin Development and Evolution of the Department of Preventive Health Services* [thesis]. Fort Sam Houston, Tex: US Army Medical Department Center and School, Carlisle Barracks Collection; 1996.

90. Oliver RT. Address delivered at the graduating exercise of the Army medical and dental schools. *Milit Dent J*. 1923;6:59–65.

91. Ashburn PM. Opening address delivered to the first class at the Medical Field Service School, Carlisle Barracks, Pa., June 1, 1921. *Mil Surg*. 1921:1.

92. Colonel Percy M Ashburn to Colonel Thomas G Tousey, MC, Medical Field Service School, Carlisle Barracks, Pennsylvania, 26 May 1939. Letter. Carlisle Barracks Collection, US Medical History Institute, Carlisle Barracks, Pa.

93. Brown PW. Draft history of the US Army Dental Corps. ND. In: Research Collections, Office of Medical History, OTSG/MEDCOM, Falls Church, Va.

94. Stone FP. Duties of a dental officer and his relation to medical officers. *Milit Dent J*. 1922;5:93–97.

95. War Department. *Official Army Register, January 1, 1923*. Washington, DC: Government Printing Office; 1923: 207.

96. Stone FP. Medical department short basic course for Reserve and National Guard officers. *Milit Dent J*. 1923;6:76.

97. Stone FP. Correspondence course for dental officers. *Milit Dent J*. 1923;6:196.

98. War Department. *Official Army Register, January 1, 1938*. Washington, DC: Government Printing Office; 1938: 820, 1050.

99. Wunderlich FR. Training for dental officers. *Milit Dent Bull*. 1927;1:7–9.

100. Training at Medical Field Service School, Carlisle, Pa. *Milit Dent J*. 1923;6:162–164.

101. US Army Service Forces. *The Medical Field Service School: Handbook of Information*. Carlisle Barracks, Pa: Army Service Forces; 1944.

102. US Department of the Army. *Military education: the Army Medical School*. Washington, DC: DA; 1926. Army Regulation 350-1000.

103. US Department of the Army. *Military education: the Army Dental School*. Washington, DC: DA; 1926. Army Regulation 350-1010.

104. US Department of the Army. *Military education: the Army Veterinary School*. Washington, DC: DA; 1926. Army Regulation 350-1020

105. US Department of the Army. *Military education: the Medical Field Service School*. Washington, DC: DA; 1926. Army Regulation 350-1030

106. US Army. Examination for Army Dental Corps. *Milit Dent J*. 1924;7:82–83.

107. Ingalls RE. The development of the Army Dental School. *Milit Dent J*. 1923;6:125–126.

108. Office of the Surgeon General. *Annual Report of the Surgeon General*. Washington, DC: OTSG; 1930: 277.

109. The Army Dental School. *Milit Dent J*. 1922;5:18–21.

110. Colonel Seibert D. Boak, 1876–1934. *Dent Bull*. 1935;6:43.

111. Colonel Seibert D. Boak. In: Biographical Files, Research Collection, Office of Medical History, OTSG/MEDCOM, Falls Church, Va.

112. Colonel Ingalls Retires. *Dent Bull*. 1934;5:240.

113. Personals. *Milit Dent J*. 1923;6:108.

114. *A History of the Army Dental School, 1 July 1929–4 August 1932*. Located at: Research Collections, Office of Medical History, OTSG/MEDCOM, Falls Church, Va.

115. A curriculum vitae of Colonel Frank LK Laflamme, December 1967. In: Colonel Frank LK Laflamme Biographical File. Research Collections, Office of Medical History, OTSG/MEDCOM, Falls Church, Va. 116. War Department. *Official Army Register, January 1, 1930*. Washington, DC: Government Printing Office; 1930: 1107.

117. Rice WS. Annual report, Army Dental School, 1927–28, 2 July 1928. In: *A History of the Army Dental School, 1927–1928*. Located at: Research Collections, Office of Medical History, OTSG/MEDCOM, Falls Church, Va.

118. Basic course, Army Dental School, seventh annual session, September 1, 1928 to January 31, 1928. In: *A History of the Army Dental School, 1927–1928*. Located at: Research Collections, Office of Medical History, OTSG/MEDCOM, Falls Church, Va.

119. Ninth annual basic course for officers, session September 3, 1929 to January 31, 1930. In: *A History of the Army Dental School, 1 July 1929–4 August 1932*. Located at: Research Collections, Office of Medical History, OTSG/MEDCOM, Falls Church, Va.

120. First annual advanced course for officers, session February 1, 1928 to May 31, 1928. In: *A History of the Army Dental School, 1927–1928*. Located at: Research Collections, Office of Medical History, OTSG/MEDCOM, Falls Church, Va.

121. Major Clyde W. Scogin (1890–1938). *Dent Bull*. 1938;9:154.

122. Major Clyde W Scogin. In: Biographical Files, Research Collection, Office of Medical History, OTSG/MEDCOM, Falls Church, Va.

123. *A History of the Army Dental School, 1927–1928*. Located at: Research Collections, Office of Medical History, OTSG/MEDCOM, Falls Church, Va.

124. Medical Field Service School, Carlisle, Pennsylvania: Graduate exercises, basic course. *Mil Surg*. 1929;65:292.

125. Major Clyde W. Scogin, D.C., retires. *Dent Bull*. 1934;5:64.

126. Fernando E. Rodriguez 1888–1932. *Dent Bull*. 1933;4:39–40.

127. Rhoades RH. Fernando E. Rodriguez, B.S., D.D.S. (1888–1932). *J Amer Dent Assoc*. 1932;19:2195.

128. Rodriguez FE. Oral lesions in tropical diseases (1) sprue (tropical scurvy). *Milit Dent Surg*. 1921;4:8-12.

129. Rodriguez FE. Studies in the specific bacteriology of dental caries. *Milit Dent J*. 1922;5:199–214.

130. Editorial Department. Etiology of dental caries. *Milit Dent J*. 1922;5:226–227.

131. Captain F.E. Rodriguez, D.C. Honored. *Milit Dent J*. 1923;6:96.

132. Major Rodriguez memorial plaque. *Dental Bulletin Supplement to the Army Medical Bulletin*. 1940;11:80–81.

133. Rodriguez FE. A method of determining, quantitatively, the incidence of lactobacillus acidophilus odontolyticus in the oral cavity. *J Amer Dent Assoc*. 1930;17:1711–1719.

134. Rodriguez FE. Quantitative incidence of lactobacillus acidophilus in the oral cavity as a presumptive index of susceptibility to dental caries. *J Amer Dent Assoc*. 1931;18:2118–2135.

135. Rodriguez General Hospital, San Juan, Puerto Rico. *Mil Surg*. 1947;101:441–442.

136. Dental Corps Medal. *Milit Dent J*. 1924;7:102–104.

137. Fairbank LC. Orthodontia in the military service. *Milit Dent J*. 1922;5:15–17.

138. Meet the general. *Oral Hygiene*. 1942;32:31.

139. Hume EE. *The Golden Jubilee of the Association of Military Surgeons of the United States: a History of Its First Half-Century: 1891–1941*. Washington, DC: The Association of Military Surgeons; 1941: 274.

140. Discontinuance of the Military Dental Journal. *Milit Dent J*. 1924;7:215–226.

141. Tingay LH. A tour of duty in China. *Milit Dent J*. 1924;7:189.

142. Boyd JL. Touring Alaska with a portable dental outfit. *Milit Dent J*. 1924;7:128–130.

143. National Archives and Records Administration. Record Group 111. Colonel John DL Hartman, Signal Corps, to chief Signal Corps, US Army, 16 May 1924. Letter. File no. 703. Box 1818. Entry 45.

144. National Archives and Records Administration. Record Group 111. Lieutenant Colonel James M Phalen, Medical Corps, to chief signal officer, US Army, 14 August 1924. Endorsement. No. 703. Box 1818. Entry 45.

145. Personals: Army. *Milit Dent J*. 1924;7:49.

146. National Archives and Records Administration. Record Group 407. Fifth endorsement, Major General MW Ireland, surgeon general, to adjutant general, April 4, 1924, to memorandum for the adjutant general, Colonel TQ Donaldson, acting assistant chief of staff, G-1; Dental service, March 11, 1924. File 703 (10-15-23). Box 1092.

147. National Archives and Records Administration. Record Group 407. War Department Circular no. 6, 4 February 1925. File 703 (1-17-25). Box 1091.

148.   National Archives and Records Administration. Record Group 112. Lieutenant Colonel Rex H Rhoades to all dental officers; "Dental attendance, February 6, 1925." Letter. File 703.1. Box 386.

149.   Fairbank LC. A resume of the dental service in war. *Dent Bull.* 1936;7:196.

150.   National Archives and Records Administration. Record Group 112. Lieutenant Colonel Rex Rhoades, Dental Corps, to dental surgeons; "Efficiency in the dental service, April 12, 1928." Letter. File no. 703.1. Box 105. Entry 29.

151.   National Archives and Records Administration. Record Group 112. Captain Craven to Colonel Bernheim, October 19, 1928. Letter. File no. 703.1. Box 105. Entry 29.

152.   National Archives and Records Administration. Record Group 112. Colonel Bernheim to Plans & Training Division, October 24, 1928. Letter. File no. 703.1. Box 105. Entry 29.

Chapter XVIII

THE DEPRESSION AND BUILDUP FOR ANOTHER WORLD WAR, 1929–1941

A depression that began with the collapse of the stock market in October 1929 soon gripped the United States and its Army. For the Dental Corps, the late 1920s had been a difficult time, with occasional glimmers of hope. Those occasional glimmers largely disappeared with the onset of the Depression and lasted until President Franklin D Roosevelt's administration (March 1933–April 1945) embarked upon its "New Deal" of social and economic relief programs after March 1933. While these fixes offered the long-term promise of getting the nation back on its feet, they took years to implement and were of little help to the Army. The US Army, its medical department, and the Dental Corps did not experience significant positive changes before the mid 1930s. Soon, the growing threat of world conflict arising from the aggressive actions of Nazi Germany, Fascist Italy, and Imperial Japan demanded heightened national security.

Dental Corps Leadership, 1929–1936

Colonel Julien R Bernheim had been chief of the dental division and the Dental Corps since mid June 1928 when the Depression plunged the nation into a downward spiral in late 1929. The Dental Corps had been in bad shape throughout the 1920s, with too few resources and too much work, and the impact of the Depression on the Army made things worse. In his report for 1930, Bernheim commended the "spirit of earnestness and zeal" that the dental service personnel had demonstrated while maintaining "a high degree of efficiency" during the year. However, he also lamented that the lack of trained oral hygienists had severely limited

> the prevention and control of pyorrhea, dental caries, and their more serious sequellae [*sic*]. . . . Here, however, as in its other efforts to furnish the required dental attendance for the Army, the Dental Service has been seriously handicapped by inadequate personnel. Each year for a number of years recommendation has been made for a substantial increase in personnel for this service and such recommendation is again earnestly renewed.[1]

In the surgeon general's "Letter of Transmission" for the 1931 annual report, Bernheim was able to insert a strong statement about the inadequacy of the dental service and a renewed request for the ratio of one dental officer per 500 soldiers that had been the Dental Corps' unrealized goal since before World War I:

requirements brought in recruits with poor dental and oral health, and the lack of dental personnel meant that a robust dental health training program and sound preventive dentistry were impossible. Higher dental enlistment requirements were needed, along with "a suitable increase in dental service personnel" to provide "a dental health training program" that would produce "a genuine health service." Rhoades concluded that "serious consideration is being given to this matter in view of placing these measures in effect," but consideration was all that could be given without additional professional personnel.[6(pp172–173)] Apparently confronted with more pressing issues, Rhoades dropped the 1-to-500 ratio and the push for more professional personnel; neither appears in his final report as chief in 1934.[7,8]

In his 1934 report, however, Rhoades was again blunt in his assessment of the Army's dental service. Now also struggling with the large new commitment of dental care for Civilian Conservation Corps (CCC) enrollees (see below, "Dental Service for the Civilian Conservation Corps, 1933–1936"), Rhoades lamented the lack of preventive dentistry that his service could perform:

> The record of dental attendance is very satisfactory when the amount of service available is considered. It should be noted, however, that results have been accomplished by corrective rather than preventive measures. This is a condition that is unsatisfactory. The requirements for corrective measures are so great that preventive measures cannot be instituted with the present personnel.[7(p164)]

One of Rhoades's lasting contributions to the professional development of Dental Corps officers was the revival of the *Dental Bulletin* in January 1933. The *Dental Bulletin* was originally compiled and published monthly (at the direction of Julien Bernheim) by the Army Dental School during 1929. It served as the Dental Corps' professional bulletin (see Chapter XVII: A Return to Normalcy: from the World War to the Depression, 1919–1929) and it was one of the first things cut during the Depression. No issues were published in 1930, two appeared in 1931 (February and July), and one in 1932 (June). Rex Rhoades realized that the *Dental Bulletin* was a valuable means for professional communication, training, and instruction within the dental service and the Dental Corps. He revived it as a quarterly publication to be printed and distributed in January, April, July, and October by the Medical Field Service School as a supplement to the *Army Medical Bulletin*. It was sent to all Dental Corps officers and dental clinics. Rhoades appointed Major Walter D Vail to be the first editor for the new publication, whose initial issue appeared in January 1933. *The Dental Bulletin Supplement to the Army Medical Bulletin* was then published on a quarterly basis until it became *The Army Dental Bulletin* in January 1942. It ceased publication in July 1943 when it was merged into the new *Bulletin of the US Army Medical Department* (whose first issue appeared in October 1943).[6,9,10] During its years of publication under various names, the *Dental Bulletin* was an important tool for tying Dental Corps members together, maintaining esprit de corps and contacts, and assuring the continued professionalization of Army dentists.

On September 17, 1934, Colonel Frank P Stone, the last of the original contract dental surgeons then on active duty, assumed the position as chief of the

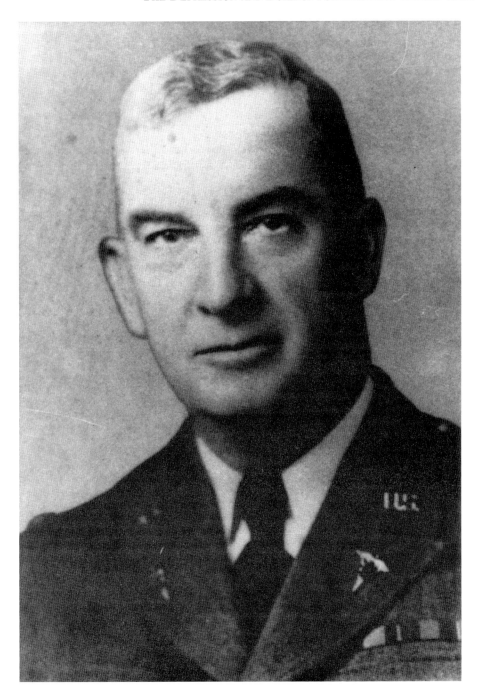

Colonel Frank P Stone was chief of the Dental Corps and dental division at the surgeon general's office from 1934 to 1938. Stone was the last of the original contract dental surgeons of 1901–1902 to serve on active duty and as chief of the Dental Corps.
Photograph: Courtesy of the National Museum of Dentistry, Major General Oscar Snyder Collection.

759

Dental Corps and dental subdivision (September 17, 1934–March 16, 1938), still a component of the professional service division of the surgeon general's office. Rex Rhoades retired on September 30th.[8]

Julien Bernheim, Rex Rhoades, and Frank Stone brought years of experience in dentistry and the Army to their labors as heads of the Dental Corps during the years from 1928 to 1938. Their experience, however, was powerless against the stark realities of the Depression, the continuing lack of fiscal resources to fund important Army programs and readiness, and an Army increasingly pushed into make-work relief programs and away from its mission of military preparedness and national defense. Bernheim, Rhoades, and Stone each struggled to juggle limited resources and competing requirements in a number of critical areas. They had to ensure that the Army's dental officers and enlisted technicians were well trained and proficient in their dental and military responsibilities, that the Army in the United States and overseas had adequate dental support in its dispensaries as well as in station and general hospitals, that dental supplies and equipment remained up to date, that dental research continued, and that the dental personnel in the Organized Reserves and National Guard were trained and ready to fulfill their wartime roles.

Strength and Distribution of the Dental Service

Short on money and personnel and overburdened with requirements, the Army's Dental Corps and dental service were severely constrained while performing their missions in the early 1930s. Constraints only worsened as a decade of change and retrenchment gave way to a decade of national depression. Even as the War Department's resources shrank, relief programs generated new requirements and the worsening global situation imposed additional strains.

The Dental Corps had been authorized a strength of 158 since 1923. In the years from 1930 through fiscal year 1936, its actual strength only reached its full authorized strength in fiscal years 1934 and 1936; in all the other years there were one to three vacancies in an already understaffed organization (Table 18-1). Further aggravating this problem was the War Department's policy of prohibiting existing vacancies to be filled during the last part of 1932–1933 because of economic pressure.[3,6] The final appointment to the Regular Army Dental Corps in fiscal year 1936 took place on April 2, 1936, when First Lieutenant Joseph LeRoy Bernier, already on voluntary extended active duty at Walter Reed General Hospital following his commissioning in the Dental Officers' Reserve Corps (DORC) in 1934, was commissioned. Lieutenant Bernier (later major general and Dental Corps chief [August 1960–August 1967]), became one of the world's leading oral pathologists during his years of service.[11]

The enlisted soldiers who filled many important roles, from chair assistants to technicians in the dental prosthetics laboratories, were just as critical to the success of the dental service as were the dental officers. In 1930 the number of enlisted personnel was 190, with 6 staff sergeants, 12 sergeants, 2 corporals, 85 privates first class, and 85 privates, and an inadequate allotment of specialist ratings.[1] The Army Dental School at Walter Reed Army Medical Center continued training students in dental hygiene and mechanics, but only 90 soldiers completed the training from 1930 through June 30, 1936 (see below, "The Army Dental School, 1930–1936").[1–3,6–8] While the training produced first-class technicians, the lack of specialist ratings resulted in the continuing loss of personnel to better paying jobs in civil practice. In his 1931 report, Bernheim noted this disquieting trend and requested additional ratings to retain these soldiers:

> Recommendation to provide for an increase in the number of specialist ratings for specially trained enlisted men has, however, been recently submitted in an effort to increase the efficiency of the dental service. In providing special technical instruction to enlisted men at the Army Dental School the Government is put to considerable expense. Without specialists' ratings commensurate with their qualifications and length of service as technicians, these men frequently become dissatisfied and are lost to the service by purchasing their discharge and engaging in more remunerative civil pursuits. It would be wise economy if this could be prevented.[2(p282)]

Nothing more was reported in the annual reports of 1932 or 1933 about increased allotments of specialist ratings for enlisted soldiers, so apparently Bernheim's initiative failed.[3,6] However, both of those reports emphasized the importance of trained enlisted technicians. In 1932 Bernheim noted that trained technicians "materially increase the general efficiency of the dental service, especially at field stations where their services can so readily be utilized."[3(p210)] The following year, Rhoades was even more emphatic in his assessment, writing that "the number of enlisted men, grades, and the ratings allotted to the dental service are inadequate. It is believed the achievement of the dental service could be increased

TABLE 18-1

REGULAR ARMY DENTAL CORPS: STRENGTH, LOSSES, APPOINTMENTS, AND VACANCIES, 1930–1936[*]

	1930	1931	1932	1933	1934	1935	1936
Authorized strength	158	158	158	158	158	158	158
Actual strength	157	157	155	156	158	156	158
Losses	6	3	3	2	2	5	3
Appointments	8	3	1	3	4	3	5
Vacancies	1	1	3	2	0	2	0

[*]As of June 30 of each fiscal year.
Data sources: (1) Office of The Surgeon General. *Annual Report of the Surgeon General.* Washington, DC: OTSG; 1930. (2) Office of The Surgeon General. *Annual Report of the Surgeon General.* Washington, DC: OTSG; 1931. (3) Office of The Surgeon General. *Annual Report of the Surgeon General.* Washington, DC: OTSG; 1932. (4) Office of The Surgeon General. *Annual Report of the Surgeon General.* Washington, DC: OTSG; 1933. (5) Office of The Surgeon General. *Annual Report of the Surgeon General.* Washington, DC: OTSG; 1934. (6) Office of The Surgeon General. *Annual Report of the Surgeon General.* Washington, DC: OTSG; 1935. (7) Office of The Surgeon General. *Annual Report of the Surgeon General.* Washington, DC: OTSG; 1936.

by 50 percent by the allotment of a suitable number of additional enlisted men to the dental service."[6(p173)]

As with the appeals for more dental officers, Rhoades's request was ignored. However, he initiated a study of dental attendance with the view of expanding the dental service. Any expansion would require more dental officers, but previous recommendations had gone nowhere. The alternative was to expand the dental service by using additional trained enlisted technicians working under dental officers. Rhoades's study concluded that a total of 364 enlisted technicians distributed throughout the Medical Department could make a significant contribution to improving the overall dental service for small additional costs. These findings formed the basis for a recommendation to the surgeon general, but it seems nothing resulted.[12] The number of enlisted soldiers in the dental service remained unchanged, at a strength of 190 authorized, from 1930 through 1935 (although 211 were noted as actually working in 1934) before dramatically bouncing up 30% to 270 at the end of fiscal year 1936.[1–3,6–8,12,13]

In the early 1930s the majority of the dental service's officer and enlisted strength was located in station hospitals at the largest posts, depots, and airfields, and in the dispensaries and general hospitals in the United States.[14] Three officers held administrative posts: the chief and an assistant at the surgeon general's office, and the dental supply and procurement officer in the medical section of the New York General Depot. Eleven others were assigned to training: three at the Army Dental School (where they also worked at the dental clinic at Walter Reed General Hospital or the Washington General Dispensary) and eight in Dental Reserve Officers' Training Corps (ROTC) units.[1,2,14] From 1930 to 1935, an average of 124 dental officers were assigned in the United States, with 110 to 113 of them serving part time or full time in the dental clinics from 1930 through 1932.[1–3,6–8] The Dental Corps officers often occupied other posts as well. For example, senior supervising dental surgeons in dental clinics located adjacent to a corps area headquarters also acted as dental advisors to the corps area surgeons, and Dental ROTC instructors often served in local dental clinics and during summers (until legislative action in the Army appropriation bill of May 1932 eliminated that program).[7,8,15]

On March 20, 1933, Congress passed an act "to maintain the credit of the United States Government" that required the Veterans Administration (VA) to withdraw its beneficiaries who were patients in Army hospitals and ceased reimbursements for their services.[6] The VA had covered the cost of placing reserve dental officers on active duty to provide dental care for its beneficiaries since 1925 (see Chapter XVII: A Return to Normalcy: from the World War to the Depression, 1919–1929). As a result of the March 20 act, the Medical Department had to release the 15 DORC officers then caring for VA patients and return them to inactive status.[6,16] Stone noted in his 1933 report that this action relieved the dental service of the burden of caring for "others."[6] In March 1934 the legislation was revised, resulting in a gradual increase in VA patients in Army hospitals, but not a return of DORC officers to care for the dental cases.[6] However, within 2 years, 6 of the 15 reservists received Regular Army commissions and were on active duty.[17–20]

Of the posts in the United States in the early 1930s, 36, with commands ranging in strength from 10 to 700 soldiers and totaling 7,000 troops, were furnished with only part time dental service because of the shortage of dental officers.[21] Once again, Army dentists were forced to undertake itinerant service to posts without assigned dental officers.[22] These installations received 1,319 days of service—or approximately 1 hour per year, per individual (not including dependents)—and the itinerant service deprived 16 other posts with a total of about 10,000 soldiers of dental service for 775 days per year.[21]

Outside the continental United States, continuous dental service was available to all military personnel in the Panama Canal, Hawaiian, and Philippine departments, except those in Alaska and at Camp John Hay and Pettit Barracks in the Philippines.[21] In 1931 31 Dental Corps officers were assigned to overseas posts—12 to Hawaii, 10 to the Philippines, 8 to the Panama Canal (7 to the department and 1 to the civil government), and 1 to American forces in China. By the end of fiscal year 1936, the distribution changed slightly to 33, with an increase to 14 assigned to Hawaii and 9 to Panama, and a decrease to 9 assigned to the Philippines.[2,13,14]

Schofield Barracks on Oahu provides a good example of the operation of an overseas dental clinic. In 1932 eight dental officers, one noncommissioned officer, and ten enlisted dental assistants on full duty were assigned to care for the 10,000-person Hawaiian Division, then the largest in the Army. A new station hospital opened in May 1929, allowing the dental personnel to be consolidated in a 10-chair clinic on the second floor of the outpatient building. The dental service was divided into operative, prosthetic, oral surgery, X-ray, and orthodontic sections. A ward surgeon referred hospital patients, accompanied by a dental consultation slip, to the dental clinic. Due to lack of personnel, however, routine dental examinations were not performed on all hospital patients.[23]

Dental Health of the Army, 1930–1935

Beginning in 1924, the Dental Corps tracked the dental health of the Army through annual examinations and surveys (see Chapter XVII: A Return to Normalcy: from the World War to the Depression, 1919–1929) that were reported and analyzed in the annual reports of the surgeon general. The annual dental survey reports for 1930–1935 indicate that the dental health record of the Army showed a steadily improving trend (Table 18-2). Rex Rhoades concluded that this was partly due to the decrease in original enlistments, which brought fewer people into the service with serious oral and dental problems, and to the fact that the dental service was able to improve dental health rates despite its personnel limitations and heavy workload.[7] Through 1935 all classifications for both officer/warrant officer and enlisted soldiers showed marked improvement, especially in classes I and IV.

"The question is, will the Army do it?": Walter D Vail on Dental Health in the Army

In the July 1933, July 1934, and January 1936 issues of the *Dental Bulletin Supplement to The Army Medical Bulletin*, Major (later Colonel) Walter D Vail, then the assistant to Rex Rhoades in the dental subdivision office and editor of the *Dental Bulletin* since its revival in January 1933, published articles on the various factors affecting dental health in the Army. As the assistant for clinical operations, Vail had intimate knowledge of all facets of the dental service. His 1933 and 1934 articles were analyses of the Army's dental health based on the 1933 annual examinations and surveys. In his first article, "A Study of Dental Conditions of Officers of the Army with Reference to the Loss of Teeth and Their Replacements," Vail looked at 6,000 reports of annual physical examinations of Army officers, ages 20 to 64. For the entire group, he calculated that each officer had lost on average 3.80 teeth and had 2.37 of them replaced, which confirmed to him the "toll exacted by dental diseases."[24] Vail concluded:

> The extent of loss of teeth shown in this study indicates the performance of a vast amount of health service and unquestionably a large portion of it was done in conjunction with, and as a part of, medical attendance for the restoration of health. The removal of dental infections is, in general, a distinct health service. On the other hand, the gross loss of teeth is evidence of failure to provide a far more valuable health service—that of preventing and controlling dental diseases which if even reasonably controlled, would afford an important and economical factor in the maintenance of health. It is more economical to perform simple operations for the prevention and control of dental diseases than it is to extract teeth and construct prosthetic appliances, which are in themselves expensive, to say nothing of the time involved, that

TABLE 18-2

DENTAL HEALTH OF THE ARMY BASED ON ANNUAL PHYSICAL EXAMINATIONS OF OFFICER PERSONNEL AND ANNUAL DENTAL SURVEYS OF ENLISTED PERSONNEL, 1930–1936[*]

Classification[†]		1930	1931	1932	1933	1934	1935	1936
I	Officers and warrant officers	3.35	3.19	2.32	14	21	16	30
	Enlisted personnel	12.76	13.46	11.14	132	110	98	98
II	Officers and warrant officers	17.84	17.50	13.68	166	144	131	153
	Enlisted personnel	31.92	32.05	29.36	284	273	268	245
III	Officers and warrant officers	8.06	6.09	7.03	61	51	50	41
	Enlisted personnel	6.68	7.16	7.43	70	67	59	56
IV	Officers and warrant officers	70.75	73.20	76.87	759	784	803	786
	Enlisted personnel	38.64	47.33	52.07	514	550	575	601

[*]Statistics are reported as a percentage of those surveyed from 1930 through 1932, and as a rate per 1,000 Army strength annually thereafter.
[†]Classifications were as follows: (I) in need of immediate treatment; (II) in need of early treatment; (III) in need of extended treatment; and (IV) no treatment needed.
Data sources: (1) Office of The Surgeon General. *Annual Report of the Surgeon General*. Washington, DC: OTSG; 1931: 285. (2) Office of The Surgeon General. Annual Report of the Surgeon General. Washington, DC: OTSG; 1932: 212. (3) Office of The Surgeon General. Annual Report of the Surgeon General. Washington, DC: OTSG; 1933: 172. (4) Office of The Surgeon General. *Annual Report of the Surgeon General*. Washington, DC: OTSG; 1934: 161. (5) Office of The Surgeon General. *Annual Report of the Surgeon General*. Washington, DC: OTSG; 1935: 154–155. (6) Office of The Surgeon General. *Annual Report of the Surgeon General*. Washington, DC: OTSG; 1936: 149.

could be more profitably employed in control service. If, however, the less expensive measures are not made available, the more expensive ones must be employed to meet the situation. . . . It is hoped that the toll exacted by dental diseases will receive the attention it deserves and that measures for the reduction of the toll will be instituted to the end that health may be conserved by preventive rather than restorative procedures.[24(pp106–107)]

In his 1934 article, "Dental Health in the Army," Vail extended his analysis to the dental health of the entire Army and the factors affecting it.[25] Vail stated that dental diseases were common to all soldiers because of low recruitment standards, and that meant that "health measures become corrective rather than preventive and, therefore, the burden of such effort rests on the dental service in so far as it has the capacity to serve."[25,26] He then named four factors that determined the capacity of the dental service to serve: "(1) the standard of dental requirements, for commission or enlistment, (2) the quota of dental service personnel, (3) the cooperation of military personnel in a dental health training program, and (4) the extension of the dental service."[25(p148)]

Currently, the Army only required an enlistee to have 12 serviceable teeth, and other existing dental and oral diseases were not considered grounds for disqualification from service. Vail believed that the adoption of a higher standard, such as the Navy's requirement of 20 serviceable teeth, could substantially alleviate this situation.[25]

Regarding the adequacy of dental service personnel, Vail noted that "there is a maximum effort a given number of dental officers can make under given conditions. Such an effort may be said to be adequate when their services are characterized by high rates of preventive measures, and relatively low extraction rates." However, the high rates of emergency treatment meant that preventive measures were not effective and took time away from the necessary corrective measures. An adequate number of trained enlisted dental assistants would allow dental officers to increase their efficiency. Vail stressed that "dental operations require close physical application and any relief that may be furnished a dental officer has an important bearing on the quality and quantity of his service." For each 1,000-person command, he proposed a dental office consisting of one dental officer and four enlisted technicians to act as the chair assistant, hygienist, dental mechanic, and record and supply clerk (who would also supervise office administration).[25]

The third factor, a sound dental health training program, required cooperation between dentists and patients. Frequent examinations, good personal habits, diet, and instruction all played parts in this area.[25] According to Vail,

In the Army a dental health training program offers great possibilities, provided it is properly planned and executed and there is sufficient dental personnel available to furnish the necessary cooperation with individual effort to make the program effective. Unfortunately individual effort is only partially successful, unless supplemented by appropriate dental examination and treatment. . . . Dental health measures should be prescribed, the necessary instruction provided, and regulations requiring reasonable compliance enforced. Dental attendance regulations should embrace the required cooperative effort of an adequate dental service. Such a program is the only practical means of applying preventive principles to dental health; otherwise, only corrective measures are applicable and these have proven ineffectual.[25(p150)]

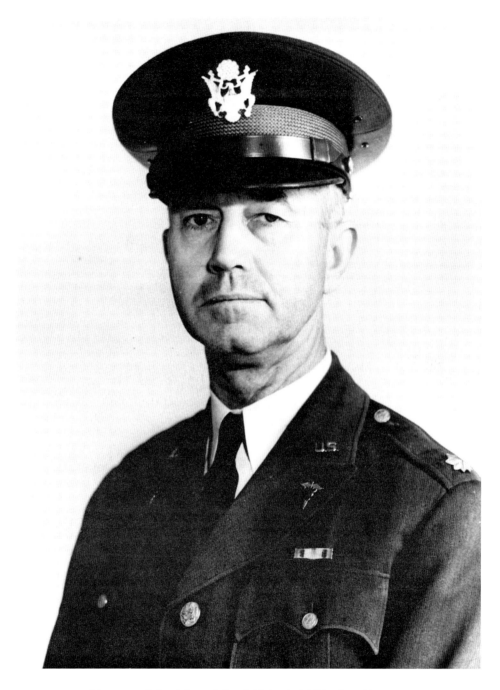

Lieutenant Colonel (later Colonel) Walter D Vail in the mid 1930s.
Reproduced from: Colonel James Vail. In: John Hyson Collection. Located at: Research Collections,
Office of Medical History, OTSG/MEDCOM, Falls Church, Virginia.

766

Vail also focused on the heavy burden imposed by the dental treatment of the "others" Army dentists treated in addition to active duty personnel. Vail noted that "inasmuch as Army Regulations provide for this character of treatment, it should be understood that the inadequacy of dental personnel is increased to that extent."[25(pp148–150)]

Vail concluded his article with the following observations:

> The wide prevalence of dental diseases in the Army is indicative that control measures have not been successfully employed. . . . The rates of extraction may be lowered and masticating function preserved with mutual benefits to health by (1) higher standards of dental requirements for admission into the Army, (2) the institution of an effective oral health training program, and (3) a suitable increase in dental service personnel.[25(p151)]

Virtually every discussion of the problems of the Army dental service came back to the inadequate number of trained dental personnel to undertake the heavy workload and develop an effective preventive dentistry program.

In his January 1936 article, "Dentistry as a Factor in Preventive Medicine in the Army," Vail stressed preventive dentistry as preventive medicine and emphasized its potential role in the conservation of strength in the Army. He contended that Army dentistry was completely involved in preventive medicine, but "that the value of dentistry as a health factor is too often discussed in terms of 'teeth.'" Army dentists prevented and removed infections that affected soldiers' health.[27] Unfortunately, because of the ongoing shortages in the Dental Corps, Vail contended that "little is being accomplished in the true prevention of dental diseases." He believed that "it would be difficult to define the limits of benefits derived by the Army through the practice of preventive dentistry." An adequate dental service could definitely be "an effective factor in the field of military medicine," though it was currently not being used to that end.[27(p4)] Going back to the arguments in his previous articles, Vail concluded "the only way to make military dentistry a more important factor in military medicine is to increase the amount of dental service. The question is, will the Army do it?"[27(p6)]

Dental Attendance and Professional Service, 1930–1935

While the annual surveys and examinations that Vail analyzed measured the current dental health of the Army, they provided no measure of dental attendance, operations, diseases treated, and overall professional service (Table 18-3, Table 18-4, Table 18-5). Unlike the US Navy Dental Corps, the Army dental service also had to care for a large number of "others entitled by regulations to dental attendance," which included the families of service members, military retirees, VA patients, and Army civilian employees.[6,25] These "others" continued to constitute a significant percent of the total workload, especially beginning in 1933 when the data included dental work that Regular Army and DORC personnel serving with the CCC completed at Army posts (see Table 18-3; see below, "Dental Service for the Civilian Conservation Corps, 1933–1936").

In his last report in 1932, Bernheim noted some positive trends in the data with satisfaction, ascribing them to the dedication of the dental service's professional personnel, better clinic management, and more and better equipment:

TABLE 18-3

ADMISSIONS FOR DENTAL TREATMENT, 1930–1936*

	1930	1931	1933		1934		1935		1936	
	Number	Number	Number	Rate	Number	Rate	Number	Rate	Number	Rate
US Army										
Routine	NR	NR	66,550	485.1	76,561	565.78	81,661	570.43	91,688	554.81
Emergency	NR	NR	33,036	240.81	33,347	246.43	37,377	261.09	39,129	236.71
Total	105,198	NR	99,586	725.91	109,908	812.21	119,038	831.52	130,817	791.58
Others[†]	45,175	NR	69,423	NR	87,545	NR	86,480	NR	81,137	NR
Total admissions	150,373	157,702	169,009	NR	197,453	NR	205,518	NR	211,954	NR
Others as percentage of total admissions	30.0	N/A	41.4	N/A	44.3	N/A	42.1	N/A	38.3	N/A

*No reports are available for 1932; beginning in 1933, rates are calculated based on cases per 1,000 Army strength annually.
†"Others" include families of active duty military personnel, civilian employees, Veterans Administration patients, retirees, and, beginning in 1933, enrollees of the Civilian Conservation Corps who were seen by Regular Army dental officers.
N/A: not applicable
NR: not reported
Data sources: (1) Office of The Surgeon General. *Annual Report of the Surgeon General*. Washington, DC: OTSG; 1931: 286–287. (2) Office of The Surgeon General. *Annual Report of the Surgeon General*. Washington, DC: OTSG; 1932: 211. (3) Office of The Surgeon General. *Annual Report of the Surgeon General*. Washington, DC: OTSG; 1933: 175. (4) Office of The Surgeon General. *Annual Report of the Surgeon General*. Washington, DC: OTSG; 1934: 164. (5) Office of The Surgeon General. *Annual Report of the Surgeon General*. Washington, DC: OTSG; 1935: 158. (6) Office of The Surgeon General. *Annual Report of the Surgeon General*. Washington, DC: OTSG; 1936: 152. (7) Office of The Surgeon General. *Annual Report of the Surgeon General*. Washington, DC: OTSG; 1937: 178.

A study of the tables included in this section of the report indicates the high degree of efficiency maintained in the dental service for the period covered. The amount of dental attendance has, in a large degree, been due to the earnest effort put forth by dental officers. Economical clinic management and the installation in many dental clinics of additional equipment, so as to provide two operating chairs for each operator, has [sic] shown the expected advantages in accomplishment.[3(pp210–211)]

In his first report as chief of the dental subdivision in 1935, Frank Stone noted that the number of duty days that dental personnel worked per 1,000 military personnel had increased from 350 in 1932 to 418 in 1934. However, he attributed most of the increase to the increased number of DORC dentists on duty with the CCC, who accounted for most of this change in cases and service. He concluded that "while there was an increase of 15 percent in the amount of dental service available, little, if any, was available for military personnel."[8(pp156–157)]

Stone also noted the data showed that preventive dentistry was not being practiced "to the extent usually considered necessary for successful results. Preventive dentistry requires that prophylaxis be furnished, teeth examined, and necessary treatment accomplished at least twice a year."[8(p157)] He concluded that:

to have accomplished the prophylactic requisites for 812.21 admissions [total admissions per 1,000 cases per annum in 1934], prophylaxis at the rate of 1,624.42 would have been necessary in 1934. This is more than seven times that accomplished (224.31). Similar but more impressive data could be cited for fillings, which are essentially preventive measures.[8(p157)]

The continuing deficiencies in preventive dentistry bothered Stone because he realized the link between them and the burden placed on the prosthetic service from the resultant loss of teeth. Although he believed that the overall prosthetic service "appears to be satisfactory with the amount of time and personnel available for this service," he also knew that loss of teeth "due to the lack of prophylactic measures requires extensive numbers of prosthetic replacements."[8(p157)] He reiterated the dilemma facing the dental service because of the lack of trained personnel, saying,

the construction of such replacements requires a great amount of time, which in turn prevents the application of preventive measures. In the meantime dental diseases are not controlled, many foci of infection are developed and health is impaired long before the teeth are extracted as the last resort in an effort to overcome the damage done.[8(p157)]

In the professional service section of his 1936 report, Stone once again concluded "that no progress is being made in the prevention of dental disease."[13(p152)] As in 1935, he noted that "when it is considered that 7,459 bridges and dentures were necessary to restore 52,564 teeth the enormous amount of work involved in restoring teeth lost from dental diseases becomes apparent."[13(p152)] He planned a study to revive and expand the prosthetic laboratory service, originally set up in the late 1920s as the "central dental laboratories," to relieve dental officers and their technicians from time-consuming prosthetic work (see Chapter XVII: A Return to Normalcy: from the World War to the Depression, 1919–1929, and "Corps Area and Central Dental Laboratories, 1930–1936" below).[8,13]

TABLE 18-4

DENTAL ATTENDANCE IN THE US ARMY, CALENDAR YEARS 1930–1936[*]

	1930		1931		1932	
	Number	Rate	Number	Rate	Number	Rate
Cases completed	NR	NR	NR	NR	NR	NR
Prophylaxis	42,743	NR	47,426	NR	30,208	227.58
Extractions	77,259	NR	77,342	NR	48,990	369.08
Fillings						
Permanent	119,571	NR	117,799	NR	87,167	656.69
Temporary	7,119	NR	6,804	NR	3,793	28.58
Root canal	1,410	NR	1,253	NR	882	6.64
Prosthetic Appliances						
Bridges	1,110	NR	1,140	NR	989	7.45
Crowns	906	NR	886	NR	825	4.71
Dentures (all)	5,358	NR	6,342	NR	4,870	36.69

[*]Numbers for 1930 and 1931 include all patients (US Army military personnel, families, civilian employees, Veterans Administration, and retirees) seen by dental officers Beginning in 1932, numbers include Army personnel only, and rates are calculated based on cases per 1,000 Army strength annually.
NR: not reported
Data sources: (1) Office of The Surgeon General. *Annual Report of the Surgeon General*. Washington, DC:

TABLE 18-5

SELECTED DENTAL DISEASES TREATED BY US ARMY DENTAL OFFICERS, 1930–1936[*]

	1930		1931		1932	
	Number	Rate	Number	Rate	Number	Rate
Abscess, periapical	30,153	N/A	29,519	N/A	21,427	161.43
Calculus	38,525	N/A	39,921	N/A	28,901	217.73
Caries	131,048	N/A	132,780	N/A	101,346	763.52
Gingivitis	8,084	N/A	8,402	N/A	6,411	48.30
Malocclusion	609	N/A	586	N/A	445	3.35
Pulpitis	18,890	N/A	17,540	N/A	13,186	99.34
Stomatitis, Vincent's	4,903	N/A	4,807	N/A	5,072	38.21
Total diseases treated	289,017	N/A	295,143	N/A	230,270	1,734.80

[*]Numbers for 1930 and 1931 include all patients (US Army military personnel, families, civilian employees, Veterans Administration, and retirees) seen by dental officers. Beginning in 1932, numbers include Army personnel only, and rates are calculated based on cases per 1,000 Army strength annually.
N/A: not applicable
Data sources: (1) Office of The Surgeon General. *Annual Report of the Surgeon General*. Washington, DC: OTSG; 1931; 284, 286, 287. (2) Office of The Surgeon General. *Annual Report of the Surgeon General*.

TABLE 18-4 *continued*

	1933		1934		1935		1936	
	Number	Rate	Number	Rate	Number	Rate	Number	Rate
Cases completed	28,612	208.56	30,775	227.42	31,917	229.93	38,662	233.95
Prophylaxis	28,872	210.46	30,354	224.31	29,882	367.17	30,090	182.08
Extractions	49,630	361.77	48,873	361.17	51,306	358.39	53,368	322.94
Fillings								
Permanent	90,765	661.61	92,278	681.92	100,610	702.79	110,294	667.40
Temporary	4,446	32.41	4,906	36.25	4,839	33.80	7,508	45.43
Root canal	864	6.30	659	4.87	593	4.14	567	3.43
Prosthetic Appliances								
Bridges	971	7.08	1,095	8.09	1,212	8.47	1,150	6.96
Crowns	540	3.92	604	4.46	595	4.16	599	3.62
Dentures (all)	5,390	39.29	5,426	40.10	6,247	43.64	5,747	34.65

OTSG; 1931: 287 (2) Office of The Surgeon General. *Annual Report of the Surgeon General*. Washington, DC: OTSG; 1932: 213. (3) Office of The Surgeon General. *Annual Report of the Surgeon General*. Washington, DC: OTSG; 1933: 176. (4) Office of The Surgeon General. *Annual Report of the Surgeon General*. Washington, DC: OTSG; 1934:164. (5) Office of The Surgeon General. *Annual Report of the Surgeon General*. Washington, DC: OTSG; 1935: 158. (6) Office of The Surgeon General. *Annual Report of the Surgeon General*. Washington, DC: OTSG; 1936: 152. (7) Office of The Surgeon General. *Annual Report of the Surgeon General*. Washington, DC: OTSG; 1937: 178.

TABLE 18-5 *continued*

1933		1934		1935		1936	
Number	Rate	Number	Rate	Number	Rate	Number	Rate
20,316	148.09	20,940	154.74	20,514	143.30	21,100	127.68
28,160	205.27	29,932	221.19	30,263	211.40	30,118	182.25
102,122	744.39	97,990	724.14	108,272	756.31	115,510	696.79
5,472	39.89	6,062	44.80	5,620	39.26	6,098	36.89
450	3.28	530	3.92	634	4.43	676	4.09
12,735	92.83	11,770	86.98	12,598	88.00	14,728	89.12
4,414	32.17	4,751	35.11	4,951	34.58	5,104	30.88
233,734	1,703.75	234,253	1,731.10	248,388	1,735.06	259,047	1,567.52

Washington, DC: OTSG; 1932.: 211, 213. (3) Office of The Surgeon General. *Annual Report of the Surgeon General*. Washington, DC: OTSG; 1933: 175, 176. (4) Office of The Surgeon General. *Annual Report of the Surgeon General*. Washington, DC: OTSG; 1934: 164, 165. (5) Office of The Surgeon General. *Annual Report of the Surgeon General*. Washington, DC: OTSG; 1935: 158, 159. (6) Office of The Surgeon General. *Annual Report of the Surgeon General*. Washington, DC: OTSG; 1936: 152, 153. (7) Office of The Surgeon General. *Annual Report of the Surgeon General*. Washington, DC: OTSG; 1937: 178–179.

Echoing Rhoades and others, Stone summed up his 1936 report on professional service with a sober analysis of the current state of the Army dental service. "Considering the amount of dental service rendered," he wrote, "the record is commendable. It is regretted, however, that the type of dental service is unsatisfactory from the standpoint of providing a genuine health service. Dental service cannot function as a true health service until progress is made in the prevention of dental disease."[13(p152)]

The Demise of the Dental Reserve Officers' Training Corps, 1930–1935

The Medical Department established Dental ROTC units at eight leading dental schools in 1920–1921 to attract dental students to serve in the Dental Reserve or even the Dental Corps after graduation. During the 1920s some notable Dental Corps officers were assigned as instructors in these units. Colonel Robert T Oliver's final active duty assignment was as assistant professor of military science and tactics at the University of Pennsylvania's School of Dentistry from 1926 until his retirement in January 1932. The units trained, graduated, and commissioned 1,165 officers into the DORC through 1929 and were a leading source for new reserve officers (see Chapter XVII: A Return to Normalcy: from the World War to the Depression, 1919–1929).

During the early 1930s Dental ROTC units continued to attract significant numbers of dental school students who were interested in the small remuneration received in the advanced course (approximately $22.50 every 3 months) and to produce graduates who were commissioned in the DORC (Table 18-6).[28] As an economy measure, Congress did not provide funds in the Army appropriation bill of May 5, 1932 (for fiscal year 1933), for new enrollments in Medical Department ROTC units, but did not terminate students already enrolled or disband the existing units.[6,28,29,30] Similar provisions were included in the appropriations bills for 1934 and 1935, effectively killing the programs at two 3-year dental schools (State University of Iowa and University of Minnesota) on June 30, 1934, and at the remaining six schools on June 30, 1935.[7,8,29,30] Through 1935, these eight dental schools had provided 2,273 trained, commissioned officers for the DORC, and all of the Medical Department ROTC program taken together produced more than 50% of the newly appointed reserve officers in the Medical Department reserve.[7,8,29,30] The Medical Department received authority to reassign its eight dental instructors from ROTC duty on June 5, 1933, and immediately dispatched them to other duties. Instruction for the remaining students was picked up by Medical Corps officers, most of whom were also reassigned by the end of fiscal year 1934.[7,31]

The demise of the Dental ROTC units presented a major problem for the Medical Department in acquiring new reserve officers for the DORC and for the entire Medical Department Officers' Reserve Corps. The Army adjutant general issued new guidance to corps area and department commanders on August 29, 1934, on policies to be used to procure officers for the Medical Department Officers' Reserve Corps. Corps area commanders were encouraged to maintain contact with the most highly rated medical, dental, and veterinary colleges and to "utilize to the fullest extent possible the appropriate personnel at their disposal to effect friendly and sympathetic contact" with these schools as well as state and county medical, dental, and veterinary societies and associations "in order to interest them in medical preparedness" and to identify potential new officers. Army Regulations were changed, waiving the requirement for a license and experience in a dental practice so select members of graduating classes could be commissioned at graduation.[30,32] What appeared to be a simple congressional cost-saving measure ended a successful and productive program for acquiring new reserve officers, and complicated the process of staffing the DORC. In August 1936, as national defense became a major concern, Congress repealed the law prohibiting funding medical ROTC units, and by the end of fiscal year 1937, 22 medical schools had reestablished their ROTC units. No dental or veterinary units were reestablished prior to World War II.[33]

Major George R Kennebeck, who later served as a major general and chief of the US Air Force Dental Corps (1949–1952), was the officer assigned to the dental ROTC unit at the College of Dentistry, State University of Iowa, in Iowa City from 1929 to 1933. In the October 1934 issue of the *Dental Bulletin*, Kennebeck wrote about his experiences with the dental ROTC and concluded:

> It is regretted that the opportunity of selecting outstanding graduates of these dental colleges for the Dental Corps, Regular Army, passes out with the units. Many of the young members of our Corps were interested in this work by officers on R.O.T.C. duty and their commission in the Regular Army can be traced back to the R.O.T.C. instruction. . . . The writer feels confident that those officers who have had the opportunity to study the R.O.T.C. at first hand will agree that the termination of this instruction is a backward step and that the advantages accruing far outweigh the cost of this activity.[28(pp213–214)]

The Dental Officers' Reserve Corps, 1930–1936

The DORC constituted a critical component of the Medical Department reserve, which the War Department required to staff the mobilization Army for future wars. The reserve dental officers were heavily concentrated in the tactical units assigned to the corps areas, especially in the infantry regiments' medical detachments, the divisional medical regiments, and various hospital units with mobilization assignments.[34,35,36] While DORC membership fluctuated during the period from 1930–1936, it was generally beyond its peacetime personnel targets and easily met the War Department procurement objectives for staffing the Organized Reserves.[1,2,6–8,13] With a strength of 4,688 in 1930, the DORC was 42% over its established quota of 3,308.[1] During the Depression, strength increased in 1931–1933 to 5,589, perhaps as dentists sought additional sources of income from reserve service to offset adverse economic times. Declining numbers in 1933–1935 were not considered problematic, despite the termination of dental ROTC, but were seen as a short-term positive trend that brought the DORC into "a much better balanced condition."[8(p139)] During these years, between 91.6% and 98.6% of the DORC were assigned to tactical units in the corps areas (Table 18-7). Beginning in 1933 a number of DORC personnel were called to active duty to serve with the CCC (see below, "Dental Service for the Civilian Conservation Corps, 1933–1936").[6–8,13,36]

TABLE 18-6

DENTAL RESERVE OFFICERS' TRAINING CORPS ENROLLMENT AND
COMMISSIONED GRADUATES, 1930–1935

	1930	1931	1932	1933	1934	1935
Enrolled in basic first year	8	8	8	8	8	0
Enrolled in basic second year	237	258	230	0	0	0
Enrolled in advanced first year	306	296	286	185	0	0
Enrolled in advanced second year	143	191	192	171	163	NR
Total enrollment	883	941	890	512	304	NR
Graduated and commissioned in DORC	277	171	211	164	163	122
Graduates commissioned since 1921	1,442	1,613	1,824	1,988	2,151	2,273

DORC: Dental Officers' Reserve Corps
NR: not reported
Data sources: (1) Office of The Surgeon General. *Annual Report of the Surgeon General*. Washington, DC: OTSG; 1930: 280. (2) Office of The Surgeon General. *Annual Report of the Surgeon General*. Washington, DC: OTSG; 1931: 346. (3) Office of The Surgeon General. *Annual Report of the Surgeon General*. Washington, DC: OTSG; 1932: 197, 198. (4) Office of The Surgeon General. *Annual Report of the Surgeon General*. Washington, DC: OTSG; 1933: 163–164. (5) Office of The Surgeon General. *Annual Report of the Surgeon General*. Washington, DC: OTSG; 1934: 152. (6) R.O.T.C. units. *Dental Bulletin Supplement to the Army Medical Bulletin*. 1936;7(January):22.

Dental Service for the Civilian Conservation Corps, 1933–1936

On March 31, 1933, Congress approved President Franklin D Roosevelt's request to form the CCC to relieve unemployment among young men. It was intended to carry out useful public works, such as reforestation, flood control, and land reclamation on federal and state lands. Encouraged by the president's sense of urgency, 250,000 men joined the CCC by July, creating an administrative challenge that only the Army was equipped to handle. Combat units provided the cadres for the CCC camps, while the quartermaster and surgeons general struggled with the logistical and medical aspects.[37,38]

War Department CCC Circular No. 3, issued May 12, 1933, required dental and medical service to be provided to CCC enrollees. It called for Dental Reserve officers or contract dental surgeons to be employed in the camps. One reserve officer or contract dentist was provided per work district or reconditioning camp. In an emergency, civilian dentists could be employed on a fee basis. The limit of one dentist could be disregarded at the discretion of the corps area commander "when special conditions warrant."[39] Major Clarence W Johnson, Dental Corps, who served for 2 years on a processing board for CCC enrollees, noted that "records of over 5,000 candidates show that more than 50% of these would be rejected for enlistment in the Regular Army because of failure to meet dental requirements."[40(p57)]

The 1934 regulations (War Department Regulations, Relief of Unemployment, Civilian Conservation Corps, September 1, 1934) for the CCC covered only authorized emergency treatment and the repair of dental injuries incurred while on duty. They did not include follow-up treatment, such as fillings, replacement of lost teeth, or repair of prosthetic appliances made necessary through injury. When dental injuries involved the restoration of tooth substance, replacement of teeth, or the repair of prosthetic devices, it was recommended that the dentist get prior authorization from the surgeon general (like Regular Army personnel) to avoid misunderstandings that might occur when "fees charged by civilian dentists" were reduced because they were "in excess of the allowed amount."[41(pp27,29)]

A CCC enrollee was entitled to necessary medical and dental treatment for an injury or disease "not the result of his own misconduct" (par. 93, War Department Regulations, CCC).[42] The surgeon general had to authorize repairs (eg, fillings or appliances) following dental injuries treated by a civilian dentist. The use of gold was not authorized, except for the "repair of traumatic injuries received in line of duty." When a CCC enrollee was hospitalized, the War Department was reimbursed $3.75 per day, which covered the entire cost of treatment, including dental. It was important that these cases be handled in Army hospitals so that the War Department could recover funds for gold used in dental treatment.[42]

In 1934, despite the successful CCC effort and the use of contract dentists and reserve dental officers, in his dental subdivision section of the *Annual Report of the Surgeon General*, Frank Stone stated "that the demand made on Regular Army Dental Corps officers in connection with C.C.C. activities has reduced the amount of dental service that otherwise would have been available to the Regular Army personnel."[7(p165)] A year later he repeated his opinion on the adverse effect of CCC work.[8] Stone presented no hard evidence to support his conclusions in the 1934 and 1935 annual reports; statistics for CCC enrollees were included within the "others" categories in the statistical tables of dental attendance and diseases treated in the annual reports of the surgeon general from 1933 through 1936.[7,8] Only two items in the *Dental Bulletin* of July 1936 provide a glimpse of the CCC workload during calendar year 1935. One piece reported on posts where only Regular Army dental officers were on duty. It reported 4,655 CCC admissions with 9,769 sittings for emergency and traumatic injuries, 108 permanent fillings, 5,358 extractions, 2,034 X-rays, 34 jaw fractures treated, and 13 prosthetic appliances repaired.[13,43] When compared to the total figures for "others" reported for 1935, these figures represented 5.4% of the admissions (86,480) and 0.02% of the permanent fillings (43,162), but 10.2% of the extractions (52,619). Another article stated that CCC enrollees accounted for 36,059 teeth extracted and 129 fractures reduced, which represented 68.5% (52,619) of all extractions for "others" and 87.2% (148) of all reduced fractures recorded for "others." Records for other posts where both regular and reserve dental officers served were incomplete and not reported.[44] It was not until the annual report of 1938 that separate statistics for CCC activities were reported for the preceding calendar year and the full workload was clearly explained.[45]

TABLE 18-7

DENTAL OFFICERS IN THE ORGANIZED RESERVES,
JUNE 30, 1930–JUNE 30, 1936

Year	Total Strength	Gross Gain/Loss	Promotions	Assigned to Corps Areas (Tactical Units)	Percent Assigned to Corps Areas
1930	4,688	477/453	221	4,297	91.6
1931	5,037	591/242	222	4,777	94.8
1932	5,557	707/187	118	5,303	95.4
1933	5,589	341/309	94	5,389	96.4
1934	5,299	538/828	110	5,144	97.1
1935	5,036	654/562	173	4,926	97.8
1936	5,128	475/370	145	5,059	98.6

Data sources: (1) Vail WD. The Dental Reserve Corps. *Dental Bulletin Supplement to the Army Medical Bulletin*. 1936;7(January):21. (2) Office of The Surgeon General. *Annual Report of the Surgeon General*. Washington, DC: OTSG; 1930: 266. (3) Office of The Surgeon General. *Annual Report of the Surgeon General*. Washington, DC: OTSG; 1931: 326. (4) Office of The Surgeon General. *Annual Report of the Surgeon General*. Washington, DC: OTSG; 1932: 192. (5) Office of The Surgeon General. *Annual Report of the Surgeon General*. Washington, DC: OTSG; 1933: 158. (6) Office of The Surgeon General. *Annual Report of the Surgeon General*. Washington, DC: OTSG; 1934: 146. (7) Office of The Surgeon General. *Annual Report of the Surgeon General*. Washington, DC: OTSG; 1935: 139–140. (8) Office of The Surgeon General. *Annual Report of the Surgeon General*. Washington, DC: OTSG; 1936: 134.

The Army Dental School, 1930–1936

Lieutenant Colonel Frank LK Laflamme's tenure as director of the Army Dental School encompassed the early years of the Depression. On August 5, 1932, Lieutenant Colonel Robert H Mills, future chief of the Dental Corps (March 17, 1942–March 16, 1946), took over as the director and Laflamme moved to Fort Sam Houston, Texas, to take Mills's former post as the dental surgeon for the Eighth Corps Area and officer in charge of the fort's dental clinic.[46,47]

Laflamme and Mills both confronted the problem arising from the paucity of new appointments in the Dental Corps (8 in 1930, 3 in 1931, and 1 in 1932), which meant that few officers required the school's basic course. With few students and an uncertain attendance, scheduling the course became difficult and the previously linked sequence with the basic course at the Medical Field Service School was no longer critical. In the 5-month basic course classes that graduated from 1930 to 1933, 19 majors, 9 captains, and 5 first lieutenants attended, and the first lieutenants were the only new Dental Corps officers undergoing the training.[1–3,6,48,49] The courses remained intense postgraduate courses. In 1929–1930, they comprised 685 hours of classroom instruction, laboratory, and clinical work focused on clinical dentistry, prosthesis, oral surgery, and preventive medicine and clinical pathology. In 1931–1932, 681 hours were required, and in 1932–1933, the number rose to 705 hours.[48,49] As fewer new officers attended the basic course, the Army Dental School opened it to Dental Corps officers who had not previously attended. In January 1933 the 12th and final basic course graduated, and the course was discontinued as a result of the War Department's change to postgraduate courses in the special service schools (such as the Army Dental School).[6,7,50,51,52]

From 1930 through 1932, six officers attended the 4-month–long advanced course that was increasingly focused on surgery and oral surgery, preventive medicine, prosthetics and clinical dentistry, and the preparation of field-grade officers with the skills needed to command a large post or hospital dental clinic.[4] Frank Laflamme intentionally designed the "gentlemen's course," as he called it, to allow the greatest possible concentration in the area of dentistry that would most benefit each student. Major (later Brigadier General) Neal A Harper, a member of the fifth advanced course class, wrote a short piece on his experiences in the only issue of the *Dental Bulletin* published in 1932.[53] Harper explained how the course worked:

> Emphasis was made by the Colonel [Laflamme] upon the fact that the session was to be conducted as a "gentlemen's course" in the sense that each student officer had the privilege of electing to major in that branch of dentistry in which he believed he would derive the greatest benefit, spending less time in the departments wherein he felt generally well qualified. Stress was laid, also, on the attitude of the faculty that better results would accrue to each member of the class if he would take all the time needed for mastery of a single problem or technique, rather than adhere to an inelastic schedule such as necessarily characterizes the intensive and wide scoped Basic Courses.[53(p20)]

The curriculum for the sixth and final advanced course session, which ran from February 1 to May 31, 1933, totaled 549 hours, with the majority of those in operative dentistry (154 hours), prosthesis (160 hours), and oral surgery (160 hours). The session began with six officers in attendance, but the dental service's need for dentists throughout the Army were so pressing that five of them were relieved and sent to new duty stations on March 1, leaving only one officer to complete the course.[54] The advanced courses recorded a total of seven graduates from 1930 to 1933.[1–3,6]

In fiscal year 1933 the War Department directed a major change in the officers' basic and advanced courses that was to be implemented in fiscal year 1934. In accordance with the new policy, the Medical Department professional special service schools (the Army Medical, Dental, and Veterinary schools) revised their basic and advanced courses into new postgraduate courses. Newly commissioned officers attended the basic course at the Medical Field Service School and later completed the postgraduate course that would constitute professional refresher training.[6,7,51,52]

The new 5-month postgraduate course for officers that replaced the basic and advanced courses in September 1933 provided 618 hours of instruction in a revised curriculum that included clinical dentistry (131 hours), prosthesis (125 hours), oral surgery (153 hours), and preventive medicine and clinical pathology (144 hours). It was first offered from September 1, 1933, to February 5, 1934.[55] Major (later Colonel) Frederic H Bockoven, who attended the initial class, remarked in a short piece

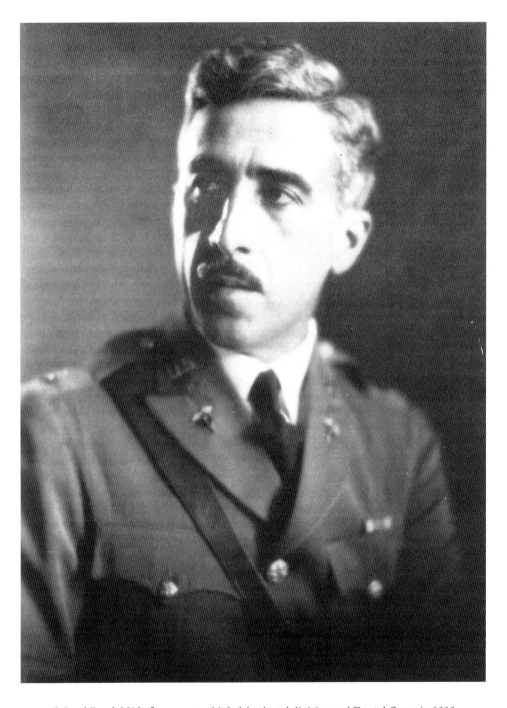

*Colonel Frank LK Laflamme was chief of the dental division and Dental Corps in 1919
and later director of the Army Dental School (1929–1932).
Photograph: Courtesy of Marie F Laflamme.*

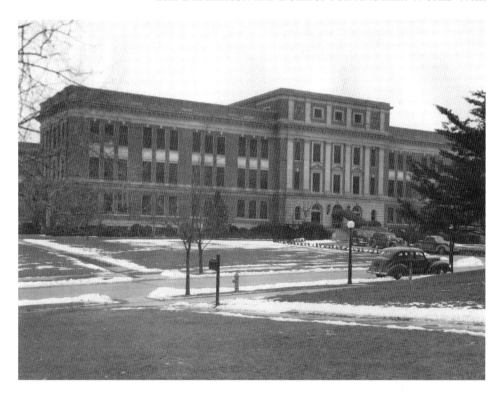

*The Army Dental School and Walter Reed Central Dental Laboratory occupied parts
of the first and second floors of the new north wing of the Army Medical Schools building,
which is just visible to the left of the south building at Walter Reed Army Medical Center,
when it opened in October 1932.*
Reproduced from: A History of the Army Dental School, March 14, 1938–Sept. 17, 1940.
Located at: Research Collections, Office of Medical History, OTSG/MEDCOM, Falls Church, Virginia.

in the *Dental Bulletin*, "I might here pause to leave the thought that the Corps is
unusually fortunate in having a school so well equipped and offering post graduate work in so many subjects. One would hardly know where to look, if it were
procurable at all, to find a course that duplicates the work that is given here."[51]

Lieutenant Colonel Leigh C Fairbank, another future Dental Corps chief and
the first brigadier general in Dental Corps history (March 17, 1938–March 16, 1942),
completed the 14th officer session from August 30, 1934, to February 5, 1935.[56] In
fiscal year 1936, the last of the postgraduate courses was offered from August 28,
1935, to February 5, 1936, and six Dental Corps officers completed it, including
then Major Oscar P Snyder, a future Dental Corps chief (1954–1956).[57]

The new advanced graduate course that was introduced in 1936 with the 16th
officer session came as a directive from the War Department. It reduced the course
to 4 months and cut the number of hours to 507. Four Dental Corps officers, all
lieutenant colonels, completed the first course offering, which ran from February
1 to May 29, 1936.[58,59]

Although the curriculum was in a constant state of flux from 1933 to 1936, the Army Dental School relocated several times. The school had been located on the Walter Reed compound in inadequate, temporary, wooden buildings from the World War I era since 1922. It moved to new quarters on June 1, 1930, when its building was condemned and scheduled for demolition, and it occupied semipermanent quarters for the next 2 years.[1,2] In October 1932 the Army Dental and Veterinary schools occupied a new, modern addition to the Army Medical School (Building 40) at Walter Reed Army Medical Center in Washington, DC.[6] The Army Dental School occupied the entire second floor of the north wing. It contained the director's office, clerk's room, executive office, clerical office, main lecture room, mimeograph room, physical laboratory and office, library, oral surgery amphitheater, bacteriology laboratory, preparation room, pathology laboratory, prosthetic laboratory (which housed the Walter Reed Central Dental Laboratory), chemical laboratory, mail room, X-ray dark room, photographic room, and oral hygiene clinic (six chairs equipped with Ritter Tri-Dent units). During a visit to the school's new facilities, Dr G Walter Dittmar, then president of the American Dental Association (ADA), "pronounced it to be one of the finest and most completely equipped that it had been his pleasure to inspect."[60]

The Army Dental School had trained enlisted dental technicians in dental mechanics, hygiene, and X-ray procedures since 1923. Centralized training of enlisted technicians was important because the instruction at the Army Dental School was much more thorough than that provided by practicing dental officers who could not be spared from their operating responsibilities. From 1930 through 1932 a total of 39 students completed the training in the 5-month (January–May) course in dental mechanics, most of whom were then sent to the various installation prosthetics laboratories or to one of the functioning central dental laboratories.[1–3] This training was even more effective because trainees were given practical instruction in the Walter Reed Central Dental Laboratory.[6,60] Two technicians completed the 4-month (January–April) dental hygiene course in April 1932.[3] Although a clear need existed for trained dental hygienists throughout the dental service, a continuing shortage of funds prevented the training of a number sufficient to meet the large demand. Thus, once again, the dental officers themselves had to train enlisted soldiers as dental hygienists, taking valuable time from their primary duties.[61]

On September 1, 1932, the Army Dental School introduced a 9-month "enlisted specialists" course for dental technicians that included instruction in dental prosthetics, radiology, and hygiene, and was intended to produce more well-rounded enlisted dental technicians. Nine students graduated from the course on May 31, 1933.[6] In January 1934, 14 enlisted soldiers were assigned to the Army Dental School for a revised course that lasted 6 months. The new course offered a total of 887 hours of instruction, with 540 hours in dental prosthetics, 225 hours in hygiene, and 87 hours in radiology.[62] The 1935 dental technicians' course that ran from January 2 to June 30 was increased to 982 hours, with a 95-hour increase in dental prosthetics instruction (a total of 635 hours).[63] Funds were only available to support travel by 10 of the 14 enlisted soldiers selected to attend, but the four other candidates came to the course school at their own expense.[64] The enlisted training program was again limited to dental mechanics from February 1 to May 29, 1936.

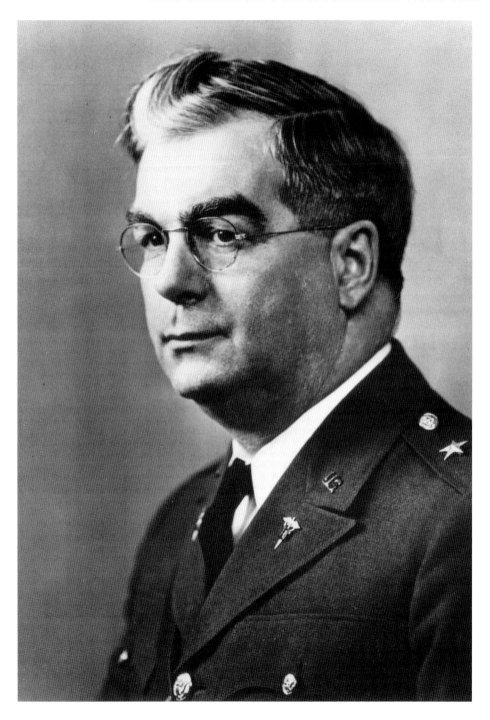

Brigadier General Leigh C Fairbank was first chief of the dental division and Dental Corps to hold the rank of general officer (March 1938). Photograph: Courtesy of the American Dental Association.

TABLE 18-8

OFFICER AND ENLISTED GRADUATES OF THE ARMY DENTAL SCHOOL, 1930–1936[*]

	1930	1931	1932	1933	1934	1935	1936	Total
Officers								
Basic course[†]	8	8	9	8	N/A	N/A	N/A	33
Advanced course[‡]	1	1	4	1	N/A	N/A	N/A	7
Postgraduate course[§]	N/A	N/A	N/A	N/A	5	6	6	17
Advanced graduate course	N/A	N/A	N/A	N/A	N/A	N/A	4	4
Total officers	9	9	13	9	5	6	10	61
Enlisted								
Mechanics course	10	14	15	N/A	N/A	N/A	12	51
Hygienists course	N/A	N/A	2	N/A	N/A	N/A	N/A	2
Technicians course[¥]	N/A	N/A	N/A	9	16	12	N/A	37
Total enlisted	10	14	17	9	16	12	12	90

[*]Figures were reported by fiscal year, ending June 30.
[†]The annual basic course for officers ended with the completion of the 12th course in January 1933.
[‡]The advanced course for officers was offered until May 1933.
[§]The postgraduate course replaced the advanced and basic courses from September 1933 until February 1936, when the advanced graduate course replaced it.
[¥]The dental technicians course offered training in dental mechanics, hygiene, and radiology.
N/A: not applicable
Data sources: (1) Office of The Surgeon General. *Annual Report of the Surgeon General*. Washington, DC: OTSG; 1930: 277, 278. (2) Office of The Surgeon General. *Annual Report of the Surgeon General*. Washington, DC: OTSG; 1931: 343, 344. (3) Office of The Surgeon General. *Annual Report of the Surgeon General*. Washington, DC: OTSG; 1932: 195, 196. (4) Office of The Surgeon General. *Annual Report of the Surgeon General*. Washington, DC: OTSG; 1933: 161, 162. (5) Office of The Surgeon General. *Annual Report of the Surgeon General*. Washington, DC: OTSG; 1934: 149, 150. (6) Office of The Surgeon General. *Annual Report of the Surgeon General*. Washington, DC: OTSG; 1935: 143, 144. (7) Office of The Surgeon General. *Annual Report of the Surgeon General*. Washington, DC: OTSG; 1936: 137, 138. (8) Army Dental School. Sixth annual advanced course for Dental Corps officers, U.S. Army, session February 1, 1933 to May 31, 1933. In: *History of the Army Dental School, August 5, 1932–August 4, 1936*. Research Collections, Office of Medical History, OTSG/MEDCOM, Falls Church, Va. (9) Army Dental School. Postgraduate course for officers, thirteenth session, September 1, 1933, to February 5, 1934. In: *History of the Army Dental School, August 5, 1932–August 4, 1936*. Research Collections, Office of Medical History, OTSG/MEDCOM, Falls Church, Va. (10) Army Dental School. Postgraduate course for officers, fourteenth session, August 30, 1934, to February 5, 1935. In: *History of the Army Dental School, August 5, 1932–August 4, 1936*. Research Collections, Office of Medical History, OTSG/MEDCOM, Falls Church, Va. (11) Army Dental School. Postgraduate course for officers, fifteenth session, August 28, 1935, to February 5, 1936. In: *History of the Army Dental School August 5, 1932–August 4, 1936*. Research Collections, Office of Medical History, OTSG/MEDCOM, Falls Church, Va. (12) Army Dental School. Advanced graduate course for officers, sixteenth session, February 1, 1936, to May 29, 1936. In: *History of the Army Dental School, August 5, 1932–August 4, 1936*. Research Collections, Office of Medical History, OTSG/MEDCOM, Falls Church, Va. (13) Army Dental School. Course for dental technicians, tenth session, January 2, 1934 to June 28, 1934. In: *History of the Army Dental School, August 5, 1932–August 4, 1936*. Research Collections, Office of Medical History, OTSG/MEDCOM, Falls Church, Va. (14) Army Dental School. Course for dental technicians, eleventh session, January 2, 1935 to June 28, 1935. In: *History of the Army Dental School, August 5, 1932–August 4, 1936*. Research Collections, Office of Medical History, OTSG/MEDCOM, Falls Church, Va. (15) Course for dental technicians, twelfth session, February 1, 1936, to May 29, 1936. In: *History of the Army Dental School, August 5, 1932–August 4, 1936*. Research Collections, Office of Medical History, OTSG/MEDCOM, Falls Church, Va.

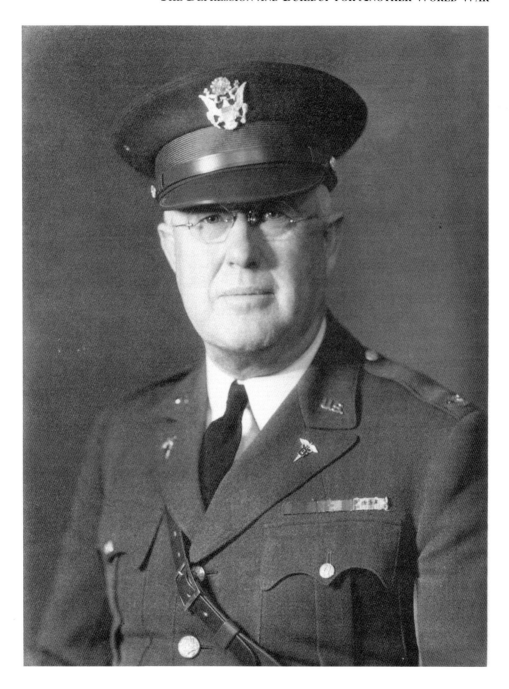

Colonel Robert H Mills, Dental Corps, director, Army Dental School,
August 5, 1932–August 4, 1936.
Reproduced from: A History of the Army Dental School, August 5, 1932–August 4, 1936.
Located at: Research Collections, Office of Medical History, OTSG/MEDCOM,
Falls Church, Virginia.

This intensive course provided 650 hours of instruction in dental prosthetics, out of a total of 658 hours.[65] The dental division's ongoing plans to expand the central dental laboratories, and the resultant requirement for a large number of trained dental mechanics to complete and supervise this prosthetics work, shaped the revival of the dental mechanics course in 1936 (Table 18-8).

A tradition began on May 30, 1935, when a group of New York dentists presented a portrait of Captain John Sayre Marshall for permanent exhibition at the Army Dental School. Lieutenant Colonel John L Peters, formerly of the Dental Reserve Corps, headed the group, which included many reservists and war veterans. They collected the necessary funds and commissioned Bernard Godwin to paint the portrait. Their purpose was to commemorate Marshall's efforts in enhancing military dentistry and the reputation of the dental profession. Officers of the Regular Army Dental Corps commissioned the same artist to render a portrait of retired Colonel Robert T Oliver, Marshall's successor. Frank P Stone, the chief of the dental subdivision, presented the Oliver portrait to Colonel Robert H Mills, director of the Army Dental School, calling Oliver a pioneer who helped lay the foundation for the present corps. For many years thereafter, officers of the Dental Corps donated toward portraits of outgoing chiefs.[66]

Training at the Medical Field Service School, 1930–1936

The Medical Field Service School at Carlisle Barracks, Pennsylvania, remained the hub of the Medical Department tactical training for all Medical Department officers. It offered a number of courses for Regular Army, Reserve, and National Guard officers and enlisted soldiers, but its most important offerings were the officers' basic and advanced courses. Of 35 new appointments in the Dental Corps from 1930 to 1936 (see Table 18-1), only five attended the basic course at the Army Dental School (all of them from 1930 to 1933, when the course was terminated) before attending the following basic course at Carlisle Barracks.[48] Most newly commissioned Dental Corps officers were sent directly to the basic course at the Medical Field Service School, which 35 officers completed in 1930–1936, including some regulars who had not previously attended (Table 18-9). Because of continuing personnel shortages and heavy demand for field grade officers, only five officers attended the advanced course at Carlisle Barracks during this time, one in 1933 and four in 1936.[6,13]

The senior Dental Corps officer assigned to Carlisle Barracks doubled as the station dental surgeon and the senior dental representative at the school.[3] This was an important assignment not only because the Medical Department's training was conducted at the Medical Field Service School, but also because medical doctrine and field organization were developed there, and the research and development of new field medical and dental equipment was concentrated at the medical equipment laboratory. Moreover, the Medical Field Service School's importance to the Medical Department meant that the faculty and staff assigned there were usually among the "best and brightest" officers of the Medical, Dental, and Veterinary corps. Major (later Colonel) Leslie D Baskin held the posts from July 1929 to July 1934 and played a critical role in the research and development of the field dental equipment that would be used during World War II (see below, "Development of Field Dental Equipment, 1930–1939"). Major Thomas L Smith (later Major General and Dental Corps chief (March 17, 1946–April 20, 1950) was then assigned to the Medical Field Service School from July 1934 to January 1939.[67,68]

Corps Area and Central Dental Laboratories, 1930–1936

In the late 1920s the dental service had organized and staffed three central dental laboratories—Walter Reed General Hospital in Washington, Letterman General Hospital at the Presidio of San Francisco, and the Fort Sam Houston Station Hospital—to provide prosthetic laboratory work for dental officers without trained dental technicians or for laboratory facilities in the various corps areas (see Chapter XVII: A Return to Normalcy: From the World War to the Depression, 1919–1929). For dentists lacking the proper laboratory equipment and technicians to fabricate and repair bridges, partials, crowns, and full dentures for their patients, the central dental laboratories were a blessing. In 1933 a new laboratory opened at Corozal to provide support to dental patients in the Panama Canal Zone and department.[7] Once the laboratories were fully operational, output rose and remained relatively steady until 1933 (Table 18-10).[1–3,6,7] A lack of trained technicians resulted in closure of the Fort Sam Houston laboratory for 6 months during 1933.[7] In 1934 the continuing lack of personnel prevented the laboratories at Letterman, Fort Sam Houston, and Corozal from functioning for much of the year. This left the prosthetics laboratory at the Army Dental School carrying most of their workloads, as well as providing prosthetic appliances to dental clinics that it already supported.[8,13]

While the laboratory at Fort Sam Houston returned to a functioning level in 1935, early in the year this deteriorating situation prompted Frank Stone to study how to establish a viable, Army-wide prosthetics laboratory structure.[8,13,69] Stone's study looked at expanding the capacity of the existing laboratories and establishing new ones for those corps areas lacking them. Once operational, these corps area dental laboratories and the central dental laboratory at Walter Reed would substantially improve the Army's dental service. At Stone's request, Patterson queried the corps area surgeons in April 1935 about the proposal and its potential costs, especially in limited dental personnel (two officers and 16 enlisted technicians).[70–72] Patterson explained:

> the purpose of these laboratories is to provide an improved and comprehensive service for the Army. It is intended that dental officers located in the respective areas to be served will send impressions or models to the designated laboratory from which the necessary teeth replacements may be fabricated and returned for use by the patient.[71]

The arguments that Patterson advanced in support of the proposal were that the laboratories' special facilities would permit the fabrication of more and better prosthetic replacements than the individual dental officers and clinics could produce, the supplies and equipment now required at individual dental clinics could be reduced, and

TABLE 18-9

DENTAL CORPS GRADUATES OF THE MEDICAL FIELD SERVICE
SCHOOL, FISCAL YEARS 1930–1936[*][†]

	1930	1931	1932	1933	1934	1935	1936	Total
Basic course	7	8	5	3	4	4	4	35
Advanced course	0	0	0	1	0	0	4	5
Total graduates	7	8	5	4	4	4	8	40

[*]Figures were reported as of June 30 of each year.
[†]The heavy demands of mobilization resulted in the cancellation of the regular 5-month Medical Field Service School Basic Course (which ran January–May or February–June) and the substitution of 3-month courses in fiscal years 1940 and 1941. Six Dental Corps officers attended the first course (December 4, 1939–March 9, 1940), 10 attended the second (March 11–June 8, 1940), and 15 attended the third (September 9–December 3, 1940). As of December 9, 1940, the basic course was replaced with an officers' course, which typically ran for 1 month.
Data sources: (1) Office of The Surgeon General. *Annual Report of the Surgeon General.* Washington, DC: OTSG; 1930: 277. (2) Office of The Surgeon General. *Annual Report of the Surgeon General.* Washington, DC: OTSG; 1931: 343. (3) Office of The Surgeon General. Annual Report of the Surgeon General. Washington, DC: OTSG; 1932: 195. (4) Office of The Surgeon General. *Annual Report of the Surgeon General.* Washington, DC: OTSG; 1933: 161. (5) Office of The Surgeon General. *Annual Report of the Surgeon General.* Washington, DC: OTSG; 1934: 149. (6) Office of The Surgeon General. *Annual Report of the Surgeon General.* Washington, DC: OTSG; 1935: 143. (7) Office of The Surgeon General. *Annual Report of the Surgeon General.* Washington, DC: OTSG; 1936: 137. (8) Office of The Surgeon General. *Annual Report of the Surgeon General.* Washington, DC: OTSG; 1937: 161. (9) Office of The Surgeon General. *Annual Report of the Surgeon General.* Washington, DC: OTSG; 1938: 168. (10) Office of The Surgeon General. *Annual Report of the Surgeon General.* Washington, DC: OTSG; 1939: 180. (11) Office of The Surgeon General. *Annual Report of the Surgeon General.* Washington, DC: OTSG; 1940: 180. (12) Office of The Surgeon General, Dental Division. History of the Army Dental Corps, personnel, 1940–1941–1942–1943. In: Research Collections, Office of Medical History, OTSG/MEDCOM, Falls Church, Va.

the time spent by station dentists constructing replacements may be more profitably employed in preventive dental operations, such as fillings, treatments and oral hygiene, on a greater number of patients. . . . Infections about the teeth necessitate careful clinical examinations, supplemented by X-ray exposures, and time consuming preventive and curative treatments in cases not too far advanced. Many teeth may be saved and disabilities prevented if the average dental officer is given more time to spend on this important work.[71]

The corps area surgeon agreed, and in 1936 the surgeon general approved the establishment of corps area dental laboratories at Fort McPherson, Georgia, for the Fourth corps area; the US Army General Dispensary, Chicago, Illinois for the Fifth, Sixth, and Seventh corps areas; Fort Sam Houston, Texas, for the Eighth corps area; and the Presidio of San Francisco, California, for the Ninth corps area. Until the new laboratories were fully equipped, staffed, and functional, the dental laboratories at Walter Reed and at Fort Sam Houston carried the burden of the prosthetic work. Once the new facilities were operational, the Walter Reed laboratory supported only the First, Second, and Third corps areas and continued to furnish special Vitallium castings for all stations in the United States.[33,73]

Turning the Corner: The Thomason Bill, 1935

On February 1, 1935, during discussion of the War Department's budget for fiscal year 1936, Representative R Ewing Thomason (1879–1973) of El Paso, Texas, introduced a bill to amend the National Defense Act of 1916. HR 5232, which came to be known as the "Thomason Bill," proposed increasing the Army by approximately 47,000 enlisted troops and the Army Air Corps by 400 officers, and recalling 2,000 reserve officers of the combat arms to active duty. No proportionate increases were called for in the services, such as the Medical Department or Quartermaster Corps, which would be required to support such increases. The Medical Department was already strained by its commitments to the expanding CCC. On February 14 Surgeon General Patterson responded to an inquiry from Representative Fontaine Maury Maverick (1895–1954) of San Antonio, Texas, on the Thomason Bill. Patterson pointed out the dire personnel situation facing the Medical Department and recommended possible changes in the bill that would help clarify and relieve some of its present problems.[74] He noted:

> While it would be much better to increase the strength of the Regular Army Medical Corps, the changes indicated in the law would give us our share of the enlisted men, which is most important, and we would be able to use a proportionate share of Reserve Officers, called to active duty, which would probably meet the needs until such time as a Bill can be sponsored by the War Department to take care of the various inequities existing in the Medical Department at the present time.[74]

TABLE 18-10

DENTAL PROSTHETIC CASES COMPLETED AT CENTRAL DENTAL LABORATORIES, 1930–1935[*][†]

Location of Laboratory	1930	1931	1931	1932	1933	1934	1935
Presidio of San Francisco, California	88	39	54	60	38	24	N/A
Fort Sam Houston, Texas	527	683	595	839	366	97	236
Walter Reed General Hospital, Washington, DC	756	828	818	1,021	1,096	1,702	1,715
Panama Canal Zone	N/A	N/A	N/A	N/A	187	35	N/A
Total	**1,371**	**1,740**	**1,467**	**1,920**	**1,687**	**1,858**	**1,941**

[*]Figures are calculated by fiscal year for 1930 and by calendar year for 1931 and after.
[†]Includes repair and construction of bridges, crowns, and all dentures.
N/A: not applicable
Data sources: (1) Office of The Surgeon General. *Annual Report of the Surgeon General*. Washington, DC: OTSG; 1930: 245. (2) Office of The Surgeon General. *Annual Report of the Surgeon General*. Washington, DC: OTSG; 1931: 286. (3) Office of The Surgeon General. *Annual Report of the Surgeon General*. Washington, DC: OTSG; 1932: 213. (4) Office of The Surgeon General. *Annual Report of the Surgeon General*. Washington, DC: OTSG; 1933: 174. (5) Office of The Surgeon General. *Annual Report of the Surgeon General*. Washington, DC: OTSG; 1934: 163. (6) Office of The Surgeon General. *Annual Report of the Surgeon General*. Washington, DC: OTSG; 1935: 156. (7) Office of The Surgeon General. *Annual Report of the Surgeon General*. Washington, DC: OTSG; 1936: 151.

The Thomason Bill also stirred the ADA into action on behalf of the Medical Department and the Dental Corps. On March 1, 1935, Dr J Ben Robinson, dean of the Baltimore College of Dental Surgery at the University of Maryland Dental School and chairman of the ADA's Committee on Dental Legislation, wrote to Surgeon General Patterson addressing his concerns that the bill would not provide "for an increased personnel of the Medical Department" that would include an increase in the size of the Dental Corps.[75] Robinson noted that "the Dental profession has felt for some time that the number of members in the Dental Corps of the United States Army is too limited for the duties which it must meet."[75] He offered his assistance in promoting a suggested amendment to the Thomason Bill "that would increase the personnel of the Medical Department to conform to the requirement of the National Defense Act, June 3, 1916."[75]

The same day, Robinson reported to the ADA's legislative committee that he had requested that an amendment be added to House Resolution (HR) 5232 to increase the size of the Dental Corps to one dentist per thousand service members. The 1922 appropriation act had limited the size of the Dental Corps to 158. Robinson believed that the Dental Corps was "stretched to its maximum capacity and can not stand the load of an additional quota as provided in the Bill," for the present Army of approximately 136,000.[76] There were now 21 posts with commands ranging in strength from 311 to 804 soldiers, and another 23 with commands ranging in size from 31 to 283 soldiers, that depended on occasional visits from dental officers. An increase in Army strength would only "make a bad situation worse." Robinson advocated a ratio of two dental officers per thousand strength (the long-sought 1-to-500 ratio), as ideal if a "satisfactory dental service" was "to be expected."[77]

On March 7, Frank Stone, the ranking Dental Corps officer in the surgeon general's office, replied for the surgeon general to Dr Robinson. He said that the surgeon general suggested Robinson contact the secretary of war and the chairmen of the military affairs committees in the Senate and House of Representatives to let them know that the Army Dental Corps was "unable to properly care for the dental needs of the military personnel of the Army with the small number of dental officers provided for such service." The surgeon general thought that "this will be useful in the future as well as directing their attention to this matter at the present time."[78]

On April 22, 1935, Secretary of War George H Dern replied to Dr Robinson's appeal to increase the size of the Dental Corps. Although he was sympathetic to the "difficulty meeting the load" they had to carry, he assured Robinson that an increase in the size of the Dental Corps would be given "careful consideration" in the future.[79] No further action was taken on HR 5232, but instead HR 6250, containing substantially the same provisions (the number of reserve officers called to active duty was 1,000 instead of 2,000), was passed by Congress. In May 1935 a companion appropriations bill for the Army, HR 5913, increased the authorized enlisted strength of the Army from 118,750 to 165,000, with no additional Medical or Dental corps officers provided for this 39% increase in the enlisted force.[80] Congress was not favorable to overtures about an increase in officers. Members thought it best to defer the bill until the next Congress convened in January 1936.[81]

On October 23, 1935, Frank Stone informed Robinson that the new surgeon general, Major General Charles R Reynolds (1877–1961; surgeon general June 1, 1935–May 31, 1939), who replaced Patterson on his retirement, had recommended to the general staff an increase of 172 officers for the Dental Corps, which was "28 officers short of one to five hundred of the whole military strength;" that is, it was "based on the enlisted strength rather than the officer and enlisted strength." Stone thought the chances of getting a "proper number of enlisted men for duty with the Dental Corps and a proper head to the Corps in the grade of Brigadier General" was favorable. The general staff drafted the bill, not the surgeon general.[82] In retrospect, the events of 1935 that were spurred by the introduction of the Thomason Bill in February changed the direction being taken by the Medical Department and the Dental Corps. The ADA was galvanized into action on behalf of the Dental Corps, and the War Department general staff came to realize that the situation in the Medical Department demanded corrective action for the Army's well being.

A Corner Turned, 1936–1939

On November 7, 1935, Frank Stone sent a memorandum to Surgeon General Reynolds outlining the results of his study of enlisted personnel assigned to the dental service. Stone, in light of a new bill to be submitted to Congress in 1936 that requested an increase in the strength of the Dental Corps, "recommended that a more or less definite number of enlisted men be provided for the dental service. An act to increase the number of dental officers naturally increases the need for enlisted assistants."[83] Stone outlined the reasons for his request and how his ongoing effort to revive a functioning prosthetics laboratory system was central to his calculations:

It is a fact that practically all the dental officers in the Army are engaged in professional work. This will also obtain in war time as well as peace time, as no provision for other than professional work is made except for a few administrative positions which would not affect the proportion of enlisted men to officer personnel. . . . In the event that an increase in dental officer personnel is provided by law, it is hoped to be able to make the dental service a real factor in the health of individuals in the military service. In order to do this it will be necessary for each dental officer to have at least two dental assistants. That is provided laboratory facilities are established to give laboratory service to the majority of dental officers; if this provision is not deemed advisable then the proportion of enlisted men to officer personnel should be three to each dental officer.[83]

Stone's proposal used the increase of 172 dental officers as the basis for his calculation of the minimum number of enlisted soldiers needed. In the attachment, he provided a detailed layout of the distribution of enlisted personnel required by corps areas, posts, grades, and functions. For an Army of 169,126 and the 330 dental officers provided by the desired increase of 172, the dental service required 636 assigned enlisted soldiers and 24 officers.[83]

Colonel James D Fife, Medical Corps, then chief of the planning and training division in the surgeon general's office, endorsed Stone's memorandum to Reynolds:

> Our practice has been to give a $5000. dentist an enlisted assistant at $24. a month. I do not believe that this is a proper division of labor. The $5000. a year man will be wasting a good deal of his time doing what should be done by trained assistants. He should be freed from the routine duties that are generally performed by a nurse or by a dental technician. The more proficient his assistants are, the more the dental surgeon's time can be spent in performing his strictly professional duties. We probably cannot provide them with nurses or female technicians except in general hospitals and larger station hospitals. The next best bet is the trained enlisted man. If we are to establish central laboratories to supply prosthetic appliances then it seems to me that the requirements for enlisted assistants stated herein are reasonable.[83]

On November 29, 1935, Surgeon General Reynolds reorganized his office, eliminating the functional subdivisions in the professional service division established in 1931 and elevating the statistical, nursing, library, veterinary, and dental subdivisions to full division status. As in the many years before 1931, the new divisions reported directly through the executive officer to the surgeon general. The assignment of two dental officers to the office, the chief and an assistant, remained unchanged.[13,84]

As the War Department negotiated with Congress and the budget bureau over the fiscal year 1937 Army appropriation, on February 13, 1936, Surgeon General Reynolds sent a detailed memorandum to the adjutant general for consideration by the general staff. Reynolds began his case as follows:

> The Medical Department of the Army is confronted with a shortage of medical and dental officers. This condition has existed for many years and has been aggravated by the advances and developments in the practice of medicine and dentistry and by the added responsibilities of the Medical Department since 1920 when the proportion of medical and dental officers was prescribed by Congress. This condition will be greatly augmented by the recent Act of Congress increasing the authorized strength of the enlisted force of the Army by nearly 40% without providing any increase in the number of medical and dental officers.[85]

Reynolds was careful to point out that the changes outlined in the attached proposal were not intended as a reorganization of the Medical Department.

> This legislation in my opinion is vitally needed in all particulars if the Medical Department of the Regular Army is to be properly organized and enabled to accomplish its main purposes, which are to care for the sick and wounded in time of peace, exercise its duties in preventive medicine and sanitation, and to make its contribution to military preparedness by the training of its own officers and those of the civilian components. The proposed legislation is so framed as to provide only the absolute and actual requirements of the medical and dental service and does not aim to effect a complete reorganization of the Medical Department as defined by the National Defense Act as amended. In other words, no violation is to be done to this Act except to make these simple provisions.[85]

Reynolds requested an increase in the authorized strength of the Medical Corps from 983 to 1,183, of the Dental Corps from 158 to 258, and in the number of brigadier generals from 2 to 7. Among the new brigadier generals would be the chief of the Dental Corps, who would serve as assistant to the surgeon general.[85]

In his detailed review of the dental service, Reynolds followed many of the lines of argument advanced by Stone and his predecessors since 1923. He proposed an increase to one dental officer for every 500 soldiers and one brigadier general, and followed the general distribution of new dental officers that Stone recommended in his November 7, 1935 study.[85] He argued that

> Dentistry can and should be made a health service. Dental survey records indicate only about 50 percent of the military personnel is receiving dental treatment. . . . To carry out the functions of a health service the Dental Corps should be provided with an enlisted force which can be trained for the dental service and retained in the dental service to obtain the benefits of training.[85]

The Army Appropriations Act for fiscal year 1937 (July 1, 1936–June 30, 1937), as finally passed and approved on May 15, 1936, provided for an increase of 50 officers in the Medical Corps and 25 officers in the Dental Corps. This brought the total strength of the Dental Corps to 183, or one dental officer per thousand service members, which included 165,000 enlisted soldiers, 12,125 officers, and approximately 6,000 Philippine scouts (a total of 183,000 members).[86] This was the first increase in the Dental Corps' authorized strength since the Act of June 30, 1922, which set its strength at 158. With two vacancies, the Dental Corps now had six colonels, 32 lieutenant colonels, 89 majors, 26 captains, and 28 first lieutenants, for a total of 181 on duty.[87]

In 1937 Surgeon General Reynolds again proposed legislation to increase the Medical Corps by 200 officers and the Dental Corps by 100 officers, and to add five brigadier generals to the Medical Department, one to be a Dental Corps officer and one to be a Veterinary Corps officer. While he was unsuccessful in gaining what he wanted, each of the appropriation acts of 1937 and 1938 provided a quarter of the proposed increase, 50 medical and 25 dental officers.[88] On January 22, 1937, Representative Ross A Collins (1880–1968) of Mississippi introduced HR 3491. It provided "that hereafter there shall be a Chief of the Dental Service with the rank of brigadier general, appointed from officers holding the grade of colonel in the Dental Corps, who shall be an assistant to The Surgeon General. Provided further, that 8 per centum of enlisted men of the Medical Department shall be assigned to duty with the Dental Corps."[88(pp85–86)] The bill also provided for "officers of the Dental Corps at a ratio of one per each five hundred enlisted strength of the Regular Army" and argued that "all contract service credited to dental officers for the purpose of promotion shall also be credited for the purpose of retirement."[88(p86)] The ADA sponsored the Collins bill through its Committee on Dental Legislation, following a study of the dental needs of the Army. The ADA encouraged its members to write their congressmen "urging vigorous support of this measure. . . . It is imperative that this be done now!"[89,90]

In March 1937 hearings on the bill were held before the House Military Affairs Committee. However, the surgeon general was not called upon to appear before the House committee because he had not initiated the legislation. Consequently, the bill was not reported out of the committee, and Congress took no further action.[88]

On January 29, 1938, the 75th Congress passed and the president signed S 2463

(Public Law No. 423), "an act to authorize an additional number of medical officers for the Army." The act authorized 1,183 medical officers, 258 dental officers, and two additional assistants for the surgeon general with the rank of brigadier general, one of whom was to be a dental officer. In other words, the 1938 act created an additional 100 officer vacancies in the Medical Corps and 50 in the Dental Corps.[88]

Public Law No. 423 was essentially the bill that Surgeon General Charles R Reynolds had recommended in February 1936 and the War Department had supported. It authorized the remaining half of the 200 medical and 100 dental officers recommended in 1936, amending the National Defense Act and increasing the strength of the Medical Corps from 983 to 1,183, and the Dental Corps from 158 to 258. The increase was based on reports and recommendations of corps area commanders, post commanders and surgeons, and the inspector general. The increase was to be effected in two increments, the first increase of 50 medical and 25 dental officers was to be commissioned on December 1, 1938, and the remainder during calendar year 1939 (Exhibit 18-1).[88]

As a result of Public Law No. 423, Colonel Leigh C Fairbank was appointed brigadier general in the Medical Department (Dental Corps) and reported to the surgeon general on March 14, 1938. He assumed duties as dental division chief and Dental Corps chief on March 17.[91] Fairbank, the Army's premier orthodontist, was the first general officer in the history of the US Army Dental Corps.

In May 1938 the *American Journal of Orthodontics and Oral Surgery* reported that Surgeon General Reynolds's broad policy gave dentistry "a useful place in the field of medicine," and that the "road is open and progress thereby assured in conjunction with medicine." It also noted that an orthodontist was the Dental Corps' first general. Fairbank was a member of the American Association of Orthodontists and was certified by the American Board of Orthodontia. He had been in charge of the orthodontic clinic at the general dispensary in Washington, DC, the past 3 years.[92] He referred to a "new concept: facial orthopedics," which "brings about the movement of bone segments, not individual teeth, restoring original occlusion or original relation of the maxillary arches." Furthermore, he stated:

> As in the larger orthopedic problems in general bone surgery, orthodontics is important in many cases of loose fibrous union, those with small loss of osseous structure, etc. In many of these cases, after slow reduction, followed by fixation, spontaneous regeneration and union will take place. There are many maxillofacial conditions where orthodontic therapy will correct the malposition without surgical interference. The principles of anchorage, fixation, stabilization, intermaxillary force, and retention are better understood by the orthodontist in the restoration of function for these mutilated faces. Developments in orthodontics during the past twenty years provide newer methods to assure the desired results today. Not only has there been splendid advancement in orthodontic technique but also there has been a great advancement in our understanding of bone repair, so essential in these maxillofacial problems. Orthodontics is recognized today as one of the most important specialties in military dentistry.[93(p314)]

On April 3, 1939, the 76th Congress increased the strength of the Regular Army Dental Corps to 316 officers in Public Law No. 18. The increase was to be attained "by equal increments over a period of 10 years from July 1, 1939."[94] The 76th Congress approved an additional increase of six officers on July 1, 1939 (Public Law No. 164).[95] Events in Europe and the Far East soon changed the national security landscape, but the authorized Regular Army Dental Corps prior to American entry into World War II only reached 269 in November 1941 (Table 18-11).

The Army Dental School, 1937–1941

After 4 busy years as the director of the Army Dental School, Colonel Robert Mills headed to his new post as supervising dental surgeon at the Presidio of San Francisco and dental surgeon for the Ninth Corps Area. He turned over command on August 5, 1936, to Lieutenant Colonel John W Scovel, who transferred from Fort Lewis, Washington. During Scovel's tenure, the new advanced graduate course for officers and the twice-yearly course for dental mechanics were both fully implemented. When Scovel left the director's position on March 14, 1938, due to his pending retirement for disability, Lieutenant Colonel Harold E Albaugh, the assistant secretary, took over until the new director, Lieutenant Colonel Terry P Bull (then the dental surgeon at Fort Myer, Virginia), assumed command on May 26, 1938.[96–99] Bull was promoted to colonel in May 1940, and on September 18, 1940, was transferred to the headquarters of the Seventh Corps Area at Fort Omaha, Nebraska, to serve as dental surgeon. He was replaced by Colonel Lowell B Wright from Tripler General Hospital in Hawaii.[98,99]

Bull oversaw the transformation of the two annual dental technicians courses offered from August 1936 through May 1938 into a single, 12-month training course in accordance with Army regulations "so that the courses could be balanced by supplementing the instruction with practical experience, under adequate supervision" and produce more highly qualified technicians.[94,100] The old 4-month course varied from 573 to 611 total hours of instruction, and each course graduated an average of 14 enlisted technicians (56 total) during its run. The new course totaled 1,789 hours, of which 1,755 were in dental prosthesis, but enrolled only 16

EXHIBIT 18-1

ROBERT B SHIRA

One of the new Regular Army Dental Corps officers commissioned in June 1938 was Robert B Shira, a graduate of Kansas City's Western Dental School in 1932 and then a captain in the Dental Officers' Reserve Corps. Shira was commissioned a first lieutenant to replace a retired officer. He served as assistant surgeon general (dental) and Dental Corps chief from November 1967 to November 1971. The Robert B Shira Dental Clinic at Fort Polk, Louisiana, is named in his honor.

Data sources: (1) Examination for appointment in the Dental Corps. *Dental Bulletin Supplement to the Army Medical Bulletin*. 1938;9(July):129,141. (2) Biographical file of Major General Robert B Shira. Research Collections, Office of Medical History, OTSG/MEDCOM, Falls Church, Va.

students from September 1938 to September 1939.[94,97,99]

To fill the requirements for highly skilled dental mechanics for the prosthetics laboratories throughout the Army, beginning in the fall of 1936 the Army Dental School expanded its course for dental laboratory technicians. Its enlisted training focused entirely on dental prosthetics after the August–December 1936 class, which had 12 students in mechanics and only one in hygiene and radiology.[101] Trained dental technicians were needed to staff the new corps area and central dental laboratories as well as the station and hospital prosthetics laboratories. Well-trained enlisted technicians who could take full advantage of the laboratories' new equipment and facilities were critical to the long success of Frank Stone's plan for relieving overworked Army dentists. The modern facilities and professional staff of the Walter Reed Central Dental Laboratory at the Army Dental School enhanced classroom instruction with large amounts of practical experience.[97,99,100] With the fiscal year 1939 enlisted class that entered in September 1938, the school began offering a 1-year course with 1,789 hours of instruction in dental mechanics to provide more practical experience and more thoroughly trained technicians for the

TABLE 18-11

REGULAR ARMY DENTAL CORPS: STRENGTH, LOSSES, APPOINTMENTS, AND VACANCIES, 1937–1941[*]

	1937	1938	1939	1940	1941
Authorized strength	183[†]	208[‡]	233[§]	264[¥]	267[¶]
Actual strength	181	208	221	253	267
Losses	0	3	2	8	1
Appointments	23	28	16	40	15
Vacancies	2	0	12	11	0

[*]Figures reported as of June 30 each fiscal year.
[†]The Army Appropriations Act of May 15, 1936 (for fiscal year 1937) increased authorized strength by 25 to 183, effective July 1, 1936.
[‡]The Military Appropriations Act of July 1, 1937 (for fiscal year 1938) increased authorized strength by 25 to 208, effective July 1, 1937.
[§]The Military Appropriations Act of January 29, 1938 (for fiscal year 1939) increased authorized strength by a total of 50, in increments of 25, to 258 as of December 1, 1939; 233 effective December 1, 1938; and 258 effective December 1, 1939.
[¥]The Military Appropriations Act of April 3, 1939 (for fiscal year 1940) increased the authorized end strength to 316 to be achieved in 10 equal increments from July 1, 1939 through June 30, 1949.
[¶]An act of July 1, 1939, increased the authorized strength by 6 to 264 effective December 1, 1939.
Data sources: (1) Office of The Surgeon General. *Annual Report of the Surgeon General*. Washington, DC: OTSG; 1937: 156. (2) Office of The Surgeon General. *Annual Report of the Surgeon General*. Washington, DC: OTSG; 1938: 162, 184. (3) Office of The Surgeon General. *Annual Report of the Surgeon General*. Washington, DC: OTSG; 1939: 172, 197. (4) Office of The Surgeon General. *Annual Report of the Surgeon General*. Washington, DC: OTSG; 1940: 167, 203–204. (5) Office of The Surgeon General. *Annual Report of the Surgeon General*. Washington, DC: OTSG; 1941: 141, 183. (6) Recent legislation for the medical department. *Dental Bulletin Supplement to the Army Medical Bulletin*. 1938;9(April):85–86. (7) Administrative notes: the Army and the Dental Corps. *The Dental Bulletin Supplement to the Army Medical Bulletin*. 1939;10(July):138–140.

prosthetics laboratories.[94,102] Two cycles of the 12-month course were completed and 36 students were trained before mounting mobilization requirements forced a change. The class that began in September 1940 was cut down to 3 months and two classes were given; 20 students completed it in December 1940 and 21 in February 1941.[103] From 1937 through 1941, the Army Dental School trained 184 new enlisted dental technicians for service in the Army's prosthetics laboratories.[33,45,94,95,103]

The requirements for dental technicians resulting from the mobilization of 1940–1941 reduced the Army Dental School's role in training enlisted dental technicians. The Medical Department's three newly opened medical replacement training centers assumed much of the responsibility for training enlisted medical, dental, and veterinary personnel beginning in 1941. That year, the centers trained 340 dental technicians.[103] The Army Medical Center and the Army and Navy, William Beaumont, Brooke, Fitzsimons, and Letterman general hospitals also set up special 4- to 12-week training courses in 1940–1941 that trained another 690 technicians and were preparing to train 115 monthly (Table 18-12).[4,103,104]

The final prewar advanced graduate course for officers was conducted from February 1 to May 27, 1939. The outbreak of war in Europe on September 1, 1939, the initial implementation of the Protective Mobilization Plan (PMP; issued in 1937 as an initial defensive mobilization plan for the War and Navy Departments that established military and industrial mobilization requirements in case of the declaration of a national emergency), the increase in the Regular Army to 280,000 soldiers, the activation of the National Guard, and the initiation of the Selection Service System (draft) all happened by the late summer of 1940. Experienced Dental Corps officers were required for critical posts on installations and with activating field medical units, and the 1940 advanced graduate course was cancelled.[95] In its place, two 3-month special graduate courses in maxillofacial surgery were given to Regular Army dental officers at the school. Fourteen officers completed the first course from September 9 to December 3, 1940, and 26 completed the second from December 9, 1940, to March 13, 1941.[103] After February 1941, the school also ran a series of refresher courses of 1 to 4 weeks "designed to train dentists in oral surgery, prosthetics, or operative dentistry in preparation for assignment as chiefs of such services in dental clinics."[4(p125)] Beginning in September 1941, the school also began another series of 4-week courses for maxillofacial plastic teams, in cooperation with the Army Medical School and Walter Reed General Hospital.[4] By the time the United States entered the war in December 1941, the Army Dental School was fully involved in extensive training programs to prepare dental officers and enlisted technicians for their wartime roles.

Training at the Medical Field Service School, 1937–1941

The attendance of Dental Corps officers in the basic course at the Medical Field Service School rose significantly with the increase in the strength of the Regular Army Dental Corps beginning in fiscal year 1937 (Table 18-13). Even the number of dental officers completing the advanced course grew in 1936–1937, before falling off as a result of the demands of mobilization after 1939. The demands of the PMP and then full mobilization after August 1940 forced the school to restructure its courses. A large number of new Medical Department officers required field

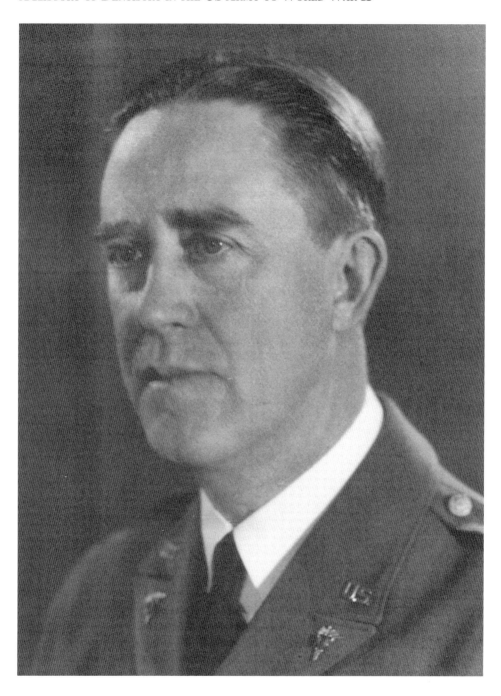

Lieutenant Colonel John W Scovel, Dental Corps, director,
Army Dental School, August 3, 1936–March 14, 1938
Reproduced from: A History of the Army Dental School, August 3, 1936–March 14, 1938.
Located at: Research Collections, Office of Medical History, OTSG/MEDCOM, Falls Church, Virginia.

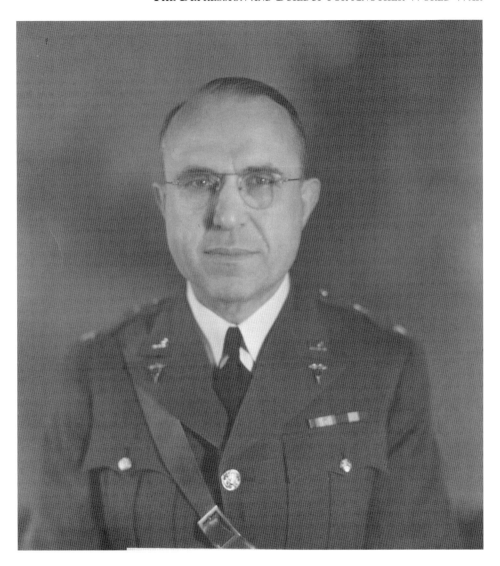

Colonel Terry P Bull, Dental Corps, director, Army Dental School,
May 26, 1938–September 17, 1940.
Reproduced from: A History of the Army Dental School, March 14, 1938–Sept. 17, 1940.
Located at: Research Collections, Office of Medical History, OTSG/MEDCOM, Falls Church, Virginia.

training, so the regular 5-month Medical Field Service School basic courses were cancelled in fiscal years 1940 and 1941 and a 3-month course was substituted. Six Dental Corps officers attended the first course (December 4, 1939–March 9, 1940), 10 attended the second (March 11–June 8, 1940), and 15 the third (September 9–December 3, 1940).[103,105] As of December 1940, the basic course was replaced with an officers' course that normally ran for 1 month. The Medical Field Service School went from training 100 officers and 100 noncommissioned officers every year to training 500 officers, 100 enlisted soldiers, and 200 officer candidates every month.[103]

Thomas L Smith remained the station dental surgeon and dental representative at the Medical Field Service School until January 1939, when Major (later Colonel) Beverley M Epes (1894–1953) replaced him. In September 1940 Lieutenant Colonel (later Brigadier General) Neal A Harper (1892–1970) took over as the director of what was then called the "department of dental field service," and remained at the Medical Field Service School at Carlisle Barracks until February 1946, when the Medical Field Service School moved to Brooke Army Medical Center at Fort Sam Houston, Texas. In this position, he was responsible for the training of 4,473 dental officers.[4,106,107]

The Dental and Oral Pathology Register

In 1933 the Army Medical Museum established a new dental and oral pathology registry, which became the first part of the American Register of Pathology formed in cooperation with the National Research Council Division of Medical Sciences in 1930. The ADA supported the development of the new registry. Within 3 years, the dental and oral pathology registry had 483 accessions, and more were being received from dental professionals through the ADA as well

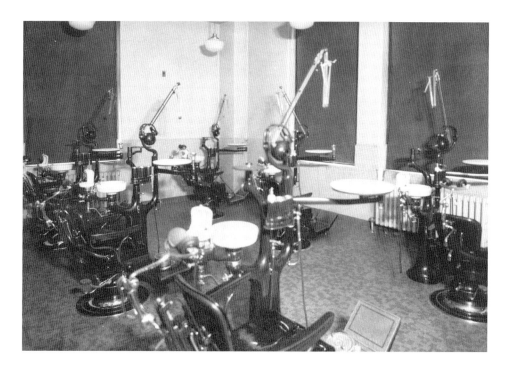

Oral hygiene classroom at the Army Dental School, 1939–1940.
Reproduced from: A History of the Army Dental School, March 14, 1938–Sept. 17, 1940.
Located at: Research Collections, Office of Medical History, OTSG/MEDCOM, Falls Church, Virginia.

798

TABLE 18-12

OFFICER AND ENLISTED GRADUATES OF THE ARMY DENTAL
SCHOOL, 1937–1941[*]

	1937	1938	1939	1940	1941	Total
Officers						
Advanced graduate course[†]	4	4	6	N/A	N/A	14
Special graduate course in maxillofacial surgery	N/A	N/A	N/A	N/A	40	40
Total officers	4	4	6	0	40	54
Enlisted						
Dental mechanics course	25[‡]	31	16[§]	20	41[¥]	184
Dental hygienists course	1					1
Total enlisted	26	31	16	20	41	236

[*]Numbers were reported by fiscal year (ending June 30).
[†]The advanced graduate course was offered from 1936 through 1939, when it was replaced with two sessions of a special graduate course in maxillofacial surgery, which ran from September 1940 through March 1941.
[‡]In fiscal year 1937 the Army Dental School began offering two 4-month courses for dental technicians heavily focused on dental mechanics to provide trained dental mechanics for the corps area and central dental laboratories that were to be established.
[§]In fiscal year 1939, with the September 1938 class, the Army Dental School began offering a 1-year course for dental technicians in dental mechanics to provide more practical experience and more thoroughly trained technicians.
[¥]In fiscal year 1941 the 12-month dental technicians course was shortened to 3 months and given to only two classes.
N/A: not applicable
Data sources: (1) Office of The Surgeon General. *Annual Report of the Surgeon General.* Washington, DC: OTSG; 1937: 161, 162. (2) Office of The Surgeon General. *Annual Report of the Surgeon General.* Washington, DC: OTSG; 1938: 168, 170. (3) Office of The Surgeon General. *Annual Report of the Surgeon General.* Washington, DC: OTSG; 1939: 173–174, 180, 182. (4) Office of The Surgeon General. *Annual Report of the Surgeon General.* Washington, DC: OTSG; 1940: 180, 182. (5) Office of The Surgeon General. *Annual Report of the Surgeon General.* Washington, DC: OTSG; 1941; 159–161, 183–184. (6) Army Dental School. Course for dental technicians, thirteenth session, August 31, 1936 to December 22, 1936. In: *History of the Army Dental School, August 5, 1936–March 14, 1938.* In: Research Collections, Office of Medical History, OTSG/MEDCOM, Falls Church, Va. (7) Army Dental School. Course for dental technicians, fourteenth session, February 1, 1937 to May 29, 1937. In: *History of the Army Dental School, August 5, 1936–March 14, 1938.* In: Research Collections, Office of Medical History, OTSG/MEDCOM, Falls Church, Va. (8) Course for dental technicians, fifteenth session, August 30, 1937 to December 22, 1937. In: *History of the Army Dental School, August 5, 1936–March 14, 1938.* In: Research Collections, Office of Medical History, OTSG/MEDCOM, Falls Church, Va. (9) Course for dental technicians, sixteenth session, January 31, 1938 to May 28, 1938. In: Research Collections, Office of Medical History, OTSG/MEDCOM, Falls Church, Va. (10) Army Dental School. Course for dental technicians, seventeenth session, September 15, 1938 to September 14, 1939. In: *History of the Army Dental School, March 14, 1938–September 18, 1940.* In: Research Collections, Office of Medical History, OTSG/MEDCOM, Falls Church, Va. (11) Course for Dental technicians, fourteenth session, February 1, 1937 to May 29, 1937. In: *History of the Army Dental School, March 14, 1938–September 18, 1940.* In: Research Collections, Office of Medical History, OTSG/MEDCOM, Falls Church, Va. (12) Course for dental technicians, eighteenth session, September 15, 1939 to September 14, 1940. In: *History of the Army Dental School, March 14, 1938–September 18, 1940.* In: Research Collections, Office of Medical History, OTSG/MEDCOM, Falls Church, Va.

as from Dental Corps officers.[7,33,108] This collection provided significant research potential and allowed the resident dental officer at the Army Medical Museum to provide consultation services and to conduct important pathological research. Lieutenant Colonel James B Mann, Dental Corps, held this post through much of the 1930s and made major strides on periodontoclasia and its surgical treatment.[109–111] Captain Joseph L Bernier, a trained oral pathologist and future chief of the Dental Corps (1960–1967), followed Mann as chief of oral pathology at the museum in 1938–1939.[11] By 1941 the registry had grown to 2,485 items.[103]

Corps Area and Central Dental Laboratories, 1936–1941

In 1936–1937 a prosthetics laboratory was reopened at Fort Clayton to provide limited service in the Panama Canal Department.[45] In 1937 the proposed corps area dental laboratory for the Fifth, Sixth, and Seventh corps areas was relocated from Chicago to Jefferson Barracks, Missouri. After several years of delay, it opened on July 1, 1939.[112–114]

In 1937–1938, however, the surgeon general had to change aspects of the plan for the new laboratories as it became clear that War Department approval was required. The resultant study had "occasioned some delay in establishing these facilities but it will assure their development in a thorough and orderly manner." However, the delay was beneficial because it allowed sufficient time to complete the design, construction, and equipping of the laboratories and to develop the dental mechanics training program at the Army Dental School.[45]

The central dental laboratories finally received official War Department approval in War Department Circular No. 42, dated August 3, 1938.[115] The corps area dental laboratories were designated "central dental laboratories," and the following five were established in 1938–1939:

1. Army Medical Center, Washington, DC, serving the First, Second, and Third corps areas;
2. Fort McPherson, Georgia, serving the Fourth and Fifth corps areas;
3. Jefferson Barracks, Missouri, serving Forts Knox, Benjamin Harrison, and Hayes and the Sixth and Seventh corps areas;
4. Fort Sam Houston, Texas, serving the Eighth Corps Area; and
5. Presidio of San Francisco, serving the Ninth Corps Area.[116]

As outlined in the Surgeon General's Circular Letter No. 9 of March 16, 1938, these laboratories were to "construct all classes of dental appliances to be supplied the military personnel within its designated area of service, leaving only the operative procedure necessary in construction of these appliances to be done at the stations served."[116] In 1939 a laboratory was established at Schofield Barracks, Hawaii, to provide limited prosthetic service to the Hawaiian Department.[95] The central dental laboratories were intended to eventually function for all posts within the continental United States except Walter Reed General Hospital, the Army and Navy Hospital, Letterman General Hospital, William Beaumont General Hospital, Fitzsimons General Hospital, the US Military Academy, Fort Benning, and the general dispensary in Washington, DC.[94,116]

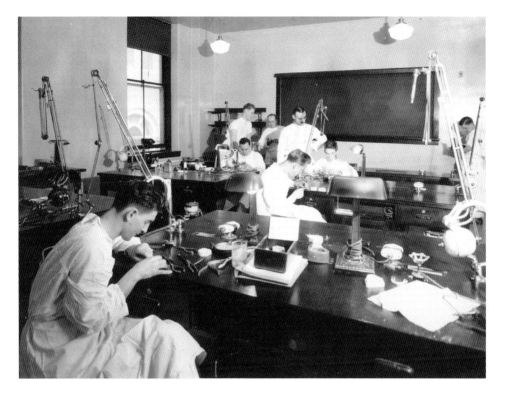

Students in the dental technicians course at the Army Dental School,
1939–1940, working in the carving room.
Reproduced from: A History of the Army Dental School, March 14, 1938–Sept. 17, 1940.
Located at: Research Collections, Office of Medical History, OTSG/MEDCOM, Falls Church, Virginia.

The central dental laboratories were exempt from the control of local post commanders, except for the purpose of "supply, inspection, and discipline." The Army Dental School trained most of the enlisted supervisors and mechanics for the central dental laboratories, the War Department assigned their personnel, and the surgeon general prescribed the number, grades, and ratings of the enlisted soldiers. The laboratory personnel could not be detailed for other duties except in case of a "definite emergency." No supplies and equipment for making dentures were to be given to other stations within the continental United States.[117]

Although Vitallium castings were only made at the central dental laboratory at the Army Dental School in Washington, Luxene dentures were fabricated by all central laboratories. In 1939 the central dental laboratories were provided with Kerr's Crystolex, a new methyl methacrylate denture base material, to replace vulcanite. DuPont worked with the LD Caulk Company for 2 years researching Kerr's Crystolex. The *Dental Bulletin* commented, "we can anticipate a new material in the near future surpassing those now on the market," and the new denture base material completely replaced vulcanite by the late 1940s (Table 18-14).[118]

TABLE 18-13

DENTAL CORPS GRADUATES OF THE MEDICAL FIELD SERVICE
SCHOOL, FISCAL YEARS 1937–1941[*]

	1937	1938	1939	1940	1941	Total
Basic course	23	4	8	0	0	35
Advanced course	9	3	1	0	0	13
Officers' course	N/A	N/A	N/A	16	172	188
Total graduates	32	7	9	16	172	236

[*]Fiscal years ended on June 30 each year.
N/A: not applicable
Data sources: (1) Office of The Surgeon General. *Annual Report of the Surgeon General.* Washington, DC: OTSG; 1938: 168. (2) Office of The Surgeon General. *Annual Report of the Surgeon General.* Washington, DC: OTSG; 1939: 180. (3) Office of The Surgeon General. *Annual Report of the Surgeon General.* Washington, DC: OTSG; 1940: 180. (4) Office of The Surgeon General, Dental Division. History of the Army Dental Corps, personnel, 1940–1941–1942–1943. In: Research Collections, Office of Medical History, OTSG/MEDCOM, Falls Church, Va.

The work of the new laboratories during their first full year of operation in 1939 indicated their success. The 7,859 cases completed were 735 more than the total completed in the years 1936 through 1938 (2,169 in 1936, 2,097 in 1937, and 2,858 in 1938).[33,45,94,95] During the first 10 months of 1939, 1,000 more prosthetic replacements were made than in any 12-month period since World War I.[114] The *Dental Bulletin* of January 1940 extolled the quality of the prosthetic work being done in the new laboratories, saying "with the facilities now provided, it is known that the quality of the replacements surpass anything ever produced in the Army at any time in the past. This marked improvement is a valuable asset to our dental service."[114(p31)] Although the "possibilities of the new laboratory provide[d] one of the most far-reaching and beneficial developments of the Dental Corps," a short information piece in the same bulletin reminded readers who was ultimately responsible for the quality of the dental service rendered:

> The completion of satisfactory replacements is contingent upon the care exercised by the individual dental officers in the preparation of mouths of patients requiring replacements, and the accuracy of impression technique and other primary steps. This is your responsibility. Take personal pride in this portion of your work for three reasons—for your own sake, for the benefit of your patient, and for your good name![114(p31)]

Speaking at a meeting of Medical Department officers at the Army Medical Center in March 1939, Leigh Fairbank noted that the dental laboratories cost almost $100,000 and were mostly functioning. Early reports, Fairbank continued, "indicate that the work is superior to anything ever produced by our dental service in the past."[119(p59)] The trained enlisted personnel coming from the Army Dental School meant that the laboratories would "become a great asset to our expanding dental service for it will permit the extension and development of the Dental Corps in the direction most necessary in relation with medicine."[119(p59)] Fairbank believed that revitalizing the dental laboratories was going to produce the results that he and Stone had hoped for. "The mechanical processes will now be delegated to properly trained enlisted men under the supervision of a few dental officers," he said, "while the great majority of dental officers can devote their entire time to the dental health problems of a greater number of our personnel."[119(p59)]

Development of Field Dental Equipment, 1930–1939

Major Leslie D Baskin, Dental Corps, the station dental surgeon and senior dental representative at the Medical Field Service School from 1929 to 1934, initially began developing new dental field equipment in the early 1930s. The new equipment was intended to replace the World War I equipment. Working at the Medical Department equipment laboratory at Carlisle Barracks, Pennsylvania, Baskin redesigned the dental outfit, which consisted of a chair, engine, instruments, and supplies, to fit into one chest instead of five. In World War I transportation for dental field equipment was problematic because the outfit weighed nearly 1,000 pounds. Its bulk made it difficult to transport and no space was assigned to it in any of the Medical Department's transportation. When troops advanced into the combat zone, dental officers did not have field kits to take with them for dental emergencies. Baskin's dental outfit, called "Medical Department Chest No. 60," fit in one chest a little larger than a standard foot locker and weighed approximately 165 pounds. It contained a chair designed by the equipment laboratory; a standard SS White Company all-cord engine with no modification; a small, collapsible instrument sterilizer heated by an alcohol burner; a portable light (which consisted of two automobile headlights mounted on cross-bars on an upright stand); a selection of operative instruments and extraction forceps; and filling materials.[120] The new chair was constructed of aluminum alloy, and some of the infrequently used instruments were discarded.[121,122]

Baskin also developed Medical Department Chest No. 61 and Medical Department Chest No. 62.[121,122] These contained the laboratory units to be used at all mobile, station, surgical, evacuation, and convalescent hospitals, preferably in buildings, not tents. They included hydrochloric acid (for pickling gold after soldering), a large Medical Field Service School alcohol lamp and boiler, a casting machine, a vulcanizer (alcohol operated), a Medical Field Service School hand lathe, Medical Field Service School Prosthetic Assortment No. 122 made by the Dentists Supply Company (Steele's facings, porcelain teeth, and stock crowns), and a selection of prosthetic instruments and supplies.[120]

Medical Department chests numbers 60, 61, and 62 provided the standard dental equipment and supplies for operating a dental service in mobile tactical units and theater of operations hospitals in field settings around the world during World War II. While some changes were made during the war to lighten and improve the chests (principally the replacement of the foot-engine with an electric dental engine in 1944), the three dental chests were used throughout the war.[4]

TABLE 18-14

DENTAL PROSTHETIC CASES COMPLETED AT CENTRAL DENTAL
LABORATORIES 1936–1941[*][†]

	1936	1937	1938	1939	1940	1941
Presidio of San Francisco, California	N/A	N/A	140	1,544	1,585	1,759
Fort Sam Houston, Texas	639	777	871	1,125	1,765	2,723
Walter Reed General Hospital, Washington, DC	1,530	1,320	1,328	1,881	2,407	2,095
Panama Canal Zone	N/A	N/A	231	513	886	1,735
San Juan Hospital, Puerto Rico	N/A	N/A	N/A	N/A	N/A	195
Fort McPherson, Georgia	N/A	N/A	204	1,304	1,435	1,814
William Beaumont General Hospital, Fort Bliss, Texas	N/A	N/A	65	756	868	767
Fitzsimons General Hospital, Arvada, Colorado	N/A	N/A	19	177	886	549
Jefferson Barracks, Missouri	N/A	N/A	N/A	550	1,348	1,784
Total	**2,169**	**2,097**	**2,858**	**7,859**	**10,658**	**13,421**

[*]Figures were calculated by calendar year.
[†]Figures include repair and construction of bridges, crowns, and all dentures.
N/A: not applicable
Data sources: (1) Office of The Surgeon General. *Annual Report of the Surgeon General.* Washington, DC: OTSG; 1937: 176. (2) Office of The Surgeon General. *Annual Report of the Surgeon General.* Washington, DC: OTSG; 1938: 187. (3) Office of The Surgeon General. *Annual Report of the Surgeon General.* Washington, DC: OTSG; 1939: 200. (4) Office of The Surgeon General. *Annual Report of the Surgeon General.* Washington, DC: OTSG; 1940: 206. (5) Office of The Surgeon General. *Annual Report of the Surgeon General.* Washington, DC: OTSG; 1941: 186. (6) Annual statistics. *The Army Dental Bulletin.* 1942;13:208.

Organization and Doctrine for the Field Dental Service in the 1930s

By 1936 the dental service in field tactical units had been well defined and had changed little since 1920. At the division level, the division dental surgeon (a Dental Corps major) was responsible to the division surgeon (a Medical Corps lieutenant colonel) for the dental health and care of the division's personnel in camp and at the front. Division dental surgeons served as staff officers to division surgeons, exercising general technical supervision over the other dentists and monitoring the dental supplies and equipment. They supervised 22 other dentists assigned to the subordinate infantry, artillery, engineer, and quartermaster units. Six of these officers were in the medical regiment, normally two in each of its three hospital companies. The dental officers in the medical regiment were "the final check against losses in his division due to dental defects."[123,124]

In combat, the dental officers in the infantry regiments were usually expected to function as additional medical officers, as they had in World War I. Those in the medical regiment also prepared maxillofacial injuries for evacuation. In an article

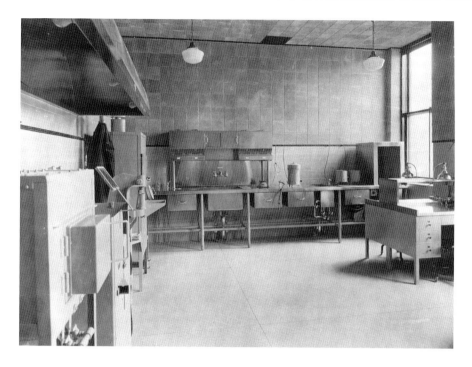

The vitallium casting laboratory at the Walter Reed Central Dental Laboratory in April 1939.
Reproduced from: A History of the Army Dental School, March 14, 1938–Sept. 17, 1940.
Located at: Research Collections, Office of Medical History, OTSG/MEDCOM, Falls Church, Virginia.

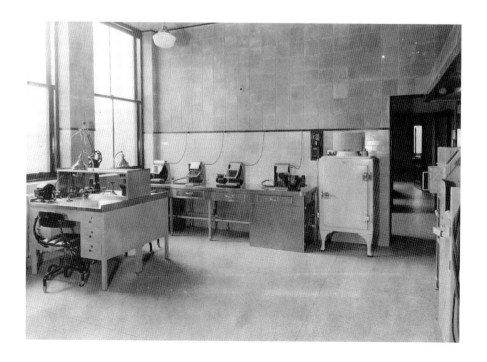

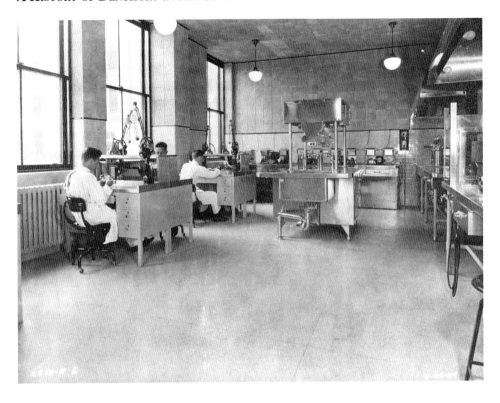

*The vulcanite section of the new Walter Reed Central Dental Laboratory in the
north wing of the Army Medical Schools building in 1939.*
Reproduced from: A History of the Army Dental School, March 14, 1938–Sept. 17, 1940.
Located at: Research Collections, Office of Medical History, OTSG/MEDCOM, Falls Church, Virginia.

on the division dental service in the July 1937 issue of the *Dental Bulletin*, Major
Leslie D Baskin, who knew the doctrine well from his 5 years at the Medical Field
Service School from 1929 to 1934, wrote that the dental surgeon's duties in the
regiment went well beyond the regimental aid station and down into the infantry
battalions:

> The dental surgeons of the regiment must be prepared to function in the capacity of
> medical officers during combat because it is perfectly apparent that after two medi-
> cal officers are assigned to each of the three battalions and to headquarters section,
> the dental officers form the only reserve within the regiment that is available for the
> reinforcement of any of these [battalion aid] stations.[124(p134)]

At the battalion aid station, the dental officer's role largely ceased to be that of a
dentist:

> . . . his greatest usefulness is as an assistant to the surgeon, either in charge of the aid
> station itself or of the collection of casualties from the field. The responsibility of the

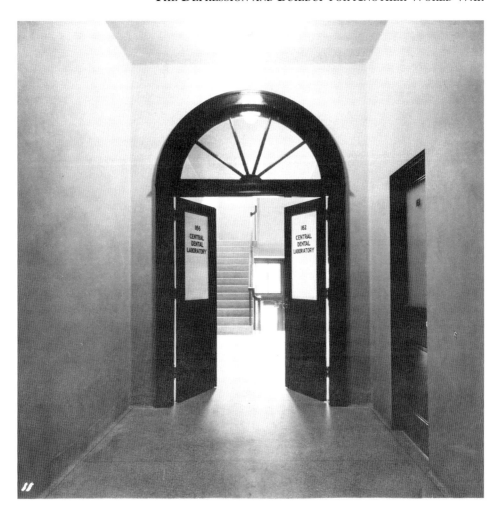

The entrance of the new Walter Reed Central Dental Laboratory in the north wing of the Army Medical Schools building in 1939.
Reproduced from: A History of the Army Dental School, March 14, 1938–Sept. 17, 1940.
Located at: Research Collections, Office of Medical History, OTSG/MEDCOM, Falls Church, Virginia.

dental service to participate in the evacuation mission of the Medical Department, becomes, for the time being, the principal duty of the dental officer.[124(p135)]

At the corps level, the dental surgeon, a Dental Corps lieutenant colonel, headed 24 dentists who performed dental duties within the corps' units. These duties were similar to those within the division. The corps dental surgeon was only concerned "with supply, evacuation, and hospitalization from and to the combat divisions" when in combat.[123(p194)]

A Dental Corps colonel acting as Army dental surgeon supervised the 113 dentists assigned to the medical units, hospitals, and tactical units of a 325,000-person

807

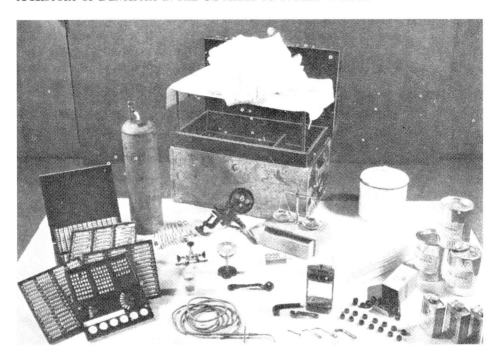

*Medical Department Chest No. 62 was the second chest of the dental field laboratory.
Reproduced from: Jeffcoat GF.* A History of the United States Army Dental Service
in World War II. *Washington, DC: Office of the Surgeon General; 1955; 186.*

officer below the grade of major on extended active duty, one enrollee as a dental assistant, and one enrollee as a truck driver and orderly (Table 18-15).[128] Each team was supplied with a truck and a dental field operating set with the three standard Medical Department dental chests. The teams visited each CCC company every 6 months and remained for a period of about 2 weeks. The dental officer treated emergency cases and provided other care commensurate with the time in camp. Some amalgam and silicate fillings were permitted, but no denture or crown and bridgework was done. In addition, the dental officer conducted a survey of the enrollees and gave a talk on oral hygiene.[128] One dental officer said of his work with the CCC, "I have found the boys in the camps to be very much interested in oral hygiene, and they listen attentively when I talk on this subject. They are vitally interested in preserving their general health, and as a rule are willing to submit to the necessary dental treatment. They are very appreciative, and many of them thank me for the work I do for them."[129]

Working with the CCC enrollees revealed much about the state of their dental health and their knowledge of dental care. One dental officer said, "we have found boys who did not know what a dentist was or that there was such a thing as a tooth brush until they came into the CCC."[129] Another commented, "I learned also that at least ninety-five percent of the boys never had any dental attention, regardless of what their need might have been."[129]

On June 16, 1939, the War Department directed that all reserve medical and dental officers on active duty be replaced by reserve officers employed in a civilian status by December 31, 1939. This change was actually completed on July 1, 1939, and there was no interruption in dental service in the CCC camps.[94,95]

The figures for dental attendance for the CCC were reported as a distinct, separate category beginning with January 1937 (Table 18-16). Over 4 years, the Army dental service admitted and treated 1,297,508 CCC enrollees, or an average of 324,377 per year, and made a significant contribution to their dental health. With the growing demands of mobilization, the War Department recalled all reserve officers employed in the CCC to active duty in September 1940.[34] The introduction of the draft reduced the need for the CCC, and with the outbreak of the war, Congress terminated the CCC in April 1942.

Dental Officers' Reserve Corps, 1937–1941

From fiscal year 1937 through fiscal year 1941, the DORC declined from 5,233 to 4,428. The major reason for the drop was that the surgeon general halted procurement of additional officers in September 1938, and the War Department suspended new appointments in October 1938 because the Dental Reserve was over its authorized peacetime strength 5,100 for mobilization.[4,94,119] Current mobilization plans in 1938 called for 4 million troops and a ratio of 1.4 dental officers per 1,000 soldiers, resulting in a Dental Corps of about 5,600 officers. With 258 Regular Army and 250 National Guard dental officers, planners concluded that the 5,197 Dental Reserve officers as of September 1938 were more than sufficient to cover the requirements for any general mobilization. The surgeon general believed "that dental officers could be procured rapidly and put on active duty with very little training," and that the Dental Reserve could even drop to 50% of its authorized strength without major concern.[4] In the Medical Department's official history, *A History of the United States Army Dental Service in World War II*, Colonel George Jeffcoat, Dental Corps, concluded that it "was certainly not foreseen that the Army would reach a strength of over 8 million men, that a drastic lowering of physical standards would be necessary, and that the 1.4 ratio, which had failed to measure up to the lesser needs during and following World War I, would be completely inadequate for this expanded force."[4]

The suspension of procurement for the Dental Reserve remained in effect for more than 2 years, until October 26, 1940, when Surgeon General Magee envisioned the "early exhaustion of the Dental Reserve" and recommended the immediate lifting of the ban on new recruitment. The War Department approved this recommendation on October 29, allowing corps area commanders to fill existing vacancies.[4] However, few vacancies existed in the dental service, "and it was found impossible in some cases to even offer commissions to those few dentists who had been inducted as enlisted men" under selective service.[4]

During these years, however, a number of reserve dental officers were called to active duty in support of the CCC or on other selective, voluntary, extended active duty tours beginning in January 1937. In 1939 under the provisions of Public Law No. 415, the Medical Department was authorized to bring on to "extended active

TABLE 18-15

DENTAL TEAM DISTRIBUTION

Corps Area	Number of Dental Teams
First	10
Second	12
Third	17
Fourth	28
Fifth	14
Sixth	18
Seventh	22
Eighth	20
Ninth	27
Total	**168**

Data source: Dental service for the Civilian Conservation Corps enrollees. *Dental Bulletin Supplement to the Army Medical Bulletin.* 1937;8(April):92–93.

duty" the reserve personnel required to support the increased enlisted strength in the build up to the 280,000-person Regular Army. The duty commitment was initially for 1 year, with indefinite extension possible "contingent upon satisfactory service, and upon Congressional appropriations." Under this authority and existing orders, a total of 157 DORC officers were on active duty on June 30, 1939 (Table 18-17).[34,95] A year later, 219 DORC officers were authorized and 101 were on duty or on orders to report as of June 30, 1940, but 121 remained to be ordered to active duty as of August 30 because of the difficulty in finding qualified junior officers who were willing to serve.[95,103]

Dentists in the Affiliated Hospital Units, 1939–1941

During World War I a number of hospitals and medical schools had sponsored, equipped, and staffed affiliated hospitals and surgical units. This system "assured a well-balanced, highly competent, professional service and coherent integrated hospital units." Although revived in 1922, War Department policies for mobilization and training reserve personnel during the 1920s and 1930s isolated these units from the surgeon general, allowing the program to die.[94] Based on his own experience in the war, Surgeon General Reynolds attached great significance to the units, which were "composed of men and women highly skilled and already trained to work together as a unit and could be quickly mobilized if needed." In March 1939 Reynolds proposed the revival of the affiliated reserve hospital units as part of the PMP.[34]

The War Department finally approved Reynolds's recommendation in August 1939, and Major General James C Magee (1883–1975; surgeon general June 1, 1939–May 31, 1943), who succeeded Reynolds, submitted a proposed list of units in October. On November 22, 1939, the secretary of war authorized the formation

TABLE 18-16

DENTAL ATTENDANCE FOR CIVILIAN CONSERVATION CORPS
ENROLLEES, 1937–1940*

	1937		1938		1939		1940	
	Number	Rate	Number	Rate	Number	Rate	Number	Rate
Admissions								
Routine	312,222	1,164.29	285,470	1,063.36	287,085	1,042.19	300,991	1,126.65
Emergency	29,068	108.40	25,233	93.99	31,228	113.36	26,211	98.06
Total	341,290	1,272.68	310,703	1,151.35	318,313	1,155.45	327,202	1,224.11
Frequent operations								
Permanent fillings	270,275	1,007.86	224,573	836.52	225,321	817.97	223,968	837.99
Extractions	169,730	632.93	117,613	438.10	141,041	512.01	134,833	504.43

*Figures were reported per calendar year; rates were calculated per 1,000 Army strength annually.
Data sources: (1) Office of The Surgeon General. *Annual Report of the Surgeon General.* Washington, DC: OTSG; 1938: 190. (2) Office of The Surgeon General. *Annual Report of the Surgeon General.* Washington, DC: OTSG; 1939: 203. (3) Office of The Surgeon General. *Annual Report of the Surgeon General.* Washington, DC: OTSG; 1940: 209. (4) Office of The Surgeon General. *Annual Report of the Surgeon General.* Washington, DC: OTSG; 1940: 189.

of 62 "affiliated" units as part of the medical PMP in accordance with existing War Department tables of organization and equipment that could be activated in time of war. The list included 32 general, 17 evacuation, and 13 surgical hospitals. This meant there were four dental officers per general hospital, two for each evacuation hospital, and one per surgical hospital. An additional 36 general, 13 evacuation, and 10 surgical hospital units were authorized in July 1940 in the first augmentation of the PMP, bringing the number of affiliated units to 68 general, 30 evacuation, and 23 surgical hospitals.[34,95,130]

In February 1941 the secretary of war "authorized the waiver of restrictions governing age and grade for the appointment of Reserve officers assigned to 'affiliated' units of the Medical Department." As a result of this action, a separate category of reserve officers was created in peacetime "whose appointment in the Reserve was contingent upon their eligibility for and assignment to specific vacancies authorized as affiliated positions in these units." Medical, dental, and nursing personnel who were "members of the staff or faculty . . . or are officially associated with the sponsoring institutions" were eligible for appointment in the Medical Department reserve and could serve with the units upon their activation for federal service. These appointments terminated upon the individual's separation from the unit or institution, and were not part of the regular Medical or Dental reserve.[95]

Affiliated medical units were organized in many of the nation's major hospitals, medical centers, and medical schools and were staffed by some of the best available medical and dental personnel. The affiliated institutions organized and staffed the units with their own personnel, who were augmented by Army personnel upon activation for federal service.[95] There were a total of 355 Dental Reserve positions in the affiliated units; 272 were in the general hospitals, 60 were in the evacuation hospitals, and 23 were in the surgical hospitals. These units began to be organized and staffed during 1941. By February 1941 72 dental officers were in affiliated units, and by June 30, 1941, 176 were assigned; there were 157 in 41 general hospitals, 15 in 11 evacuation hospitals, and 4 in 4 surgical hospitals.[34,103] During the war, affiliated hospitals accounted for a total of 52 general and 20 evacuation hospitals that were activated for service and deployed to theaters of operation around the world.[130,131]

The Dental Internship Program, 1939–1941

In the April 1939 issue of the *Dental Bulletin*, the dental division announced what it called "one of the most significant developments in recent months." The War Department and surgeon general had authorized eight dental internships at Army general hospitals to augment the dental service and "provide suitable candidates for appointment in the Dental Corps, Regular Army," effective July 1, 1939. Interns would receive a salary of $60 a month plus maintenance.[94,132,133] In Circular Letter No. 6 of February 14, 1939, the surgeon general clarified the status of dental interns in Army hospitals. Interns were to be considered "civilian employees," but were unofficially to be "recognized and treated" as if they were commissioned officers. Three interns were assigned to Walter Reed General Hospital, Washington, DC, and one was assigned to each Letterman General Hospital, San Francisco, California; Fitzsimons General Hospital, Denver, Colorado; Army and Navy General Hospital, Hot Springs, Arkansas; William Beaumont General Hospital, El Paso, Texas; and the Station Hospital, Fort Sam Houston, Texas.[133,134]

TABLE 18-17

DENTAL OFFICERS IN THE ORGANIZED RESERVES, 1937–1941[*]

Year	Total Strength	Gross Gain/Loss	Promotions	Assigned to Corps Areas (Tactical Units)	Percent Assigned to Corps Areas
1937	5,233	475/370	145	5,175	98.9
1938	5,199	516/550	137	5,150	99.0
1939	5,063	221/357	127	5,018	99.1
1940	4,665	0/398	NR	NR	NR
1941	4,428	722/959	327	4,207	95.0

[*]Figures were reported as of June 30 of each year.
NR: not reported
Data sources: (1) Office of The Surgeon General. *Annual Report of the Surgeon General.* Washington, DC: OTSG; 1937: 159. (2) Office of The Surgeon General. *Annual Report of the Surgeon General.* Washington, DC: OTSG; 1938: 165. (3) Office of The Surgeon General. *Annual Report of the Surgeon General.* Washington, DC: OTSG; 1939: 175. (4) Office of The Surgeon General. *Annual Report of the Surgeon General.* Washington, DC: OTSG; 1940: 170. (5) Office of The Surgeon General. *Annual Report of the Surgeon General.* Washington, DC: OTSG; 1941: 146–147.

At each general hospital, the dental interns were under the supervision of a "training officer" and the commanding officer of the hospital.[133,134] The Army Dental School developed a standardized training program that was "comprehensive and methodical in character embracing clinical dentistry and oral surgery, as well as the relation of dental diseases to the more generalized diseases with which they are commonly associated."[133,134] According to the *Dental Bulletin*, the dental interns served as an important "new source of supply for the annual requirements of the Dental Corps by providing a group of adequately trained candidates, familiar with military dentistry."[133] Looking ahead to the completion of the dental internships, the War Department requested and the 76th Congress approved Public Law No. 517 on May 15, 1940, which amended the existing entrance requirements. In the past, dental candidates had to be graduates of "acceptable dental Schools" who had been engaged in practice for at least 2 years; Public Law No. 517 added "or must have, after such graduation, satisfactorily completed a dental internship of not less than 1 year in a hospital or dispensary."[95,135] The first eight interns successfully completed their training programs on June 30, 1940, and were commissioned.[95] In fiscal year 1941, the program was expanded to 10 interns, with three each at Walter Reed and Fort Sam Houston, two at Fitzsimons, and one each at Letterman and Army and Navy General hospitals, and William Beaumont was dropped. All the interns in this group completed their training on June 30, 1941, and were subsequently commissioned.[103,136] One of them was Edwin H Smith, Jr (May 3, 1916–June 19, 2001), a 1940 graduate of the dental school at the University of Pennsylvania, who went on to become a major general and assistant surgeon general for dental service and Dental Corps chief (December 1971–August 1975).[137,138]

Mobilization and Expansion of the Dental Corps, 1938–1941

At the end of 1939 the Regular Army numbered 224,252 soldiers, had two new, activated infantry divisions, and had an authorized strength of 264 dental officers.[95] Within 6 months under the PMP, it had grown to 264,118 and was on its way to 375,000 with the activation of four infantry and two armored divisions during 1940, bringing the number of Regular Army divisions in active service to 13.[139] Looking ahead to the planned federalization of the National Guard, the beginning of selective service, and the addition of four more divisions to the Regular Army in 1941, Surgeon General Magee reported in July that the Medical Department lacked the medical and dental officers necessary to sustain such an expansion. He was short 391 dental officers, would be short 1,259 with the activation of the National Guard, and would need 2,044 additional officers with the implementation of selective service.[34]

For the first time since World War I, the DORC "was called upon to fulfill its real function—to furnish the additional officer personnel required for an extensive increase in the individuals and units of the Army of the United States" in fiscal year 1941. It was evident early on that the number of reserve officers needed for the rapidly expanding Army in the summer of 1941 could not be obtained on a "purely voluntary basis." In order to furnish the necessary personnel to solve the

TABLE 18-18

GROWTH OF THE DENTAL CORPS ON ACTIVE DUTY SERVICE,
JANUARY 1941–JANUARY 1942*

	January 1941	February 1941	March 1941	April 1941	May 1941	June 1941	July 1941	August 1941
Regular Army	267	267	267	267	267	267	267	267
Reserve	449	565	705	1,024	1,360	1,693	1,844	2,090
National Guard	202	273	304	307	308	309	310	305
Total	918	1,105	1,276	1,598	1,935	2,269	2,421	2,662

*These numbers, reported on the first of each month, include Regular Army, Reserve, and National Guard soldiers. Data sources: (1) Jeffcoat GF. *A History of the United States Army Dental Service in World War II*. Washington, DC: Office of The Surgeon General, Department of the Army; 1955: 48–49.

maneuvers where adequate dental care was not provided (Table 18-19).[95] The rates for fiscal year 1941 showed a marked decline in all categories for enlisted personnel, as much as 47.5% in Class I cases requiring immediate care.[103] The cause for the increases lay in the increase in the size of the Army, especially during the January to June 1941 period. The 1941 annual report concluded:

> Although the facilities for rendering dental care and the personnel of the dental service have been increased proportionately with the increase in the size of the Army, it will be some time before the dental health of the new troops can be brought up to that of the Army before the present emergency. . . . during periods when the Army is growing rapidly, the need for immediate and early dental treatment is greater than the need for extended treatment.[103(pp185–186)]

Dental Attendance and Professional Service, 1937–1941

In his section of the 1937 annual report, Frank Stone noted that the record for dental attendance in fiscal year 1937 was "very satisfactory when the amount of service available is considered."[33(p177)] He went on to say:

> results have been accomplished, though, through corrective rather than preventive measures, a condition that is unsatisfactory from the standpoint of a health service. Without adequate personnel the requirements of corrective measures is so great that no progress can be made in the prevention of dental diseases.[33(p177)]

For 1938 the general improvement in the amount of dental service available and provided was attributed to the additional Regular Army personnel on duty. The number of those seeking dental treatment had also increased, so the rates did not "indicate a corresponding improvement."[94(p203)] Within 2 years, however, the large numbers of soldiers entering the Army with poor dental and oral health and requiring treatment, many of them under emergency conditions, increased

TABLE 18-18 *continued*

	September 1941	October 1941	November 1941	December 1941	January 1942
Regular Army	267	267	269	269	267
Reserve	2,231	2,354	2,441	2,531	2,566
National Guard	301	301	301	301	291
Total	2,779	2,922	3,011	3,101	3,124

(2) Historical report 1940–1943, The Army Dental Corps: Personnel. In: Office of The Surgeon General, Dental Division. History of the Army Dental Corps (unpublished manuscript). Research Collection. Office of Medical History, OTSG/MEDCOM, Falls Church, Va.

the rates for fillings and extractions and dropped those for prosthetic restorations. The number of "others" treated decreased as the Medical Department focused on improving the troops' dental health (Table 18-20, Table 18-21, Table 18-22).[103]

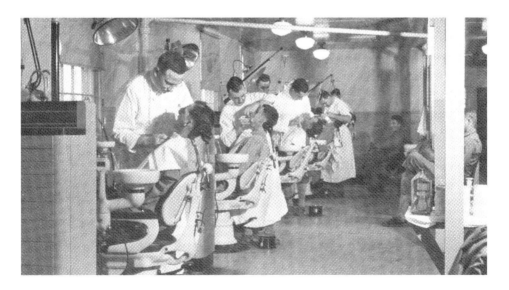

The DC-1 dental clinic had a 14-chair general operating room.
Reproduced from: Jeffcoat GF. A History of the United States Army Dental Service in World War II. *Washington, DC: Office of the Surgeon General; 1955; 258.*

With Some Help from Your Friends:
the American Dental Association and the Army, 1939–1941

As the state of national emergency grew, Dr Arthur H Merritt, president of the ADA, appointed a committee on national defense in December 1939 that he charged with organizing the dental profession to meet a national emergency. The committee met on February 29, 1940, in Washington, DC, and requested the state dental societies appoint committees on military affairs to work in conjunction with the ADA committee. During 1940 the ADA Committee on National Defense required the certification of qualified dentists, dental hygienists, and dental technicians by the American Red Cross. It also cooperated with the surgeons general of the Army and Navy in procuring professional personnel for the service dental corps.[143]

On July 19, 1940, the ADA committee met to discuss the deferment of predental and dental students. They also discussed a recommendation of the surgeons general that a questionnaire be sent to all members of the dental profession to survey their status. The information was to be used if full mobilization occurred.

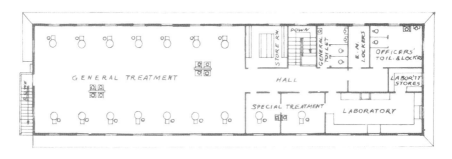

SECOND FLOOR PLAN

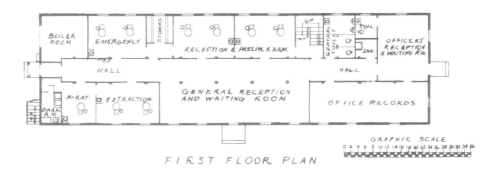

FIRST FLOOR PLAN

The 25-chair Dental Clinic-1 (DC-1) of 1940, with a staff of 25 dentists and 42 dental technicians, could provide full dental support for a 15,000-person division. Reproduced from: Jeffcoat GF. A History of the United States Army Dental Service in World War II. Washington, DC: Office of the Surgeon General; 1955; 258.

TABLE 18-19

DENTAL HEALTH OF THE ARMY BASED ON ANNUAL PHYSICAL
EXAMINATIONS OF OFFICER PERSONNEL AND ANNUAL DENTAL
SURVEYS OF ENLISTED PERSONNEL, 1936–1941[*]

Classification[†]		1936	1937	1938	1939	1940	1941
I	Officers and warrant officers	30	10	21	14	8	NR
	Enlisted personnel	98	84	82	77	80	118
II	Officers and warrant officers	153	144	141	103	125	NR
	Enlisted personnel	245	268	284	282	307	373
III	Officers and warrant officers	41	36	41	34	23	NR
	Enlisted personnel	56	55	51	52	41	52
IV	Officers and warrant officers	786	810	797	849	844	NR
	Enlisted personnel	601	593	583	589	572	457

[*]Statistics are reported as a percentage of those surveyed from 1930 through 1932 and as a rate per 1,000 per annum thereafter.
[†]Classifications were as follows: (I) in need of immediate treatment; (II) in need of early treatment; (III) in need of extended treatment; and (IV) no treatment needed.
NR: not reported
Data sources: (1) Office of The Surgeon General. *Annual Report of the Surgeon General*. Washington, DC: OTSG; 1937: 175. (2) Office of The Surgeon General. *Annual Report of the Surgeon General*. Washington, DC: OTSG; 1938: 186. (3) Office of The Surgeon General. *Annual Report of the Surgeon General*. Washington, DC: OTSG; 1939: 199. (4) Office of The Surgeon General. *Annual Report of the Surgeon General*. Washington, DC: OTSG; 1940: 205. (5) Office of The Surgeon General. *Annual Report of the Surgeon General*. Washington, DC: OTSG; 1941: 185.

On September 11, 1940, the ADA House of Delegates approved the questionnaire and it was sent out to all practicing dentists in the United States. The same day, the committee's name was changed to the Committee on Dental Preparedness.[143]

On October 28, 1940, the Army closed applications for appointments in the DORC, except for inducted dentists and those with low call numbers. In early November, the surgeon general recommended that priority be given to "applicants who had been placed in Class 1-A by local draft boards." However, in January 1941, "contrary to the wishes of the Surgeon General's Office," appointments were completely suspended in the Dental Reserve Corps. As a result of the War Department's decision and the failure of selective service to defer dentists, approximately 100 dentists were inducted into the Army as privates. All dentists with low call numbers were in jeopardy. Despite the committee's appeal, the War Department stood firm on the issue. Their argument was that there were "sufficient dentists already in the Reserve Corps to serve the tables of organization for two years, and therefore the reserve could not be opened for additional appointments."[143(pp82–83)]

On May 5, 1941, the War Department adjutant general issued a directive to all commanding generals that individuals qualified for appointment in the Dental Reserve Corps and inducted by the Selective Service Act of 1940 should be "encouraged

TABLE 18-20

ADMISSIONS FOR DENTAL TREATMENT IN THE US ARMY, 1937–1941

	1937		1938		1939		1940		1941	
	Number	Rate*	Number	Rate*	Number	Rate*	Number	Rate*	Number	Rate*
Routine admissions[†]	96,983	550.29	101,910	555.47	114,618	596.24	184,890	548.82	NR	754.43
Emergency admissions[†]	41,724	236.74	42,865	233.64	42,664	221.94	88,322	262.17	NR	364.94
Total[†]	138,707	787.03	144,775	789.11	157,282	818.18	273,212	810.99	NR	1,119.37
Others[‡]	73,469	NR	77,878	NR	77,280	NR	77,890	NR	NR	NR
Total admissions	212,176	NR	222,653	NR	234,562	NR	351,121	NR	NR	NR
Others as percentage of total admissions	34.6	NR	35.0	NR	32.9	NR	22.1	NR	NR	NR

*Rates are calculated per 1,000 total Army strength annually.
[†]US Army personnel only.
[‡]"Others" includes families of active duty military personnel, civilian employees, Veterans Administration patients, retirees, and enrollees of the Civilian Conservation Corps who were treated by Regular Army dental officers.
NR: not reported
Data sources: (1) Office of The Surgeon General. *Annual Report of the Surgeon General.* Washington, DC: OTSG; 1938: 188. (2) Office of The Surgeon General. *Annual Report of the Surgeon General.* Washington, DC: OTSG; 1939: 201. (3) Office of The Surgeon General. *Annual Report of the Surgeon General.* Washington, DC: OTSG; 1940: 208. (4) Office of The Surgeon General. *Annual Report of the Surgeon General.* Washington, DC: OTSG; 1941: 207. (5) Statistics: summary of dental attendance, 1941. *The Army Dental Bulletin.* 1943;14:38.

TABLE 18-21

DENTAL ATTENDANCE, US ARMY PATIENTS ONLY, 1937–1941[*][†]

	1937		1938		1939		1940		1941	
	Number	Rate	Number	Rate	Number	Rate	Number	Rate	Number	Rate
Cases completed	43,105	244.58	47,923	261.21	46,666	242.76	76,153	226.06	NR	299.35
Prophylaxis	31,982	181.47	35,311	192.47	35,471	184.52	53,777	159.63	NR	187.86
Extractions	55,594	315.44	62,060	338.26	67,697	352.16	124,438	369.38	614,143	457.27
Fillings										
Permanent	115,256	653.97	138,849	756.81	143,789	747.99	257,453	764.21	1,544,166	1,149.74
Temporary	6,060	34.88	6,385	34.80	5,682	29.56	11,853	35.18	75,815	56.45
Root canal	668	3.79	752	4.10	594	3.09	826	2.45	3,103	2.31
Prosthetic appliances constructed										
Bridges	1,037	5.88	1,328	7.24	1,284	6.68	1,603	4.76	2,970	2.21
Crowns	607	3.44	698	3.80	618	3.21	820	2.43	1,787	1.33
Dentures (all)	5,776	32.77	6,715	36.60	8,059	41.92	8,788	26.09	18,953	14.11

[*]Numbers were gathered per calendar year.
[†]Rates are figured per 1,000 total Army strength annually.
NR: not reported
Data sources: (1) Office of The Surgeon General. *Annual Report of the Surgeon General.* Washington, DC: OTSG; 1938: 188. (2) Office of The Surgeon General. *Annual Report of the Surgeon General.* Washington, DC: OTSG; 1939: 201. (3) Office of The Surgeon General. *Annual Report of the Surgeon General.* Washington, DC: OTSG; 1940: 207. (4) Office of The Surgeon General. *Annual Report of the Surgeon General.* Washington, DC: OTSG; 1941: 187. (5) Annual statistics. *The Army Dental Bulletin.* 1942;13:210. (6) Statistics: summary of dental attendance, 1941. *The Army Dental Bulletin.* 1943;14:38.

TABLE 18-22

SELECTED DENTAL DISEASES TREATED BY US ARMY DENTAL OFFICERS, 1937–1940[*][†]

	1937		1938		1939		1940	
	Number	Rate	Number	Rate	Number	Rate	Number	Rate
Abscess, periapical	19,556	111.02	18,913	103.09	22,325	116.13	52,540	155.98
Calculus	35,115	199.24	32,821	178.89	35,844	186.46	53,291	158.19
Caries	130,751	741.89	145,611	793.66	157,004	816.73	283,842	842.55
Gingivitis	6,530	37.05	6,791	37.01	7,463	38.82	13,986	41.52
Malocclusion	548	3.11	639	3.48	802	4.17	1,160	3.44
Pulpitis	17,375	98.59	18,161	98.99	16,748	87.12	35,282	104.73
Stomatitis, Vincent's	5,400	30.64	5,304	28.91	4,656	24.22	9,042	26.81
Total diseases treated	**286,702**	**1,626.76**	**309,283**	**1,685.77**	**329,877**	**1,716.01**	**560,370**	**1,663.38**

[*]Figures include US Army cases only.
[†]Rates were calculated per 1,000 total Army strength annually.
Data sources: (1) Office of The Surgeon General. *Annual Report of the Surgeon General.* Washington, DC: OTSG; 1938: 189. (2) Office of The Surgeon General. *Annual Report of the Surgeon General.* Washington, DC: OTSG; 1939: 202. (3) Office of The Surgeon General. *Annual Report of the Surgeon General.* Washington, DC: OTSG; 1940: 208. (4) Office of The Surgeon General. *Annual Report of the Surgeon General.* Washington, DC: OTSG; 1941: 189–190.

to apply for appointment in order that they may serve in a professional capacity." After April 1941 dentists were commissioned as officers in the AUS. In August 1942 dental students "in good standing" were being deferred and dentists inducted as privates were gradually commissioned.[143] The quick reaction of the ADA, Congress, and the War Department was a reflection of the lessons learned from the previous war, the increased status of dentistry, and a new appreciation for its wartime role.

Dental Field Service in a Changing Army, 1939–1941

From 1939 to 1941, the Army was in an almost constant state of flux as PMP and then full mobilization hit. At the same time, the Army's tactical organization underwent an equally swift and turbulent transformation to the mechanized Army needed to fight World War II. For the Dental Corps, that meant a significant change in the number of dental officers and their responsibilities in the divisions, corps, field armies, and communication zones in potential theaters of operations around the world. Much of the medical structure changed as the infantry division was restructured from the former "square division" of four infantry regiments into the more flexible "streamlined" or "triangular division" of three infantry regiments for mobile, mechanized operations. A large part of the divisional support structure was pushed back to the corps, army, and communication zone levels. The divisional medical regiment was reduced to a medical battalion, with three collecting companies aligned with the regiments and a clearing company for holding and moving the sick and wounded to the rear.[95,103,139,144]

The division's dental service remained under the command of a major as division dental surgeon, but the number of Dental Corps officers dropped from 23 in the 1930s to 12 in the new infantry division. The medical detachment of the infantry regiment had two dental officers, who often acted as assistant battalion surgeons because of a lack of dental work while in combat. Two other dental officers were assigned to the divisional clearing station, where they generally performed emergency dental work and prepared maxillofacial casualties for evacuation. During the interwar years, a ratio of 1 dental officer to a thousand soldiers was the standard for allocation, and that ratio remained the yardstick during restructuring; it even rose to 1 officer to 1,200 soldiers in many allocations.[4]

The missions of the corps and Army became more focused on hospitalization and evacuation, and the corps medical regiment was reorganized and eventually replaced by the medical group, with separate medical battalions to treat corps troops and evacuate the front line divisions. All of these changes had consequences for the dental service in the field army. As the hospitalization and evacuation functions were pushed back, so too were many of the assigned dental officers.[301]

A Dental Corps Ready for War

When the Japanese struck Pearl Harbor on December 7, 1941, Leigh C Fairbank presided over an Army Dental Corps that was preparing, but not yet ready, for war. The Army Dental School led a network of training facilities intended to provide qualified "clinicians, prosthetists and oral surgeons." Dental officers supervised fully equipped clinics at 46 new camps and posts, and 60 dental laboratories served the various clinics. Each of the 35 combat divisions in training and a number of additional tactical and service units had a full complement of dental personnel, and plans were underway to supply the dental needs of units envisioned for future activation. The dental division in the surgeon general's office, aware of the hit-and-miss approach of 1917–1918, was staffed to deal adequately with the problems of personnel, training, equipment, and doctrine. It sustained a close relationship with the dental profession to maintain its interest and support and to assure the greatest technical currency.[103,145] On December 1, 1941, as Japanese carriers steamed toward the Hawaiian Islands, the Dental Corps stood trained and ready, with 3,101 officers of the Regular Army, National Guard, and DORC who staffed an Army dental service that was still expanding to meet the demands of the growing Army.

On the 21st anniversary of dentistry in the Army in 1922, the editor of *The Military Dental Journal* likened the growth of the Dental Corps to that of a person. Prior to 1911, like any growing individual, it had experienced numerous disappointments from which it had developed and learned. Army dentists were recognized with commissioned status for what they contributed to the well-being of the Army. Between 1911 and 1917, the corps matured and became increasingly accepted as other members of the Army and Medical Department came to value the contributions it made to conserving fighting strength. World War I completed the process of maturation and acceptance, and the Dental Corps itself learned all the requirements necessary for a full wartime dental service. The editor concluded that the corps had passed its probationary period and "with the support of a progressive dental profession . . . the Dental Corps has reached the age of full citizenship, prepared to carry on and perform the full functions of an integral part of the Medical Department."[146] The lessons of the First World War were fully absorbed during the lean times of the 1920s and 1930s, when problems steeled the Dental Corps and brought forth new and creative solutions that helped it prepare to meet the great challenges of a world war.

When Robert H Mills succeeded Brigadier General Leigh C Fairbank as director of the dental division in the surgeon general's office on March 17, 1942, the United States was again at war. By this time, 267 Regular Army, 2,777 reserve, and 287 National Guard dental officers were already on duty, with more to come in a concerted dental system capable of serving the expanded force. The Dental Corps had matured and grown in stature within the Medical Department and the US Army, as well as in its profession, in the 31 years since its establishment in March 1911. Dentistry in the US Army had come a long way from its predecessors in the nation's earlier conflicts. Under Robert Mills's leadership, it expanded to provide dental service to a US Army and Army Air Force that grew to more than 8.2 million in fighting a world war.

The change in the status of the dental profession in such a relatively short period was a reflection of a growing modernization of many professions to assure standards and the social and economic status related to them. Educational and training requirements were clarified, along with the criteria of acceptable professional performance. One of the symbols essential to the completion of this process was public recognition of a profession's practitioners as highly skilled profession-als. Many people thought that the dental profession had not been legitimized until dentists achieved the same status as their medical counterparts as commissioned military officers in a career progression. This explains the tenacity and high degree of interest that the dental profession displayed in achieving this goal. The valida-tion of their objective lay partly in the support of the numerous military veterans in Congress who also persevered until the Dental Corps became a reality. Their vindication was in the improved health of the Army and the alleviation of suffer-ing through their skills.[147]

References

1. Office of The Surgeon General. *Annual Report of the Surgeon General*. Washington, DC: OTSG; 1930.

2. Office of The Surgeon General. *Annual Report of the Surgeon General*. Washington, DC: OTSG; 1931.

3. Office of The Surgeon General. *Annual Report of the Surgeon General*. Washington, DC: OTSG; 1932.

4. Jeffcoat GF. *A History of the United States Army Dental Service in World War II*. Washington, DC: Office of The Surgeon General, Department of the Army; 1955.

5. National Archives and Records Administration. Record Group 112. Major General Robert U Patterson, surgeon general, to the adjutant general, "Medical department bill," October 6, 1931. Memo. Document file no. 333.9 Med Dept (4)10-6-31, File 011.-1 (Enactment of Laws, General), 1928–1931. Box 2. Entry E29B.

6. Office of The Surgeon General. *Annual Report of the Surgeon General*. Washington, DC: OTSG; 1933.

7. Office of The Surgeon General. *Annual Report of the Surgeon General*. Washington, DC: OTSG; 1934.

8. Office of The Surgeon General. *Annual Report of the Surgeon General*. Washington, DC: OTSG; 1935.

9. An announcement. *Dental Bulletin Supplement to the Army Medical Bulletin*. 1933;4:1.

10. Office of The Surgeon General, Dental Division. History of the Army Dental Corps (unpublished manuscript). Research Collection. Office of Medical History, OTSG/MEDCOM, Falls Church, Va.

11. Biographical file on Joseph L Bernier. Research Collections, Office of Medical History, OTSG/MEDCOM, Falls Church, Va.

12. Enlisted personnel for the dental service. *Dental Bulletin Supplement to the Army Medical Bulletin*. 1934;5(April):99–103.

13. Office of The Surgeon General. *Annual Report of the Surgeon General*. Washington, DC: OTSG; 1936.

14. Distribution of dental service. *Dental Bulletin Supplement to the Army Medical Bulletin*. 1935;6(April):81–88.

15. Office of The Surgeon General. *Annual Report of the Surgeon General*. Washington, DC: OTSG; 1929.

16. Dental reserve officers relieved. *Dental Bulletin Supplement to the Army Medical Bulletin*. 1933;4(July):123–124.

17. Appointments in the Dental Corps. *Dental Bulletin Supplement to the Army Medical Bulletin*. 1933;4(October):175.

18. Appointment in the Dental Corps. *Dental Bulletin Supplement to the Army Medical Bulletin*. 1934;5(January):55.

19. Appointment in the Dental Corps. *Dental Bulletin Supplement to the Army Medical Bulletin*. 1935;6(January):33.

20. Appointment in the Dental Corps. *Dental Bulletin Supplement to the Army Medical Bulletin* 1935;6(October):218.

21. Distribution of Dental Service. *Dental Bulletin Supplement to the Army Medical Bulletin*. 1933;4(April): 88.

22. Smalley HE. Itinerary dental service. *Dental Bulletin Supplement to the Army Medical Bulletin*. 1935;6(January):13–15.

23. Harper NA. The dental service of Schofield Barracks, T.H. *Dental Bulletin Supplement to the Army Medical Bulletin*. 1933;4(July):108–109.

24. Vail WD. A study of dental conditions of officers of the Army with reference to the loss of teeth and their replacements. *Dental Bulletin Supplement to the Army Medical Bulletin*. 1933;4(July):103–107.

25. Vail WD. Dental health in the Army. *Dental Bulletin Supplement to the Army Medical Bulletin*. 1934;5(July):144–151.

26. Annual sanitary report (an extract). *Dental Bulletin Supplement to the Army Medical Bulletin*. 1933;4(January):20–23

27. Vail WD. Dentistry as a factor in preventive medicine in the Army. *Dental Bulletin Supplement to the Army Medical Bulletin*. 1936;7(January):4–6.

28. Kennebeck GR. The Dental R.O.T.C. *Dental Bulletin Supplement to the Army Medical Bulletin*. 1934;5(October):210–214.

29. R.O.T.C. units. *Dental Bulletin Supplement to the Army Medical Bulletin*. 1934;5(July):164.

30. R.O.T.C. units. *Dental Bulletin Supplement to the Army Medical Bulletin*. 1936;7(January):22.

31. Dental officers with R.O.T.C. units released. *Dental Bulletin Supplement to the Army Medical Bulletin*. 1933;4(July):124–125.

32. Conley ET. Officers' Reserve Corps, Medical Department. *Dental Bulletin Supplement to the Army Medical Bulletin.* 1934;5(October):228.

33. Office of The Surgeon General. *Annual Report of the Surgeon General.* Washington, DC: OTSG; 1937.

34. McMinn JH, Levin M. *Personnel in World War II.* Washington, DC: Office of The Surgeon General; 1963: 111–124.

35. Gaynor CJ. The Organized Reserve Corps: procurement, training, distribution and purpose of the medical section. *Dental Bulletin Supplement to the Army Medical Bulletin.* 1937;8(July):111–121.

36. Vail WD. The Dental Reserve Corps. *Dental Bulletin Supplement to the Army Medical Bulletin.* 1936;7(January):25.

37. Salmond JA. *The Civilian Conservation Corps, 1933–1942: a New Deal Case Study.* Durham, NC: Duke University Press; 1967.

38. Risch E. *Quartermaster Support of the Army: A History of the Corps, 1775–1939.* Washington, DC: Government Printing Office; 1962: 728–729.

39. Dental service for the Civilian Conservation Corps. *Dental Bulletin Supplement to the Army Medical Bulletin.* 1933;4(July):130.

40. Johnson CW. Dental problems in the present mobilization scheme. *Dental Bulletin Supplement to the Army Medical Bulletin.* 1936;7(April):57.

41. Civilian dental attendance. *Dental Bulletin Supplement to the Army Medical Bulletin.* 1935;6(January):27,29.

42. Repair of dental injuries for Civilian Conservation Corps enrollees involving the use of precious metals, gold, etc. *Dental Bulletin Supplement to the Army Medical Bulletin.* 1936:7(January):36–37.

43. Dental attendance furnished C.C.C. enrollees (calendar year, 1935). *Dental Bulletin Supplement to the Army Medical Bulletin.* 1936:7(July):163.

44. Summary of dental attendance (Dental Corps, U.S. Army, 1935). *Dental Bulletin Supplement to the Army Medical Bulletin.* 1936:7(July):158,159.

45. Office of The Surgeon General. *Annual Report of the Surgeon General.* Washington, DC: OTSG; 1938.

46. A curriculum vitae of Colonel Frank L.K. Laflamme, December 1967. In: Biographical file of Frank LK Laflamme. Research Collections, Office of Medical History, OTSG/MEDCOM, Falls Church, Va.

47. Biographical file of Robert H Mills. Research Collections, Office of Medical History, OTSG/MEDCOM, Falls Church, Va.

48. *A History of the Army Dental School, 1 July 1929–4 August 1932*. Research Collections, Office of Medical History, OTSG/MEDCOM, Falls Church, Va.

49. *A History of the Army Dental School, Aug. 5, 1932–August 4, 1936*. Research Collections, Office of Medical History, OTSG/MEDCOM, Falls Church, Va.

50. Army Dental School. Twelfth annual basic course for officers, session: August 29, 1932 to January 27, 1933. In: *History of the Army Dental School, Aug. 5, 1932–August 4, 1936*. Research Collections, Office of Medical History, OTSG/MEDCOM, Falls Church, Va.

51. Bockoven FH. The post graduate course for dental officers. *Dental Bulletin Supplement to the Army Medical Bulletin*. 1934;5(April):85.

52. Rhoades RH. Army Dental School, thirteenth session. *Dental Bulletin Supplement to the Army Medical Bulletin*. 1933;4(October):181.

53. Harper NA. The advanced course. *Dental Bulletin Supplement to the Army Medical Bulletin*. 1932;3(June):20–22.

54. Army Dental School. Sixth annual advanced course for Dental Corps officers, U.S. Army, session February 1, 1933 to May 31, 1933. In: *History of the Army Dental School, August 5, 1932–August 4, 1936*. Research Collections, Office of Medical History, OTSG/MEDCOM, Falls Church, Va.

55. Army Dental School. Postgraduate course for officers, thirteenth session, September 1, 1933, to February 5, 1934. In: *History of the Army Dental School, August 5, 1932–August 4, 1936*. Research Collections, Office of Medical History, OTSG/MEDCOM, Falls Church, Va.

56. Army Dental School. Postgraduate course for officers, fourteenth session, August 30, 1934, to February 5, 1935. In: *History of the Army Dental School, August 5, 1932–August 4, 1936*. Research Collections, Office of Medical History, OTSG/MEDCOM, Falls Church, Va.

57. Army Dental School. Postgraduate course for officers, fifteenth session, August 28, 1935, to February 5, 1936. In: *History of the Army Dental School August 5, 1932–August 4, 1936*. Research Collections, Office of Medical History, OTSG/MEDCOM, Falls Church, Va.

58. Army Dental School. Advanced graduate course for officers, sixteenth session, February 1, 1936, to May 29, 1936. In: *History of the Army Dental School, August 5, 1932–August 4, 1936*. Research Collections, Office of Medical History, OTSG/MEDCOM, Falls Church, Va.

59. Summary of personnel activities for 1936. *Dental Bulletin Supplement to the Army Medical Bulletin*. 1937;8(January):33.

60. Rohde SJ. Annual local clinic of the District of Columbia Dental Society and formal opening of the new Army Dental School building. *Dental Bulletin Supplement to the Army Medical Bulletin*. 1933;4(April):60,64–66.

61. Enlisted personnel for the dental service. *Dental Bulletin Supplement to the Army Medical Bulletin*. 1934;5 (1934):99–100.

62. Army Dental School. Course for dental technicians, tenth session, January 2, 1934 to June 28, 1934. In: *History of the Army Dental School, August 5, 1932–August 4, 1936*. Research Collections, Office of Medical History, OTSG/MEDCOM, Falls Church, Va.

63. Army Dental School. Course for dental technicians, eleventh session, January 2, 1935 to June 28, 1935. In: *History of the Army Dental School, August 5, 1932–August 4, 1936*. Research Collections, Office of Medical History, OTSG/MEDCOM, Falls Church, Va.

64. Enlisted men's class, Army Dental School. *Dental Bulletin Supplement to the Army Medical Bulletin*. 1935;6(January):33.

65. Course for dental technicians, twelfth session, February 1, 1936, to May 29, 1936. In: *History of the Army Dental School, August 5, 1932–August 4, 1936*. Research Collections, Office of Medical History, OTSG/MEDCOM, Falls Church, Va.

66. The presentation of the portraits of Captain John S. Marshall and Colonel Robert T. Oliver to the Army Dental School. *Dental Bulletin Supplement to the Army Medical Bulletin*. 1935;6(July):124–134.

67. Tousey TG. *Military History of Carlisle and Carlisle Barracks*. Richmond, Va: The Dietz Press; 1939: 433, 436, 438.

68. Biographical file of Thomas L Smith. Research Collections, Office of Medical History, OTSG/MEDCOM, Falls Church, Va.

69. Central (or corps area) dental laboratories. *Dental Bulletin Supplement to the Army Medical Bulletin*. 1935;6(April):89.

70. National Archives and Records Administration. Record Group 112. Lieutenant Colonel Robert C McDonald, executive officer, surgeon general's office, to corps area surgeons, "Dental service," April 27, 1935, letter with attachments. Decimal file no. 703.1 (dental attendance) 1935, in Office of The Surgeon General, Correspondence, 1928–1937. Box 105. Entry 29.

71. National Archives and Records Administration. Record Group 112. Major General RU Patterson, surgeon general, to the adjutant general, "Corps area dental laboratories." Draft letter. Decimal file no. 703.1 (dental attendance) 1935, in Office of The Surgeon General, Correspondence, 1928–1937. Box 105. Entry 29.

72. National Archives and Records Administration. Record Group 112. "Dental laboratories." Draft circular letter. Decimal file no. 703.1 (dental attendance) 1935, in Office of The Surgeon General, Correspondence, 1928–1937. Box 105. Entry 29.

73. Corps Area Dental Laboratories. *Dental Bulletin Supplement to the Army Medical Bulletin*. 1936;7(July):152.

74. National Archives and Records Administration. Record Group 112. Major General Robert U Patterson, surgeon general, to Honorable Maury Maverick, February 14, 1935, letter with attached comments on the Thomason Bill. Document File No. SGO 011-1 (Enactment of Laws), 1933–1935. Box 2. Entry E29B.

75. Dr J Ben Robinson, dean, Baltimore College of Dental Surgery, to Surgeon General Patterson, March 1, 1935, letter. In: Robinson Papers, National Museum of Dentistry Archives, Baltimore, Md.

76. Dr J Ben Robinson, dean, Baltimore College of Dental Surgery, to ADA Legislative Committee, March 1, 1935, letter. In: Robinson Papers, National Museum of Dentistry Archives, Baltimore, Md.

77. House Resolution 5232, report. In: Robinson Papers, National Museum of Dentistry Archives, Baltimore, Md.

78. Frank P Stone to Dr J Ben Robinson, March 7, 1935, letter. In: Robinson Papers, National Museum of Dentistry Archives, Baltimore, Md.

79. George H Dern, secretary of war, to Dr J Ben Robinson, April 22, 1935, letter. In: Robinson Papers, National Museum of Dentistry Archives, Baltimore, Md.

80. Kreidberg MA, Henry MG. *History of Military Mobilization in the United States Army, 1775–1945*. Washington, DC: Department of the Army, 1955: 451.

81. Frank P Stone to Dr J Ben Robinson, August 29, 1935, letter. In: Robinson Papers, National Museum of Dentistry Archives, Baltimore, Md.

82. Frank P Stone to Dr J Ben Robinson, October 23, 1935, letter. In: Robinson Papers, National Museum of Dentistry Archives, Baltimore, Md.

83. National Archives and Records Administration. Record Group 112. Memorandum for the surgeon general, Frank P Stone, "Assignment of enlisted men to the dental service," November 7, 1935, with attachment, "Distribution of dental personnel," and comment, Colonel James D Fife, "Increase enlisted strength for Dental Corps." Document File No. SGO 011.-1 (Enactment of Laws), 1933–1935. Box 2. Entry E29B.

84. Office of The Surgeon General, Dental Division. Reorganization, surgeon general's office. *Dental Bulletin Supplement to the Army Medical Bulletin*. 1936;7(January):34.

85. National Archives and Records Administration. Record Group 112. Memorandum, Major General CR Reynolds, surgeon general, to the adjutant general, "Proposed legislation to increase the efficiency of the medical department," February 13, 1936, with attachment, "Proposed legislation to increase the efficiency of the medical department." Document File No. SGO 011.-1 (Enactment of Laws), 1936. Box 2. Entry E29B.

86. Vail WD. The Army and the Dental Corps. *Dental Bulletin Supplement to the Army Medical Bulletin*. 1936;7(July):145.

87. Summary of personnel activities for 1936. *Dental Bulletin Supplement to the Army Medical Bulletin*. 1937;8(January):33.

88. Dabney AS. Recent legislation for the Medical Department. *Dental Bulletin Supplement to the Army Medical Bulletin*. 1938;9(April):85–86.

89. Patterson AB. Committee on legislation report. *Illinois Dental Journal*. 1937;6(March):85.

90. The Army Dental Corps. *J Amer Dent Assoc*. 1937;24(July):1176.

91. Administrative notes. *Dental Bulletin Supplement to the Army Medical Bulletin*. 1938;9(April):88.

92. Pollock HC. The new Army dental bill. *Amer J Orthod Oral Surg*. 1938;24(May):596.

93. Fairbank LC. Orthodontics: its place in military dentistry. *Amer J Orthod Oral Surg*. 1940;26(April):314.

94. Office of The Surgeon General. *Annual Report of the Surgeon General*. Washington, DC: OTSG; 1939.

95. Office of The Surgeon General. *Annual Report of the Surgeon General*. Washington, DC: OTSG; 1940.

96. Colonel John W. Scovel Retires. *Dental Bulletin Supplement to the Army Medical Bulletin*. 1938;9(July):158.

97. Army Dental School. *History of the Army Dental School, August 5, 1936–March 14, 1938*. In: Research Collections, Office of Medical History, OTSG/MEDCOM, Falls Church, Va.

98. US War Department, The Adjutant General's Office. *Official Army Register January 1, 1941*. Washington, DC: US Government Printing Office; 1941: 1195.

99. Amy Dental School. *History of the Army Dental School, March 14, 1938–Sept 18, 1940*. In: Research Collections, Office of Medical History, OTSG/MEDCOM, Falls Church, Va.

100. Richeson V. Dental technicians' course. *Dental Bulletin Supplement to the Army Medical Bulletin*. 1938;9(January):22–26.

101. Army Dental School. Course for dental technicians, thirteenth session, August 31, 1936 to December 22, 1936. In: *History of the Army Dental School, August 5, 1936–March 14, 1938*. In: Research Collections, Office of Medical History, OTSG/MEDCOM, Falls Church, Va.

102. Army Dental School. Course for dental technicians, seventeenth session, September 15, 1938 to September 14, 1939. In: *History of the Army Dental School, March 14, 1938–September 18, 1940*. In: Research Collections, Office of Medical History, OTSG/MEDCOM, Falls Church, Va.

103. Office of The Surgeon General. *Annual Report of the Surgeon General*. Washington, DC: OTSG; 1941.

104. Office of The Surgeon General, Dental Division. Historical report, 1940–1943: the Army Dental Corps: personnel. In: *History of the Army Dental Corps* (unpublished). In: Research Collections, Office of Medical History, OTSG/MEDCOM, Falls Church, Va.

105. Office of The Surgeon General, Dental Division. History of the Army Dental Corps, personnel, 1940–1941–1942–1943. In: Research Collections, Office of Medical History, OTSG/MEDCOM, Falls Church, Va.

106. Biographical file of Beverley M Epes. Research Collections, Office of Medical History, OTSG/MEDCOM, Falls Church, Va.

107. Biographical file of Neal A Harper. Research Collections, Office of Medical History, OTSG/MEDCOM, Falls Church, Va.

108. Henry RS. *The Armed Forces Institute of Pathology, its First Century, 1862–1962*. Washington, DC: Office of The Surgeon General; 1964: 220.

109. Fairbank LC. An address (New York State Dental Society, May 11, 1938). *Dental Bulletin Supplement to the Army Medical Bulletin*. 1938;9(July):114.

110. Mann JB. The purpose and value of the registry of dental and oral pathology. *Dental Bulletin Supplement to the Army Medical Bulletin*. 1939;10(July):109–114.

111. Bernier JL. The registry of dental and oral pathology. *Dental Bulletin Supplement to the Army Medical Bulletin*. 1938;9(October):193–194.

112. Office of the Surgeon General, Dental Division. Corps area dental laboratories. *Dental Bulletin Supplement to the Army Medical Bulletin*. 1937;8(April):95.

113. Central dental laboratories. *Dental Bulletin Supplement to the Army Medical Bulletin*. 1939;10(January):30.

114. Central dental laboratories. *Dental Bulletin Supplement to the Army Medical Bulletin*. 1940;11(January):31.

115. Central dental laboratories. *Dental Bulletin Supplement to the Army Medical Bulletin*. 1938;9(October):195.

116. Central dental laboratories. *Dental Bulletin Supplement to the Army Medical Bulletin*. 1938;9(April):89.

Corps Chiefs
U.S. Army Dental Corps

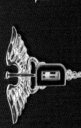

John Sayre Marshall
1901-1911

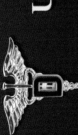

William H. G. Logan
1917-1919

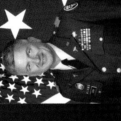

Frank L. K. LaFlamme
1919

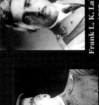

Robert T. Oliver
1919-1924

Rex H. Rhoades
1924-1928
1932-1934

Julien R. Bernheim
1928-1932

Russell J. Czerw
2006 –

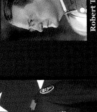

Frank P. Stone
1934-1938

Leigh C. Fairbank
1938-1942

Robert H. Mills
1942-1946

Thomas L. Smith
1946-1950

Walter D. Love
1950-1954

Oscar P. Snyder
1954-1956

James M. Epperly
1956-1960

Joseph L. Bernier
1960-1967

Robert B. Shira
1967-1971

Edwin H. Smith
1971-1975

Surindar N. Bhaskar
1975-1979

George Kuttas
1979-1982

H. Thomas Chandler
1982-1986

Bill B. Lefler
1986-1990

Thomas R. Tempel
1990-1994

John J. Cuddy
1994-1998

Patrick D. Sculley
1999-2002

Joseph G. Webb, Jr.
2002-2006

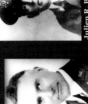

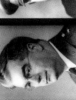
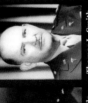

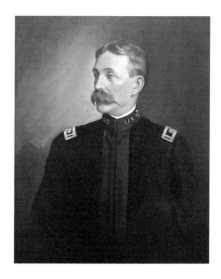

John Sayre Marshall
June 26, 1846–November 20, 1922.

Education
University of Syracuse, 1876.

Assignments
1864–1865: Enlisted and served in New York Volunteer Cavalry.
1869–1901: Civilian career in dentistry, including establishing the Northwestern University Dental Department and serving as its dean, reorganizing the American College of Dental Surgery, and publishing two textbooks.
1901–1905 : Served as one of original contract dental surgeons; appointed to dental examining board; sent to the Presidio of San Francisco.
1901–1911: President of the Board of Examining and Supervising Dental Surgeons, senior contract dental surgeon.
1905–1906 : Duty at San Francisco's General Hospital.
1906–1907: Served temporarily in Honolulu, Hawaii, before returning to San Francisco; served as sanitary inspector of refugee camp at Point Lobos.
1907: Served at Camp Yosemite, Yosemite Valley, California.
1908–1910: Served at Manila, Philippine Islands.
1910: Served to Columbus Barracks, Ohio.
1911: Retired from active service.

Distinctions
Viewed as the father of the Dental Corps, instructor in dental and oral surgery at Northwestern University, reorganized the American College of Dental Surgery, wrote several books on dentistry and diseases of the mouth, and received an honorary Doctor of Science degree from the University of Syracuse.

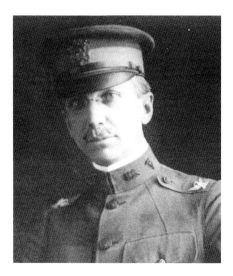

Colonel William HG Logan
October 14, 1872–April 6, 1943.

Education:
DDS, Chicago College of Dental Surgery, 1896.
MD, Chicago College of Medicine and Surgery, 1905.

Assignments:
1917: Chairman of the Committee of Dentistry of the General Medical Board of the Council of National Defense.
1917–1919: Chief of the Dental Service at the Surgeon General's Office.
1920: Became dean and chief of oral surgery at the Chicago College of Dental Surgery, Dental Department of Loyola University.
1922–1933: Colonel in the Medical Reserve Corps.
1935: Became chairman of the Foundation for Dental Research of the Chicago College of Dental Surgery.

Distinctions:
1970: The Logan Army Dental Clinic at Fort Belvoir, Virginia, was dedicated in Colonel Logan's honor.

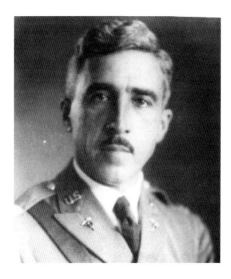

Lieutenant Colonel Frank LK Laflamme
December 7, 1879–June 6, 1966.

Education:
DDS, Baltimore College of Dental Surgery, 1907.

Assignments:
1909–1911: Contract dental surgeon.
1910–1913: Dental surgeon, Fort Mills and other stations, Philippine Islands.
1911: Received commission as a first lieutenant, Dental Corps.
1913–1915: Dental surgeon, Fort Hamilton, New York.
1915–1917: Dental surgeon, US Military Academy, West Point, New York.
1917–1918: Temporary duty to examine Dental Corps candidates, Camp Meade, Maryland.
1918–1919: Dental surgeon 79th Division, Camp Meade, Maryland.
1919: Chief, Dental Section, Office of The Surgeon General.
1919–1925: Assistant dental surgeon until 1924, then chief dental surgeon, US Military Academy.
1925–1928: Chief, Dental Service, Tripler General Hospital, Hawaii.
1919–1929: Dental surgeon, General Dispensary, US Army, Washington, DC.
1929–1932: Commandant of the Army Dental School, US Army Medical Center, Washington, DC.
1932–1938: Post dental surgeon, Fort Sam Houston, Texas.
1938–1942: Chief, Dental Service, Fort Jay, New York.
1942: Dental surgeon, Stark General Hospital, Charleston, South Carolina.
1942–1943: Chief, Dental Service, Moore General Hospital, Swannanoa, North Carolina.

Distinctions:
On December 1, 1969, the new dental clinic at Fort Bragg, North Carolina, was dedicated as the Laflamme Army Dental Clinic.

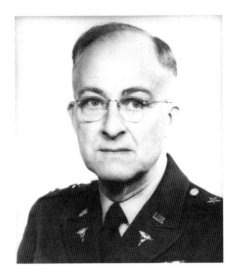

Major General Oscar P Snyder
January 6, 1895–February 21, 1983.

Education:
DDS, Ohio State University, 1916.

Assignments:
1916: Dental surgeon, Columbus Barracks, Ohio.
1917–1918: Dental surgeon, 28th Infantry Division.
1918: Participated in four campaigns in France, including the Meuse-Argonne Offensive.
1919: Assistant to the base dental surgeon, Base Section No. 2, France; served as camp dental surgeon, Camp Dodge, Iowa.
1920–1922: Camp dental surgeon, Camp Grant, Illinois.
1923–1924: Post dental surgeon, Camp Sheridan, Illinois.
1924: Dental surgeon, Camp Stotsenberg, Philippine Islands.
1925–1927: Assistant to the chief, Dental Service, Sternberg General Hospital, Manila.
1927–1931: Served at Walter Reed General Hospital, Washington, DC.
1931–1935: Post dental surgeon, Fort Thomas, Kentucky.
1936–1941: Dental officer, General Dispensary, Washington, DC; dental surgeon, US Military Academy, West Point, New York.
1941–1942: Chief, Dental Service, Lawson General Hospital, Atlanta, Georgia.
1942–1944: Chief dental surgeon, Southwest Pacific Theater, Melbourne, Australia.
1945: Chief, Dental Service, England General Hospital, Atlantic City, New Jersey.
1945–1948: Chief, Dental Service, Fitzsimons General Hospital, Denver, Colorado.
1948–1953: Director of dental activities, Walter Reed Army Medical Center, Washington, DC.
1953–1954: Director of dental activities, Brooke Army Medical Center, Fort Sam Houston, Texas.
1954–1956: Chief, US Army Dental Corps.

Distinctions:
Awarded the Legion of Merit, Mexican Border Medal, World War I Victory Medal (with four bronze stars), Army of Occupation Germany, American Defense Medal, American Theater Medal, Asiatic-Pacific Theater Medal (with one bronze star), and World War II Victory Medal.

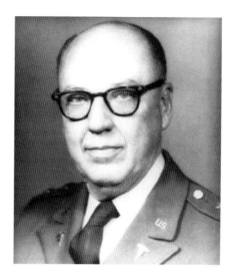

Major General James M Epperly
July 5, 1900–November 14, 1973.

Education:
DDS, Saint Louis University School of Dentistry, 1923.

Assignments:
1924: Served at Fitzsimons Army Hospital, Denver, Colorado.
1926: Attended the Army Dental School and Medical Field Service School.
1926–1928: Served in the Philippines.
1928–1935: Served at the Presidio of San Francisco and Letterman Army Hospital, California.
1935–1942: Served in Panama and at the US Military Academy.
1942–1944: Chief of dental service at Camp Breckinridge, Kentucky.
1944: Named dental surgeon of the Ninth Army at Fort Sam Houston, Texas, and served with the Ninth in England, France, and Germany.
1945: Dental surgeon of the Second Army in Memphis, Tennessee.
1946: Trained at Walter Reed Army Medical Center and was appointed chief of the Dental Service Branch in the surgeon general's office.
1951–1953: Served at Fitzsimons Army Hospital.
1953: Appointed temporary advisor on dental service to the Greek army.
1954–1956: Director of dental activities at Brooke Army Medical Center, Fort Sam Houston, Texas.
1956–1960: Chief, US Army Dental Corps.

Distinctions:
Awarded the Legion of Merit and the Bronze Star Medal..

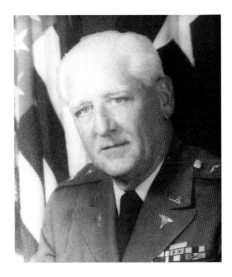

Major General Joseph L Bernier
April 5, 1909–January 4, 1989.

Education:
DDS, University of Illinois, 1932.

Assignments:
1934–1938: Served at Walter Reed General Hospital, Washington, DC.
1938–1939: Chief, Oral Pathology Branch, Armed Forces Institute of Pathology, Washington, DC.
1939–1941: Chief, Department Dental Laboratory, Panama Canal Zone.
1941–1942: Chief, Oral Pathology Branch, Armed Forces Institute of Pathology.
1942–1943: Dental coordinator, 15th Hospital Center.
1943: Dental surgeon, Camp Polk, Louisiana.
1943–1944: Director, Dental Division, McCloskey General Hospital, Temple, Texas.
1944–1945: Dental surgeon, 254th General Hospital, European Theater.
1945–1960: Chief, Oral Pathology Branch, Armed Forces Institute of Pathology.
1960–1967: Chief, US Army Dental Corps.

Distinctions:
Awarded the American Defense Medal, American Campaign Medal, European African Mediterranean Medal, World War II Victory Medal, Army of Occupation Medal (Germany), Meritorious Service Medal, and National Defense Service Medal.

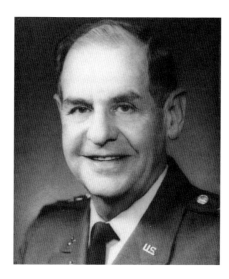

Major General Robert Bruce Shira
December 2, 1910–November 22, 2002.

Education:
DDS, Kansas City Western Dental College, 1932.

Assignments:
1938: Commissioned first lieutenant.
1938–1941: Dental officer, Barksdale Field, Louisiana.
1941–1947: Chief, Dental Activities, Gorgas Hospital, Ancon, Canal Zone.
1947–1954: Chief, Oral Surgery, Letterman General Hospital, San Francisco,
California.
1954–1964: Chief, Dental Service and chief, Oral Surgery, Walter Reed General Hospital,
Washington, DC.
1964–1966: Dental surgeon, US Army, Europe.
1966–1967: Director of dental activities, Walter Reed General Hospital,
Washington, DC.
1967–1971: Chief, US Army Dental Corps.

Distinctions:
Awarded the Legion of Merit (with two oak leaf clusters); Army Commendation Medal;
American Defense Medal; American Campaign Medal; World War II Victory Medal; National Defense Service Medal (with oak leaf cluster); Hinman Award; "Sword of Hope
Award" of Pennsylvania Division, American Cancer Society; "Man of the Year Award" of
University of Missouri at Kansas City; Jarvie-Burkhart Medal, Dental Society of State of
New York; Pierre Fauchard Medal; and Distinguished Alumni Award, University of Missouri at Kansas City.

854

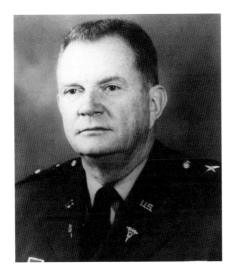

Major General Edwin Howell Smith, Jr
May 3, 1916–June 19, 2001.

Education:
DDS, University of Pennsylvania, 1940.

Assignments:
1941–1941: Dental officer, surgery, Walter Reed General Hospital.
1941–1943: Chief, Prosthodontics, Brooke General Hospital.
1943: Dental surgeon, Station Hospital, San Juan, Puerto Rico; chief, Dental Service, Henry Barracks, Puerto Rico; dental surgeon, Station Hospital, Camp Sutton.
1943–1944: Chief, Prosthetics Section, Glennan General Hospital.
1944–1946: Chief, Prosthetics, and assistant chief, Dental Service, Valley Forge General Hospital.
1947–1948: Chief, Prosthetics Section, Walter Reed General Hospital.
1948–1949: Dental officer, Operations Section, and assistant chief, Prosthetics Section, Tripler General Hospital; chief, Prosthetics Section, Tripler General Hospital.
1949–1956: Chief, Prosthetics Section, Dental Service, Walter Reed General Hospital.
1956–1959: Assistant chief, Dental Career and Assignments Brigade, Dental Division, Office of The Surgeon General.
1959–1960: Chief, Dental Career and Assignment Brigade, Dental Division, Office of The Surgeon General.
1960–1963: Deputy dental surgeon, chief, Dental Clinic No. 1, and consultant to chief, Army Dental Corps, 89th Medical Detachment.
1963–1965: Chief, Dental Service, Headquarters Company.
1965–1967: Dental surgeon and director of dental education, US Army Infantry Center, Fort Benning.
1967–1971: Chief, Department of Dentistry, and consultant on removable prosthetics to the surgeon general, Walter Reed General Hospital.
1971–1975: Chief, US Army Dental Corps.

Distinctions:
Awarded the Legion of Merit, Meritorious Service Medal, Army Commendation Medal (with oak leaf cluster), American Defense Service Medal, American Campaign Medal, World War II Victory Medal, and National Defense Service Medal.

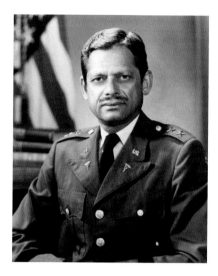

Major General Surindar N Bhaskar
Born January 7, 1923.

Education:
DDS, University of Punjab, 1942.
DDS, Northwestern University, 1946.

Assignments:
1962–1970: Chief, Department of Dental and Oral Pathology, and consultant to the surgeon general on oral pathology, US Army Institute of Dental Research, Washington, DC.
1970–1973: Director, US Army Institute of Dental Research, and consultant on oral pathology to the surgeon general, Walter Reed Army Medical Center, Washington, DC.
1973–1975: Director of personnel and training, Office of The Surgeon General.
1975–1978: Chief, US Army Dental Corps.

Distinctions:
Awarded the Legion of Merit and the Meritorious Service Medal.

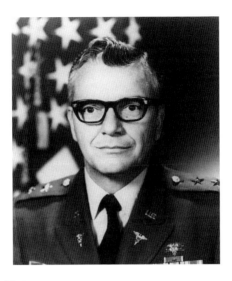

Major General George Kuttas
Born February 24, 1927.

Education:
DDS, University of Pennsylvania School of Dentistry, 1951.

Assignments:
1968–1971: Assistant chief, Dental Corps Branch, Military Personnel Division, Personnel and Training Directorate; later assistant chief, Professional Branch, Office of the Assistant for Dental Services, Office of The Surgeon General.
1971–1972: Attended US Army War College, Carlisle Barracks, Pennsylvania.
1972–1973: Chief, Operations, Programming and Planning Branch, Office of the Assistant Surgeon General (Dental), Office of The Surgeon General.
1973–1975: Senior Dental Corps staff officer, Office of The Surgeon General.
1975–1979: Deputy commander, US Army Medical Command, Europe; dental surgeon, US Army Europe.
1979–1982: Chief, US Army Dental Corps.

Distinctions:
Awarded the Distinguished Service Medal, Legion of Merit (with oak leaf cluster), and the Bronze Star Medal.

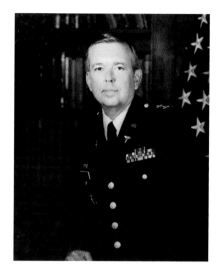

Major General H Thomas Chandler
Born December 8, 1933.

Education:
DDS, University of Maryland, 1957.

Assignments:
1968–1969: Commander, 518th Medical Department, Vietnam.
1979–1973: Chief, Prosthetic Department, Regional Dental Activity, Walter Reed Army Medical Center, Washington, DC.
1973–1974: Attended US Army War College, Carlisle Barracks, Pennsylvania.
1974–1975: Management and studies officer, Office of The Surgeon General.
1975–1979: Senior Dental Corps staff officer, Office of The Surgeon General.
1979–1982: Dental surgeon, US Army Medical Command, Europe.
1982–1986: Chief, US Army Dental Corps.

Distinctions:
Awarded the Distinguished Service Medal, Bronze Star Medal, Meritorious Service Medal, and Army Commendation Medal.

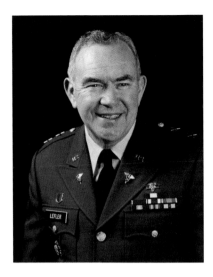

Major General Bill B Leffler
Born October 20, 1933.

Education:
DDS, University of Tennessee, 1956.

Assignments:
1956–1959: Dental officer, Dental Detachment, US Army Garrison, Fort Chaffee, Arkansas.
1959–1960: Dental officer, 469th Medical Detachment, 2nd Brigade, 4th Cavalry, Korea; dental officer, US Army Dental Detachment, Fort Hood, Texas.
1961–1963: Dental officer, Dispensers A, US Army Garrison, Fort Benning, Georgia.
1963–1965: Dental officer, later chief, Crown and Bridge Section, 196th Station Hospital, US Army Europe.
1965–1966: Chief, Fixed Prosthodontic Section, US Army Dental Unit, Fort Bragg, North Carolina.
1968–1972: Chief, Fixed Prosthodontics, US Army Armor Center Dental Detachment, Fort Knox, Kentucky.
1972–1976: Chief, Fixed Prosthodontia Service, Department of Dentistry, Walter Reed Army Medical Center, Washington, DC.
1976–1979: Commander, US Army Dental Activity, Fort Jackson, South Carolina.
1979–1984: Deputy commanding general/assistant chief surgeon (dental), US Army Health Services Command, Fort Sam Houston, Texas.
1984–1986: Deputy commanding general/assistant chief surgeon (dental), 7th Medical Command Europe.
1986–1990: Chief, US Army Dental Corps.

Distinctions:
Awarded the Distinguished Service Medal (with oak leaf cluster), Legion of Merit, Meritorious Service Medal, Army Commendation Medal, and Expert Field Medical Badge.

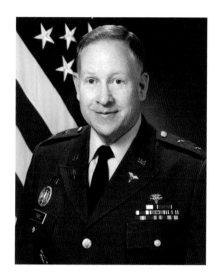

Major General Thomas Robert Tempel
Born March 12, 1939.

Education:
DDS, University of Pennsylvania, Dental Surgery, 1963.

Assignments:
1964: Dental officer, 768th Medical Detachment, United States Army Europe, Germany.
1964–1966: Dental officer, 8th Medical Battalion, 8th Infantry Division, United States Army Europe, Germany.
1966–1967: Chief, United States Army Dental Clinic, Coleman Barracks, US Army Europe, Germany.
1968–1970: Guest scientist, Immunology Section, Laboratory of Microbiology, National Institute of Health.
1971–1974: Research periodontist, Maxillofacial Sciences Division, Letterman Army Institute of Research, Presidio of San Francisco, California.
1976–1977: Deputy commander, United States Army Institute of Dental Research, Walter Reed Army Medical Center, Washington, DC.
1977–1979: Chief, Periodontics Service, Walter Reed Army Medical Center, Washington, DC.
1979–1981: Dental education advisor, and later dental education coordinator, United States Army Medical Department Personnel Support Agency, Washington, DC.
1982–1983: Commander, 123rd Medical Detachment (dental), United States Army Europe, Germany.
1983–1987: Senior Dental Corps staff officer, Office of The Surgeon General, Falls Church, Virginia.
1987–1990: Deputy commander/assistant chief surgeon (dental), 7th Medical Command, United States Army Europe, Germany.
1990–1994: Chief, US Army Dental Corps.

Distinctions:
Awarded the Distinguished Service Medal, Legion of Merit (with oak leaf cluster), Meritorious Service Medal, Army Commendation Medal (with oak leaf cluster), Army Achievement Medal, and Expert Field Medical Badge.

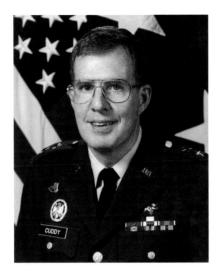

Major General John J Cuddy
Born August 19, 1942.

Education:
DDS, Marquette University, 1969.

Assignments:
1969–1972: General dental officer, US Army Dental Detachment, Fort Hood, Texas; dental officer, Darnall Army Hospital, Fort Hood, Texas.
1972–1973: Team leader, instructor, and general dentistry officer, Dental Company, Fort Hood, Texas.
1973–1975: General dentistry resident, Student Detachment, Dental Company, Fort Ord, California.
1975–1977: Chief, Dental Activity, US Army Medical Activity, Tehran, Iran.
1977–1981: Dental instructor, Academy of Health Sciences, Fort Sam Houston, Texas.
1981–1984: Commander, US Army Dental Activity, 7th Medical Command, Vicenza, Italy.
1984–1986: Chief, Graduate Dental Education Branch, Office of The Surgeon General, US Army Medical Department Personnel Support Activity, Washington, DC.
1987–1991: Assistant chief of staff, Dental Services, 7th Medical Command, US Army Europe and Seventh Army, Germany.
1991: Deputy commanding general/assistant chief surgeon (dental), 7th Medical Command, US Army Europe and Seventh Army, Germany.
1991–1994: Deputy commanding general, US Army Health Services Command, Fort Sam Houston, Texas.
1994–1996: Chief, Dental Corps/commanding general, US Army Medical Department Center and School, Fort Sam Houston, Texas.
1994–1998: Chief, US Army Dental Corps.

Distinctions:
Awarded the Distinguished Service Medal, Legion of Merit (with oak leaf cluster), Meritorious Service Medal (with three oak leaf clusters), Army Commendation Medal, and Expert Field Medical Badge.

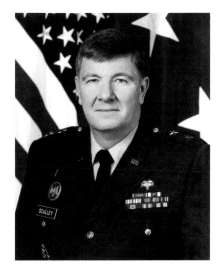

Major General Patrick D Sculley
Born September 12, 1947.

Education:
DDS, State University of New York, Buffalo, 1973.

Assignments:
1974–1976: General dental officer, McAfee United States Army Health Clinic, White Sands Missile Range, New Mexico.
1976–1977: General dental officer/assistant director, Hospital Dental Clinic, Dental Company, United States Army Medical Department Activity, Fort Knox, Kentucky.
1977–1979: Resident, US Army Dental Activity, Fort Knox, Kentucky.
1979–1981: Chief dentist, Dental Clinic No. 3, United States Army Dental Activity, Fort Riley, Kansas.
1982–1985: Commander, 576th Medical Detachment, 7th Medical Command, US Army Europe and Seventh Army, Germany.
1985–1988: Dental staff officer, later assistant inspector general, United States Army Health Services Command, Fort Sam Houston, Texas.
1988–1990: Dental requirements officer, United States Health Professional Support Agency, Falls Church, Virginia.
1991–1992: Commander, US Army Dental Activity, Fort Bragg, North Carolina.
1992–1993: Director of dental services, US Army Health Services Command, Fort Sam Houston, Texas.
1993–1996: Commander, US Army Dental Command, Fort Sam Houston, Texas.
1996–1998: Commanding general, US Army Center for Health Promotion and Preventive Medicine, Aberdeen Proving Ground, Maryland.
1998–2002: Chief, US Army Dental Corps.

Distinctions:
Awarded the Legion of Merit (with three oak leaf clusters), Meritorious Service Medal (with oak leaf cluster), Joint Service Commendation Medal, Army Commendation Medal, Army Achievement Medal (with oak leaf cluster), and Expert Field Medical Badge.

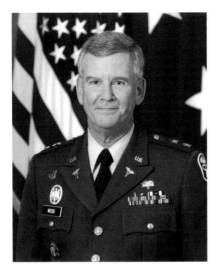

Major General Joseph G Webb, Jr
Born December 18, 1945.

Education:
DMD, Medical University of South Carolina, 1971.

Assignments:
1971–1974: Dental officer, US Army Dental Activity, Fort Benning, Georgia.
1974: Clinic chief, US Army Dental Activity, Bangkok, Thailand.
1975–1976: Chief, Oral Medicine, US Army Dental Activity, Fort Meade, Maryland.
1976–1979: Resident, Oral Pathology, later research dental officer, US Army Institute of Dental Research, Walter Reed Army Medical Center, Washington, DC.
1979–1984: Chief, Oral Pathology and Oral Medicine, US Army Dental Activity, Fort Ord, California.
1985–1986: Staff officer resident/dental augmentee to the inspector general, 7th Medical Command, United States Army Europe and Seventh Army, Germany.
1986–1988: Assistant division commander, 8th Infantry Division, US Army Europe and Seventh Army, Germany; Commander, 766th Medical Detachment, 7th Medical Command, US Army Europe and Seventh Army, Germany.
1988–1992: Commander, US Army Dental Activity-Alaska, Fort Wainwright, Alaska.
1992–1995: Dental consultant to the deputy surgeon general/assistant surgeon general for Dental Services, US Health Professional Support Agency, Falls Church, Virginia.
1995–1997: Senior Dental Corps staff officer, Office of The Surgeon General, Falls Church, Virginia.
1997–1999: Commander, US Army Dental Command, Fort Sam Houston, Texas.
1999–2002: Assistant surgeon general for Force Development and Sustainment, US Army Medical Command, Fort Sam Houston, Texas.
2002–2006: Chief, US Army Dental Corps, Deputy Surgeon General.

Distinctions:
Awarded the Distinguished Service Medal, Defense Superior Service Medal, Legion of Merit (with four oak leaf clusters), Meritorious Service Medal (with two oak leaf clusters), Army Commendation Medal, Army Achievement Medal, and Expert Field Medical Badge.

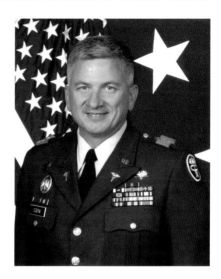

Major General Russell J Czerw
Born April 7, 1961.

Education:
DDS, State University of New York, 1987.

Assignments:
1987–1988: Dental resident, US Army Medical Department Activity, Fort Jackson, South Carolina.
1988–1991: Dental officer, later general dentist officer-in-charge, Muenchweiler Dental Clinic, 124th Medical Detachment, 7th Medical Command, US Army Europe and Seventh Army, Germany.
1992–1994: Resident, US Army Dental Activity, Fort Hood, Texas.
1994–1997: Professional development officer, later chief professional development officer, Dental Corps Branch, Officer Personnel Management Directorate, US Total Army Personnel Command, Alexandria, Virginia.
1997–1999: Commander, 464th Medical Company (Dental Service), 30th Medical Brigade, V Corps, US Army Europe and Seventh Army, Germany, and Operation Joint Guard, Bosnia-Herzegovina.
1999–2001: Chief, Dental Corps Branch, Officer Personnel Management Directorate, US Total Army Personnel Command, Alexandria, Virginia.
2002–2004: Commander, 93rd Medical Battalion (Dental Service), 30th Medical Brigade, V Corps, US Army Europe and Seventh Army, Germany, and Operation Iraqi Freedom, Iraq.
2004–2005: Dental Corps staff officer, Office of The Surgeon General, Falls Church, Virginia.
2005–2006: Commander, US Army Dental Command, Fort Sam Houston, Texas.
2006– : Commander, US Army Medical Department Center and School and Fort Sam Houston; chief, US Army Dental Corps.

Distinctions:
Awarded the Legion of Merit, Bronze Star Medal, Meritorious Service Medal (with five oak leaf clusters), Army Commendation Medal (with oak leaf cluster), Army Achievement Medal (with two oak leaf clusters), and the Expert Field Medical Badge.

INDEX

A

Abbott, Captain George N., 630
Abbott, Dr. Frank, 100
Account books, 129
Acklin, Murray, 107
ADA. *See* American Dental Association
Adair, Colonel George, 85
Adams, Captain Waldo J., 630
AEF. *See* American Expeditionary Forces
Affiliated hospital units
    dentists in, 1939-1941, 812–814
AFG. *See* American Forces in Germany
African Americans
    training camp at Fort Des Moines, Iowa,
        449–451
Agnew, Dr. Hayes, 46
Ainsworth, Major General Fred, 307
Alaska
    dental care to Army units, 273, 277
    Washington-Alaska Military Cable and
        Telegraph System, 735
Albaugh, Lieutenant Colonel Harold E., 793
Allen, Major General Henry T., 673
Allied Intervention, 659
Allied Powers, 361
Allied Young Men's Christian Association, 660,
    662
Allport, Dr. Walter Web, 95, 99
Aluminum dentures, 507–508, 509
AMA. *See* American Medical Association
Amalgam
    invention of, 18
Ambelang, First Lieutenant Lisle P., 635
Ambulances, 435–441
American Academy of Dental Surgery, 90
American Ambulance, Paris, France, 361–364,
    367
American College of Dentists, 730
American Dental Association
    Committee on Dental Preparedness, 821–825
    Committee on National Defense, 820–821
    Committee on State Dental Laws and the
        Appointment of Dentists in the Army and
        Navy, 103
    dental amalgam issue, 18
    efforts to secure dentists in the Union Army,
        40–41
    meeting, 1881, 94–95
    reaction to the Thomason Bill, 788
    support of the American Register of
        Pathology, 798
American Dental Convention, 18, 39
American Expeditionary Forces
    awards for heroism, 621–638
    combat dental care in France, 1917-1919,
        587–648

deaths due to disease, accident and other
    causes, 644–647
dental assistant casualties, 636–638
Dental Corps Officers killed in action, 635,
    644
dental officers at the front, 587–600, 610–621
dental personnel allocation, 410–411, 639–640
Dental Reserve Corps Officers who died prior
    to entering active service, 648
dental service, 1917-1919, 475–520, 574
dental service, January 1919-May 1919, 573
dental service, November 1918-March 1919,
    641–642
dental supplies and equipment, 410–411, 427,
    431–435, 499–506, 639
dental surgeon shortage, 513–517, 666
dentists with the 2nd Division, 1917-1918,
    604–610
dentists with the 1st Division, 1917-1918,
    600–604
diseases of concern, 546–551
foreign excursions, 659–674
initial echelon in France, 1917, 475–477
line of communications, 479–480, 510–513
maxillofacial surgery service, 554–565,
    570–572
oral and dental care in France, 1917-1919,
    535–575
prosthetic treatment policy, 509–510
structure of dental support, 1917, 479–481
American Expeditionary Forces University,
    517–518
American Forces in Germany, 666, 669–674
American Institute of Dental Teachers, 364–366
American Journal of Dental Science, 13
American Medical Association, 95, 97–99, 178,
    302, 304
American Military Supply Depot, 666
American Red Cross, 364, 425–426, 499, 667, 820
American Red Cross Military Hospital, 554, 558,
    560
American Register of Pathology, 798, 800
American Society of Dental Surgeons, 13
American Women's Hospital Group, 429–430
Ames, Dr. G.F., 123
Amex Dentures, 507–508
AMSUS. *See* Association of Military Surgeons of
    the United States
Anderson, Major General James Patton, 71
Annual examinations, 712–715
Annual Report of the Surgeon General, 695–696,
    731, 735–736, 739
AOCP. *See* Army of Cuban Pacification
Apothecary general, 11
Appointment books, 129
AR. *See* Army Regulations

Philippines, 273
Philippines' assignment and schedule, 228, 230
as president of the Association of Military Dental Surgeons of the United States, 375, 380, 430–431
Millington, First Lieutenant Robert E.F., 631
Mills, Colonel Robert H., 690, 776, 783, 793, 826, 848
Mills, Dr. G.A., 94
Mississippi Valley Association of Dental Surgeons, 16
Mitchell, Captain William S., 666
Mitchell, L.P., 347
Modie, First Lieutenant Clyde R., 632
Moore, L.C., 154–155
Moore, Surgeon General Samuel Preston, 60, 61, 63, 72, 75
Morale issues, 735–743
Morgan, Captain David R., 602
Morgan, Dr. W.H., 59
Morgan, H.W., 155
Morgan, Robert, 148, 170, 172, 203, 204
Morgan Riflemen, 18
Morrison, Dr. Frank, 91
Morrison, Private Harry P., 636
Morrissey, First Lieutenant Howard M., 635
Morse, Captain C.F., 329
Morton, Dr. William T.G., 16, 41, 43
Motley, First Lieutenant Robert E., 625
Mount, Lieutenant Colonel James R., 502
Mullins, Private First Class Grover C., 663
Murdock, First Lieutenant Reginald S., 501
Murphy, John, 88
Musgrave, First Lieutenant Charles A., 632
Musketeers, 2
Myers, Dr. Helen E., 499
Myers, Henry, 379
Myers, Private First Class William C., 627, 632

N

Nash, First Lieutenant C.H., 501
National Army, 442
National Defense Act amendments, 417–422, 792
National Defense Act of 1916, 377–381, 384, 404, 787
National Defense Act of 1920, 686, 693
National Dental Association
  annual meeting, Ashville, North Carolina, 1903, 213–215
  annual meeting, Niagara Falls, New York, 1899, 157–158
  annual meeting, Old Point Comfort, Virginia, 1900, 165
  annual meeting, Omaha, Nebraska, 1898, 150–151
  Committee on Army and Navy Dental Legislation, 161

Ireland's address, 688
renewed campaign for Dental Corps reorganization, 1915-1916, 371–376
support for legislation to create a commissioned corps, 243–247
National Guard, 377, 384–386, 718, 816
National Research Council, 730, 798
National Security Act of 1916, 382
NDA. *See* National Dental Association
Neuilly, Paris, France
  American Ambulance, 361–364
Nevin, Dr. Sophie, 496
New Deal, 755
New Orleans Dental College, 56
Nichols, Major Henry J., 729
Nitrous oxide
  discovery of use as an anesthetic, 16
Noble, Dr. Henry Briss, 103, 105, 179
Noble, Major General Robert, 373
Noel, Dr. L.G., 213
North Russia Expedition, 660–663

O

Occupation of Germany, 665–666
O'Connell, Private Phillip J., 636
O'Connor, Corporal John, 88
O'Donnell, Major Frederick W., 600
Oeder, Private Lambert, 387
Officer training, 451–452
Officers Reserve Corps, 380, 404
O'Hara, First Lieutenant Mortimer J., 633
Ohio Dental Journal, 107
Ohio State Dental Society, 105
Oliver, Colonel Robert T.
  Army Dental School portrait, 784
  assignment to France, 1917, 477–481
  assignment to the Philippines, 192–195, 298
  biography, 843
  as chief of Dental Corps, 407, 413, 421, 437, 504–505, 516, 556, 572, 603–604
  as chief of the dental section of the surgeon general's office, 687–688, 690, 698–699
  comments on dental care for Spanish-American soldiers, 131–132
  concept of an Army dental school, 720–722, 727–728
  death of, 690
  dental organization proposal, 404–405
  Distinguished Service Medal, 634, 637
  establishment of dental school, 388–389
  as member of dental examining board, 163, 170, 172, 203
  portraits, 131, 171, 691
  presentations to the National Dental Association meetings, 1905, 220–222
  as professor of military science and tactics, 772